Cystic Fibrosis: A Genetic Disorder

Cystic Fibrosis: A Genetic Disorder

Editor: Tamzin Gillespie

FOSTER
ACADEMICS

www.fosteracademics.com

www.fosteracademics.com

FOSTER ACADEMICS

Cataloging-in-Publication Data

Cystic fibrosis : a genetic disorder / edited by Tamzin Gillespie.
p. cm.
Includes bibliographical references and index.
ISBN 978-1-63242-537-9
1. Cystic fibrosis. 2. Genetic disorders. I. Gillespie, Tamzin.
RC858.C95 C97 2018
616.37--dc23

Foster Academics,
118-35 Queens Blvd., Suite 400,
Forest Hills, NY 11375, USA

ISBN 978-1-63242-537-9 (Hardback)

Printed and bound in China.

Contents

Preface

It is often said that books are a boon to mankind. They document every progress and pass on the knowledge from one generation to the other. They play a crucial role in our lives. Thus I was both excited and nervous while editing this book. I was pleased by the thought of being able to make a mark but I was also nervous to do it right because the future of students depends upon it. Hence, I took a few months to research further into the discipline, revise my knowledge and also explore some more aspects. Post this process, I begun with the editing of this book.

Cystic fibrosis is a disease which affects the lungs, liver, kidneys and pancreas. It is caused by mutations in the genes. Sinus infections, clubbing of the fingers, fatty stool, etc. are some of the symptoms of cystic fibrosis. It is very important to diagnose this disorder at an early age to avoid further complications. Some of the diagnostic methods include sweat testing, newborn screening and genetic testing. This book presents researches and studies performed by experts across the globe. The extensive content of this book provides the readers with a thorough understanding of the disorder.

I thank my publisher with all my heart for considering me worthy of this unparalleled opportunity and for showing unwavering faith in my skills. I would also like to thank the editorial team who worked closely with me at every step and contributed immensely towards the successful completion of this book. Last but not the least, I wish to thank my friends and colleagues for their support.

Editor

High Variability in Oral Glucose Tolerance among 1,128 Patients with Cystic Fibrosis: A Multicenter Screening Study

Nicole Scheuing[1*¶], Reinhard W. Holl[1¶], Gerd Dockter[2], Julia M. Hermann[1], Sibylle Junge[3], Cordula Koerner-Rettberg[4], Lutz Naehrlich[5], Christina Smaczny[6], Doris Staab[7], Gabriela Thalhammer[8], Silke van Koningsbruggen-Rietschel[9], Manfred Ballmann[4]

1 Institute of Epidemiology and Medical Biometry, Central Institute for Biomedical Technology, University of Ulm, Ulm, Germany, **2** Cystic Fibrosis Centre, Saarland University Hospital for Pediatric and Adolescent Medicine, Homburg/Saar, Germany, **3** Clinic for Pediatric Pneumology and Neonatology, Hannover Medical School, Hannover, Germany, **4** Department of Pediatric Pulmonology, St. Josef Hospital Pediatric Clinic, Ruhr University Bochum, Bochum, Germany, **5** Department of Pediatrics, Justus-Liebig University Giessen, Giessen, Germany, **6** Medical Clinic I, Pneumology and Allergology, University Hospital Frankfurt/Main, Goethe University, Frankfurt/Main, Germany, **7** Division of Pulmonology and Immunology, Department of Pediatrics, Charité Berlin, Berlin, Germany, **8** Department for Pediatric Pulmonology and Allergology, Medical University of Graz, Graz, Austria, **9** Cystic Fibrosis Centre Cologne, Childrens Hospital, University of Cologne, Cologne, Germany

Abstract

Background: In cystic fibrosis, highly variable glucose tolerance is suspected. However, no study provided within-patient coefficients of variation. The main objective of this short report was to evaluate within-patient variability of oral glucose tolerance.

Methods: In total, 4,643 standardized oral glucose tolerance tests of 1,128 cystic fibrosis patients (median age at first test: 15.5 [11.5; 21.5] years, 48.8% females) were studied. Patients included were clinically stable, non-pregnant, and had at least two oral glucose tolerance tests, with no prior lung transplantation or systemic steroid therapy. Transition frequency from any one test to the subsequent test was analyzed and within-patient coefficients of variation were calculated for fasting and two hour blood glucose values. All statistical analysis was implemented with SAS 9.4.

Results: A diabetic glucose tolerance was confirmed in 41.2% by the subsequent test. A regression to normal glucose tolerance at the subsequent test was observed in 21.7% and to impaired fasting glucose, impaired glucose tolerance or both in 15.2%, 12.0% or 9.9%. The average within-patient coefficient of variation for fasting blood glucose was 11.1% and for two hour blood glucose 25.3%.

Conclusion: In the cystic fibrosis patients studied, a highly variable glucose tolerance was observed. Compared to the general population, variability of two hour blood glucose was 1.5 to 1.8-fold higher.

Editor: Dominik Hartl, University of Tübingen, Germany

Funding: The study was funded by the German and French CF associations (Mukoviszidose e.V. and its regional group Saarland-Pfalz, Vaincre de la Mucoviszidose), and by Novo Nordisk. The funders had no role in study design, data collection and analysis, decision to publish, or preparation of the manuscript.

Competing Interests: The study was partly funded by Novo Nordisk. There are no patents, products in development or marketed products to declare. Mukoviszidose e.V. - the German CF association - is a registered not-for-profit charity with tax-exempt status under German tax law. It is by no means a "commercial funder".

* Email: nicole.scheuing@uni-ulm.de

¶ Shared first authorship.

Introduction

Cystic fibrosis (CF) is a life-limiting autosomal recessive illness occurring in about one of 2,500 newborns in Europe. As the life expectancy for CF patients has increased due to earlier diagnosis and improved care, CF-related comorbidities became more frequent over the last decades. A growing comorbidity with impact on the course of CF is cystic fibrosis-related diabetes (CFRD). The latest comprehensive guidelines for CFRD recommend yearly screening for abnormal glucose metabolism by oral glucose tolerance test (OGTT) in CF patients aged ≥10 years [1]. A small study suspected that CF patients have a high variation in glucose tolerance over time [2].

Therefore, we aimed to investigate in this short report the variability of glucose tolerance in a large cohort of CF patients. For the first time, a within-patient coefficient of variation (CV) for 2-hour blood glucose was calculated in CF.

Materials and Methods

Ethics statement

The ethical committees of Ulm University and Hannover Medical School approved the study, and patients or their parents provided written informed consent.

Study subjects

Between 2001 and 2010, 1,778 CF patients aged 10 years or older were screened serially by OGTT in a multicenter screening program carried out by 43 German/Austrian specialized centers (Trial No. NCT00662714). All patients had a physician-based diagnosis of CF according to the latest German guidelines [3]. OGTTs were performed and interpreted in line with recommendations of the World Health Organization modified by the American Diabetes Association as described in detail previously [4,5].

In total, 5,765 OGTTs among clinically stable CF patients were carried out until the end of the study (Figure 1). As mentioned in reference [4], all patients screened had to be without symptoms of acute infections or exacerbations of chronic infections and should not have a reduced carbohydrate intake. Moreover, patients with respiratory failure (FEV1<40%) or with enteral tube feeding were excluded. In case of a confirmed diagnosis of CFRD or the use of anti-hyperglycemic treatment, patients were also excluded from screening.

For the present analysis, only OGTTs of non-pregnant patients with no prior systemic steroid therapy or lung transplantation were considered (Figure 1). If patients awaited lung transplantation, OGTTs were also excluded. Furthermore, at least two OGTTs had to be performed per patient (Figure 1). The final study population comprised 4,643 OGTTs of 1,128 CF patients. For each patient included, test results were classified as normal glucose tolerance (NGT), impaired fasting glucose (IFG), impaired glucose tolerance (IGT), IFG and IGT combined, or diabetic glucose tolerance (DGT). The detailed cut-offs are described in reference [4]. As there are some CF patients with isolated IFG [4] and the pathophysiology between IFG and IGT is at least in part different [6], we introduced an IFG group in this analysis. CFRD was defined as a diabetic OGTT confirmed by a consecutive OGTT in the DGT range [1]. Body mass index standard deviation score (BMI-SDS) was calculated using data from the German Health Interview and Examination Survey for Children and Adolescents (KiGGS study, [7]) as national reference. The KiGGS study was used as a reference in a number of previous publications by our group to calculate BMI-SDS in CF patients [4,8,9] and is the best currently available reference data for healthy German children. Data to calculate BMI-SDS on the basis of CF-specific anthropometric reference percentiles are currently not available.

Statistical analysis

To analyze the variation in glucose tolerance, transition frequency from any one test to the subsequent test was studied. As there is no subsequent test for the last test in each patient, 3,515 pairs of consecutive OGTTs were available in the study population (the number of OGTT pairs therefore equals the total number of OGTTs minus the number of patients). For each pair of OGTTs, the first test was categorized in one of the five glucose

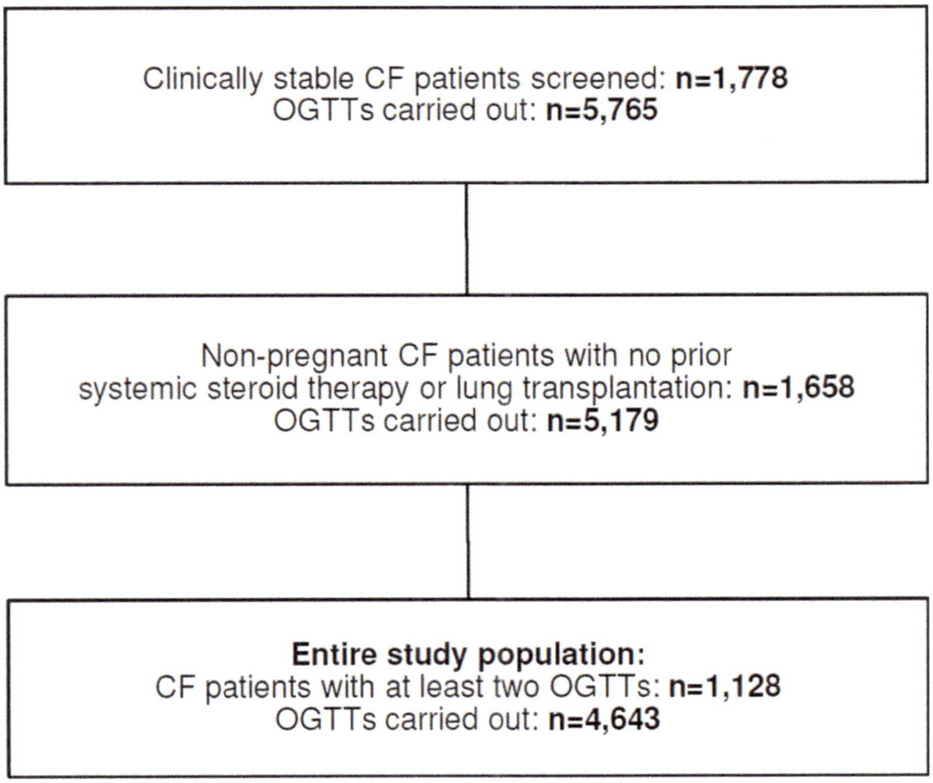

Figure 1. Selection of study population. Abbreviations: *CF* cystic fibrosis, *OGTT* oral glucose tolerance test.

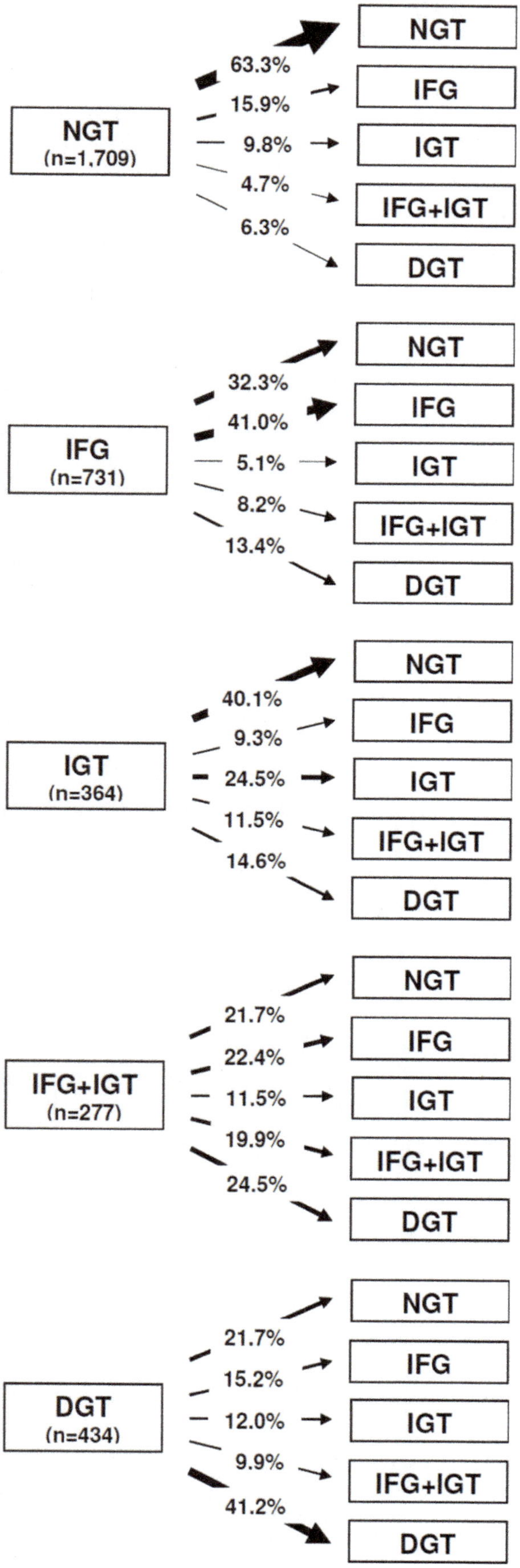

Figure 2. Transition from any one test to a subsequent test. In total, 3,515 pairs of consecutive OGTTs are summarized. For each pair, the first test was categorized in one of the five glucose tolerance classes (NGT, IFG only, IGT only, IFG+IGT, DGT). The figure shows the percentage of subsequent test results for each glucose tolerance category. The number in parentheses indicates the number of OGTTs available for analysis. Abbreviations: *NGT* normal glucose tolerance, *IFG* impaired fasting glucose, *IGT* impaired glucose tolerance, *DGT* diabetic glucose tolerance, *OGTT* oral glucose tolerance test.

tolerance classes (NGT, IFG only, IGT only, IFG+IGT, DGT) and the percentage of subsequent test results was calculated. Moreover, the variation in glucose tolerance is depicted in three individual patients who had seven consecutive OGTTs with at least one diabetic result. To assess the degree of variability of serially measured fasting and 2-hour blood glucose values in CF patients, within-patient CVs (defined as ratio between within-subject standard deviation and mean) were calculated and compared to the general population. CVs were calculated as they are normalized measures of the variability and independent of the mean level.

To evaluate gender or age differences in the deterioration of glucose tolerance from test to test, a logistic mixed regression model was applied. Deterioration of glucose metabolism was defined as worsening of glucose tolerance in a subsequent test compared to the pretest or as confirmation of a diabetic OGTT. Sex and age were entered as independent fixed effects. Age was categorized as 10–<15 years, 15–<20 years and ≥20 years. To account for repeated OGTTs per patient, random effects with first-order autoregressive covariance structure were used. Results are given as odds ratios (OR) with lower and upper confidence limit (CL).

Statistical analyses were performed with SAS 9.4. The level of significance was set at 0.05. To compare demographics between patients included and excluded, Kruskal-Wallis test was applied for continuous parameters and χ^2-test for dichotomous parameters.

Results

48.8% of patients included were female and 28.9% were >20 years. Median [Q_1;Q_3] (mean±SD) age at first OGTT was 15.5 [11.5; 21.5] (18.0±8.4) years and at last OGTT 18.6 [15.3; 25.4] (21.3±8.5) years. At baseline OGTT, the youngest patient aged 10.0 years and the oldest patient 63.9 years. On average, median (mean) duration between two consecutive OGTTs was 1.0 [0.7; 1.2] (1.1±0.7) year. A diabetic OGTT was repeated within a median (mean) time of 6.9 [4.9; 12.9] (9.1±6.2) weeks. As published previously [4], the median duration between two consecutive OGTTs in the DGT range (confirmed diagnosis of CFRD) was 8.1 [5.1; 27.9] weeks. All patients with suspected CFRD (i.e. one OGTT in the DGT range) at the end of the study were followed-up outside the context of the screening study. Each patient with a confirmed diagnosis of CFRD was invited to participate in a randomized controlled trial investigating the use of repaglinide in comparison to insulin therapy. CFRD patients not participating in the clinical trial received insulin therapy and CF-specific nutritional counseling as recommended by guidelines.

Baseline characteristics of the 650 patients excluded are depicted in table 1. Excluded patients were older and had on average a lower BMI-SDS.

Figure 2 displays the transition frequency from any one test to a subsequent test. For example, an OGTT in the DGT range was confirmed in 41.2% by the subsequent test.

Table 1. Demographics of patients included and patients excluded at baseline OGTT.

	Patients included	Patients excluded	p-value
Number, n	1,128	650	-
Age, years	15.5 [11.5; 21.5] (18.0±8.4)	17.4 [12.3; 25.2] (20.0±9.3)	<0.001
Female sex, %	48.8	45.1	NS
Weight, kg	47.8 [34.5; 57.8] (47.8±15.4)	50.2 [35.5; 59.0] (49.0±15.2)	0.04
Height, cm	160.0 [145.6; 170.0] (157.8±15.6)	162.0 [147.0; 172.0] (159.8±15.9)	0.008
BMI, kg/m^2	18.4 [16.2; 20.4] (18.6±3.3)	18.6 [16.2; 20.7] (18.7±3.3)	NS
BMI-SDS	−0.76 [−1.42;−0.11] (−0.80±1.08)	−0.87 [−1.65;−0.18] (−0.99±1.26)	0.005

Data are given as median with quartiles (mean with standard deviation) or as percentage. Abbreviations: *BMI* body mass index, *SDS* standard deviation score, *NS* not significant.

Until the end of the screening study, a total of 136 CF patients revealed a confirmed diagnosis of CFRD i.e. two consecutive OGTTs revealing DGT. Despite the fact that two consecutive OGTTs in the DGT range are sufficient to diagnose CFRD, 54 out of the 136 patients had additional OGTTs. In 42.6% (n = 23) of patients, all subsequent tests were diabetic. In 20.4% (n = 11) of cases, at least one of the subsequent tests revealed NGT.

Figure 3 indicates that independent of age, glucose tolerance varied highly from test to test in three individual patients.

Overall, in CF patients the average within-patient CV for fasting blood glucose values was 11.1% and for 2-hour blood glucose 25.3%. Analyzing patients with (n = 339) and without (n = 789) at least one OGTT in the DGT range separately, patients without an OGTT in the diabetic range had lower CVs for both fasting and 2-hour blood glucose values (fasting: 8.9 vs. 16.1%, p<0.001; 2-hour: 22.2 vs. 32.4%, p<0.001).

Logistic regression analysis revealed for girls a 1.18-fold [lower CL: 1.03; upper CL: 1.36] higher risk for the deterioration of

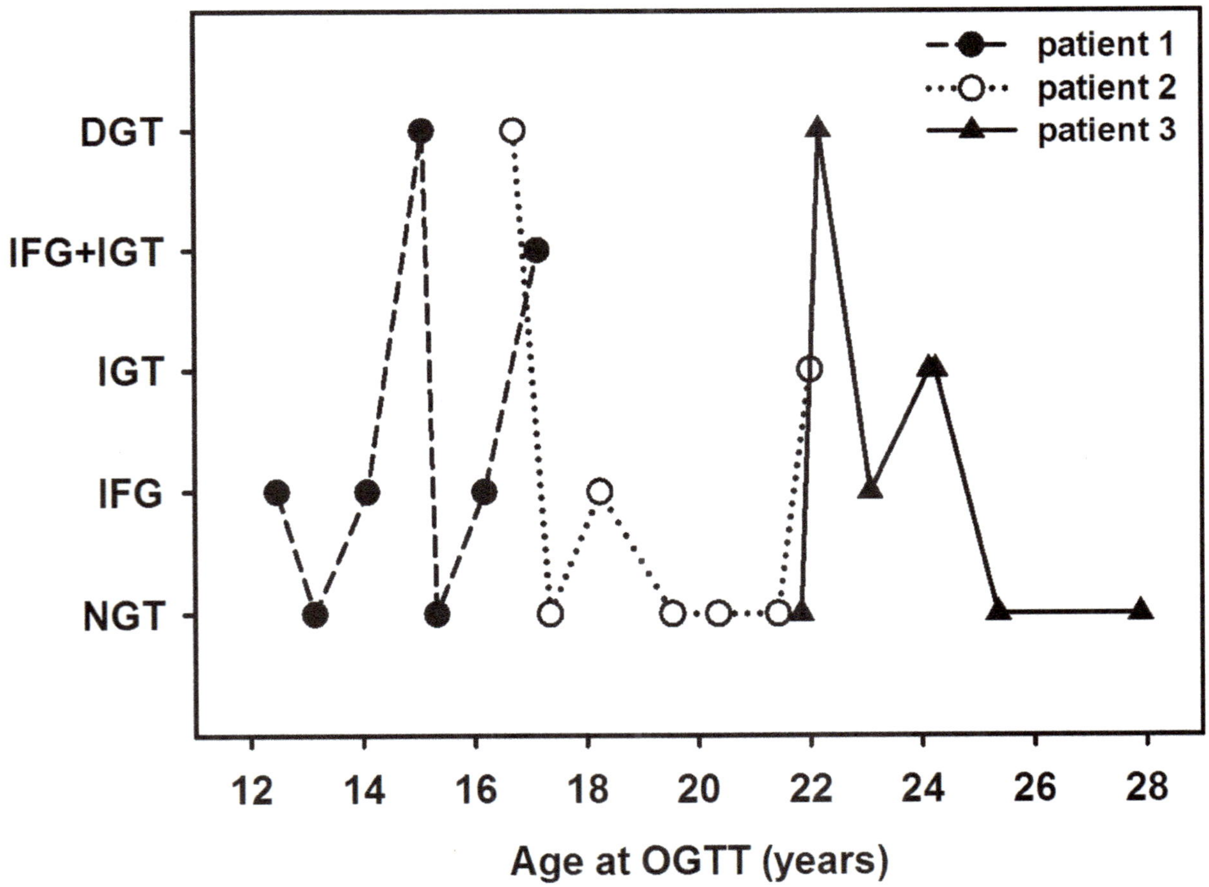

Figure 3. Variation of glucose tolerance in three patients of different age. Each patient had seven consecutive OGTTs with at least one diabetic result. Abbreviations: *DGT* diabetic glucose tolerance, *IFG* impaired fasting glucose, *IGT* impaired glucose tolerance, *NGT* normal glucose tolerance, *OGTT* oral glucose tolerance test.

glucose tolerance compared to boys ($p = 0.015$). In addition, patients aged 15–<20 years (OR: 1.23 [1.04; 1.47], $p = 0.019$) or ≥20 years (OR: 1.22 [1.03; 1.44], $p = 0.024$) had a higher risk than patients aged 10–<15 years. In 15 to <20 year old patients, risk was comparable to patients aged ≥20 years (OR: 1.01 [0.86; 1.19], $p = 0.867$).

Analyzing the influence of sex in the subgroup of older patients (>20 years at baseline OGTT; n = 326 patients with 1,276 OGTTs), revealed also an increased risk in females compared to males, even though the influence was no longer significant due to the lower number of patients studied (OR: 1.23 [0.92; 1.63], $p = 0.162$).

Discussion

Our analysis among asymptomatic CF patients revealed a high variability in glucose tolerance over time, even though patients without DGT seem to be more stable with respect to glucose tolerance. Compared to the general population [10–12], overall within-patient variability of 2-hour blood glucose is 1.5 to 1.8-fold higher in CF. The NHANES III Second Examination revealed a within-patient CV of 16.6% for 2-hour blood glucose [12] and the Hoorn study of 16.7% [11]. In a general practice [10], a within-patient CV of 14.3% was observed. Fluctuating levels of insulin resistance due to acute and chronic infections or CF-related inflammatory cytokines may explain the highly variable glucose tolerance in CF.

The fluctuation in glucose tolerance observed in this study implicates regular control of glucose metabolism in CF. Future guidelines should provide recommendations regarding an adequate time frame for repeating OGTTs in patients with abnormal glucose tolerance as well as for the confirmation interval of a diabetic test result. As outlined by the study protocol and described previously [4], a diabetic OGTT had to be repeated within 4 to 6 weeks in the present study and an OGTT revealing IFG or IGT after 6 months. According to guidelines, all patients with a confirmed CFRD diagnosis or with a diabetic OGTT and classical symptoms of diabetes should receive insulin treatment immediately [1]. Oral antidiabetic agents are not advised until sufficient data become available regarding their efficiency.

Reasons for performing additional OGTTs in patients with already confirmed CFRD are unknown. Maybe patients requested an additional OGTT in the context of intensifying therapy. Especially, asymptomatic CF patients often have problems starting insulin treatment besides numerous CF-related therapies. Another possibility might be that patients with a confirmed CFRD diagnosis were not totally clinically stable at the time of the confirmation test and the medical team therefore decided to repeat the test at a later time point. As OGTT results depend also on the supplementation of pancreatic enzymes, the medical team may have repeated the confirmation test after adjusting pancreatic enzyme substitution.

Although the OGTT revealed a high degree of within-patient variance in CF, it is the best screening tool for abnormalities in glucose tolerance currently available. Fasting plasma glucose, hemoglobin A1c or other classical methods applicable for type 1 or type 2 diabetes are not recommended in CF [1]. In the future, continuous glucose monitoring or standardized test meals might be a useful alternative to OGTT. However, there are no reference values for continuous glucose monitoring so far. To minimize the variability of OGTTs in CF patients, CF-adapted standardization might be one possibility. At the moment, criteria for the performance and interpretation of OGTT are identical to other diabetes types. However, pancreatic enzyme substitution and the grade of inflammation (e.g. C-reactive protein measurement) should be considered before performing an OGTT in CF, and when interpreting OGTT results. More advanced interpretation criteria that take into account dynamics in oral glucose challenge in CF patients might be appropriate. As CFRD is less common compared to the more frequent type 1 or type 2 diabetes, other measures of ß-cell function (e.g. C-peptide) or calculation of indices for insulin secretion and sensitivity might be practicable in clinical settings that may result in better assessment of glucose tolerance in CF patients.

The higher risk for deterioration of glucose tolerance in girls confirms previous studies indicating an earlier onset and a higher prevalence of CFRD in females [4,13,14]. The lower risk in patients younger than 15 years compared to older patients might be explained by the rare occurrence of CFRD in patients <10 years and the increasing prevalence of abnormal glucose tolerance with age [4,15,16].

Selection biases might be one limitation of the present study. Not all centers or CF patients participated, although all German/Austrian medical facilities providing care for CF patients were invited for participation in written form. Moreover, some CF-related therapies (e.g. steroids, lung transplantation) led to exclusion of patients and the complexity of CF itself made study participation often difficult. The higher age and the lower BMI-SDS of patients excluded may point to a more severe progression of the disease compared to patients included. Exclusion criterion for the majority of the 650 patients not analyzed was the availability of solely one OGTT. This might be due to termination of the study or occurrence of exclusion criteria after the first OGTT. Moreover, each patient could withdraw from the study at any time.

In summary, in the asymptomatic CF patients studied, one diabetic OGTT seems not sufficient to diagnose CFRD due to the existing high variability of glucose tolerance. A normal glucose tolerance after a confirmed CFRD diagnosis (i.e. two consecutive OGTTs revealing DGT) cannot be excluded. Despite improvement of glucose tolerance, these patients are classified as diabetic [1], although this labelling may be contra-intuitive for patients and physicians. It is still a debate whether solely a persistently diabetic glucose tolerance is associated with an increased risk of clinical decline in CF or even a pre-diabetic condition.

Acknowledgments

The authors thank all participating centers for performing OGTTs and providing data for the present analysis. A detailed list of centers was recently published [4].

Author Contributions

Conceived and designed the experiments: RWH MB. Performed the experiments: GD SJ CKR LN CS DS GT SVKR MB. Analyzed the data: NS JMH RWH. Contributed reagents/materials/analysis tools: GD SJ CKR LN CS DS GT SVKR MB. Contributed to the writing of the manuscript: NS. Revision of manuscript: RWH GD JMH SJ CKR LN CS DS GT SVKR MB. Final approval of the version to be published: NS RWH GD JMH SJ CKR LN CS DS GT SVKR MB.

References

1. Moran A, Brunzell C, Cohen RC, Katz M, Marshall BC, et al. (2010) Clinical care guidelines for cystic fibrosis-related diabetes: A position statement of the American Diabetes Association and a clinical practice guideline of the Cystic Fibrosis Foundation, endorsed by the Pediatric Endocrine Society. Diabetes Care 33: 2697–2708.

2. Sterescu AE, Rhodes B, Jackson R, Dupuis A, Hanna A, et al. (2010) Natural history of glucose intolerance in patients with cystic fibrosis: Ten-year prospective observation program. J Pediatr 156: 613–617.
3. Naehrlich L, Stuhrmann-Spangenberg M, Barben J, Bargon J, Blankenstein O, et al. (June 2013) S2 consensus-guideline: diagnostic of mucoviscidosis. AWMF 026–023.Available: www.awmf.org/uploads/tx_szleitlinien/026-023 m_S2k_Diagnostik_der_Mukoviszidose_ 2013-07.pdf. Accessed 2014 June 4.
4. Scheuing N, Holl RW, Dockter G, Fink K, Junge S, et al. (2013) Diabetes in cystic fibrosis: Multicenter screening results based on current guidelines. PLoS One 8: e81545.
5. Schmid K, Fink K, Holl RW, Hebestreit H, Ballmann M (2014) Predictors for future cystic fibrosis-related diabetes by oral glucose tolerance test. J Cyst Fibros 13: 80–85.
6. Nathan DM, Davidson MB, DeFronzo RA, Heine RJ, Henry RR, et al. (2007) Impaired fasting glucose and impaired glucose tolerance: implications for care. Diabetes Care 30: 753–759.
7. Rosario AS, Kurth BM, Stolzenberg H, Ellert U, Neuhauser H (2010) Body mass index percentiles for children and adolescents in Germany based on a nationally representative sample (KiGGS 2003–2006). Eur J Clin Nutr 64: 341–349.
8. Scheuing N, Berger G, Bergis D, Gohlke B, Konrad K, et al. (2014) Adherence to clinical care guidelines for cystic fibrosis-related diabetes in 659 German/Austrian patients. J Cyst Fibros [Epub]. DOI:10.1016/j.jcf.2014.05.006.
9. Scheuing N, Badenhoop K, Borkenstein M, Konrad K, Lilienthal E, et al. (2014) Why is insulin pump treatment rarely used in adolescents and young adults with cystic fibrosis-related diabetes? Pediatr Diabetes [Epub]. DOI:10.1111/pedi.12158.
10. Feskens EJ, Bowles CH, Kromhout D (1991) Intra- and interindividual variability of glucose tolerance in an elderly population. J Clin Epidemiol 44: 947–953.
11. Mooy JM, Grootenhuis PA, de Vries H, Kostense PJ, Popp-Snijders C, et al. (1996) Intra-individual variation of glucose, specific insulin and proinsulin concentrations measured by two oral glucose tolerance tests in a general Caucasian population: The Hoorn study. Diabetologia 39: 298–305.
12. Selvin E, Crainiceanu CM, Brancati FL, Coresh J (2007) Short-term variability in measures of glycemia and implications for the classification of diabetes. Arch Intern Med 167: 1545–1551.
13. Ode KL, Frohnert B, Laguna T, Phillips J, Holme B, et al. (2010) Oral glucose tolerance testing in children with cystic fibrosis. Pediatr Diabetes 11: 487–492.
14. Konrad K, Thon A, Fritsch M, Fröhlich-Reiterer E, Lilienthal E, et al. (2013) Comparison of cystic fibrosis-related diabetes with type 1 diabetes based on a German/Austrian pediatric diabetes registry. Diabetes Care 36: 879–886.
15. Lanng S, Thorsteinsson B, Lund-Andersen C, Nerup J, Schiøtz PO, et al. (1994) Diabetes mellitus in Danish cystic fibrosis patients: prevalence and late diabetic complications. Acta Paediatr 83: 72–77.
16. Moran A, Dunitz J, Nathan B, Saeed A, Holme B, et al. (2009) Cystic fibrosis-related diabetes: current trends in prevalence, incidence, and mortality. Diabetes Care 32: 1626–1631.

2

Advances toward the Elucidation of Hypertonic Saline Effects on *Pseudomonas aeruginosa* from Cystic Fibrosis Patients

Anne-Laure Michon[1,2]*, Estelle Jumas-Bilak[1,3], Raphaël Chiron[4], Brigitte Lamy[1,2], Hélène Marchandin[1,2]

1 UMR 5119 ECOSYM, Equipe Pathogènes et Environnements, U.F.R. des Sciences Pharmaceutiques et Biologiques, Université Montpellier 1, Montpellier, France, **2** Laboratoire de Bactériologie, Hôpital Arnaud de Villeneuve, Centre Hospitalier Régional Universitaire de Montpellier, Montpellier, France, **3** Laboratoire d'Hygiène hospitalière, Centre Hospitalier Régional Universitaire de Montpellier, Montpellier, France, **4** Centre de Ressources et de Compétences pour la Mucoviscidose, Hôpital Arnaud de Villeneuve, Centre Hospitalier Régional Universitaire de Montpellier, Montpellier, France

Abstract

Objectives: Nebulized hypertonic saline (HTS) has beneficial effects including reducing pulmonary exacerbations in Cystic Fibrosis (CF) patients. Several mechanisms may explain these effects but antimicrobial activity of NaCl remains largely unexplored. We aimed to measure the antimicrobial effect of NaCl on *Pseudomonas aeruginosa* isolated from the respiratory tract in CF patients.

Methods: NaCl minimal inhibitory concentration (MIC) and minimal bactericidal concentration (MBC) were determined for strains characterized for mucoidy, antimicrobial resistance, and ability to form biofilm using 0,9% to 15% NaCl solutions. NaCl effects on biofilm formation, preformed biofilm, and mobility were evaluated. Kinetics of antimicrobial effects was studied.

Results: The growth of all isolates (n = 85) from 34 patients was inhibited by 6% NaCl solution. A 10% concentration had a bactericidal activity on 90% of the isolates. Mucoid and multidrug resistant (MDR) isolates displayed lower MICs compared to non-mucoid and to non-MDR isolates, respectively. Time-kill kinetics showed that NaCl exhibited a rapid, dose and growth phase dependent bactericidal effect. Three percent or more of NaCl inhibited biofilm formation for 69% of strongly adherent isolates. A dose-dependent decrease of preformed biofilm viability and an inhibitory activity on bacterial motility were observed.

Conclusions: NaCl inhibited the growth of all isolates and killed 38% of tested isolates within concentration range currently used in therapeutics. Our results suggest that anti-pseudomonal activity is another mechanism of action of HTS to add to those already established. Clinical trials are needed to compare diverse HTS conditions of use (rhythm, dose and mode of delivery) to obtain efficient and optimized anti-*P. aeruginosa* effects. More generally, NaCl effect on other opportunistic pathogens as well as on global microbiotae recovered during polymicrobial diseases warrants further investigations.

Editor: Michael Tunney, Queens University Belfast, Ireland

Funding: This work was supported by the Ministère de l'enseignement supérieur et de la recherche, France. The funders had no role in study design, data collection and analysis, decision to publish, or preparation of the manuscript.

Competing Interests: The authors have declared that no competing interests exist.

* E-mail: al-michon@chu-montpellier.fr

Introduction

Cystic fibrosis (CF) is the most common inherited disease in Caucasians. The disorder is initiated by a defect in the CF transmembrane conductance regulator (CFTR) gene coding for an apical membrane chloride channel mediating transepithelial salt and liquid movement [1]. CF lung disease is characterized by a persistent inflammation and polymicrobial infectious disease evolving throughout life [2]. The chronic persistence of *Pseudomonas aeruginosa* is linked to lung function decline [3]. The consequences of hydro-electrolytic imbalance in the lung have been controversial in the past [1]. Currently, the volume of the airway surface liquid hypothesis suggesting that CFTR defect leads to water loss related to sodium chloride (NaCl) depletion in the mucus remains the main hypothesis [1,4]. According to this hypothesis, immotile dehydrated plugs are formed leading to inefficient mucociliary clearance that allows bacteria to cause lung infection [4]. This mechanism suggested that hypertonic saline (HTS) nebulization could favor mucociliary clearance [5]. Clinical trials confirmed beneficial effects on lung function and rate of pulmonary exacerbations but no effect on bacterial density was observed [6–11]. Testing HTS on a large population of *P. aeruginosa* CF isolates should elucidate the anti-microbial effect of NaCl.

The aim of this study was to characterize the effects of NaCl on 85 *P. aeruginosa* isolates from CF respiratory tract in 34 patients. Results were interpreted according to strains characteristics, i.e., mucoidy, multidrug resistance, and biofilm biomass formation.

Materials and Methods

Bacterial strains and collected data

Eighty-five clinical isolates of *P. aeruginosa* have been retrospectively studied (Pa1 to Pa85). Four reference strains, *P. aeruginosa* ATCC 27853, *P. aeruginosa* ATCC 15442, *P. aeruginosa* ATCC 9027, and *P. aeruginosa* CIP A22 were included in the study. Clinical isolates have been recovered over a 6-year period (from 2006 to 2011) from 36 respiratory tract samples in 34 CF patients attending our local CF center (Centre de Ressources et de Compétences de la Mucoviscidose) of Montpellier, France. Patient age ranged from two-month to 61-year old (median, 19 year-old). Chronic colonization was noted for 19 patients with a median period of colonization of 5 years (1 to 14 years). A single isolate was included for 12 patients and multiple colonial morphotypes, i.e., two to six isolates collected either from one or two samples, were tested for 22 patients. Species identification, mucoid status, and antimicrobial susceptibility were retrieved from routine bacteriological sputum analysis. A multidrug-resistant isolate was defined according to the Cystic Fibrosis Consensus Conference of 1994 as an organism resistant to all of the agents in at least of the following groups of antibiotics (ß-lactam agents, amino-glycosides, fluoroquinolones) [12]. HTS nebulization during the study period was noted for each patient.

Dilution methods used for bacteriostatic and bactericidal activity testing of NaCl

Inoculums for bacteria in stationary and logarithmic growth phases were prepared from MH agar and broth cultures, respectively, by visual comparison to MacFarland standards followed by dilution steps depending on the assay as previously recommended [13]. Minimal Inhibitory Concentration (MIC) determination was performed by 2 different methods, agar (MICa) and microbroth (MICb) dilution methods with bacteria in stationary phase. For MICa, Mueller-Hinton (MH) plates containing 0%, 0.9%, 1%, 2%, 3%, 4%, 5%, 6%, 7%, 8%, 9%, 10%, 12%, and 15% of NaCl were inoculated with a final inoculum of 10^4 colony forming units (CFU) per spot and incubated one night at 37°C as described previously [13] before reading. For MICb, MH broth containing 0%, 0.9%, 1%, 2%, 3%, 4%, 5%, 6%, 7%, 8%, 9% and 10% of NaCl were inoculated with a final inoculum of $5*10^5$ CFU/ml and incubated one night at 37°C as described previously [13] before reading. Minimal Bactericidal Concentration (MBC) corresponding to the lowest antimicrobial concentration reducing the inoculum by 99.99% within 24 h was determined from MICb assay by subculturing wells, which had no visible growth and the growth control well as described previously [14]. Each inoculum was confirmed by colony count and all assays were performed in duplicate. When different results were obtained in the two independent tests, the higher MIC or MBC value was taken as the result. Time-kill kinetic study of NaCl was performed with a macrobroth dilution method using final inoculum of $5*10^5$ CFU/ml with bacteria in stationary and/or in logarithmic growth phases according to the assay. Inoculation of NaCl-containing broth was performed as described previously [13]. The final test volume was 10 ml of MH and bacterial suspension loads were determined by subculturing serial dilutions of the inoculum after different incubation periods, i.e., 10 min, 30 min, 1 h, 2 h, 3 h, and 24 h, at 4°C or 37°C according to the assay.

Biofilm formation

The ability to form biofilm biomass was tested according to the crystal violet method [15] and strains were categorized as non-adherent, weakly, moderately, or strongly adherent [15,16]. The measurement of HTS effect on biofilm biomass formation was performed as described above using a final bacterial inoculum of $5*10^5$ CFU/ml in MH broth containing 0%, 0.9%, 1%, 2%, 3%, 4%, 5%, 6%, 7%, 8%, 9% and 10% of NaCl. All tests were carried out at least three times and results were averaged. The reduction in biofilm biomass formation and hypertonic saline activity on preformed biofilm were evaluated according to the modified method of Pompilio and colleagues [17].

Evaluation of bacterial motility

Motility of strains in presence of different concentrations of NaCl was globally estimated from diameter of spotted cultures on MH plates used for MICa. A strain was considered as motile when overnight cultures had increased diameter compared to the spot initial size. Motility has been estimated for all isolates for NaCl concentrations lower than MICs obtained by the agar dilution method.

Statistical analysis

MIC, MBC, and killing quotient (KQ) distributions were analyzed according to the mucoid status, the multidrug resistance, and the ability to produce biofilm. Differences between groups were assessed by Mann-Whitney's test, with the exception of the evaluation depending on biofilm producer groups, assessed by the Kruskal-Wallis' test and Spearman correlation coefficient when Kruskal-Wallis' test was positive. Data were analyzed at the total population level and at a restricted level defined by one isolate type per patient to avoid biased results due to possible clonal relatedness of isolates in a patient because strains have not been genotyped in this study. Statistical analysis of results was done with R project software (http://www.r-project.org). A P value ≤ 0.05 was considered to reflect significance.

Ethics statements

This in vitro study required neither the agreement of the ethical committee of our institution nor the patient informed consent because it involved only bacterial strains. The study does not involve the sample collection or patient data, and no patient intervention occurred with the obtained results. Only general data patients (age, type of colonization by P. aeruginosa) were reported but no patient-related data were analyzed. No primary human sample materials were used, only bacterial isolates from routine diagnostic procedures or strain collections. All analyzed clinical strains were acquired during routine diagnostic procedures. Accordingly, no acquisition of patient samples for the study was undertaken. We did not conduct research outside of our country of residence.

Results

Antibacterial effect of NaCl on the *P. aeruginosa* population

MIC and MBC results are presented in Table 1. Intra and inter-method variability is given in Table S1. For the 85 CF isolates, MIC values ranged from 0.9 to 6%. Depending on the method considered, MIC_{50} and MIC_{90} values were 4 or 5% and 5 or 6%, respectively. The growth of all the isolates was inhibited after a 24 h-incubation with 6% NaCl solution whatever the method considered. Moreover, NaCl displayed a bactericidal effect, 38% of the CF isolates being killed by a 7% NaCl solution, concentration currently used in therapeutics, 50% and 90% of the isolates being killed by 8% and 10% of NaCl, respectively. The effect of NaCl varied depending on the isolate, differences between

MICb and MBC value observed for a strain ranging from 1% to up to 7%. No correlation between MICb and MBC values was observed, some isolates displaying low MIC values of 1 or 3% and high MBC values of 7% or 10%, respectively and conversely (data not shown). This resulted in KQ values < 4 for the 83 strains exhibiting MBC values within tested range supporting a bactericidal activity of NaCl on a large majority of strains (Table 1).

NaCl activity varied according to relevant sub-populations of *P. aeruginosa*

Considering strains recovered in patients with multiple isolates, differences between MICb and/or MBC values ranging from 0 to 3% were observed. Variable response to NaCl with MICb and/or MBC values differing by 3% of NaCl were observed for the isolates recovered from four patients.

Table 2 exhibits MIC, MBC and KQ values of relevant sub-populations. MICb values obtained for mucoid CF isolates were significantly lower than the ones obtained for non-mucoid isolates when the total population ($P<0.0001$) and a subgroup defined by one isolate type, mucoid and/or non-mucoid, per patient ($P=0.0003$) were considered. MBC distribution did not significantly differ between mucoid and non-mucoid isolate groups when the subpopulation defined by one isolate type per patient was considered ($P=0.07$) but did when the whole population (n = 85) was considered ($P=0.01$), which may be related to a lower statistical power in relation to a limited number of strains in the subpopulation (n = 48). KQs for mucoid isolates were consequently higher than those for non-mucoid isolates ($P=0.0002$ and $P=0.0008$ for the whole population and the defined subpopulation, respectively) (Table 2). Twenty-two isolates recovered from eleven samples obtained from eleven patients were multidrug resistant (MDR). Considering the whole population (n = 85), non-MDR isolates displayed significantly higher MICb than did the MDR isolates ($P=0.0005$) while no difference was observed for MBC values. Consequently, KQs were higher for MDR isolates than for non-MDR isolates ($P=0.002$). A similar trend was observed when considering one randomly selected isolate type, MDR and/or non-MDR, per patient (n = 40) (MICb: $P=0.005$, KQ: $P=0.001$) (Table 2).

Five strains were recovered (Pa17 to Pa21) from one patient under 6% HTS treatment administered once or twice daily for 4 years. These isolates displayed low MICb values (3%, 3%, 2%, 3%, and 3%, respectively) and high MBC values (>10%, >10%, 8%, >10%, and >10%, respectively).

NaCl mechanism of action

Time-kill kinetics. Time-kill kinetics was performed on two strains selected for divergent phenotype, i.e., strain Pa1 (mucoid, MICb of 3%, MBC of 7%) and strain Pa71 (non-mucoid, MICb of 2%, MBC of 5%). Inoculum in logarithmic phase of growth was tested for isolate Pa71 against various concentrations of NaCl (Figure 1). Time-kill curves highlighted that a rapid decrease in inoculum size was observed from 30 min and before 3 h of contact with NaCl. NaCl antibacterial activity under *in vitro* conditions was shown to be both concentration- and time-dependent. Impact of both growth phase and temperature on time-kill kinetics of NaCl was evaluated on isolate Pa1 (Figure 2). The Pa1-time-kill curve also showed a rapid NaCl effect when bacteria in logarithmic phase of growth were incubated at 37°C in presence of NaCl at the MBC. With bacteria in stationary phase of growth tested in the same conditions, the killing effect was also observed but was drastically delayed (Figure 2) and the bactericidal effect of 4-log reduction of the inoculum was absent within 24h when the assay was performed at 4°C (Figure 2). Altogether, these results suggested that anti-*P. aeruginosa* activity of NaCl might be different than a mere osmotic effect because it depended on temperature conditions and physiological bacterial state.

Effects of NaCl on biofilm. All reference strains were able to form biofilm biomass, being either strongly, moderately, or weakly adherent. The majority of the 85 CF *P. aeruginosa* isolates were able to form biofilm biomass (n = 76) but most of these isolates were weakly adherent (n = 42) (Table 2). Most mucoid isolates were weakly adherent (Table 2). Among the 22 patients colonized by two or more *P. aeruginosa* colony types, five harbored isolates showing a unique adherence type and 13 had isolates showing two adherence types. More rarely, isolates recovered from a same patient may present three or four adherence types (two patients each).

We found that MICb values were correlated to the ability to form biofilm biomass, the strongly adherent isolates being associated with higher MICb values when both the whole population and a subgroup defined by one randomly selected isolate per type per patient were considered ($P<0.0001$ and $P=0.0004$, respectively) (Table 2). There was no significant trend between the MBC value and the level of adherence ($P=0.14$ and 0.12 respectively) (Table 2).

A reduction of at least 25% of biofilm biomass formation was highlighted for 23% to 69% of strongly adherent strains depending on the NaCl concentration with a dose-dependent effect, and for 27% to 53% of moderately adherent isolates (Figure 3). Twenty percent of weakly adherent isolates showed a decrease in their ability to form biofilm biomass independently of the NaCl concentration tested. With 2 and 3% of NaCl, rates of isolates

Table 1. NaCl Minimal Inhibitory Concentration (MIC), Minimal Bactericidal Concentration (MBC) and Killing quotient (KQ) distributions for the 85 CF isolates and the 4 reference strains of *P. aeruginosa*.

	NaCl MIC values (in %)											
	Agar dilution method			Broth dilution method			NaCl MBC values (in %)			Killing quotient (KQ)[a]		
Strains or isolates (n)	MIC_{50}	MIC_{90}	Range	MIC_{50}	MIC_{90}	Range	MBC_{50}	MBC_{90}	Range	KQ_{50}	KQ_{90}	Range
All strains (n = 89)	4	5	2–6	5	6	0.9–6	8	10	4->10	1.8	2.7	1.2–7.8
Reference strains (n = 4)	5	5	5	5	6	5–6	7	9	7–9	1.4	1.6	1.4–1.6
CF isolates (n = 85)	4	5	2–6	4	6	0.9–6	8	10	4->10	1.8	3	1.2–7.8

MIC_{50} and MIC_{90} values were defined as the lowest concentration of NaCl at which 50% and 90% of the isolates were inhibited, respectively.
[a]Only isolates exhibiting MBC values within tested range were considered.

Table 2. Comparison of NaCl Minimal Inhibitory Concentration (MIC), Minimal Bactericidal Concentration (MBC) and Killing quotient (KQ) distributions for subgroups of *P. aeruginosa* CF isolates according to mucoid characteristic, antimicrobial susceptibility pattern, ability to form biofilm and patient under HTS treatment.

			NaCl MIC values (in %)															
			Agar dilution method				Broth dilution method				NaCl MBC values (in %)				Killing quotient (KQ)[a]			
Population	Subgroup	Isolate type (n)	MIC_{50}	MIC_{90}	Range	*P* value [d]	MIC_{50}	MIC_{90}	Range	*P* value [d]	MBC_{50}	MBC_{90}	Range	*P* value[d]	KQ_{50}	KQ_{90}	Range	*P* value [d]
Total CF isolates	Mucoid characteristic	Mucoid (25)	3	4	2–4	**<0.0001**	3	5	0.9–5	**<0.0001**	7	9	6–>10	**0.01**	2.3	3.5	1.4–7.8	**0.0002**
		Non-mucoid (60)	5	5	2–6		5	6	2–6		8	10	4–>10		1.6	2.3	1.2–4	
	Antimicrobial susceptibility pattern	Multidrug resistance (22)	3	4	2–5	**<0.0001**	3	5	2–5	**0.0005**	8	>10	7–>10	0.3	2.3	3.5	1.4–4	**0.002**
		Non-multidrug resistance (63)	4	5	2–6		5	6	0.9–6		8	9	4–>10		1.8	2.3	1.2–7.8	
	Ability to form biofilm	No (9 of which 3 mucoid)	3	5	2–5	**<0.0001 Rs = 0.44**	3	5	2–5	**<0.0001 Rs = 0.48**	7	9	4–9	0.14	2.3	4	1.4–4	**0.0009 Rs = −0.37**
		Weak (42 of which 16 mucoid)	4	5	2–5		4	5	0.9–6		8	10	5–>10		1.8	3.5	1.2–7.8	
		Moderate (18 of which 3 mucoid)	5	5	2–5		5	6	2–6		8	>10	7–>10		1.8	2.3	1.2–3.5	
		Strong (16 of which 3 mucoid)	5	6	3–6		5	6	3–6		8	9	6–10		1.5	2	1.2–2.7	
	Patient under HTS treatment	Yes (5) [b]	2	3	2–3	ND	3	3	2–3	ND	>10	>10	8–>10	ND	ND	ND	ND	ND
		No (80)	4	5	2–6		5	6	0.9–6		8	9	4–>10		1.8	2.7	1.2–7.8	
One isolate per type, per patient [c]	Mucoid characteristic	Mucoid (18)	3	4	2–4	**<0.0001**	3	5	2–5	**0.0003**	7	9	7–>10	0.07	2.3	3.5	1.4–4.5	**0.0008**
		Non-mucoid (30)	5	5	2–6		5	6	2–6		8	9	5–>10		1.5	2.3	1.2–3.3	
	Antimicrobial susceptibility pattern	Multidrug resistance (11)	3	4	2–5	**0.002**	3	5	2–5	**0.005**	8	10	7–>10	0.6	2	3.5	1.6–3.5	**0.001**
		Non-multidrugresistance (29)	5	5	2–6		5	6	0.9–6		8	9	5–>10		1.5	2.3	1.2–7.8	
	Ability to form biofilm	No (7 of which 1 mucoid)	3	5	2–5	**<0.0001 Rs = 0.5**	3	5	2–5	**0.0004 Rs = 0.46**	7	9	4–9	0.12	2.3	4	1.4–4	0.056
		Weak (24 of which 8 mucoid)	4	5	2–5		4	6	2–6		8	10	5–>10		1.6	2·5	1.3–3.5	
		Moderate (15 of which 3 mucoid)	5	5	2–5		5	6	2–6		8	>10	7–>10		1.8	2·3	1.3–3.5	
		Strong (11 of which 2 mucoid)	5	6	4–6		5	6	4–6		9	9	7–10		1.5	2	1.3–2	
	Patient under HTS treatment	Yes (1)	ND	ND	2	ND	ND	ND	3	ND	ND	ND	>10	ND	ND	ND	ND	ND
		No (33)	5	5	2–6		5	6	2–6		8	9	5– >10		1.6	2.5	1.2–3.5	

MIC_{50} and MIC_{90} values were defined as the lowest concentration of NaCl at which 50% and 90% of the isolates were inhibited, respectively.

[a]Only isolates exhibiting MBC values within tested range were considered.

[b]5 isolates recovered in one patient.

[c]isolates were randomly selected.

[d]Comparison of MIC, MBC and KQ distribution between subgroups was performed with Mann-Whitney's test, with the exception of the evaluation depending on biofilm producer groups, assessed by the Kruskal-Wallis' test, and Spearman correlation coefficient (Rs) when Kruskal-Wallis' test was positive. A *P* value ≤0.05 was considered to reflect significance and was indicated in bold type.

ND, not determined either because only one isolate or one patient was included in the sub-population, or because one isolate exhibiting a MBC value within the tested range.

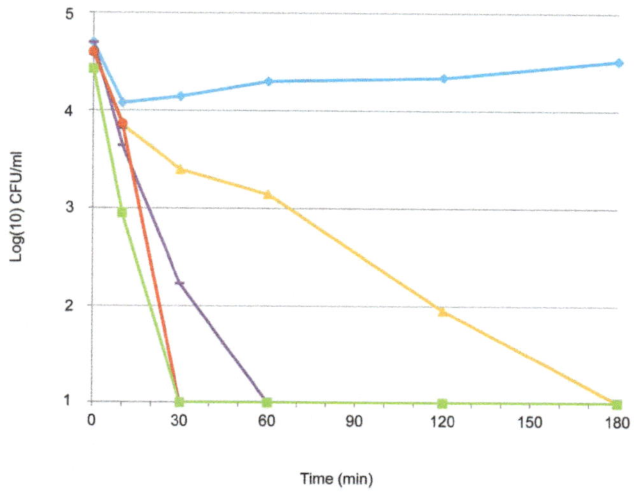

Figure 1. Time-kill kinetics of different NaCl concentrations against *P. aeruginosa* isolate Pa71. 3% NaCl solution (orange line, filled triangles), 5% NaCl solution - corresponding to the MBC value (violet line, dash), 7% NaCl solution (red line, filled circles), and 10% NaCl solution (green line, filled squares). Control (blue line, filled lozenges) was not exposed to NaCl. Time-kill curves of 15% (not shown) and 10% NaCl solution were similar.

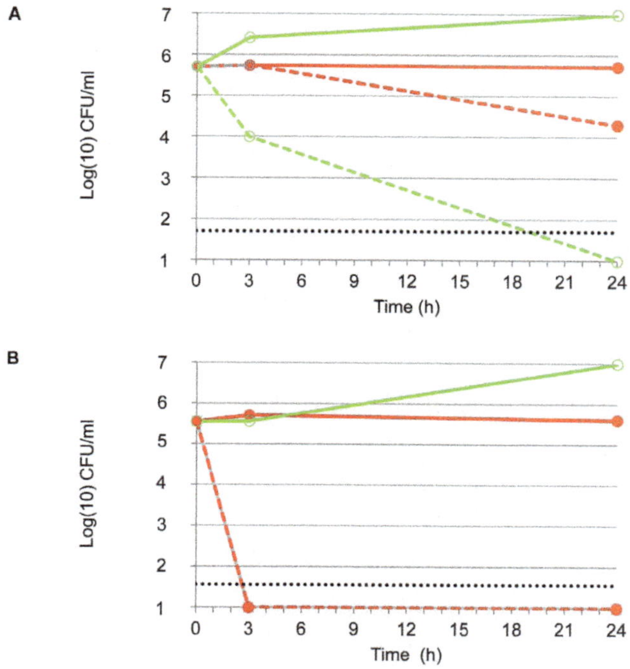

Figure 2. Time-kill kinetics of NaCl against *P.aeruginosa* Pa1 according to bacterial phase of growth and incubation temperature. Inoculum in stationary phase of growth (A) and in logarithmic phase of growth (B) for Pa1 (NaCl MBC: 7%). Bacterial suspension in NaCl at the MBC value were incubated at 37°C (green dotted line, open circles) or 4°C (red dotted line, filled circles). Controls (full lines) were not exposed to NaCl and were incubated at 37°C (green line, open circles) or 4°C (red line, filled circles). The horizontal dotted line indicates a 4-log reduction in viability. B: dotted green (open circles) and red (filled circles) lines are superposed.

showing reduction in biofilm biomass formation increased with the adherence level. Analysis conducted on subgroups defined by one isolate per type of adherence per patient showed similar results (data not shown).

In vitro activity of NaCl solution (7% and 10%) was evaluated on preformed biofilm for Pa28, Pa29, and Pa31, three strongly adherent, non-mucoid, non-MDR isolates with identical MICb and MBC values (MICb = 6%, MBC = 9%) recovered from three patients. Biofilm viability was reduced and this appeared to be dose dependent (Figure 4).

Time-kill kinetics showed a killing effect on preformed biofilm resulting in at least a 10^{-3} decrease in bacterial load and occurring between 1 h and 4 h of contact with 10% of NaCl (Figure 5).

Evaluation of NaCl activity on motility. For NaCl concentration above 2%, none of the 46 isolates displaying motility in the absence of NaCl were motile anymore (Figure 6), suggesting that NaCl inhibited isolate motility at concentrations lower than those inhibiting bacterial growth.

Discussion

Short-term and long-term clinical randomized trials in CF patients showed beneficial effects of HTS nebulization on lung function in reducing exacerbations or on the perception of effectiveness of chest physiotherapy [6,8,9,11]. Positive effects were explained by mucus rehydration and mucociliary clearance improvement, anti-inflammatory activity and indirect effects by activation of antimicrobial peptides [4,5,18]. No report investigated antimicrobial activity of NaCl as a possible explanation supporting beneficial effects of such a treatment.

We proposed the first study evaluating *in vitro* NaCl activity on a large population of *P. aeruginosa* isolated from CF patients. Multiple antimicrobial effects of NaCl on CF *P. aeruginosa* are demonstrated with NaCl concentrations used in therapeutics. Indeed, we showed that: i) 6% NaCl solution inhibits bacterial growth for all the tested isolates, ii) a killing effect was observed from 4% NaCl solution, and iii)10% NaCl solution had a bactericidal activity on 90% of the isolates. We also demonstrated that NaCl had effects on bacterial biofilm being able to alter biofilm biomass formation of strongly adherent isolates at sub-inhibitory concentrations and to have a killing effect on preformed biofilm. However, according to

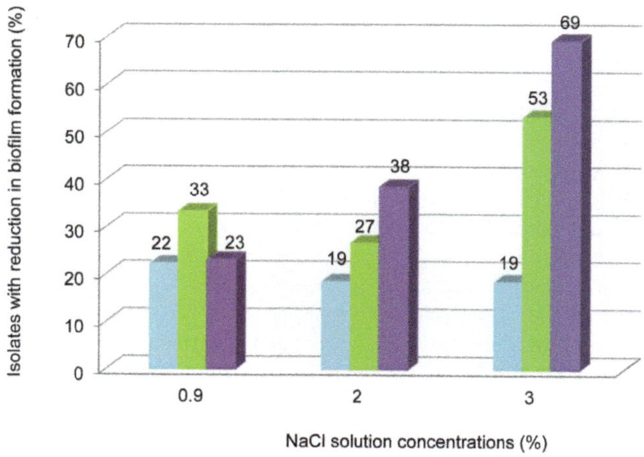

Figure 3. Effect of three sub-inhibitory concentrations of NaCl against *P. aeruginosa* CF isolate biofilm biomass formation. Tested for 55 adherent CF isolates of *P. aeruginosa* with MIC values > 3% distributed as follows: strongly adherent (n = 13, violet bars), moderately adherent (n = 15, green bars), weakly adherent phenotype (n = 27, blue bars). Prevention of biofilm biomass formation is presented as percentage of strains for which ability to form biofilm biomass was decreased by at least 25% compared to controls (not exposed).

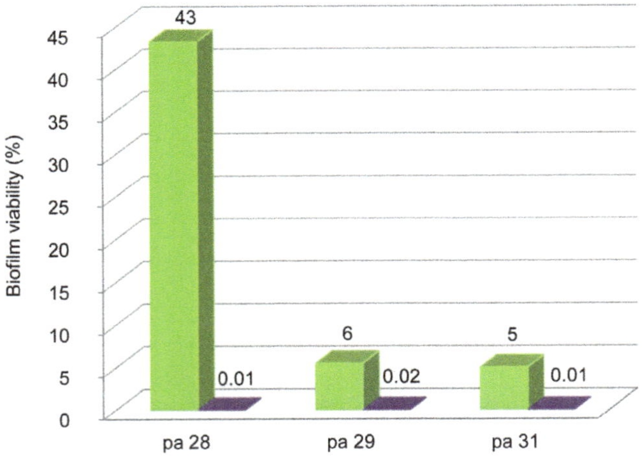

Figure 4. Activity of 7% and 10% NaCl solution against preformed biofilm for three strongly adherent isolates. 7% (green bars) and 10% (violet bars) NaCl solution was tested against preformed biofilm for the three *P. aeruginosa* CF isolates Pa28, Pa29, and Pa31. Results are expressed as percentage of biofilm viability compared to non-exposed control after 24 h of NaCl exposure.

MIC values, isolates with strong biofilm biomass production abilities were more resistant to NaCl action suggesting that the mature biofilm acts as a protection against inhibitory effect of NaCl. Finally, although the method used in this study did not allow study of the type of motility, i.e., swarming, swimming or twitching motility, affected by NaCl, we showed that NaCl inhibited the strain global motility as previously suggested for four *P. aeruginosa* strains [19]. Since bacterial motility and loss of motility are known to play a role in biofilm formation by *P. aeruginosa* [20], the specific impact of the motility inhibition by NaCl on biofilm formation has still to be evaluated. Time kill kinetics evaluated *in vitro* for 2 selected isolates suggested that NaCl antibacterial activity was both concentration- and time-dependent. Of note, these results were observed even though using the most stringent definition of the MBC, i.e., the lowest antimicrobial concentration reducing the inoculum by 99.99% within 24 h and bacterial growth conditions, i.e., bacteria in stationary phase of growth, which could have led to overestimation of MBC for some isolates. Of particular interest is the higher susceptibility to NaCl observed for clinically relevant subpopulations of *P. aeruginosa*, i.e., mucoid and/or multidrug resistant isolates. We found that the growth of mucoid isolates was inhibited by significantly lower NaCl concentrations than the one of non-mucoid isolates, as described for a *mucA22* mutant that was significantly more sensitive to osmotic stress than the isogenic parental *P. aeruginosa* PAO1 strain [21]. These results suggested that the reduction in exacerbation rate following prolonged treatment with HTS nebulization resulted from a population shift from mucoid to non-mucoid *P. aeruginosa* [21,22]. MICs were also significantly lower for MDR isolates than non-MDR isolates. Although not further investigated here, this could be related to a fitness cost of multidrug resistance [23] that could impair osmotic stress response. Altogether, active antimicrobial activity of NaCl against CF *P. aeruginosa* isolates might contribute to the *in vivo* global positive effect of HTS treatment. In addition, indirect effects may also enhance NaCl antimicrobial effect *in vivo* like disruption of inhibitory interactions between glycosaminoglycans present within the mucus and antimicrobial peptides [24].

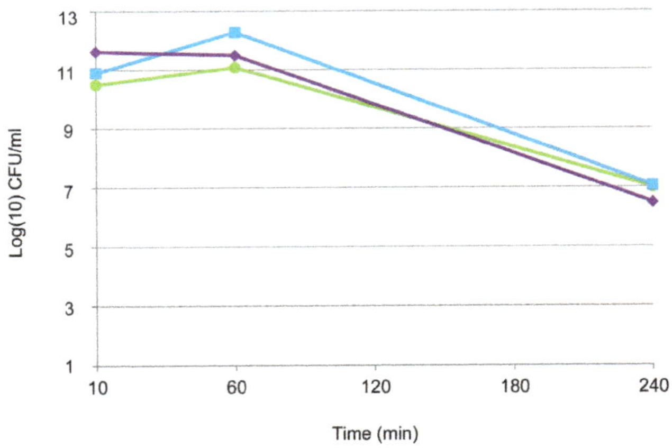

Figure 5. Time-kill kinetics of 10% NaCl solution against preformed biofilm for three strongly adherent CF isolates. *P. aeruginosa* CF isolates: Pa28 (green line, filled circles), Pa29 (blue line, filled squares), Pa31 (violet line, filled lozenges).

HTS treatment is currently not standardized and varies according to the study in the volume of aerosolized HTS (4, 5, or 10 ml), the rhythm of administration (twice or four times daily), the mode of administration (via jet or positive expiratory pressure nebulizers), and the HTS concentration (5.85%, 6%, or 7%) [6,8,9,11,25]. The effect of HTS appeared to be both dose-dependent [26] and time-dependent [27]. Considering the absence of significant change in the density of *P. aeruginosa* observed in a previous study [6], it could be assumed that the conditions of treatment, i.e., 4 ml of 7% HTS twice daily, were not bactericidal but only inhibitory against *P. aeruginosa in vivo*. Our results open important areas of research by suggesting that optimization of HTS conditions of use (rhythm, dose, mode of delivery) in CF may contribute to enhance anti-*P.aeruginosa* effects and thereby treatment clinical efficacy. However, studies that use *in vivo* models and randomized clinical trials are needed to evaluate the performances of diverse HTS administration conditions and to determine the more appropriate and efficient conditions of HTS use in CF patients. More largely our study highlights the potential use of NaCl as a basic but important component of the therapeutic arsenal used in the management of infectious diseases. Hyperosmotic stress is known for reducing biofilm growth and for being bactericidal on *Escherichia coli*, *P. aeruginosa*, and *Enterococcus faecalis*

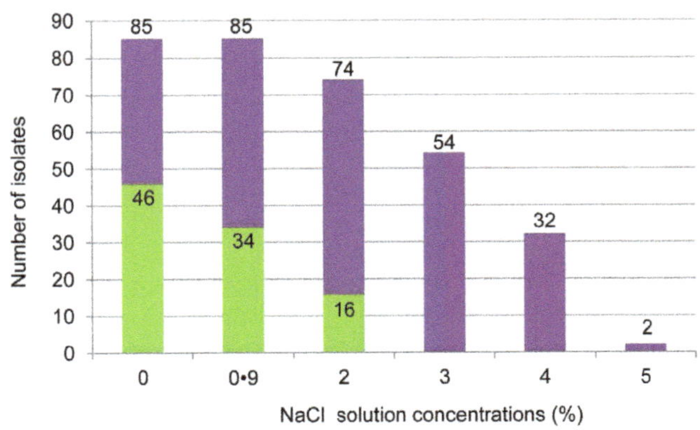

Figure 6. Rate of motile isolates according to NaCl concentration. Green bars show the number of motile isolates among isolates with non-inhibited growth (full bars).

when NaCl is used at 13% to 35% and could be used for treatment of root canal infection [28] or for locking tunneled hemodialysis catheters [29]. Considering the lower NaCl concentrations used in this study, the antimicrobial effect was probably not related to a direct hyperosmotic lysis. We presented arguments for an antimicrobial activity linked to an active biological process: i) NaCl was efficient mainly on bacteria in logarithmic phase of growth independently of the temperature and to a lesser extent on bacteria in stationary phase of growth at 37°C, ii) in stationary phase of growth at 4°C, which could be considered as metabolic standby conditions, HTS produced slight antimicrobial effects on *P. aeruginosa*, iii) variable response to HTS was observed among the population, and iv) loss of motility occurred from 2% NaCl solution. In summary, because the response to NaCl depended on the bacterial physiological status and varied among the population of *P. aeruginosa*, we assumed that NaCl bactericidal effect could be due to complex regulated mechanisms rather than to a mere hyperosmotic effect.

Several bioclinical answers remain to be addressed. Particularly, longitudinal studies are needed to monitor the evolution of NaCl MICs and MBCs of *P. aeruginosa* isolates recovered from the respiratory tract in patients under HTS treatment. In this study, only one patient was under HTS treatment for 4 years and isolates displayed high MBC and low MIC values. For this purpose, methods first proposed in this study for NaCl antimicrobial activity evaluation appeared suitable because of their good reproducibility. In addition, evaluating the NaCl action on several other CF pathogens including viruses, yeast, and fungi would be of interest because recent studies suggested NaCl-altered growth beyond NaCl concentration used in therapeutics for some viruses and yeasts not involved in CF [30,31]. The effect of HTS on polymicrobial community of the CF respiratory tract should be investigated not only because halotolerant bacteria may be favored by such a treatment but also because any modification of the relative composition of this complex microbiota will impact intercellular interactions and communication involved in this polymicrobial disease with unknown consequences [2,32]. Finally, the antimicrobial mechanism of action of NaCl warrants further investigation because it is still not fully elucidated, particularly the hypothesis of the possible induction of lytic activity of *P. aeruginosa* bacteriophages by NaCl has to be explored. Indeed, several environmental factors such as temperature or pH but also salinity could influence the transition from lysogenic to lytic phage [33,34].

Over the last decade, treatment strategies have shifted from controlling chronic infection to attempting to eradicate *P. aeruginosa* in the early stages of infection. Whatever the strategy, the antibiotic resistance makes the need for alternative approaches obvious and non-antibiotic treatments may expand the therapeutic repertoire. NaCl, as a simple and basic compound, may become a pivotal resource in CF care and in fighting *P. aeruginosa*. Beside polyvalent effects on the CF respiratory tract, we gave insights into antimicrobial activities of NaCl. NaCl kills *P. aeruginosa* but also acts on a range of its core eco-physiological functions such as biofilm formation and motility. Future studies should go further toward evaluating the role of NaCl in bacteriophage predation. Taken together, results and hypotheses on NaCl effects open research paths to treat CF as an eco-pathology of the respiratory tract. More widely, the efficacy of NaCl alone or in association with current available therapeutics should be more deeply investigated in infectious diseases.

Supporting Information

Table S1 Reproducibility and inter-method variability of Minimal Inhibitory Concentration (MIC) and Minimal Bactericidal Concentration (MBC) measurements.

Author Contributions

Conceived and designed the experiments: ALM HM EJB. Performed the experiments: ALM. Analyzed the data: ALM HM EJB BL. Wrote the paper: ALM. Acquisition of data: ALM RC. Performed statistical analyses: ALM BL. Critically revised the manuscript: HM RC BL EJB.

References

1. Clunes MT, Boucher RC (2007) Cystic Fibrosis: the mechanisms of pathogenesis of an inherited lung disorder. Drug Discov Today Dis Mech 4: 63–72.
2. Sibley CD, Rabin H, Surette MG (2006) Cystic fibrosis: a polymicrobial infectious disease. Future Microbiol 1: 53–61.
3. Emerson J, Rosenfeld M, McNamara S, Ramsey B, Gibson RL (2002) *Pseudomonas aeruginosa* and other predictors of mortality and morbidity in young children with cystic fibrosis. Pediatr Pulmonol 34: 91–100.
4. Boucher RC (2007) Evidence for airway surface dehydration as the initiating event in CF airway disease. J Intern Med 261: 5–16.
5. Reeves EP, Molloy K, Pohl K, McElvaney NG (2012) Hypertonic saline in treatment of pulmonary disease in cystic fibrosis. Scientific World Journal 465230.
6. Elkins MR, Robinson M, Rose BR, Harbour C, Moriarty CP, et al. (2006) A controlled trial of long-term inhaled hypertonic saline in patients with cystic fibrosis. N Engl J Med 354: 229–240.
7. Dmello D, Nayak RP, Matuschak GM (2011) Stratified assessment of the role of inhaled hypertonic saline in reducing cystic fibrosis pulmonary exacerbations: a retrospective analysis. BMJ Open 1:e000019.
8. Eng PA, Morton J, Douglass JA, Riedler J, Wilson J, et al. (1996) Short-term efficacy of ultrasonically nebulized hypertonic saline in cystic fibrosis. Pediatr Pulmonol 21: 77–83.
9. Ballmann M, Von der Hardt H (2002) Hypertonic saline and recombinant human DNase: a randomised cross-over pilot study in patients with cystic fibrosis. J Cyst Fibros 1: 35–37.
10. Wark P, McDonald V (2009) Nebulised hypertonic saline for cystic fibrosis. Cochrane Database Syst Rev CD001506.
11. Donaldson SH, Bennett WD, Zeman KL, Knowles MR, Tarran R, et al. (2006) Mucus clearance and lung function in cystic fibrosis with hypertonic saline. N Engl J Med 354: 241–250.
12. Cystic Fibrosis Consensus Conference May 17–18, 1994. Microbiology and infectious disease in cystic fibrosis. Bethesda, MD, Cystic Fibrosis Foundation, 1994; Vol. 5, Section 1, pp. 1–26.
13. Patel JB, Tenover FC, Turnidge JD, Jorgensen JH (2011) Susceptibility test methods: dilution and disk diffusion methods. In: Versalovic J, Carroll KC, Funke G, Jorgensen JH, Landry ML, Warnock DW, editors. Manual of Clinical Microbiology, 10th edn. Washington, DC: American Society for Microbiology press, pp 1122–1143.
14. Courvalin P, Leclercq R, Rice L (2009) Antibiogram, 3rd edn. Washington, DC: American Society for Microbiology press.
15. Stepanovic S, Vukovic D, Dakic I, Savic B, Svabic-Vlahovic M (2000) A modified microtiter-plate test for quantification of staphylococcal biofilm formation. J Microbiol Methods 40: 175–179.
16. Deligianni E, Pattison S, Berrar D, Ternan NG, Haylock RW, et al. (2010) *Pseudomonas aeruginosa* Cystic Fibrosis isolates of similar RAPD genotype exhibit diversity in biofilm forming ability *in vitro*. BMC Microbiol 10: 38.
17. Pompilio A, Crocetta V, Scocchi M, Pomponio S, Di Vincenzo V, et al. (2012) Potential novel therapeutic strategies in cystic fibrosis: antimicrobial and anti-biofilm activity of natural and designed α-helical peptides against *Staphylococcus aureus*, *Pseudomonas aeruginosa*, and *Stenotrophomonas maltophilia*. BMC Microbiol 12: 145.
18. Bye PT, Elkins MR (2007) Other mucoactive agents for cystic fibrosis. Paediatr Respir Rev 8:30–39.
19. Havasi V, Hurst CO, Briles TC, Yang F, Bains DG, et al. (2008) Inhibitory effects of hypertonic saline on *P. aeruginosa* motility. J Cyst Fibros 7: 267–269.
20. O'Toole GA, Kolter R (1998) Flagellar and twitching motility are necessary for *Pseudomonas aeruginosa* biofilm development. Mol Microbiol 30: 295–304.
21. Behrends V, Ryall B, Wang X, Bundy JG, Williams HD (2010) Metabolic profiling of *Pseudomonas aeruginosa* demonstrates that the anti-sigma factor MucA modulates osmotic stress tolerance. Mol Biosyst 6: 562–569.
22. Williams HD, Behrends V, Bundy JG, Ryall B, Zlosnik JE (2010) Hypertonic saline therapy in cystic fibrosis: do population shifts caused by the osmotic sensitivity of infecting bacteria explain the effectiveness of this treatment? Front Microbiol 1: 120.

23. Abdelraouf K, Kabbara S, Ledesma KR, Poole K, Tam VH (2011) Effect of multidrug resistance-conferring mutations on the fitness and virulence of *Pseudomonas aeruginosa*. J Antimicrob Chemother 66: 1311–1317.
24. Bergsson G, Reeves EP, McNally P, Chotirmall SH, Greene CM, et al. (2009) LL-37 complexation with glycosaminoglycans in cystic fibrosis lungs inhibits antimicrobial activity, which can be restored by hypertonic saline. J Immunol 183: 543–551.
25. O'Connell OJ, O'Farrell C, Harrison MJ, Eustace JA, Henry MT, et al. (2011) Nebulized hypertonic saline via positive expiratory pressure versus via jet nebulizer in patients with severe cystic fibrosis. Respir Care 56: 771–775.
26. Robinson M, Hemming AL, Regnis JA, Wong AG, Bailey DL, et al. (1997) Effect of increasing doses of hypertonic saline on mucociliary clearance in patients with cystic fibrosis. Thorax 52: 900–903.
27. Tarran R, Grubb BR, Parsons D, Picher M, Hirsh AJ, et al. (2001) The CF salt controversy: *in vivo* observations and therapeutic approaches. Mol Cell 8: 149–158.
28. Van der Waal SV, Van der Sluis LWM, Özok AR, Exterkate RA, van Marle J, et al. (2011) The effects of hyperosmosis or high pH on a dual-species biofilm of *Enterococcus faecalis* and *Pseudomonas aeruginosa*: an in vitro study. Int Endod J 44: 1110–1117.
29. Oguzhan N, Pala C, Sipahioglu MH, Cilan H, Durmaz S, et al. (2012) Locking tunneled hemodialysis catheters with hypertonic saline (26% NaCl) and heparin to prevent catheter-related bloodstream infections and thrombosis: a randomized, prospective trial. Ren Fail 34: 181–188.
30. Parmar JH, Bhartiya S, Venkatesh KV (2011) Characterization of the adaptive response and growth upon hyperosmotic shock in *Saccharomyces cerevisiae*. Mol Biosyst 7: 1138–1148.
31. Seo K, Lee JE, Lim MY, Ko G (2012) Effect of temperature, pH, and NaCl on the inactivation kinetics of murine norovirus. J Food Prot 75: 533–540.
32. Peters BM, Jabra-Rizk MA, O'May GA, Costerton JW, Shirtliff ME (2012) Polymicrobial interactions: impact on pathogenesis and human disease. Clin Microbiol Rev 25: 193–213.
33. Williamson SJ, Paul JH (2006) Environmental factors that influence the transition from lysogenic to lytic existence in the phiHSIC/Listonella pelagia marine phage-host system. Microb Ecol 52: 217–225.
34. Shkilnyj P, Koudelka GB (2007) Effect of salt shock on stability of lambdaimm434 lysogens. J Bacteriol 189: 3115–3123.

3

Chemically Modified Peptide Scaffolds Target the CFTR-Associated Ligand PDZ Domain

Jeanine F. Amacher[1], Ruizhi Zhao[2,3], Mark R. Spaller[2,3,4], Dean R. Madden[1]*

1 Department of Biochemistry, Geisel School of Medicine at Dartmouth, Hanover, New Hampshire, United States of America, 2 Department of Chemistry, Dartmouth College, Hanover, New Hampshire, United States of America, 3 Norris Cotton Cancer Center, Dartmouth-Hitchcock Medical Center, Lebanon, New Hampshire, United States of America, 4 Department of Pharmacology and Toxicology, Geisel School of Medicine at Dartmouth, Hanover, New Hampshire, United States of America

Abstract

PDZ domains are protein-protein interaction modules that coordinate multiple signaling and trafficking pathways in the cell and that include active therapeutic targets for diseases such as cancer, cystic fibrosis, and addiction. Our previous work characterized a PDZ interaction that restricts the apical membrane half-life of the cystic fibrosis transmembrane conductance regulator (CFTR). Using iterative cycles of peptide-array and solution-binding analysis, we targeted the PDZ domain of the CFTR-Associated Ligand (CAL), and showed that an engineered peptide inhibitor rescues cell-surface expression of the most common CFTR disease mutation ΔF508. Here, we present a series of scaffolds containing chemically modifiable side chains at all non-motif positions along the CAL PDZ domain binding cleft. Concordant equilibrium dissociation constants were determined in parallel by fluorescence polarization, isothermal titration calorimetry, and surface plasmon resonance techniques, confirming robust affinity for each scaffold and revealing an enthalpically driven mode of inhibitor binding. Structural studies demonstrate a conserved binding mode for each peptide, opening the possibility of combinatorial modification. Finally, we diversified one of our peptide scaffolds with halogenated substituents that yielded modest increases in binding affinity. Overall, this work validates our approach and provides a stereochemical foundation for further CAL inhibitor design and screening.

Editor: Jeffrey L. Brodsky, University of Pittsburgh, United States of America

Funding: This work was supported by National Institutes of Health (NIH): http://grants.nih.gov/grants/oer.htm, 1. R01-DK101541 to DRM, 2. P30-GM106394 to DRM, 3. T32-DK007301 to JFA, 4. R01-CA150190 to MRS, and The Hitchcock Foundation: http://med.dartmouth-hitchcock.org/hitchcock_foundation.html, Program Project Grant (PPG) to DRM. The funders had no role in study design, data collection and analysis, decision to publish, or preparation of the manuscript.

Competing Interests: Dr. Madden is a co-inventor on patent filings covering the therapeutic use of CAL inhibitor peptides. Patent number is 8,415,292, issued 4/9/13.

* Email: drm0001@dartmouth.edu

Introduction

One of the key goals of drug development is selectivity. Without it, side effects can overwhelm even highly promising therapeutic effects [1]. It has proven especially difficult to design selective inhibitors of a common class of targets, the protein-protein interaction PDZ domains, named after the founding members PSD-95, Dlg, and ZO-1 [2,3,4,5]. PDZ domains generally recognize the extreme C-termini of target proteins, and engage only a limited set of motif residues [6,7]. As a result, they frequently exhibit considerable overlap in their binding profiles. Furthermore, PDZ interactions are transient, and affinities are typically in the micromolar range [8]. Thus, despite over a decade of research, there are currently no reports of PDZ domain inhibitors in clinical trials or late stages of drug development.

In previous work, we have investigated the binding preferences of a PDZ domain that is known to interact with the C-terminus of the cystic fibrosis transmembrane conductance regulator (CFTR). The CFTR-associated ligand (CAL) controls the apical membrane half-life of CFTR and is a validated therapeutic target for the disease cystic fibrosis [5,9,10]. We have previously described a peptide array-based approach that enabled us to design a selective inhibitor for the CAL PDZ (CALP) domain. The result was iCAL36, a decameric peptide with sequence ANSRWPTSII [5,9].

Despite this success, the micromolar CALP-binding affinity of iCAL36 remains weak by pharmacological standards. To address this limitation we sought a platform that would enable us to expand the chemical space available for inhibitor optimization. Given the dearth of high-affinity small-molecule PDZ inhibitors and the inherent propensity of such domains to bind peptides, we decided to focus on peptidomimetic strategies, which include the addition of lipids, chemical moieties, cycles, non-natural amino acids and backbone chemistries [2,3,4,5,11,12]. Such modifications can increase the contact surface area of the interaction, and thus potentially enhance its affinity. In addition, since non-natural moieties can reach surfaces outside the peptide-binding cleft, these peptides may be more specific than those derived from naturally occurring amino acids [13,14]. As a result, iterative rounds of stereochemical refinement may provide opportunities to develop higher affinity, more selective inhibitors.

Indeed, CALP provides an ideal system to investigate the biochemistry of chemically modified peptides. We know peptide inhibitors are efficacious in cells [5,9,15], and we can use X-ray

Table 1. Comparison of binding affinities measured by various techniques.

Peptide	Sequence	K_D from FP (μM)	K_D from ITC (μM)[a]	K_D from SPR (μM)[a]
iCAL36	ANSRWPTSII	22.6±8.0[b]	42.2±4.0	44.2±0.3
			(1.9)[c]	(2.0)[c]
Ac-iCAL36	Ac-ANSRWPTSII[d]	22.6±1.7	73.2±12.9	74.0±2.6
			(3.2)	(3.3)
iCAL36$_{Ac\text{-}K^{-1}}$	ANSRWPTS[Ac-K]I[e]	14.9±5.8	26.4±4.5	39.5±3.2
			(1.8)	(2.7)
iCAL36$_{Ac\text{-}K^{-3}}$	ANSRWP[Ac-K]SII[e]	180±110	91.9[f]	122±10
			(0.5)	(0.7)
iCAL36$_{Ac\text{-}K^{-4}}$	ANSRW[Ac-K]TSII[e]	32.3±6.2	49.4[f]	64.6±4.0
			(1.5)	(2.0)
iCAL36$_{Ac\text{-}K^{-5}}$	ANSR[Ac-K]PTSII[e]	550±400	ND	298±5
				(0.5)
iCAL36$_{BB\text{-}K^{-1}}$	ANSRWPTS[BB-K]I[g]	11.1±3.9	20.7±2.0	20.0±0.4
			(1.9)	(1.8)
iCAL36$_{FB\text{-}K^{-1}}$	ANSRWPTS[FB-K]I[h]	11.4±3.7	12.8±1.7	27.9±3.6
			(1.1)	(2.4)
iCAL36$_{Tfa\text{-}K^{-1}}$	ANSRWPTS[Tfa-K]I[i]	14.1±2.0	34.5±8.8	22.3±4.2
			(2.4)	(1.6)

[a] K_D values as reported in ref. [20].
[b] Value previously reported in ref. [17].
[c] Value in parentheses indicates fold-deviation from the value obtained by FP.
[d] Ac- indicates N-terminal acetylation.
[e] [Ac-K] indicates N_ζ-acetyl-lysine.
[f] n = 1.
[g] [BB-K] indicates N_ζ-4-bromobenzoyl-lysine.
[h] [FB-K] indicates N_ζ-4-fluorobenzoyl-lysine.
[i] [Tfa-K] indicates N_ζ-trifluoroacetyl-lysine.

crystallography to investigate the stereochemistry of the interactions at high resolution [16,17]. We have previously explored dirhodium modification of CALP peptide inhibitors and seen a robust effect; however, crystallization efforts with those peptides have so far been unsuccessful due to solubility limits of the peptides [18]. Here, we describe another strategy, with the goal of testing the suitability of a set of iCAL36-based scaffolds, each carrying a lysine side-chain acceptor for chemical modifications at one of the non-motif positions along the peptide-binding cleft. In addition, we use structural and biochemical techniques to directly investigate the hypothesis that side-chain modification can regulate the affinity of peptide-based inhibitors for a PDZ target without disrupting the binding pose of the complex.

Materials and Methods

Protein and Peptide Synthesis

CALP protein was expressed and purified as previously described [19]. The peptides described in Table 1, with the exception of iCAL36 used in FP studies (which was synthesized by the Tufts Core Facility), were prepared at room temperature (RT) using standard Fmoc-based solid-phase peptide synthesis protocols, with modifications to accelerate preparation. Pre-loaded Fmoc-Ile-Wang resin was swollen 30 min in dimethylformamide (DMF), drained, deprotected with piperidine/DMF (shaken 1 min; drained; repeated once), and washed with DMF (shaken 15 sec; drained; repeated twice). During sequential coupling of the remaining residues, the appropriate Fmoc amino acid was precombined with peptide coupling reagent 2-(6-chloro-1H-benzotriazole-1-yl)-1,1,3,3-tetramethylaminium hexafluorophosphate (5 equivalents each/mol bound resin) in DMF and added to the resin. After mixing for 20 seconds, *N,N′*-diisopropylethylamine (DIEA) was added and allowed to react for 3 min, followed by an additional DMF wash (shaken 15 sec, drained; repeated twice). These steps were iterated for each standard amino acid. For modified residues, Lys with side chain 4-methyltrityl (Mtt) protection was incorporated at the appropriate position. Introduction of the desired organic acid was effected through selective Mtt removal (2% [*v/v*] trifluoroacetic acid [TFA] at RT for 1 h), after which the specific organic acid was coupled (*N,N′*-diisopropylcarbodiimide and DIEA in DMF, 30 min). Remaining residues were added using the conditions described above. After final Fmoc deprotection, the resin mixture was pipetted into a vessel, and the resin was sequentially washed with DMF and dichloromethane (twice each). Peptide removal from the resin and global deprotection were accomplished by addition of resin cleavage solution (5× resin volume of TFA and scavenger mixture triisopropylsilane/thioanisole/anisole [90:4:3:3]), using microwave heating at 38°C for 30 minutes (Discover S-Class microwave synthesizer; CEM Corporation).

All peptides were purified using reverse-phase HPLC. Masses were confirmed by either liquid chromatography/mass spectrometry (Shimadzu LCMS-2020) or matrix-assisted laser desorption/ionization time-of-flight mass spectrometry (Voyager DE), and peptides were then lyophilized to white solids.

Table 2. Data collection and refinement statistics for iCAL36 acetylated peptide derivatives in complex with CALP.

	$iCAL36_{Ac\text{-}K^{-1}}$	$iCAL36_{Ac\text{-}K^{-3}}$	$iCAL36_{Ac\text{-}K^{-4}}$	$iCAL36_{Ac\text{-}K^{-5}}$
Data Collection				
Space Group	$P\ 2_1\ 2_1\ 2_1$	$P\ 2_1\ 2_1\ 2_1$	$P\ 2_1\ 2_1\ 2_1$	$P\ 2_1\ 2_1\ 2_1$
Unit cell dimensions				
a,b,c (Å)	36.3,47.7,97.8	35.9,47.7,97.2	36.2,47.8,98.1	36,47.5,100.5
Resolution[a] (Å)	19.5-1.4 (1.52-1.4)	19.5-1.3 (1.37-1.3)	19.7-1.4 (1.46-1.4)	19.5-1.55 (1.6-1.55)
R_{sym}[b] (%)	7.2 (55.7)	8.4 (67.2)	6.3 (59.4)	8.0 (50.9)
I/σ_I	30.16 (4.83)	29.31 (4.93)	23.23 (3.73)	23.85 (3.73)
Completeness (%)	99.8 (99.2)	99.6 (98.7)	99.9 (100)	99.2 (96.6)
Crystallization conditions	37% (*w/v*) PEG 8000	34% (*w/v*) PEG 3350	40% (*w/v*) PEG 3350	31% (*w/v*) PEG 8000
	0.15 M NaCl	0.2 M NaCl	0.15 M NaCl	0.15 M NaCl
	0.1 M Tris pH 7.5	0.1 M Tris pH 7.5	0.1 M Tris pH 7.5	0.1 M Tris pH 7.5
Refinement				
Total # of reflections	34,123	41,732	32,997	25,711
Reflections in the test set	1,716	2,094	1,660	1,310
R_{work}[c]/R_{free}[d]	18.4/20.3	18.1/20.0	18.1/19.9	18.8/21.9
Number of atoms:				
Protein	1343	1367	1342	1314
Water	203	214	199	265
Ramachandran plot[e] (%)	97.4/2.6/0/0	95.3/4.7/0/0	96.1/3.9/0/0	97.3/2.7/0/0
B_{av} (Å^2)				
Protein	12.22	11.09	13.79	12.59
Solvent	24.92	22.36	24.24	24.80
Bond length RMSD (Å)	0.012	0.006	0.014	0.006
Bond angle RMSD (°)	1.221	1. 076	1.314	1.060

[a]Values in parentheses are for data in the highest-resolution shell.
[b]$R_{sym} = \Sigma_h \Sigma_i |I(h) - I_i(h)| / \Sigma_h \Sigma_i I_i(h)$, where $I_i(h)$ and $I(h)$ values are the *i*-th and mean measurements of the intensity of reflection *h*.
[c]$R_{work} = \Sigma || F_{obs}|_h - |F_{calc}||_h / \Sigma |F_{obs}|_h$, h ∈ {working set}.
[d]R_{free} is calculated as R_{work} for the reflections h ∈ {test set}.
[e]Core/allowed/generously allowed/disallowed.

Fluorescence Polarization (FP)

FP competition experiments were performed as previously described [16,17]. The reporter peptide for CALP was *F**-iCAL36 (fluorescein coupled via an amino-hexanoic acid linker to the N-terminus of ANSRWPTSII; $K_D = 0.97$ μM), and the CALP concentration was $1.5 \times K_D$. Experiments were performed in triplicate using separate protein-reporter and peptide stock solutions, and K_I values were determined using least-squares fitting of the set of competitive binding equilibria.

Isothermal Titration Calorimetry (ITC)

ITC experiments were performed and analyzed in a manner similar to that described previously [14,20]. Titrations were performed with a Nano ITC 2G (TA Instruments). In brief, for a typical titration, 100–320 μM CALP was loaded into the 943 μL sample cell, and 2–3 mM peptide placed in a 250 μL injector syringe. For $iCAL36_{BBK\text{-}K^{-1}}$, titrations were performed with polyhistidine-tagged CALP. Peptide concentrations were adjusted based on the amount of protein, so the final ratio of peptide to protein ranged between 3:1–4:1. Each titration included an initial 1 or 2 μL injection followed by 5 or 10 μL injections performed at 180 s intervals, for a total of 25–50 injections. The stirring speed was 250 rpm, and experimental temperature was 25°C. Thermograms were analyzed using NanoAnalyze software (TA Instruments). Experiments were performed in duplicate (n = 2), except as indicated in Table 1. Details are described in ref. [21].

Surface Plasmon Resonance (SPR)

SPR experiments were performed on a Biacore X100 Plus (GE Healthcare Life Sciences), with CALP covalently immobilized on a CM5 sensor chip. Peptide solutions were prepared using HBS-EP buffer, and a series of dilutions from approximately $10 \times K_D$ to $0.1 \times K_D$. SPR experiments were conducted for each peptide dilution, and the equilibrium analysis mode of the instrument was used to determine the dissociation constant. Sensorgrams were analyzed using the Biacore evaluation software. Experiments were performed in duplicate or triplicate (n≥2). A detailed description is provided in ref. [21].

Crystallization and Structure Determination

CALP was co-crystallized with each of the 7 side-chain modified peptides as previously described [16,17,19]. Crystallization conditions for all complexes were similar and are listed in Tables 2 and 3. Crystals appeared in 1–2 d and grew for up to 2 weeks before harvest and flash-cooling. Cryoprotectant solutions were also similar (35% [*w/v*] PEG 8000 or PEG 3350, 100–200 mM sodium chloride, 100 mM Tris pH 7.5, 20% [*w/v*] glycerol).

Table 3. Data collection and refinement statistics for chemically-modified iCAL36 peptide derivatives, bound to CALP.

	$iCAL36_{FB-K^{-1}}$	$iCAL36_{Tfa-K^{-1}}$	$iCAL36_{BB-K^{-1}}$
Data Collection			
Space Group	$P\,2_1\,2_1\,2_1$	$P\,2_1\,2_1\,2_1$	$P\,2_1\,2_1\,2_1$
Unit cell dimensions			
a,b,c (Å)	36.3,47.7,97.8	36.2,47.9,97.4	36.0,47.9,97.5
Resolution[a] (Å)	19.5-1.7 (1.76-1.7)	19.5-1.4 (1.52-1.4)	19.5-1.4 (1.46-1.4)
R_{sym}[b] (%)	8.9 (60.0)	7.6 (56.4)	7.8 (68.6)
I/σ_I	16.33 (3.46)	17.6 (3.72)	25.63 (4.29)
Completeness (%)	99.9 (99.9)	96.3 (94.2)	99.6 (99.1)
Crystallization conditions	33% (*w/v*) PEG 3350	33% (*w/v*) PEG 3350	31% (*w/v*) PEG 3350
	0.2 M NaCl	0.2 M NaCl	0.1 M NaCl
	0.1 M Tris pH 7.5	0.1 M Tris pH 7.5	0.1 M Tris pH 7.5
Refinement			
Total # of reflections	19,345	32,898	33,913
Reflections in the test set	980	1,636	1,720
R_{work}[c]/R_{free}[d]	17.3/20.7	18.0/19.9	18.2/20.1
Number of atoms:			
Protein	1314	1368	1342
Water	181	228	204
Ramachandran plot[e] (%)	96.7/3.3/0/0	96.7/3.3/0/0	96.7/3.3/0/0
B_{av} (Å^2)			
Protein	14.94	12.15	11.96
Solvent	26.47	25.35	24.35
Bond length RMSD (Å)	0.007	0.0008	0.008
Bond angle RMSD (°)	1.100	1.129	1. 139

[a]Values in parentheses are for data in the highest-resolution shell.
[b]$R_{sym} = \Sigma_h \Sigma_i |I(h) - I_i(h)| / \Sigma_h \Sigma_i I_i(h)$, where $I_i(h)$ and $I(h)$ values are the *i*-th and mean measurements of the intensity of reflection *h*.
[c]$R_{work} = \Sigma || F_{obs}|_h - |F_{calc}||_h / \Sigma |F_{obs}|_h$, h ∈ {working set}.
[d]R_{free} is calculated as R_{work} for the reflections h ∈ {test set}.
[e]Core/allowed/generously allowed/disallowed.

Diffraction data were collected on beamline X6A at the National Synchrotron Light Source at $\lambda = 0.8856$ Å. The crystal-to-detector distance varied from 120–180 mm. 0.3° oscillation images were collected over a range of 360° for all crystals, with the exception of CALP : $iCAL36_{Ac\text{-}K^{-4}}$ (180° range). Data were processed using the XDS and CCP4 programs, as previously described [16].

Phases were calculated using molecular replacement in PHENIX [22], with the CAL PDZ domain as a search model (A-protomer of PDB entry 4E34). Since no ligand was included in the search model, the observation of clear electron density for the bound peptide was used to assess initial phase quality. Representative F_O-F_C electron density starting 'omit' maps are shown in the panels in Figure 1A for each of the three halogenated moieties. Models were built from composite omit maps and refined using PHENIX. The electron density following refinement is shown for each of the three modified side chains in separate panels in Figure 1B. Structure geometries were validated using MOLPROBITY and the PDB Validation Server [23,24]. PYMOL was used to render figures [25]. Electrostatic potential surface maps were determined using APBS [26]. AREAIMOL, part of the CCP4 suite of programs, was used to calculate solvent accessible surface area [27,28]. Data collection and refinement statistics are reported in Tables 2 and 3. All structures have been deposited in the Protein Data Bank, with accession codes 4NMO, 4NMP, 4NMQ, 4NMR, 4NMS, 4NMT, and 4NMV.

Results

A set of scaffolds for chemical modification

As a first step in developing peptidomimetic acceptor scaffolds, we investigated the importance of the chemistry at the peptide N-terminus. Specifically, since native binding partners of the CAL PDZ domain are not short peptides, but rather intact proteins, we tested whether N-terminal acetylation (Ac-) would enhance binding affinity by neutralizing the charged peptide amino-terminal moiety at the P^{-9} position. In head-to-head fluorescence polarization (FP) displacement assays, Ac-iCAL36 (sequence: Ac-ANSRWPTSII) showed no significant change in binding affinity compared to iCAL36 (sequence: ANSRWPTSII; Figure 2A and Table 1). For subsequent experiments, we therefore used peptides with native N-termini.

Recent work from our lab revealed that positions along the entire length of the CALP binding cleft can contribute to peptide affinity [17]. We therefore considered substituting lysine residues at non-motif positions along the iCAL36 backbone, to provide primary amino groups for facile downstream modification. A previously published substitutional analysis of the iCAL36

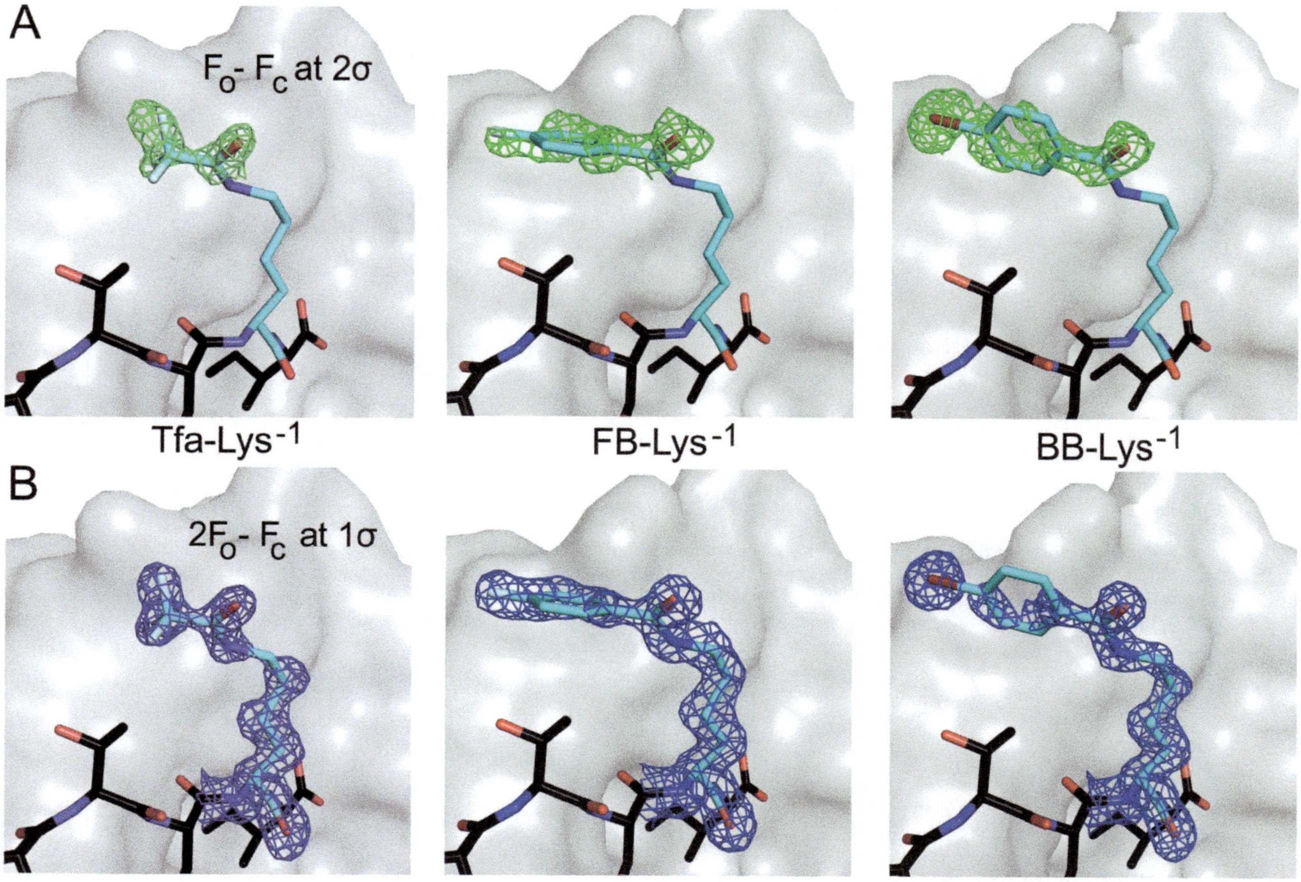

Figure 1. Electron density of chemically modified peptides. A) Prior to ligand modeling, positive electron density was observed in $F_O - F_C$ difference maps, as illustrated here (contour level: 2σ) for the halogenated substituents attached to the Lys side chain at P^{-1}. B) After iterative rounds of refinement and model building, final $2F_O - F_C$ electron density maps (contour level: 1σ) showed excellent agreement with the model, as shown here for the corresponding P^{-1} side chains. The final refined peptide structures are shown as stick figures and colored by atom/position (C = light blue for P^{-1} or black for other positions, O = blue, F = sky blue, N = red, Br = dark red). The van der Waals surface of CALP is shown in gray. The substituents are indicated as follows: Tfa, trifluoroacetic acid; FB, 4-fluorobenzoic acid; BB, 4-bromobenzoic acid.

sequence by peptide array [9,17] suggested that replacement with lysine should yield baseline or enhanced affinity at the P^{-1} or P^{-4} positions, but weaker binding at the P^{-3} or P^{-5} positions. However, analysis of SubAna arrays based on alternative starting sequences suggested that lysine substitution at the P^{-3} and P^{-5} positions might not be detrimental [17]. In order to test which positions can accommodate a modified lysine residue without a substantial loss in peptide binding affinity, we substituted residues at the P^{-1}, P^{-3}, P^{-4}, and P^{-5} positions of the iCAL36 peptide. Each substituted lysine was capped with an acetyl group, to more closely mimic the electrostatic character that would be present following modification with an organic acid (here: acetic acid).

The sequences of the resulting peptides $iCAL36_{Ac\text{-}K^{-1}}$, $iCAL36_{Ac\text{-}K^{-3}}$, $iCAL36_{Ac\text{-}K^{-4}}$, and $iCAL36_{Ac\text{-}K^{-5}}$, are listed in Table 1, along with binding affinities determined by FP displacement assays (Figure 2B). Consistent with our SubAna data, modifications at the P^{-1} and P^{-4} positions yielded the highest affinities, comparable to or slightly better than the affinity of the template sequence. Substitution of an acetylated lysine at the P^{-3} and P^{-5} positions yielded binding constants weaker by ~8-fold and ~24-fold, respectively. Thus, while each of the substituted peptides retained binding affinity, different positions exhibited differential sensitivity, consistent with our previous evaluation of 'modulator' stereochemical preferences at non-motif positions [17].

Structural analysis of acetyl-lysine scaffolds along CALP peptide binding cleft

We next wanted to test the hypothesis that the lysine substitutions were accommodated without significant changes to the backbone geometry. The structures of CALP bound to each of the substituted peptides were determined by X-ray crystallography, for comparison with the structure in complex with iCAL36 [16]. Overall data collection and refinement statistics are reported in Table 2. As in previous analyses, co-crystals contained two protomers in the asymmetric unit. The A- and B-protomers are superimposable for all crystals, except for the $iCAL36_{Ac\text{-}K^{-1}}$ complex, in which the P^{-1} side-chain amino group is oriented towards solvent in protomer A, but forms a hydrogen bond with CALP-Ser^{302} in protomer B (distance: 2.9 Å), suggesting a dynamic interaction. In the following descriptions, we will use the B-protomers of each complex for our analyses. The refined structures reveal similar peptide conformations in the binding cleft (Figure 3). When compared to the CALP:iCAL36 structure, the root mean squared deviation (RMSD) for the main chain atoms in

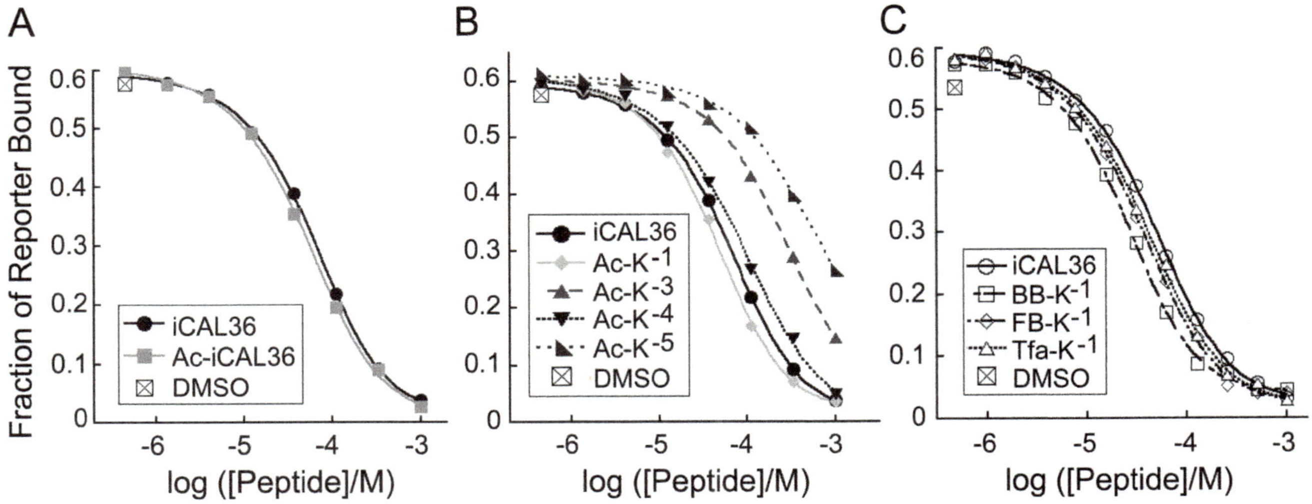

Figure 2. Fluorescence polarization binding studies of modified peptides. Representative FP isotherms are shown for the displacement of CALP:reporter binding by (A) Ac-iCAL36, (B) scaffold peptides containing acetylated lysine substitutions at each non-motif position, or (C) peptides containing halogenated substituents at the P^{-1} position (C). In each panel, iCAL36 displacement is also shown for reference. A fluoresceinated iCAL36 peptide (*F**-iCAL36) was used as the reporter for all measurements. For illustrative purposes, a logistic curve-fit is shown, but K_I values and fractional reporter occupancy values were determined by least-squares fitting of the complete binding equation. Summary values of independent experiments (n = 3) are reported in Table 1.

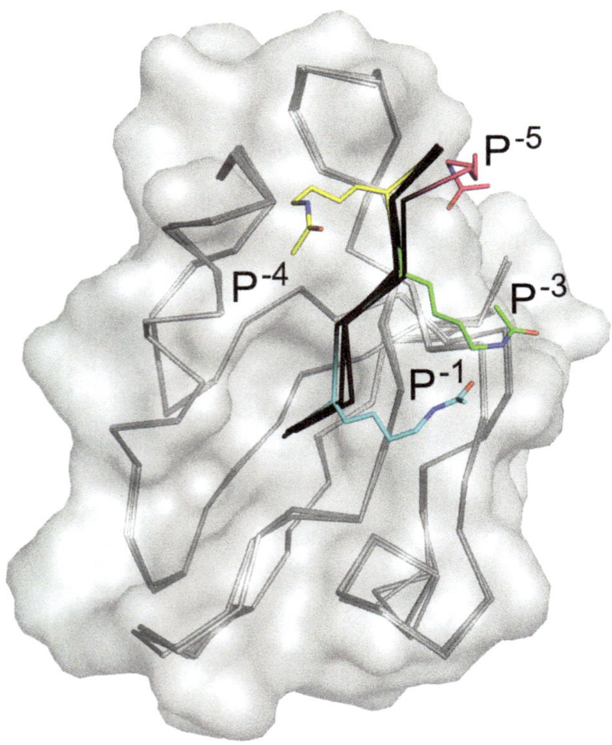

Figure 3. Chemically modifiable scaffolds at each non-motif position in the CALP binding cleft. The C_α trace (gray) shows all CALP structures, aligned by main chain atoms (RMSD ≤0.3 Å compared to CALP:iCAL36, PDB ID: 4E34). CALP is also shown as a transparent surface (gray). The peptides are shown as black C_α traces, with the acetylated lysine residue of each respective peptide highlighted (carbon atoms colored by position, as indicated). Peptide positions are labeled, and non-carbon atoms are colored separately: O = blue, N = red.

the B-protomers was ≤0.1 Å in all cases, except $iCAL36_{Ac\text{-}K^{-5}}$ (RMSD = 0.3 Å).

We also wished to assess the stereochemical environment surrounding the terminal acetyl moiety at each position. Thus, although an acetylated lysine substitution is slightly more disruptive at P^{-3} than at P^{-1}, there may be hydrophobic pocket accessible from P^{-3}, for example, which could represent a target for further peptidomimetic engineering. Indeed, alignment of the structures of our acetylated complexes reveals different stereochemical environments for each substituted position. For example, a P^{-4} acetylated lysine interacts with the CALP α2 helix, whereas a P^{-1} or P^{-3} acetylated lysine faces the opposite side of the peptide binding cleft, and a P^{-5} acetylated lysine can access either side of the interaction pocket (Figure 3). Furthermore, the electrostatic potential surface of CALP reveals that the site interacting with the P^{-4} acetylated lysine residue (S^{-4}) is positive. The other three sites are negative, and S^{-1} and S^{-3} are more negative than S^{-5} (Figure 4). Taken together, all four positions are potential sites for targeted differential modification.

Chemically-modified peptides increase binding affinity for CALP

For proof-of-principle studies, we chose to further diversify the position with the highest baseline affinity, i.e., P^{-1} in $iCAL36_{Ac\text{-}K^{-1}}$, by introducing three halogenated substituents. Halogenated organic moieties are found in a disproportionate number of biologically active substances of both natural and synthetic origin, and halogenated aromatic residues can significantly contribute to binding affinity [29]. Further, hundreds of aromatic organic acids, halogenated and otherwise, are commercially available. Thus, our initial set of ligands enables us to test the feasibility of affinity modification by preparing and screening a larger library of chemically-modified peptides [14]. At the P^{-1} position, we coupled trifluoroacetic acid ($iCAL36_{Tfa\text{-}K^{-1}}$), 4-fluorobenzoic acid ($iCAL36_{FB\text{-}K^{-1}}$), or 4-bromobenzoic acid ($iCAL36_{BB\text{-}K^{-1}}$) to the side-chain terminal amino group, as illustrated in Figure 5A. The binding affinities of the resulting

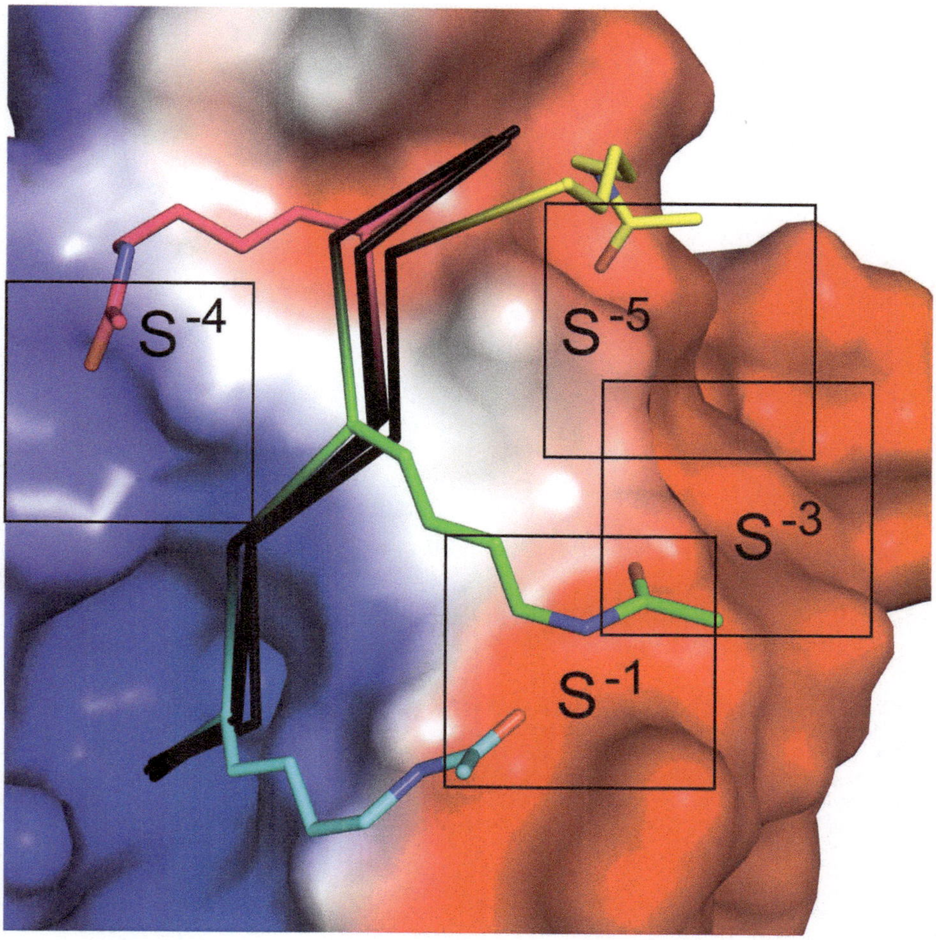

Figure 4. Differential stereochemical and electrostatic environments at each modifiable position. The electrostatic potential surface map of CALP is shown, rendered at ±10 k_BT/e (negative surface in red, positive surface in blue). Boxes and labels (S^{-1}, S^{-2}, etc.) indicate an approximate area that chemical modifications could bind when attached to the lysine N_ζ moiety at that position. Overlap in accessible area suggests a possible region for side-chain cyclization. Peptide backbones are shown as black C_α traces, with acetyl-lysine residues shown as sticks and colored by position. Non-carbon atoms are colored separately: O = blue, N = red.

peptides were determined by FP displacement (Figure 2C) and are listed in Table 1. All three peptides reveal modestly enhanced binding affinity. Overall, the largest increase is for $iCAL36_{BB\text{-}K^{-1}}$ and $iCAL36_{FB\text{-}K^{-1}}$, which are each ~2-fold stronger than iCAL36.

To explore the stereochemistry of these interactions, we also solved the complex structures of CALP bound to each of these three peptides. All data collection and refinement statistics are in Table 3. The modified lysine and the terminal moieties are oriented similarly in the complexes with $iCAL36_{Ac\text{-}K^{-1}}$ and with the additional P^{-1} substituted peptides (Figures 1B and 5B). Furthermore, the distal functional groups overlap with the surface on CALP contacted by the acetyl group of the P^{-3} lysine in $iCAL36_{Ac\text{-}K^{-3}}$ (Figure 5B). Thus, S^{-1} and S^{-3} can intersect and could potentially be bridged using a cyclic peptide, a strategy previously employed in targeting PSD-95 [11].

$iCAL36_{Tfa\text{-}K^{-1}}$, $iCAL36_{FB\text{-}K^{-1}}$, and $iCAL36_{BB\text{-}K^{-1}}$ bind CALP with affinities modestly higher than the value observed for iCAL36 (Table 1). In addition, the substituents increase the contact surface area of the modified P^{-1} lysine residue by 69, 32, and 40 Å^2, respectively. Finally, they can serve as chemical scaffolds for additional elaboration. Indeed, the availability of high-resolution stereochemical information for each of the complexes with CALP (Figure 5B) will facilitate *in silico* docking screens to identify candidates for more detailed biochemical and structural characterization.

Comparison of binding constants determined by multiple techniques

There are a number of techniques used to measure PDZ domain:peptide binding affinities [as discussed, e.g., in ref. 20]. In some cases, significant technique-dependent differences have been reported for PDZ ligands (e.g., [30,31]). Here, we directly compare the three most prevalent techniques and investigate the affinities of these singly substituted peptides, as well as to an unmodified iCAL36 peptide, in parallel by FP, ITC, and SPR (Table 1). Across techniques, the rank order of affinities is largely conserved. The P^{-1}-substituted peptides are the four highest-affinity ligands, and rank-order switches are found largely within experimental uncertainties. Relative to iCAL36, there is little change in affinity for the P^{-4}-substituted peptide, and the P^{-3}- and P^{-5}-substituted peptides are the weakest ligands. The most significant rank-order reversal involves the Ac-iCAL36 peptide, for which the ITC and SPR values are ~3-fold larger than the FP

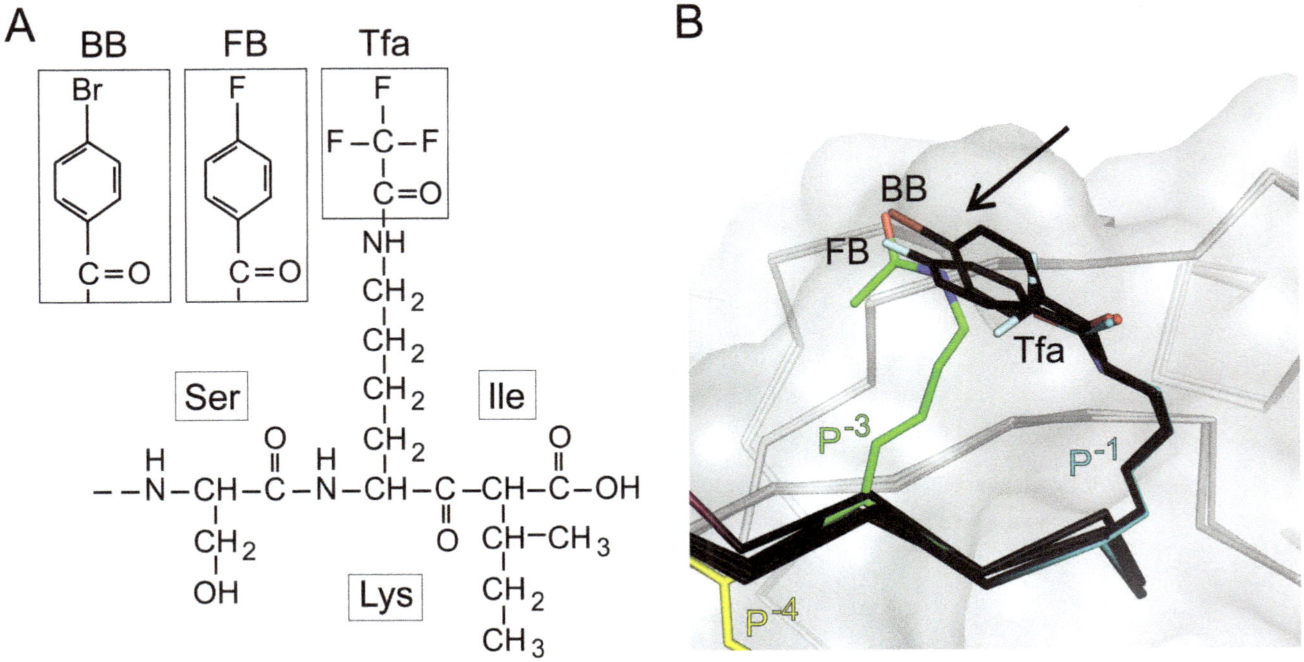

Figure 5. Chemical modifications at the P^{-1} position reveal similar modes of binding to CALP. A) Schematic representations of the three additional chemically modified peptides are shown for reference and labeled by modification: BB = $iCAL36_{BB\text{-}K^{-1}}$, FB = $iCAL36_{FB\text{-}K^{-1}}$, Tfa = $iCAL36_{Tfa\text{-}K^{-1}}$. B) The structures of CALP (gray C_α trace and van der Waals surface) in complex with these peptides (stick figures, black carbons), or in complex with peptides bearing acetylated lysines at P^{-1} (blue carbons), P^{-3} (green carbons), and P^{-4} (yellow carbons) are shown following alignment. Superposition of these structures reveals that all halogenated substituents interact with a similar region (arrow) at the edge of the CALP peptide-binding cleft, in close proximity to the P^{-3} binding site. Non-carbon atoms are colored by element: O = blue, F = sky blue, Br = dark red, N = red.

value. Indeed, with the exception of the two weakest ligands with larger uncertainties, the SPR values are generally 2–3-fold higher than the FP values. The ITC values are somewhat more variable, but mostly fall at or between the FP and SPR values (Table 1). Overall, despite modest differences, the results are largely concordant, with the highest affinities seen for $iCAL36_{BB\text{-}K^{-1}}$ (FP and SPR) and $iCAL36_{FB\text{-}K^{-1}}$ (ITC).

Discussion

As regulators of important intracellular trafficking and scaffolding processes, PDZ domains are potentially attractive therapeutic targets [32]. However, despite promising new approaches such as fragment-based design, attempts to develop small-molecule inhibitors have so far faced limits of druggability common to protein-protein interactions [33]. High-affinity ($K_D \leq 20$ nM) peptides have been engineered, which could serve as competitive inhibitors [34,35]. However, as therapeutics, native peptides are susceptible to proteolysis and often have low inherent membrane permeability, which has led to an increasing interest in peptidomimetic strategies [36–39]. Here, we have tested the feasibility of developing competitive inhibitors of the CAL PDZ domain by chemically modifying a series of peptides carrying lysine acceptor residues at non-motif positions.

A limited set of four organic acid modifications of the iCAL36 P^{-1} side chain revealed modest enhancements of affinity. In evaluating these inhibitor leads, we performed a direct comparison of estimates of PDZ domain binding affinities determined by ITC, SPR, and FP. For specific peptide:PDZ complexes, the precise values showed some variation between binding methods. Since all three methods were performed under equilibrium binding conditions, it is unclear what caused the ~3-fold discrepancy in K_D values observed, e.g. for the N-terminally acetylated iCAL36 peptide (Table 1). Each technique does involve different incubation times and temperatures, as well as the presence or absence of stirring, shaking, or laminar flow, suggesting the need for care in evaluating the significance of subtle affinity shifts, both within and across techniques. Nevertheless, the ranking of strong, modest, and weak binders was concordant across techniques, suggesting that each method can each be reliably used to monitor changes in affinity substantial enough to affect ultimate *in vivo* therapeutic potency.

The approach described here is similar to the strategy used in the design of chemically modified peptides to inhibit both the PDZ3 domain of postsynaptic density protein 95 (PSD-95) for the treatment of stroke, and the PDZ domain of the GAIP-interacting protein, C-terminus (GIPC) for cancer therapy [13,14]. In the PSD-95 PDZ3 study, binding affinities for the chemically modified peptides were measured, and the stereochemistry of binding was analyzed using NMR footprinting [13]. For GIPC inhibitors, cellular efficacy was confirmed, although data were not available for binding affinities or complex stereochemistry [14]. Our investigation of chemically modified peptide binding to CALP combines both thermodynamic and crystallographic evaluation of a series of chemically modified peptide scaffolds binding to a shared PDZ domain target.

In particular, our structural studies confirm that even modified peptides bind to the CAL PDZ domain in a common conformation, such that each peptide side chain interacts with a defined stereochemical environment [17]. As a result, our acetylated lysine peptide structures provide templates for future screening efforts. They can also be aligned to previously determined CAL PDZ domain structures. Thus, together with our previous studies of natural and metallated CALP inhibitor peptides [5,9,15,18], these data help to establish an extensive framework for future peptidomimetic development. By combining multiple modifications to an already refined starting peptide sequence, we may achieve the chemical complexity necessary for truly selective CALP inhibition. If successful, such studies will provide additional proof-of-principle data for targeting of PDZ trafficking pathways in cystic fibrosis, as well as stereochemical leads to support the ultimate goal of therapeutic design.

Acknowledgments

We would like to thank all members of the Madden and Spaller labs for helpful discussions and suggestions. We would also like to thank Edwin Lazo, Dr. Jean Jakoncic and Dr. Vivian Stojanoff (NSLS) for assistance with data collection and analysis. This work was supported in part by grants from the NIH (R01-DK101541, P30-GM106394, T32-DK007301, R01-CA150190) and from the Hitchcock Foundation.

Author Contributions

Conceived and designed the experiments: JFA RZ MRS DRM. Performed the experiments: JFA RZ. Analyzed the data: JFA RZ MRS DRM. Contributed reagents/materials/analysis tools: JFA RZ MRS DRM. Contributed to the writing of the manuscript: JFA MRS DRM.

References

1. Craik DJ, Fairlie DP, Liras S, Price D (2013) The future of peptide-based drugs. Chem Biol Drug Des 81: 136–147.
2. Zhang Y, Appleton BA, Wiesmann C, Lau T, Costa M, et al. (2009) Inhibition of Wnt signaling by Dishevelled PDZ peptides. Nat Chem Biol 5: 217–219.
3. Chen X, Longgood JC, Michnoff C, Wei S, Frantz DE, et al. (2007) High-throughput screen for small molecule inhibitors of Mint1-PDZ domains. Assay Drug Dev Technol 5: 769–783.
4. Thorsen TS, Madsen KL, Rebola N, Rathje M, Anggono V, et al. (2010) Identification of a small-molecule inhibitor of the PICK1 PDZ domain that inhibits hippocampal LTP and LTD. Proc Natl Acad Sci U S A 107: 413–418.
5. Vouilleme L, Cushing PR, Volkmer R, Madden DR, Boisguerin P (2010) Engineering peptide inhibitors to overcome PDZ binding promiscuity. Angew Chem Int Ed Engl 49: 9912–9916.
6. Songyang Z (1999) Recognition and regulation of primary-sequence motifs by signaling modular domains. Prog Biophys Mol Biol 71: 359–372.
7. Songyang Z, Fanning AS, Fu C, Xu J, Marfatia SM, et al. (1997) Recognition of unique carboxyl-terminal motifs by distinct PDZ domains. Science 275: 73–77.
8. Davey NE, Van Roey K, Weatheritt RJ, Toedt G, Uyar B, et al. (2012) Attributes of short linear motifs. Mol Biosyst 8: 268–281.
9. Cushing PR, Vouilleme L, Pellegrini M, Boisguerin P, Madden DR (2010) A stabilizing influence: CAL PDZ inhibition extends the half-life of DeltaF508-CFTR. Angew Chem Int Ed Engl 49: 9907–9911.
10. Wolde M, Fellows A, Cheng J, Kivenson A, Coutermarsh B, et al. (2007) Targeting CAL as a negative regulator of DeltaF508-CFTR cell-surface expression: an RNA interference and structure-based mutagenetic approach. J Biol Chem 282: 8099–8109.
11. Piserchio A, Salinas GD, Li T, Marshall J, Spaller MR, et al. (2004) Targeting specific PDZ domains of PSD-95; structural basis for enhanced affinity and enzymatic stability of a cyclic peptide. Chem Biol 11: 469–473.
12. Li T, Saro D, Spaller MR (2004) Thermodynamic profiling of conformationally constrained cyclic ligands for the PDZ domain. Bioorg Med Chem Lett 14: 1385–1388.
13. Patra CR, Rupasinghe CN, Dutta SK, Bhattacharya S, Wang E, et al. (2012) Chemically modified peptides targeting the PDZ domain of GIPC as a therapeutic approach for cancer. ACS Chem Biol 7: 770–779.
14. Udugamasooriya DG, Sharma SC, Spaller MR (2008) A chemical library approach to organic-modified peptide ligands for PDZ domain proteins: a synthetic, thermodynamic and structural investigation. Chembiochem 9: 1587–1589.
15. Roberts KE, Cushing PR, Boisguerin P, Madden DR, Donald BR (2012) Computational Design of a PDZ Domain Peptide Inhibitor that Rescues CFTR Activity. PLoS Comput Biol 8: e1002477.
16. Amacher JF, Cushing PR, Bahl CD, Beck T, Madden DR (2013) Stereochemical Determinants of C-terminal Specificity in PDZ Peptide-binding Domains: a novel contribution of the carboxylate-binding loop. J Biol Chem 288: 5114–5126.
17. Amacher JF, Cushing PR, Brooks L, 3rd, Boisguerin P, Madden DR (2014) Stereochemical preferences modulate affinity and selectivity among five PDZ domains that bind CFTR: comparative structural and sequence analyses. Structure 22: 82–93.
18. Kundu R, Cushing PR, Popp BV, Zhao Y, Madden DR, et al. (2012) Hybrid organic-inorganic inhibitors of a PDZ interaction that regulates the endocytic fate of CFTR. Angew Chem Int Ed Engl 51: 7217–7220.
19. Amacher JF, Cushing PR, Weiner JA, Madden DR (2011) Crystallization and preliminary diffraction analysis of the CAL PDZ domain in complex with a selective peptide inhibitor. Acta Crystallogr Sect F Struct Biol Cryst Commun 67: 600–603.
20. Saro D, Li T, Rupasinghe C, Paredes A, Caspers N, et al. (2007) A thermodynamic ligand binding study of the third PDZ domain (PDZ3) from the mammalian neuronal protein PSD-95. Biochemistry 46: 6340–6352.
21. Zhao R (2012) Synthesis and biophysical characterization of peptide ligands targeting PDZ domains [Dartmouth College, M.S. Thesis]. Ann Arbor: UMI Dissertations Publishing. 128 pp.
22. Adams PD, Afonine PV, Bunkoczi G, Chen VB, Davis IW, et al. (2010) PHENIX: a comprehensive Python-based system for macromolecular structure solution. Acta Crystallogr D Biol Crystallogr 66: 213–221.
23. Chen VB, Arendall WB 3rd, Headd JJ, Keedy DA, Immormino RM, et al. (2010) MolProbity: all-atom structure validation for macromolecular crystallography. Acta Crystallogr D Biol Crystallogr 66: 12–21.
24. Feng J, Westbrook J, Berman H (1998) PDB Validation Server. Rutgers University, New Brunswick, NJ NDB-407.
25. DeLano W (2008) The PyMOL molecular graphics system. The PyMOL molecular graphics system DeLano Scientific LLC, Palo Alto, CA.
26. Baker NA, Sept D, Joseph S, Holst MJ, McCammon JA (2001) Electrostatics of nanosystems: application to microtubules and the ribosome. Proc Natl Acad Sci U S A 98: 10037–10041.
27. Saff E, Kuijlaars A (1997) ArealMol. *The Mathematical Intelligencer* 19: 5–11.
28. Collaborative Computational Project N (1994) The CCP4 suite: programs for protein crystallography. Acta Crystallogr D Biol Crystallogr 50: 760–763.
29. Memic A, Spaller MR (2008) How do halogen substituents contribute to protein-binding interactions? A thermodynamic study of peptide ligands with diverse aryl halides. Chembiochem 9: 2793–2795.
30. Lim IA, Hall DD, Hell JW (2002) Selectivity and promiscuity of the first and second PDZ domains of PSD-95 and synapse-associated protein 102. J Biol Chem 277: 21697–21711.
31. Cushing PR, Fellows A, Villone D, Boisguerin P, Madden DR (2008) The relative binding affinities of PDZ partners for CFTR: a biochemical basis for efficient endocytic recycling. Biochemistry 47: 10084–10098.
32. Dev KK (2004) Making protein interactions druggable: targeting PDZ domains. Nat Rev Drug Discov 3: 1047–1056.
33. Higueruelo AP, Jubb H, Blundell TL (2013) Protein-protein interactions as druggable targets: recent technological advances. Curr Opin Pharmacol 13: 791–796.
34. Reina J, Lacroix E, Hobson SD, Fernandez-Ballester G, Rybin V, et al. (2002) Computer-aided design of a PDZ domain to recognize new target sequences. Nat Struct Biol 9: 621–627.
35. Yan X, Zhou H, Zhang J, Shi C, Xie X, et al. (2009) Molecular mechanism of inward rectifier potassium channel 2.3 regulation by tax-interacting protein-1. J Mol Biol 392: 967–976.
36. Bach A, Eildal JN, Stuhr-Hansen N, Deeskamp R, Gottschalk M, et al. (2011) Cell-permeable and plasma-stable peptidomimetic inhibitors of the postsynaptic density-95/N-methyl-D-aspartate receptor interaction. J Med Chem 54: 1333–1346.
37. Whitby LR, Boger DL (2012) Comprehensive peptidomimetic libraries targeting protein-protein interactions. Acc Chem Res 45: 1698–1709.
38. Drew K, Renfrew PD, Craven TW, Butterfoss GL, Chou FC, et al. (2013) Adding diverse noncanonical backbones to rosetta: enabling peptidomimetic design. PLoS One 8: e67051.
39. Lohan S, Bisht GS (2013) Recent approaches in design of peptidomimetics for antimicrobial drug discovery research. Mini Rev Med Chem 13: 1073–1088.

4

Emergence of Carbapenem Resistance Due to the Novel Insertion Sequence IS*Pa*8 in *Pseudomonas aeruginosa*

Randal C. Fowler, Nancy D. Hanson*

Creighton University School of Medicine, Department of Medical Microbiology and Immunology, Center for Research in Anti-Infectives and Biotechnology, Omaha, Nebraska, United States of America

Abstract

Chronic lung infections due to the persistence of *Pseudomonas aeruginosa* in cystic fibrosis patients are typically associated with the emergence of antibiotic resistance. The purpose of this study was to investigate the mechanisms responsible for the emergence of carbapenem resistance when a clinical isolate of *P. aeruginosa* collected from a patient with cystic fibrosis was challenged with meropenem. Nine carbapenem-resistant mutants were selected with subinhibitory concentrations of meropenem from a clinical isolate of *P. aeruginosa* and characterized for carbapenem resistance. Increased carbapenem MICs were associated with the identification of the novel insertion sequence IS*Pa*8 within *oprD* or its promoter region in all the mutants. The position of IS*Pa*8 was different for each of the mutants evaluated. In addition, Southern blot analyses identified multiple copies of IS*Pa*8 within the genomes of the mutants and their parent isolate. These data demonstrate that transposition of IS elements within the *Pseudomonas* genome can influence antibiotic susceptibility. Understanding the selective pressures associated with the emergence of antibiotic resistance is critical for the judicious use of antimicrobial chemotherapy and the successful treatment of bacterial infections.

Editor: Ruth Hall, The University of Sydney, Australia

Funding: This work was supported in part by a research grant from Johnson and Johnson Pharmaceutical Research and Development and by Creighton University. The funders had no role in study design, data collection and analysis, decision to publish, or preparation of the manuscript.

Competing Interests: This work was supported in part by a research grant from Johnson and Johnson Pharmaceutical Research. There are no patents, products in development, or marketed products to declare.

* E-mail: ndhanson@creighton.edu

Introduction

Carbapenems such as imipenem, meropenem, and doripenem are frequently used as last resort drugs for the treatment of multidrug-resistant *P. aeruginosa* infections. *P. aeruginosa* is the predominate pathogen in chronic respiratory infections in patients with cystic fibrosis. The most formidable characteristic of *P. aeruginosa* is the rapid development of resistance during therapy to multiple antibiotics including the carbapenems, making eradication of this microorganism from the airways of cystic fibrosis patients difficult if not impossible [1,2]. Although the carbapenems remain a viable therapeutic option, their usage carries an increased risk for developing carbapenem resistance thereby reducing their efficacy [3–9].

P. aeruginosa can employ a combination of plasmid-encoded and/or chromosomally-encoded mechanisms to evade carbapenem therapy. However, in non-carbapenemase-producing *P. aeruginosa*, meropenem and doripenem resistance is associated with the overexpression of the *mexAB-oprM* efflux pump with concomitant loss of the carbapenem-specific porin OprD [10,11], while imipenem resistance has only been associated with the down-regulation of OprD [10,12]. Mutations such as nucleotide substitutions, deletions, and insertion sequence (IS) elements within the *oprD* gene or its promoter region can decrease or cause a loss of OprD production, resulting in significant reductions in susceptibility of *P. aeruginosa* to carbapenem antibiotics [13–17]. Furthermore, IS21 disruption of the efflux regulator *mexR* has been associated with decreased β-lactam susceptibility due to increased expression of the efflux pump *mexAB-oprM* [18]. These data in addition to other studies highlight the various roles IS elements play in promoting the emergence of antibiotic resistance [19].

In this study, we challenged a carbapenem susceptible *P. aeruginosa* isolate collected from a cystic fibrosis patient with subinhibitory concentrations of meropenem and investigated the molecular mechanisms associated with the emergence of carbapenem resistance.

Methods

Strains and Culture Conditions

P. aeruginosa isolate PA42 was isolated from a sputum culture of a 20 year-old patient with cystic fibrosis from the Pediatrics Pulmonology Cystic Fibrosis Clinic at the University of Nebraska Medical Center. Gram staining revealed that PA42 had a rounded cell morphology compared to the laboratory isolate PAO1 (Figure S1). PA42 was identified as *P. aeruginosa* using the Vitek 2 System. In addition, the sequence data for *oprF* and *oprD* showed 100% and 92% identities to the sequenced strain *P. aeruginosa* PAO1 (GenBank Accession No. AE004091.2).

Bacterial Susceptibility

PAO1 and PA443, an isolate collected from a cystic fibrosis patient, were susceptible to all anti-pseudomonal agents tested and were used as comparator isolates. Susceptibility of the *P. aeruginosa* isolates to imipenem, meropenem, and doripenem was determined using agar dilution methodology according to the Clinical Laboratory Standards Institute (CLSI) [20]. Quality control strains *E. coli* ATCC 25922, *E. coli* ATCC 35218, and *P. aeruginosa* ATCC 27853 were included in susceptibility testing experiments.

Generation of Isogenic Mutants

Parent isolate PA42 was challenged with subinhibitory concentrations of meropenem during log-phase growth to generate an isogenic panel of carbapenem-resistant mutants. *P. aeruginosa* cells were harvested by centrifugation, resuspended in sterile saline, and diluted to achieve populations of 10^7, 10^8, and 10^9 cfu/mL. Diluted cultures were inoculated into sets of Mueller-Hinton agar plates containing 0.25 μg/mL or 0.5 μg/mL of meropenem. After 24 h of incubation at 37°C, individual colonies were selected at random from each meropenem plate and putative mutants were evaluated for a ≥4-fold increase in meropenem MIC by agar dilution in accordance with CLSI guidelines [20].

PCR and Sequencing

Genomic DNA was prepared from all bacterial isolates as previously described [21]. PCR was conducted in a final volume of 50 μL with 2 units of High-Fidelity Platinum® Taq Polymerase (Invitrogen, Carlsbad, CA), 3% DMSO, and primers that flanked either *oprD* or *oprF* (Table S1). The amplification conditions were 95°C for 5 min followed by 25 cycles at 95°C for 30 s, 56°C for 30 s, and 72°C for 3 min. A combination of primers specific for *oprD* and IS*Pa8* were used in a PCR using a 52°C annealing temperature to determine the location of IS*Pa8* with respect to the *oprD* gene in the isogenic mutants (Table S1). PCR products were column purified using a Millipore Amicon® Ultra Ultracel® 50 K filter (Millipore, Billerica, MA, USA) and sequenced by ACGT, Inc. (Wheeling, IL).

Real Time RT-PCR

RNA was isolated from cultures grown to mid-log phase and gene expression was evaluated by real time RT-PCR as previously described [22]. The expression of *mexA* for PA42 and its isogenic mutants was compared to PAO1 and represented as a ratio (fold-change). Expression studies were performed in triplicate with independent bacterial cultures and the relative expression of *mexA* was determined by averaging the results from three independent RNA extractions.

Outer Membrane Protein Analysis

Outer membrane proteins were isolated and resolved in an 11% SDS–PAGE with a constant current of 25 mA [23]. Proteins were stained with coomassie blue R-250 and photographed using the Molecular Imager® Gel Doc XR+ System with Image Lab Software.

Pulsed Field Gel Electrophoresis and Southern Hybridization

Pulsed field gel electrophoresis (PFGE) analysis was performed on *P. aeruginosa* genomic DNA digested with *Spe*I as previously described [24]. Southern hybridizations were performed on restricted genomic DNA using methods described by Sambrook and Russell [25]. A 182 bp DIG-labeled probe specific for IS*Pa8* was synthesized with primers ISPa8F2 and ISPa8R2 (Table S1) using a Roche PCR DIG Probe Synthesis Kit (Roche, Penzberg, Germany) and column purified. The restricted genomic DNA was vacuum blotted to a positively charged nylon membrane and hybridization was carried out with a Roche DIG Nucleic Acid Detection Kit (Roche, Penzberg, Germany) as instructed by the manufacturer.

Results

In vitro Meropenem Mutant Selection and Susceptibilities

Clinical isolate PA42 was challenged with subinhibitory levels of meropenem. Mutants were isolated from meropenem agar plates and evaluated for carbapenem susceptibilities and mechanisms of carbapenem resistance. The mutational frequency of PA42 challenged with 0.25 μg/mL (⅛ the MIC) of meropenem ranged from 1×10^{-7} to 9×10^{-7}, while the mutational frequency was 8×10^{-9} with 0.5 μg/mL (¼ the MIC) of meropenem. In comparison to PA42, the MICs of imipenem and doripenem were 32-fold and 16-fold higher for the selected mutants 711M, 714M, 811M, 812M, 925M, and 927M, while a 4- to 8-fold increase in doripenem MICs and an 8- to 16-fold increase in imipenem MICs were observed for mutants 922M and 924M, respectively. In addition, all the isogenic mutants had a meropenem MIC of 16 μg/mL (Table 1).

Mechanisms Associated with Carbapenem Resistance

Previous studies have shown that a loss of the OprD porin is the most common mechanism associated with reduced susceptibility to the carbapenems in *P. aeruginosa* [2,13,14]. It is possible that the elevated carbapenem MICs for the isogenic mutants was associated with mutations within *oprD* that were selected during meropenem exposure (Table 1). To determine whether nucleotide changes within *oprD* had occurred, the *oprD* gene and its flanking regions were amplified by PCR and sequenced. Parent isolate PA42 generated a PCR product of the predicted size (1586 bp) (Figure 1) and sequence analysis of the *oprD* gene from PA42 showed 99% similarity to *oprD* from *P. aeruginosa* LESB58 (GenBank Accession No. FM209186.1) and 92% similarity to *oprD* from *P. aeruginosa* PAO1 (GenBank Accession No. AE004091.2). Surprisingly, the PA42 mutants amplified a much larger PCR product (~3000 bp) than the PCR product for PA42, which suggested the presence of a large insertion within the *oprD* gene (Figure 1). Sequence analysis of mutant 712M revealed the presence of a 1324 bp IS element located within the *oprD* gene (Accession No. KC710194). The IS element was identified as having 96% similarity to IS*Pa8* (http://www-IS.biotoul.fr) and was flanked by 19 bp imperfect terminal inverted repeats. An open reading frame within IS*Pa8* was found to encode a 364 amino acid protein having 84% identity to a putative transposase in *Pseudoxanthomonas suwonensis* (GenBank Accession No. CP002446.1). PCR analysis using a combination of IS*Pa8* and *oprD*-specific primer sets listed in Table S1 revealed that IS*Pa8* had also inserted within *oprD* or its promoter region in the other isogenic mutants (Figure 1). To identify the insertion site and confirm the IS element was IS*Pa8*, a single sequence reaction was performed using primers listed in Table S1. PCR and sequence analysis determined that the disruption of *oprD* in eight mutants was due to IS*Pa8* insertion, while the insertion of IS*Pa8* was found 57 bp upstream of the translational start codon of *oprD* in mutant 922M. Although inactivation of the *oprD* gene in the isogenic mutants was due to IS*Pa8*, the position and orientation of this IS element was different with respect to *oprD* (Figure 2).

Meropenem and doripenem resistance can emerge through a combination of down-regulation or loss of OprD in the outer membrane and an up-regulation of MexAB-OprM in non-metallo-β-lactamase producing *P. aeruginosa* isolates [2,11]. To account for the higher MICs of meropenem and doripenem in the isogenic mutants, we compared the relative transcript levels of

Table 1. Carbapenem susceptibility and gene expression data for *P. aeruginosa* isolates.

Isolate	Phenotype[a]	Selective Agent[b]	Mutant Frequency	MIC (μg/mL)[c]			Relative *mexA* expression ± SD
				IPM	MEM	DOR	
PAO1	WT	–	–	2	0.5	0.5	1.00
PA443	CF	–	–	2	0.25	0.25	0.85±0.20
PA42	P	–	–	0.5	2	0.25	3.99±1.23
711M	M	0.25	9×10^{-7}	16	16	4	3.57±1.10
712M	M	0.25	9×10^{-7}	8	16	8	3.62±0.74
714M	M	0.25	9×10^{-7}	16	16	4	5.46±1.35
811M	M	0.25	1×10^{-7}	16	16	4	4.95±0.85
812M	M	0.25	1×10^{-7}	16	16	4	4.14±1.99
922M	M	0.5	8×10^{-9}	4	16	1	3.12±0.38
924M	M	0.5	8×10^{-9}	8	16	2	4.89±1.48
925M	M	0.5	8×10^{-9}	16	16	4	4.02±1.73
927M	M	0.5	8×10^{-9}	16	16	4	4.57±1.32

[a]WT, wild-type isolate; CF, clinical isolate from cystic fibrosis patient; P, parent isolate; M, mutant of PA42.
[b]Subinhibitory concentration (μg/mL) of meropenem used for mutant selection.
[c]IPM, imipenem; MEM, meropenem; DOR, doripenem.

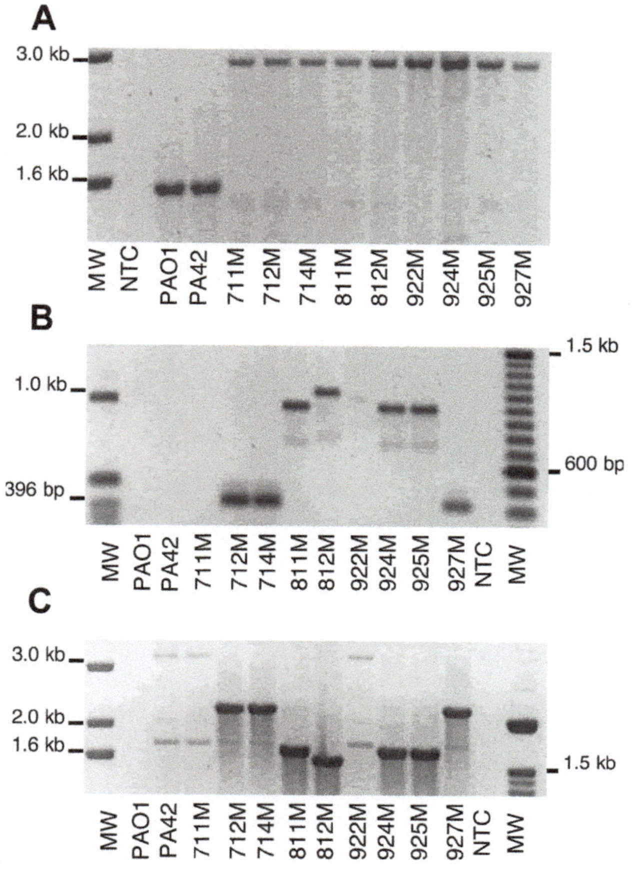

Figure 1. PCR amplification of *oprD* and IS*Pa8* from carbapenem-resistant mutants of *P. aeruginosa.* (A) Primers that flanked the *oprD* gene were used to PCR-amplify the *oprD* gene giving an expected PCR product size is 1586 bp. Each lane is labeled with its respective DNA ladder (1 kb DNA ladder, Invitrogen), no template control (NTC), or *P. aeruginosa* isolate. (B) PCR amplification of IS*Pa8* within the *oprD* gene in the nine carbapenem-resistant mutants. Primers ISPa8F1 and OprDRTR3 were used to map the approximate location of the IS*Pa8* within the *oprD* gene. The smaller PCR products indicate IS*Pa8* has inserted near the 3′ end of *oprD*, while larger PCR products indicate IS*Pa8* is inserted near the 5′ end. No PCR product was observed for mutant 711M. (C) Primers OprDRTF2 and ISPa8R2 were used to confirm the location of IS*Pa8* within the *oprD* gene in the nine isogenic mutants. Non-specific bands were amplified in PA42, mutant 711M, and mutant 922M suggesting that multiple IS*Pa8* elements may be present within the genome. To confirm that IS*Pa8* had inserted within the *oprD* gene or its flanking regions in mutants 711M and 922M, PCR products for these mutants shown in (A) were sequenced using primers OprDRTF2 or ISPa8F1.

mexA in the isogenic mutants, their parent PA42, and a fully susceptible cystic fibrosis isolate PA443 to *mexA* transcript levels in PAO1. *mexA* expression was 4-fold higher in PA42 than PAO1 and PA443, indicating that *mexA* expression was already elevated above "wild-type" levels observed for PAO1 and PA443. However, *mexA* transcript levels were similar among the isogenic mutants and their parent, PA42 suggesting that *mexA* expression did not change upon meropenem selection (Table 1).

Outer Membrane Profiles of PA42 and Isogenic Mutants

The inactivation of *oprD* by IS*Pa8* suggested that the OprD protein was no longer produced. Therefore, the presence of OprD in the outer membrane was analyzed in the isogenic mutants. The outer membrane profiles for PA42 and its mutants showed that OprD was produced in PA42 but not in the isogenic mutants (Figure 3). The loss of OprD correlated with the insertional inactivation of the *oprD* gene by IS*Pa8* and the reduced carbapenem susceptibility in the isogenic mutants. In addition to the loss of OprD in the mutants, parent isolate PA42 and the isogenic mutants did not produce the major outer membrane protein OprF (Figure 3). To investigate the potential source of IS*Pa8* on the chromosome of PA42, we sought to identify whether the loss of OprF was also the result of IS*Pa8* insertion within the *oprF* gene. To test this hypothesis, the *oprF* gene and its flanking regions were PCR amplified and sequenced. PCR amplification of *oprF* from PA42 generated a much larger product (~3000 bp) than the predicted 1672 bp product from PAO1 (Figure 4). Sequence analysis of *oprF* for PA42 identified the insertion of IS*Pa8* 31 nucleotides upstream of the translational start codon of *oprF* (Accession No. KC710195). The disruption of the *oprF* promoter region by IS*Pa8* in parent isolate PA42 correlated with a 50-fold decrease in *oprF* expression compared to *oprF* expression in PAO1 (data not shown). Additionally, the rounded cell shape observed for PA42 could be linked to the loss of OprF as previously reported [26–28]. Subsequently, amplification of the *oprF* gene in the isogenic mutants resulted in PCR products that were ~1,400 bp larger than expected (Figure 4). OprF was absent or produced at low levels in the outer membranes of PA42 and its mutants (Figure 3). Taken together, these data indicated that IS*Pa8* remained upstream of *oprF* during meropenem exposure and was responsible for the lack of OprF production in PA42 and the isogenic mutants.

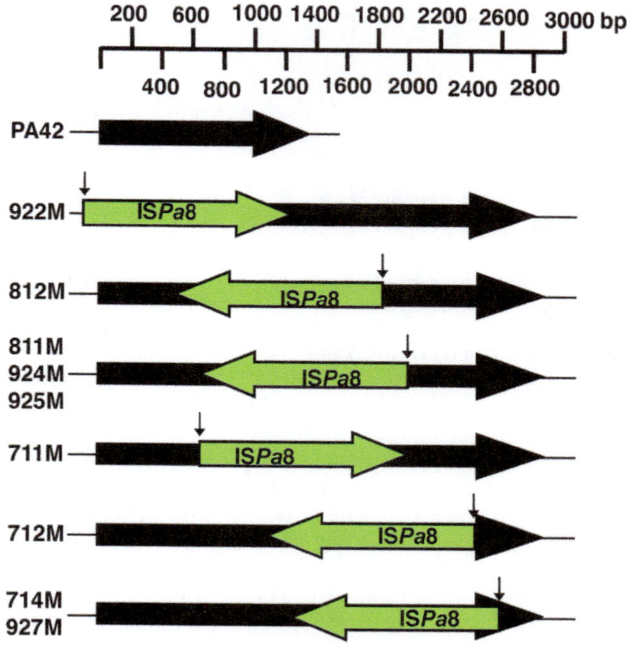

Figure 2. Insertion sites of IS*Pa8* with respect to the *oprD* gene in PA42 and nine isogenic mutants. The solid black arrows represent the *oprD* gene while the green arrows represent the location and orientation of IS*Pa8* within *oprD*. The downward arrow indicates the predicted insertion site of IS*Pa8* within *oprD* as determined by sequence analysis.

PFGE Patterns and IS*Pa8* Copy Number

To determine the copy number of IS*Pa8* in PA42 and its mutants, PFGE and Southern blot experiments were performed.

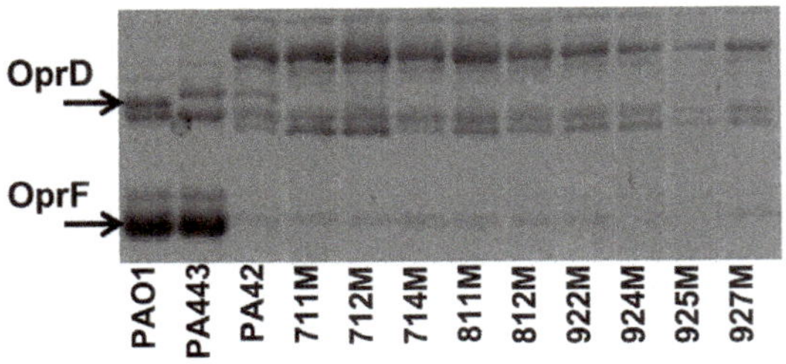

Figure 3. Outer membrane analysis of *P. aeruginosa* PA42 and nine isogenic mutants. Outer membrane profiles were analyzed for the presence of the porin, OprD. PAO1 and a fully susceptible cystic fibrosis isolate, PA443, were included as positive controls. The locations of OprD and OprF proteins are indicated.

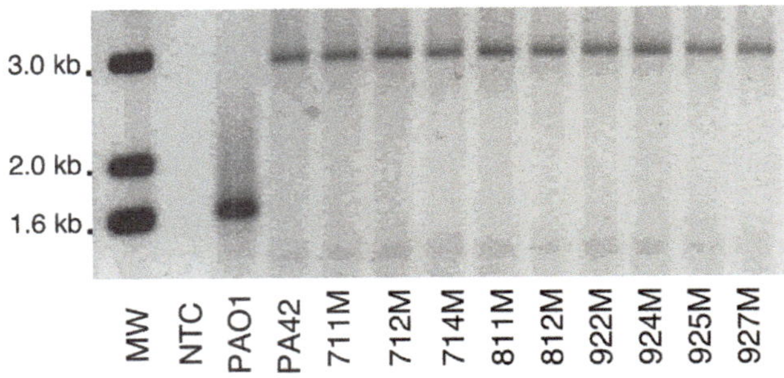

Figure 4. PCR amplification of the *oprF* gene in PAO1, PA42, and nine isogenic mutants. The expected PCR product size is 1,672 bp. Each lane is labeled with its respective DNA ladder (1 kb DNA ladder, Invitrogen), no template control (NTC), or *P. aeruginosa* isolates.

As anticipated, PA42 and its mutants were highly related by PFGE as indicated by their indistinguishable PFGE patterns (Figure 5, Figure S2). Surprisingly, Southern blot analysis revealed multiple hybridization signals for IS*Pa8* in PA42 and mutant 812M demonstrating that multiple copies of IS*Pa8* exist in their genomes (Figure 5). Note that in Figure 5 the DIG-probe was highly specific for IS*Pa8* as no hybridization signal was observed in the IS*Pa8*-negative control PAO1. Multiple copies of IS*Pa8* were also observed in the genomes of the other mutants (Figure S2). However, we could not differentiate the number of hybridization signals between PA42 and each mutant due to the high copy number (>20 copies) of the IS*Pa8* within their genomes as illustrated in the analysis of PA42 and mutant 812M (Figure 5).

Discussion

Carbapenem resistance poses a major therapeutic challenge for the treatment of *P. aeruginosa* infections, particularly in patients with cystic fibrosis. Our current understanding of the mechanisms responsible for carbapenem resistance consists of an interplay between the over-expression of *mexAB-oprM* and the down-regulation of the porin, OprD [2,10,11]. The most common mechanism of imipenem resistance is the absence of OprD production which can result from mutations, insertions, and/or deletions in the *oprD* gene as well as the down-regulation of *oprD* transcription [13–17]. In this study, the insertion of a novel IS element, identified as IS*Pa8*, within the *oprD* gene was associated with the emergence of carbapenem resistance in *P. aeruginosa* mutants selected with subinhibitory levels of meropenem. These findings are in agreement with other investigations where IS element insertion has been linked to a decrease in carbapenem susceptibility and loss of OprD production. These observations indicate that the *oprD* gene and/or its promoter region may serve as a hot spot in the genome for IS element insertion [15–17,29].

The loss of OprD in the outer membrane has been shown to decrease the susceptibility of *P. aeruginosa* by 4- to 16-fold for imipenem, compared to 4- to 32-fold for meropenem and 8- to 32-fold for doripenem [11,30], while up-regulation of *mexAB-oprM* expression increased the MICs of meropenem and doripenem from 0.12–0.5 μg/mL to 4 μg/mL [11]. However, a concomitant loss of OprD and up-regulation of this efflux pump can increase the MIC of meropenem above "wild-type" levels (~16 μg/mL) [10]. In this study, meropenem resistance (16 μg/mL) among the isogenic mutants resulted from increased *mexA* transcript levels that preceded meropenem exposure in addition to a loss of OprD through insertional disruption by IS*Pa8* allowing for the selection of the meropenem mutants. Interestingly, the parent isolate from which carbapenem-resistant mutants were selected showed a 4-fold increase in *mexA* expression compared *mexA* expression in PAO1 which correlated with the MIC of meropenem (2 μg/mL). However, meropenem selection did not modify the expression of *mexA* in the isogenic mutants compared to the parent isolate PA42, suggesting that *mexA* expression may have reached an expression threshold sufficient to achieve high meropenem MICs (Table 1). However, as previous described [10], it is the combination of increased *mexA* expression and loss of OprD as displayed in these isogenic mutants that resulted in the MICs of doripenem and meropenem to increase above the resistance breakpoint, while the loss of OprD alone was responsible for the reduction in susceptibility to imipenem in these mutants. These data demonstrate that OprD-mediated resistance is not always the first step

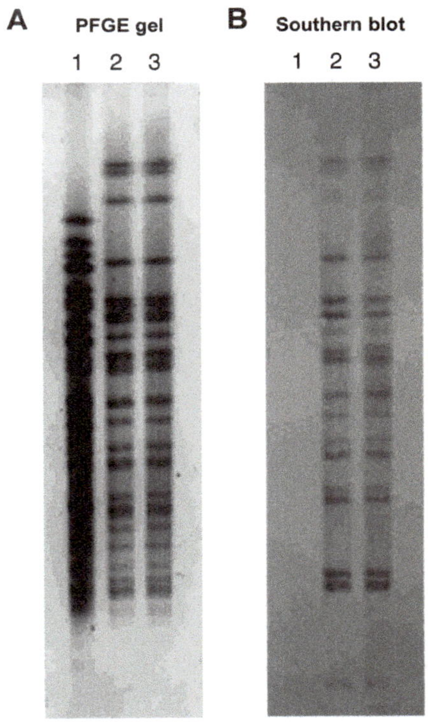

Figure 5. Pulsed Field Gel Electrophoresis and Southern blot analyses using IS*Pa8*-specific probe. (A) PFGE gel of *Spe*I chromosomal digests of wild-type strain PAO1, parent isolate PA42, and mutant 812M visualized using SYBR gold. (B) Southern blot of the gel depicted in Figure 5(A) using an IS*Pa8*-specific probe. Lane 1, PAO1 (negative control); lane 2, parent isolate PA42; lane 3, mutant 812M.

toward carbapenem resistance as has been previously suggested [10,11]. Taken together, these data further support that a combination of chromosomally-encoded resistance mechanisms are necessary to achieve meropenem and/or doripenem MICs above the resistance breakpoint.

Transposable elements such as IS elements can promote the adaptation and survival of Gram-negative bacteria under different environmental niches through the disruption of genes and genomic rearrangements. This form of adaptation has been well documented in clinical isolates of *P. aeruginosa* that have developed resistance to β-lactam antibiotics [15–19]. Moreover, IS elements modulate genomic plasticity and participate in the evolution of *P. aeruginosa* isolates within the lung environment of patients with cystic fibrosis through genetic rearrangements [31]. The presence of multiple copies of IS*Pa*8 in the host chromosome of PA42 suggests that it may have played an important role in the evolution of this clinical isolate. Recently, Doumith *et al* suggested that bacterial chromosomes may contain multiple copies of IS elements and their insertion into porin genes may be selected under antibiotic pressure [32]. To our knowledge, our study is the first to provide support that when a selective pressure is applied to a bacteria with multiple copies of an IS element, antibiotic-resistant mutants with insertional disruptions in porin genes will be selected for within the bacterial population. Interestingly, multiple insertion events of IS*Pa*8 occurred within the *oprD* gene or promoter region among the meropenem selected mutants, which may be a reflection of the host genome containing several copies of the IS*Pa*8 element (Figure 2). These data suggest that *P. aeruginosa* isolates with a high copy number of IS elements within its genome could lead to the emergence of antibiotic resistance. This observation could have serious implications in clinical practice where carbapenem monotherapy is used as the primary treatment of *P. aeruginosa* infections. Ruiz-Martinez *el al* reported a similar finding where imipenem monotherapy was used to treat a fully susceptible *P. aeruginosa* infection in a patient, which resulted in the selection of an imipenem-resistant variant due to the inactivation of the *oprD* gene by IS*Pa*133 [29]. Taken together, these data indicate that the selective pressure exerted by a carbapenem can select mutants from *P. aeruginosa* isolates that contain multiple copies of IS element in the genome thereby allowing for the rapid development carbapenem resistance.

This study serves as an important reminder that monotherapy, particularly with a carbapenem, may not always be appropriate for treating *P. aeruginosa* infections as it can readily develop resistance to antibiotics. Although IS elements have been shown to influence the genetic and phenotypic characteristics of bacteria as described in this study, little is known about what stimulates their transposition. Therefore, future studies looking to identify factors that influence the mobilization and insertion of IS elements could contribute significantly to our current knowledge of mechanisms involved in the emergence of antibiotic resistance and the evolution of *P. aeruginosa.*

Supporting Information

Figure S1 Macroscopic and microscopic analysis of *P. aeruginosa* isolates PAO1 and PA42. Macroscopic analysis of PAO1 grown on blood agar shows a non-mucoid phenotype while PA42 was mucoid when grown on blood agar. Gram-staining revealed characteristic Gram-negative rods for PAO1 and unique Gram-negative cocci for PA42 at 40X and 100X objectives.

Figure S2 Pulsed Field Gel Electrophoresis and Southern blot analyses using IS*Pa*8-specific probe. (A) PFGE gel of *Spe*I chromosomal digests of wild-type strain PAO1, parent isolate PA42, and eight carbapenem-selected mutants visualized using SYBR gold. Lane 1, size standard *Staphylococcus aureus* NCTC 8325; lane 2, negative control PAO1; lane 3, parent isolate PA42; lane 4, mutant 711M; lane 5, mutant 712M; lane 6, mutant 714M; lane 7, mutant 811M; lane 8, mutant 922M; lane 9, mutant 924M; lane 10, mutant 925M; lane 11, mutant 927M. (B) Southern blot of the gel depicted in Figure S2(A) using an IS*Pa*8-specific probe. Lane 1, size standard *Staphylococcus aureus* NCTC 8325; lane 2, negative control PAO1; lane 3, parent isolate PA42; lane 4, mutant 711M; lane 5, mutant 712M; lane 6, mutant 714M; lane 7, mutant 811M; lane 8, mutant 922M; lane 9, mutant 924M; lane 10, mutant 925M; lane 11, mutant 927M.

Table S1 Primers used in this study.

Acknowledgments

We thank Richard Goering for his contribution to the collection and interpretation of data.

Author Contributions

Conceived and designed the experiments: RCF NDH. Performed the experiments: RCF. Analyzed the data: RCF NDH. Contributed reagents/materials/analysis tools: NDH. Wrote the paper: RCF NDH.

References

1. George AM, Jones PM, Middleton PG (2009) Cystic fibrosis infections: Treatment strategies and prospects. FEMS Microbiol Lett. 300: 153–164. doi: 10.1111/j.1574-6968.2009.01704.x.
2. Lister PD, Wolter DJ, Hanson ND (2009) Antibacterial-resistant *Pseudomonas aeruginosa*: Clinical impact and complex regulation of chromosomally encoded resistance mechanisms. Clin Microbiol Rev. 22: 582–610. doi:10.1128/CMR.00040-09.
3. Carmeli Y, Troillet N, Eliopoulos GM, Samore MH (1999) Emergence of antibiotic-resistant *Pseudomonas aeruginosa*: Comparison of risks associated with different antipseudomonal agents. Antimicrob Agents Chemother 43: 1379–1382.
4. Lepper PM, Grusa E, Reichl H, Hoqel J, Trautmann M (2002) Consumption of imipenem correlates with beta-lactam resistance in *Pseudomonas aeruginosa*. Antimicrob Agents Chemother 46: 2920–2925. doi: 10.1128/AAC.46.9.2920-2925.2002.
5. Andrade SS, Jones RN, Gales AC, Sader HS (2003) Increasing prevalence of antimicrobial resistance among *Pseudomonas aeruginosa* isolates in latin american medical centres: 5 year report of the SENTRY antimicrobial surveillance program (1997–2001). J Antimicrob Chemother 52: 140–141. doi: 10.1093/jac/dkg270.
6. Cao B, Wang H, Sun H, Zhu Y, Chen M (2004) Risk factors and clinical outcomes of nosocomial multi-drug resistant *Pseudomonas aeruginosa* infections. J Hosp Infect 57: 112–118. doi:10.1016/j.jhin.2004.03.021.
7. Hsueh PR, Chen WH, Luh KT (2005) Relationships between antimicrobial use and antimicrobial resistance in Gram-negative bacteria causing nosocomial infections from 1991–2003 at a university hospital in Taiwan. Int J Antimicrob Agents 26: 463–472. doi:10.1016/j.ijantimicag.2005.08.016.
8. Fujimura S, Nakano Y, Sato T, Shirahata K, Watanabe A (2007) Relationship between the usage of carbapenem antibiotics and the incidence of imipenem-resistant *Pseudomonas aeruginosa*. J Infect Chemother 13: 147–150. doi: 10.1007/s10156-007-0507-x.
9. Pluss-Suard C, Pannatier A, Kronenberg A, Muhlemann K, Zanetti G (2013) Impact of antibiotic use on carbapenem resistance in *Pseudomonas aeruginosa*: Is there a role for antibiotic diversity? Antimicrob Agents Chemother doi:10.1128/AAC.01348-12.
10. Kohler T, Michea-Hamzehpour M, Epp SF, Pechere JC (1999) Carbapenem activities against *Pseudomonas aeruginosa*: Respective contributions of OprD and efflux systems. Antimicrob Agents Chemother 43: 424–427.
11. Livermore DM (2002) Of *Pseudomonas*, porins, pumps and carbapenems. J Antimicrob Chemother. 47: 247–250.

12. Ochs MM, McCusker MP, Bains M, Hancock REW (1999) Negative regulation of the *Pseudomonas aeruginosa* outer membrane porin OprD selective for imipenem and basic amino acids. Antimicrob Agents Chemother 43: 1085–1090.
13. Pai H, Kim J-W, Kim J, Lee JH, Choe KW, et al. (2001) Carbapenem resistance mechanisms in *Pseudomonas aeruginosa* clinical isolates. Antimicrob Agents Chemother 45: 480–484.
14. Pirnay JP, De Vos D, Mossialos D, Vanderkelen A, Cornelis P, et al. (2002) Analysis of the *Pseudomonas aeruginosa oprD* gene from clinical and environmental isolates. Environ Microbiol 4: 872–882.
15. Wolter DJ, Hanson ND, Lister PD (2004) Insertional inactivation of *oprD* in clinical isolates of *Pseudomonas aeruginosa* leading to carbapenem resistance. FEMS Microbiol Lett 236: 137–143.
16. Evans JC, Segal H (2007) A novel insertion sequence, ISPA26, in *oprD* of *Pseudomonas aeruginosa* is associated with carbapenem resistance. Antimicrob Agents Chemother 51: 3776–3777.
17. Diene SM, L'homme T, Bellulo S, Stremler N, Dubus J, et al. (2013) IS*Pa*46, a novel insertion sequence in the *oprD* porin gene of an imipenem-resistant *Pseudomonas aeruginosa* isolate from a cystic fibrosis patient in marseille, France. Int J Antimicrob Agents 42: 268–271.
18. Boutoille D, Corvec S, Caroff N, Giraudea C, Espaze E, et al. (2004) Detection of an IS21 insertion sequence in the *mexR* gene of *Pseudomonas aeruginosa* increasing beta-lactam resistance. FEMS Microbiol Lett. 230: 143–146.
19. Depardieu F, Podglajen I, Leclercq R, Collatz E, Courvalin P (2007) Modes and modulations of antibiotic resistance gene expression. Clin Microbiol Rev 20: 79–114. doi: 10.1128/CMR.00015-06.
20. Clinical and Laboratory Standards Institute (2012) Performance Standards for Antimicrobial Susceptibility Testing: Twenty-Second Informational Supplement. CLSI document M100-S22. CLSI, Wayne, PA, USA.
21. Schmidtke AJ, Hanson ND (2006) Model system to evaluate the effect of *ampD* mutations on AmpC-mediated beta-lactam resistance. Antimicrob Agents Chemother 50: 2030–2037. doi:10.1128/AAC.01458-05.
22. Wolter DJ, Black JA, Lister PD, Hanson ND (2009) Multiple genotypic changes in hypersusceptible strains of *Pseudomonas aeruginosa* isolated from cystic fibrosis patients do not always correlate with the phenotype. J Antimicrob Chemother 64: 294–300. doi: 10.1093/jac/dkp185. Epub 2009 May 25.
23. Wolter DJ, Smith-Moland E, Goering RV, Hanson ND, Lister PD (2004) Multidrug resistance associated with *mexXY* expression in clinical isolates of *Pseudomonas aeruginosa* from a Texas hospital. Diagn Microbiol Infect Dis 50: 43–50.
24. Goering R, Ribot E, Gerner-Smidt P (2011) Pulsed-field gel electrophoresis: Laboratory and epidemiologic considerations for interpretation of data. In: Persing D, Tenover F, Tang Y, et al, editors. Molecular Microbiology. Washington, DC: ASM. p. 167–177.
25. Sambrook J, Russell D (2001) Molecular Cloning – A Laboratory Manual. Cold Spring Harbor, NY: Cold Spring Harbor Laboratory Press.
26. Woodruff WA, Hancock RE (1989) *Pseudomonas aeruginosa* outer membrane protein F: Structural role and relationship to the *Escherichia coli* OmpA protein. J Bacteriol 171: 3304–3309.
27. Rawling EG, Brinkman FS, Hancock RE (1998) Roles of the carboxy-terminal half of *Pseudomonas aeruginosa* major outer membrane protein OprF in cell shape, growth in low-osmolarity medium, and peptidoglycan association. J Bacteriol 180: 3556–3562.
28. Freulet-Marriere MA, El Hamel C, Chevalier S, Dé E, Molle G, et al. (2000) Evidence for association of lipopolysaccharide with *Pseudomonas fluorescens* strain MF0 porin OprF. Res Microbiol 151: 873–876. doi.org/10.1016/S0923-2508(00)01154-2.
29. Ruiz-Martinez L, Lopez-Jimenez L, d'Ostuni V, Fuste E, Vinuesa T, et al. (2011) A mechanism of carbapenem resistance due to a new insertion element (ISPa133) in *Pseudomonas aeruginosa*. Int Microbiol 14: 51–58.
30. Sakyo S, Tomita H, Tanimoto K, Fujimoto S, Ike Y (2006) Potency of carbapenems for the prevention of carbapenem-resistant mutants of *Pseudomonas aeruginosa*: The high potency of a new carbapenem doripenem. J Antibiot (Tokyo) 59: 220–228. doi:10.1038/ja.2006.31.
31. Kresse AU, Blocker H, Romling U (2006) ISPa20 advances the individual evolution of *Pseudomonas aeruginosa* clone C subclone C13 strains isolated from cystic fibrosis patients by insertional mutagenesis and genomic rearrangements. Arch Microbiol 185: 245–254. doi: 10.1007/s00203-006-0089-5.
32. Doumith M, Ellington MJ, Livermore DM, Woodford N (2009) Molecular mechanisms disrupting porin expression in ertapenem-resistant *Klebsiella* and *Enterobacter spp.* clinical isolates from the UK. J Antimicrob Chemother 63: 659–667. doi: 10.1093/jac/dkp029.

5

The Tumor Necrosis Factor α (-308 A/G) Polymorphism Is Associated with Cystic Fibrosis in Mexican Patients

Celia N. Sanchez-Dominguez[1], Miguel A. Reyes-Lopez[2], Adriana Bustamante[3], Ricardo M. Cerda-Flores[4], Maria del C. Villalobos-Torres[1], Hugo L. Gallardo-Blanco[5], Augusto Rojas-Martinez[1,6], Herminia G. Martinez-Rodriguez[1], Hugo A. Barrera-Saldaña[1], Rocio Ortiz-Lopez[1,6]*

1 Departamento de Bioquimica y Medicina Molecular, Facultad de Medicina, Universidad Autonoma de Nuevo Leon, Monterrey, Nuevo Leon, Mexico, **2** Laboratorio de Medicina de Conservacion, Centro de Biotecnologia Genomica, Instituto Politecnico Nacional, Reynosa, Tamaulipas, Mexico, **3** Clinica de Fibrosis Quistica, Centro de Prevencion y Rehabilitacion de Enfermedades Pulmonares Cronicas (CEPREP), Facultad de Medicina y Hospital Universitario "Dr. Jose Eleuterio Gonzalez", Universidad Autónoma de Nuevo Leon, Monterrey, Nuevo Leon, Mexico, **4** Facultad de Enfermeria, Universidad Autonoma de Nuevo Leon, Monterrey, Nuevo Leon, Mexico, **5** Departamento de Genetica, Facultad de Medicina, Universidad Autonoma de Nuevo Leon, Monterrey, Nuevo Leon, Mexico, **6** Centro de Investigacion y Desarrollo en Ciencias de la Salud, Universidad Autonoma de Nuevo Leon, Monterrey, Nuevo Leon, Mexico

Abstract

Environmental and genetic factors may modify or contribute to the phenotypic differences observed in multigenic and monogenic diseases, such as cystic fibrosis (CF). An analysis of modifier genes can be helpful for estimating patient prognosis and directing preventive care. The aim of this study is to determine the association between seven genetic variants of four modifier genes and CF by comparing their corresponding allelic and genotypic frequencies in CF patients (n = 81) and control subjects (n = 104). Genetic variants of MBL2 exon 1 (A, B, C and D), the IL-8 promoter (−251 A/T), the TNFα promoter (TNF1/TNF2), and SERPINA1 (PI*Z and PI*S) were tested in CF patients and control subjects from northeastern Mexico by PCR-RFLP.

Results: The TNF2 allele ($P = 0.012$, OR 3.43, 95% CI 1.25–9.38) was significantly associated with CF under the dominant and additive models but was not associated with CF under the recessive model. This association remained statistically significant after adjusting for multiple tests using the Bonferroni correction ($P = 0.0482$). The other tested variants and genotypes did not show any association with the disease.

Conclusion: An analysis of seven genetic variants of four modifier genes showed that one variant, the TNF2 allele, appears to be significantly associated with CF in Mexican patients.

Editor: Amit Gaggar, University of Alabama-Birmingham, United States of America

Funding: This work was supported by grants from the Consejo Nacional de Ciencia y Tecnología CONACyT (62291 and 48497) and UANL's PAICyT (1648-07) for ROL, Fondo Mixto de Fomento a la Investigación Científica y Tecnológica CONACYT – Gobierno del Estado de Tamaulipas (73578) and SIP-IPN (20080682) for MARL. The authors gratefully acknowledge scholarships from CONACyT, PIFI-IPN and Universia Santander for CNSD. The funders had no role in study design, data collection and analysis, decision to publish, or preparation of the manuscript.

Competing Interests: The authors have declared that no competing interests exist.

* E-mail: rortizlopez@gmail.com

Introduction

Gene-environment and gene-gene interactions play a role in the phenotypic expression of genetic diseases in individuals harboring the same genotype [1]. Cystic fibrosis (CF) has an estimated incidence of one in 3000 in the Caucasian population, although its frequency may vary in specific subgroups. A newborn screening study conducted in Mexico City revealed two CF-affected newborns among 7193 screened (1:3597) participants, suggesting a high frequency of CF among Mexicans [2]. Approximately 1900 mutations and variants have been reported in the CF transmembrane conductance regulator (CFTR) gene, with ΔF508 being the most prevalent mutation (50%–60%, http://www.genet.sickkids.on.ca/app). CF primarily involves epithelial cells in the respiratory tract, intestine, pancreas, bladder, and sweat glands; respiratory failure, however, is the major cause of death in CF patients [3].

Variants in genes that are involved in the inflammatory response have been studied in CF patients based on their potential effects on inflammation and host defense mechanisms. The mannose binding lectin (MBL2) gene encodes a serum acute-phase protein secreted by the liver, resembling the complement component C1q, that leads to opsonization and activation of the complement system through the classical pathway [4]. The serum concentration and complement-triggering activity of MBL depend on single-base mutations in the MBL2 gene [5–7]. These mutations may increase the susceptibility of carriers to colonization by bacterial and viral pathogens [8]. The best known genetic variants in exon 1 of the MBL2 gene are Gly54Asp (the B allele, rs1800450), Gly57Glu (the C allele, rs1800451) and Arg52Cys (the D allele, rs5030737), which are together referred to as the O allele. The interleukin 8 (IL-8) gene codes for a member of the CXC chemokine family and is mainly involved in the initiation and amplification of acute inflammatory reactions [9]. IL-8 is

Table 1. Mutations included in the kits used for the molecular diagnosis of CF patients.

Kit	Detected mutations
ASO16 Roche	DF508, G542X, G551D, R553X, W1282X, N1303K, R117H, 621+1G >T, R334W, R347P, A455E, DI507, 1717-1G >A, S549N, R560T, 3849+10Kb C >T
ASO26 Roche	DF508, G542X, G551D, R553X, W1282X, N1303K, R117H, 621+1G >T, R334W, R347P, A455E, DI507, 1717-1G >A, R560T, 3849+10KbC>T, G85E, 2307insA, G480C, A559T, R1162X, 3659delC, S1255X, R347H, 2789+5G>A, 405+3 A>C, 3120+1G>A
INNOLiPA CFTR36 Innogenetics	F508del, G542X, G551D, R553X, W1282X, N1303K, R117H, 621+1G>T, R334W, R347P, A455E, I507del, 1717-1G>A, R560T, 3849+10KbC>T, G85E, R1162X, 3659delC, 2789+5G>A, 3120+1G>A, 711+1G>T, 3905insT, S1251N, Q552X, I148T, 1898+1G>A, 394delTT, 1078delT, 2183AA>G, 2184delA, E60X, 2143delT, 711+5G>A, 3199del6, 3272-26A>G, dele2,3

produced by a wide range of cell types, such as monocytes, macrophages, and fibroblasts; it primarily mediates the activation and migration of neutrophils from peripheral blood into pathogen-infected tissue, initiating and amplifying inflammatory processes [10]. A polymorphism in position −251 of the IL-8 gene (rs4073) is associated with increased IL-8 expression [11–12]. The tumor necrosis factor alpha (TNFα) gene expresses a multifunctional pro-inflammatory cytokine secreted in response to numerous specific stimuli, such as lipopolysaccharides. This molecule induces the release of cytokines IL-6 and IL-8 and increases airway mucus production [13–14]. The −308 A TNFα promoter polymorphism (TNF2, rs1800629) has been associated with increased TNFα transcription activity relative to the normal TNF1 allele (−308 G) [15–17]. The Alpha-1-antitrypsin (AAT, SERPINA1) gene codes for an acute-phase serine protease glycoprotein that limits tissue self-damage during the inflammatory immune response. AAT deficiency, caused by the S (p.E264V, rs17580) and Z (p.E342K, rs28929474) alleles in the SERPINA1 gene, may induce liver and pulmonary disease [18]. Severe AAT deficiency is a co-dominant autosomal hereditary disorder that clinically resembles early onset pulmonary emphysema, particularly in smokers [19].

In our Cystic fibrosis clinic, we have a broad range of severity of the CF disease, even with patients carrying the same genotype. No reports on variations in modifier genes in Mexican CF patients have been previously published. Our goal was to explore polymorphisms in genes related to host defense in healthy controls and CF patients from northeastern Mexico to find differences in allelic distribution between both groups. In this study, we report the genotype and allele frequencies of seven genetic variants in four previously reported CF modifier genes: MBL, IL-8, TNFα and AAT.

Materials and Methods

Biological Samples

The study was approved by the Research and Ethics Committee of the Universidad Autonoma de Nuevo Leon University Hospital (Registry number BI09-003). After signing written informed consent, blood samples were drawn from 81 CF patients attending the Chronic Lung Disease Prevention and Rehabilitation Center (CEPREP, in Spanish) and from control subjects recruited from the University Hospital and School of Medicine (Universidad Autonoma de Nuevo Leon). Also we collected blood samples from 104 control subjects that met the following inclusion criteria: they agreed to informed consent, they were born in northeastern Mexico (the states of Nuevo Leon, Tamaulipas, Coahuila, and San Luis Potosi), and they belonged to a family with at least three ascending Mexican generations. Genomic DNA was isolated from peripheral venous blood using the phenol–chloroform method, precipitated in ethanol, and finally suspended in Tris-EDTA (pH 7.8).

Screening for the CFTR Gene Mutations

Mutation screening was performed according to the availability of resources and kits along the time. For previously screened CF patients: direct detection of ΔF508 mutation, and Roche ASO16 and 27 mutations kits, for new CF patients: direct detection of ΔF508 mutation, INNOLiPA CFTR36 probe kit and Exon

Table 2. Modifier genes analysis by PCR-RFLP adapted from previously published techniques [21–24].

Gene	Polymorphism	Primers	Enzyme	Mutant allele, bp	Normal allele, bp
MBL	Arg52Cys (D)	F: CAT CAA CGG CTT CCC AGG GCA AGA TGG G	*Mwo* I	134	109+25
	Gly54Asp (B)	R: GTC TCC TCA TAT CCC CAG GC	*Ban* I	134	95+39
	Gly57Glu (C)		*Mbo* II	78+56	134
IL-8	−251 T/A	F: GAT TCT GCT CTT ATG CCT CCA	*Mfe* I	816	520+296
		R: CCC AAG CTT GTG TGC TCT GCT GTC			
TNFα	−308 G/A	F: GGG ACA CAC AAG CAT CAA GG	*Nco* I	142	126+16
		R: AAT AGG TTT TGA GGG CCA TG			
AAT	PI*S Glu264Val	F: GAG GGG AAA CTA CAG CAC CTC G	*Taq* I$^{\alpha}$	98	78+20
		R: ACC CTC AGG TTG GGG AAT CAC C			
	PI*Z Glu342Lys	F: TAA GGC TGT GCT GAC CAT CGT C	*Taq* I$^{\alpha}$	144	123+21
		R: GGA GAC TTG GTA TTT TGT TCA ATC			

11-specific PCR and sequencing. Short descriptions of the methodologies are presented below.

PCR and electrophoresis to detect the ΔF508 mutation: PCR product was analyzed in polyachrylamide gels and the diagnosis was established comparing to molecular marker and DNAs of previously ΔF508 diagnosed patients and control subjects (98 bp band for normal allele or 95 bp band for ΔF508 mutation) [20].

Roche ASO16 and 27 kits (Roche Molecular Systems, Alameda CA, USA) or the INNOLiPA CFTR36 probe kit (Innogenetics, Ghent, Belgium). Methodology consisted of multiplex PCR reactions with biotinylated primers. After verifying the amplification in an agarose gel of 2%, the products were hybridized to membrane bound probes. A positive result was expressed as the appearance of a purple band. Both kits detected normal and mutated versions to report homozygous or heterozygous status for the CF patients. Complete list of mutations is shown in Table 1.

Exon 11- specific PCR and sequencing. Exon 11 PCR fragment was amplified and sequenced in one patient with absence of hybridization of PCR product on the normal and mutated versions of the G551D probe in the CFTR36 probe kit.

Modifier Genes Analysis

DNA from CF patients and control subjects was tested for the Gly54Asp (B allele, rs1800450), Gly57Glu (C allele, rs1800451), Arg52Cys (D allele, rs5030737), and A (wild type) alleles in exon 1 of the MBL2 gene; the −251 T/A (rs4073) allele of the IL-8 gene; the −308 G/A (TNF1/2, rs1800629) alleles of the TNFα gene; and the PI*S Glu264Val (rs17580), PI*Z Glu342Lys (rs28929474), and PI*M (wild type) alleles of the SERPINA1 gene. PCR-RFLP protocols were adapted from previously reported methods. More details are explained in Table 2 and Figure 1 [21–24].

Statistical Analysis

The SNP & Variation Suite (SVS) 7 (Golden Helix Inc., Bozeman, MA, USA) software program was used to perform all statistical analyses. The association between the tested genotypes

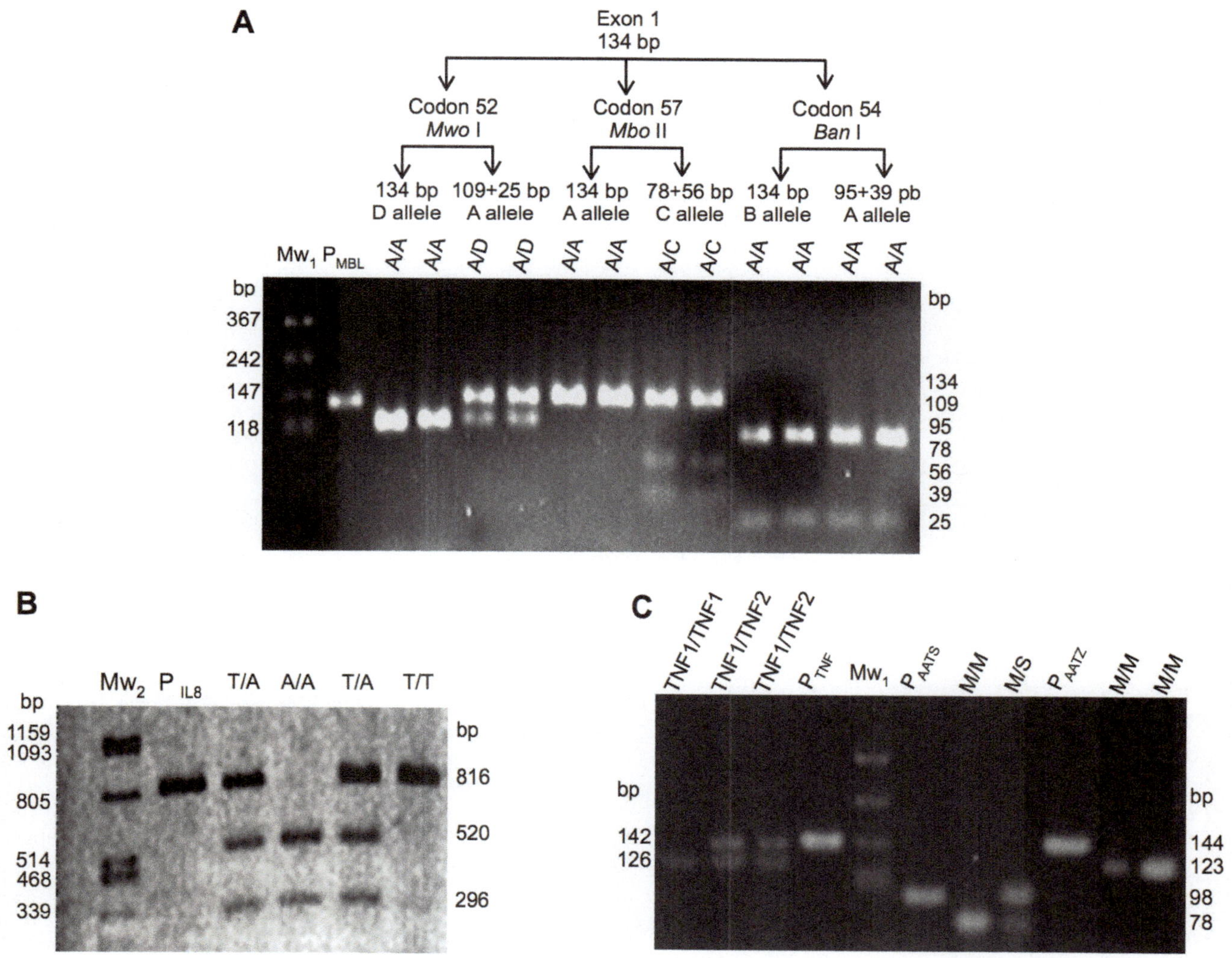

Figure 1. PCR-RFLP for the modifier genes analysis. 1A: the 134 bp PCR product from exon 1 of the MBL1 gene was digested with *Mwo* I, *Ban* I and *Mbo* II for detection of polymorphisms in the 52, 54 and 57 codons. 1B: the 816 bp PCR product from promoter region of the IL-8 gene was digested with *Mfe* I for detection of the −251 polymorphism. 1C: the 142 bp PCR product from promoter region of the TNFα gene was digested with *Nco* I for detection of the −308 polymorphism (TNF2); the 98 bp PCR product from the SERPINA1 gene was digested with *Taq* I^{α} for detection of the S genetic variant; the 144 bp PCR product from the SERPINA1 gene was digested with *Taq* I^{α} enzyme for detection of the Z genetic variant. Mw1 is the molecular marker pBs+*Msp* I, Mw2 is the molecular marker λ+*Pst* I. P_{MBL}, P_{IL8}, P_{TNF}, P_{AATS} and P_{AATZ} are undigested PCR products. The Z allele was not detected.

and CF was analyzed by correlation/trend and chi-squared (χ^2) tests under three different models (dominant, recessive, and additive) and was confirmed with the Bonferroni correction to detect the false discovery rate. Odds ratios were estimated within 95% confidence intervals. Values of $P<0.05$ were considered statistically significant. The Hardy–Weinberg Equilibrium (HWE) *P*-values were assessed using a chi-square test.

Results

Eighty-one CF patients and 104 control subjects were recruited for this study. Genotype frequencies for the CFTR gene are described in Table 3. A complete genotype characterization was achieved in 55.6% (n = 45) of the CF patients; in 39.5% (n = 32) of the CF patients, only one mutation was identified, and in 4.9% (n = 4) of the CF patients, both mutations remained undetected. The most prevalent genotypes were ΔF508/other (46.9%, n = 38) and ΔF508/ΔF508 (35.8%, n = 29). The overall frequency of the ΔF508 allele among CF patients was 59.3%. Ten additional mutations were detected: G542X (4.9%), S549N (3.1%), 2789+5G>A (2.5%), 3849+10 kb (1.9%), G85E, R1162X, I148T, R334W, ΔI507, and L206W (0.6% each one). Mutations in the CFTR gene were not detected in 24.7% of the total CFTR alleles.

The PCR-RFLP patterns of the seven genetic variants in the four modifier genes are shown in the Figure 1. The Z allele, and the homozygote TNF2 and AATS genotypes were not found. The genotype frequencies of modifier genes in CF patients and control subjects are shown in Table 4. The B, C, and D alleles of the MBL2 gene were grouped together and reported as the O allele. The polymorphisms were in Hardy-Weinberg equilibrium. The frequencies of the mutant alleles for CF patients and controls were: the MBL-O allele 0.231 and 0.233, the IL-8 -251T allele 0.576 and 0.569, AATS allele 0.012 and 0.014, and TNF2 allele 0.087 and 0.029, respectively. The TNF2 allele ($P=0.012$, Odds Ratio (OR) 3.43, 95% CI 1.25–9.38) was significantly associated with CF patients using the dominant model. This association remains statistically significant after adjusting for multiple testing using the Bonferroni correction ($P=0.0482$). The association value and the OR of the TNF2 allele were statistically significant when assessed using the additive model (Dd vs. dd) but not the recessive model (Table 5). The other genetic variants tested did not show any association.

Table 3. CFTR genotype frequencies from 81 Mexican CF patients.

Genotype	N	%
ΔF508/ΔF508	29	35.8
ΔF508/X	26	32.1
ΔF508/G542X	5	6.2
ΔF508/3849+10 kb	3	3.7
S549N/S549N	2	2.5
G542X/X	2	2.5
ΔF508/S549N	1	1.2
ΔF508/L206W	1	1.2
ΔF508/2789+5G>A	1	1.2
ΔF508/G85E	1	1.2
2789+5G>A/2789+5G>A	1	1.2
G542X/R1162X	1	1.2
2789+5G>A/X	1	1.2
ΔI507/X	1	1.2
I148T/X	1	1.2
R334W/X	1	1.2
X/X	4	4.9
Total	81	100

X: unknown allele.

Discussion

In the present study, the ΔF508 mutation accounted for 59.3% of the mutated CFTR alleles, a frequency that resembles the mutation frequencies of European Mediterranean countries. In this regard, this work may be comparable with modifier genes studies performed in those countries. Two previous CFTR mutation reports in the Mexican population showed ΔF508 frequencies of 40.72% [25], 45% [26] and 44.6% [27]. Differences could be explained by the clinical criteria, geographic origin and the analytical methods available at that time. The Spanish federation reported a frequency of 45%. Previous studies in the Hispanic population reported a ΔF508 allele frequency ranging from 29 to 46% [28–30]. The frequencies of the G542X, R1162X and R334W alleles reflect the Spanish heritage in the Mexican population, but the S549N and 2789+5 G>A alleles are not among the most frequent in Spain [31–32]. In this study we previously detected homozygote S549N and ΔF508/S549N genotypes with the ASO16 kit. A second patient was detected by exon 11 direct sequencing because she presented an abnormal pattern of the INNOLiPA CFTR36 kit with the normal and mutant G551D probes. This kit along with the ASO27 excluded the S549N mutation from the mutation panel, hindering the CFTR molecular diagnosis in our population. CFTR gene sequencing should be performed for new or rare CFTR mutations in Mexican population as S549N, and those mutations obtained from central Mexico patients (P750L, 846delT, 4160insGGGG and 297–1 G>A) [25], as well as for those mutations that remained undetected. It is necessary to establish an adequate diagnosis strategy based in Mexican genetic profile, considering that available commercial kits are designed mainly for Caucasian mutations profile.

In northeastern Mexico, medical care for CF patients is offered at the Cystic Fibrosis Clinic of the CEPREP (http://www.ceprep.edu.mx). Since 1987, approximately 200 patients have been diagnosed with CF based on clinical and molecular analyses. Once the diagnosis of CF is established, the rate of adherence to medical treatment and long-term medical monitoring is low, making investigations into the genetic and environmental factors that influence the outcome in CF Mexican patients difficult.

In this study, we analyzed seven variants in four modifier genes previously reported in CF patients and we found an association between CF and the TNF2 allele.

The proinflammatory role of the TNF2 allele has been demonstrated in B cell line cultures, where the TNF2 allele was more potent transcriptional activator compared to the normal TNF1 [17]. TNF2 allele has been implicated as a potent immunomediator and pro-inflammatory cytokine in the pathogenesis of several human diseases, including pulmonary diseases as CF and asthma. Patients with genotypes related to higher TNFα production had increased frequency of asthma [33]. In Mexican population TNF2 allele was found in 6.0% of asthmatic compared to 2.9% of the controls [34]. These results are similar that those we found in our study (2.9% for controls and 8.9% for CF patients).

Table 4. Modifier gene genotype frequencies (%) in CF patients and control subjects; OR, Hardy–Weinberg Equilibrium (HWE) and results of the association test with Dominant Model *P*-values.

Gene	Genotypes	Genotype Frequency in CF Patients	HWE P in CF Patients	Genotype Frequency in Controls	HWE P in Controls	OR (95% CI) Dominant Model	P-Value Dominant Model	
		N (%)		N (%)			X^2	X^2 Bonf. P
MBL2	AA	46 (57.5)	0.4210	63 (61.2)	0.1843	A 1.01 (0.62–1.65)	0.6163	1.0000
	AO	31 (38.8)		32 (31.1)		O 0.99 (0.61–1.61)		
	OO	3 (3.8)		8 (7.8)				
IL-8	AA	13 (16.5)	0.5786	19 (18.6)	0.9937	T 1.03 (0.68.1.57)	0.9194	1.0000
	AT	41 (51.9)		50 (49.0)		A 0.97 (0.64–1.48)		
	TT	25 (31.6)		33 (32.4)				
TNFα	TNF1/TNF1	66 (82.5)	0.3911	97 (94.2)	0.7608	[a]TNF1 0.30 (0.11–0.80)	0.0120	0.0482
	TNF1/TNF2	14 (17.5)		6 (5.8)		[b]TNF2 3.43 (1.25–9.38)		
	TNF2/TNF2	0 (0.0)		0 (0)				
AAT	MM	79 (97.5)	0.9104	101 (97.1)	0.8814	M 1.17 (0.19–7.01)	0.8627	1.0000
	MS	2 (2.5)		3 (2.9)		S 0.85 (0.14–5.17)		
	M/Z, S/Z, S/S, Z/Z	0 (0)		0 (0)				

CF, cystic fibrosis; OR, Odds Ratio; CI, confidence interval.
[a]TNF1 −308 G: (dd) vs. (DD, Dd),
[b]TNF2 −308 A: (DD, Dd) vs. (dd).
HW-P: *P*-value for the Hardy-Weinberg equilibrium.
X^2 Bonf. P = Chi squared test with a Bonferroni-corrected *P*-value.

By the other hand, recent studies in Mexican population reported a higher frequency of the TNF2 allele in healthy unrelated Mexican individuals (7.3%) [35]. Another report related TNF2 allele to breast cancer in Mexican patients compared to healthy women (7.5 and 24.5% respectively) [36]. Differences in TNF1 allele frequency in control subjects could be explained by sample size, methodology and characteristics of the studied group. Our study included population from Northeastern Mexico, while the other studies had different criteria as gender, living in Mexico City or been born in Mexico.

Previous studies in CF patients have shown that TNF2 is associated with a lower percentage of predicted forced expiratory volume in one second (FEV_1) and weight z scores [37]. In Mexican population, the TNF2 allele has been associated with rheumatoid arthritis [38], geriatric lipid profile [39] and spondyloarthritis [40]. This variant has also been reported to be associated with obesity and asthma [41–42]. The high frequency of the TNF2 allele in Mexican CF patients could suggest a heterozygote advantage. In Colombia, an inverse association between the TNF polymorphism and autoimmunity and TB has been reported; this association suggests the existence of a heterozygote advantage and is consistent with the hypothesis that autoimmune diseases are a consequence of natural selection for enhanced TB resistance [43–44].

Table 5. TNF1/TNF2 association values using dominant, additive and recessive models.

Model	TNFα −308 G/−308 A OR[1] (95% CI)	*P*-value	
Dominant	TNF1 = 0.29 (0.11–0.79)	0.012[2]	0.048[3]
	TNF2 = 3.43 (1.25–9.38)		
Additive	TNF1 = NA	0.012[4]	0.049[3]
	TNF2 = 3.429 (1.25–9.38)		
Recessive	NA	NA	NA

[1]odds ratio.
[2]Chi-Squared P.
[3]Bonf. P.
[4]Correl/Trend P.

MBL2, IL-8 and AAT did not show an association with the CF genotype. MBL2 had previously shown associations with different disturbances in the lung function, infection risk, and survival of CF patients [6,45–48]. In asthma, MBL has been associated with *Chlamydia pneumoniae*-specific IgG and a greater risk of developing asthma, especially in children with chronic or recurrent infection [49]. MBL levels in asthmatic children positively correlate with peripheral blood eosinophils [50]. MBL therapy may be useful in MBL-deficient patients; it may reduce the susceptibility to or enhance the recovery from bacterial infection or modify the natural history of the disease [51–53]. The IL-8 −251 polymorphism has been associated with CF lung disease severity and the differential expression of IL-8, suggesting that the IL-8 variant modifies CF lung disease severity [54]. The −251 variant has been associated with asthma, infection by respiratory syncytial virus, and chronic obstructive pulmonary disease (COPD) [10,55–56]. Finally, despite the association between AAT deficiency and COPD, studies of AAT variants and infection in CF patients have been inconclusive [57–60]. The incidence of AAT deficiency for all five phenotypic classes of the Pi*S and Pi*Z deficiency alleles is 1 in 9.8 for Canada and 1 in 11.3 for the United States. However, a previous report from our group showed very low allele frequencies of Pi*S and Pi*Z variants in a Mexican population (1.5% and 0%, respectively) [61].

In summary, the frequencies of genetic variants in the MBL2, IL-8, and AAT genes of CF patients did not show significant differences when compared to control subjects, but the TNF2 allele was significantly associated with CF patients. More studies are needed to identify the role of inflammatory mediators in the pathophysiology of CF, as emphasized in previous studies. This information is relevant because clinical trials of drugs targeting TNFα activity [62] have shown outstanding efficacy in treating chronic inflammatory diseases.

Acknowledgments

We especially acknowledge the volunteers, whose cooperation made these studies possible. The authors gratefully acknowledge Dr. Sergio Lozano for his critical reading of the manuscript and his contribution in editing the manuscript.

Author Contributions

Conceived and designed the experiments: CNSD AB ROL MARL. Performed the experiments: CNSD MCVT. Analyzed the data: HLGB RMCF. Contributed reagents/materials/analysis tools: ROL MARL HLGB. Wrote the paper: CNSD. Helped to design and revised the manuscript: HGMR HABS ARM.

References

1. Collaco JM, Cutting GR (2008) Update on gene modifiers in cystic fibrosis. Curr Opin Pulm Med 14: 559–566.
2. Velázquez A, Vela-Amieva M, Naylor EW, Chace DH (2000) Tamiz neonatal ampliado. Rev Mex Pediatr 67: 206–213.
3. Rowntree RK, Harris A (2003) The phenotypic consequences of CFTR mutations. Ann Hum Genet 67: 471–485.
4. Turner MW (1996) Mannose-binding lectin: the pluripotent molecule of the innate immune system. Immunol Today 17: 532–540.
5. Madsen HO, Satz ML, Hogh B, Svejgaard A, Garred P (1998) Different molecular events result in low protein levels of mannan-binding lectin in populations from southeast Africa and South America. J Immunol 161: 3169–3175.
6. Yarden J, Radojkovic D, De Boeck K, Macek M Jr, Zemkova D, et al. (2004) Polymorphisms in the mannose binding lectin gene affect the cystic fibrosis pulmonary phenotype. J Med Genet 41: 629–633.
7. Garred P, Larsen F, Seyfarth J, Fujita R, Madsen HO (2006) Mannose-binding lectin and its genetic variants. Genes Immun 7: 85–94.
8. Eisen DP (2010) Mannose-binding lectin deficiency and respiratory tract infection. J Innate Immun 2: 114–122.
9. Harada A, Sekido N, Akahoshi T, Wada T, Mukaida N, et al. (1994) Essential involvement of interleukin-8 (IL-8) in acute inflammation. J Leukoc Biol 56: 559–564.
10. Puthothu B, Krueger M, Heinze J, Forster J, Heinzmann A (2006) Impact of IL8 and IL8-receptor alpha polymorphisms on the genetics of bronchial asthma and severe RSV infections. Clin Mol Allergy 4: 2.
11. Hull J, Thomson A, Kwiatkowski D (2000) Association of respiratory syncytial virus bronchiolitis with the interleukin 8 gene region in UK families. Thorax 55: 1023–1027.
12. Mizunoe S, Shuto T, Suzuki S, Matsumoto C, Watanabe K, et al. (2012) Synergism between interleukin (IL)-17 and toll-like receptor 2 and 4 signals to induce IL-8 expression in cystic fibrosis airway epithelial cells. J Pharmacol Sci 118: 512–520.
13. Cowan MJ, Huang X, Yao XL, Shelhamer JH (2000) Tumor necrosis factor alpha stimulation of human Clara cell secretory protein production by human airway epithelial cells. Ann N Y Acad Sci 923: 193–201.
14. Lora JM, Zhang DM, Liao SM, Burwell T, King AM, et al. (2005) Tumor necrosis factor-alpha triggers mucus production in airway epithelium through an IkappaB kinase beta-dependent mechanism. J Biol Chem 280: 36510–36517.
15. Hajeer AH, Hutchinson IV (2000) TNF-alpha gene polymorphism: clinical and biological implications. Microsc Res Tech 50: 216–228.
16. Gambari R, Borgatti M, Lampronti I, Fabbri E, Brognara E, et al. (2012) Corilagin is a potent inhibitor of NF-kappaB activity and downregulates TNF-alpha induced expression of IL-8 gene in cystic fibrosis IB3–1 cells. Int Immunopharmacol 13: 308–315.
17. Wilson AG, Symons JA, McDowell TL, McDevitt HO, Duff GW (1997) Effects of a polymorphism in the human tumor necrosis factor alpha promoter on transcriptional activation. Proc Natl Acad Sci U S A 94: 3195–3199.
18. Kok KF, te Morsche RH, van Oijen MG, Drenth JP (2010) Prevalence of genetic polymorphisms in the promoter region of the alpha-1 antitrypsin (SERPINA1) gene in chronic liver disease: a case control study. BMC Gastroenterol 10: 22.
19. Miravitlles M, Vila S, Jardi R, de la Roza C, Rodriguez-Frias F, et al. (2003) Emphysema due to alpha-antitrypsin deficiency: familial study of the YBARCELONA variant. Chest 124: 404–406.
20. Araujo FG, Novaes FC, Santos NP, Martins VC, Souza SM, et al. (2005) Prevalence of deltaF508, G551D, G542X, and R553X mutations among cystic fibrosis patients in the North of Brazil. Braz J Med Biol Res 38: 11–15.
21. Sandford AJ, Chagani T, Spinelli JJ, Pare PD (1999) alpha1-antitrypsin genotypes and the acute-phase response to open heart surgery. Am J Respir Crit Care Med 159: 1624–1628.
22. Tin SK, Lee LY, Thumboo J, Koh DR, Fong KY (2005) PCR-RFLP genotyping for exon 1 and promoter region mutations of the human mannose binding lectin (MBL-2) gene. J Immunol Methods 303: 148–151.
23. Lee WP, Tai DI, Lan KH, Li AF, Hsu HC, et al. (2005) The −251T allele of the interleukin-8 promoter is associated with increased risk of gastric carcinoma featuring diffuse-type histopathology in Chinese population. Clin Cancer Res 11: 6431–6441.
24. Chen YP, Pfab T, Slowinski T, Richter CM, Godes M, et al. (2006) Impact of genetic variation of tumor necrosis factor-alpha on gestational hypertension. Chin Med J (Engl) 119: 719–724.
25. Orozco L, Velazquez R, Zielenski J, Tsui LC, Chavez M, et al. (2000) Spectrum of CFTR mutations in Mexican cystic fibrosis patients: identification of five novel mutations (W1098C, 846delT, P750L, 4160insGGGG and 297–1G–>A). Hum Genet 106: 360–365.
26. Villalobos-Torres C, Rojas-Martinez A, Villareal-Castellanos E, Cantu JM, Sanchez-Anzaldo FJ, et al. (1997) Analysis of 16 cystic fibrosis mutations in Mexican patients. Am J Med Genet 69: 380–382.
27. Chavez-Saldana M, Yokoyama E, Lezana JL, Carnevale A, Macias M, et al. (2010) CFTR allelic heterogeneity in Mexican patients with cystic fibrosis: implications for molecular screening. Rev Invest Clin 62: 546–552.
28. Grebe TA, Seltzer WK, DeMarchi J, Silva DK, Doane WW, et al. (1994) Genetic analysis of Hispanic individuals with cystic fibrosis. Am J Hum Genet 54: 443–446.
29. Sugarman EA, Rohlfs EM, Silverman LM, Allitto BA (2004) CFTR mutation distribution among U.S. Hispanic and African American individuals: evaluation in cystic fibrosis patient and carrier screening populations. Genet Med 6: 392–399.
30. Schrijver I, Ramalingam S, Sankaran R, Swanson S, Dunlop CL, et al. (2005) Diagnostic testing by CFTR gene mutation analysis in a large group of Hispanics: novel mutations and assessment of a population-specific mutation spectrum. J Mol Diagn 7: 289–299.
31. Aliño-Pellicer SF, Antelo-Landeira MC, Baamonde-Vidarte A, Beltrán-Bengoechea B, Berná-Torres N, et al. (2003) Federación Española contra la Fibrosis Quística. Libro Blanco de atención a la fibrosis quística; Consumo MdSy, editor. Madrid, España.
32. Alonso MJ, Heine-Suner D, Calvo M, Rosell J, Gimenez J, et al. (2007) Spectrum of mutations in the CFTR gene in cystic fibrosis patients of Spanish ancestry. Ann Hum Genet 71: 194–201.
33. Shmarina G, Pukhalsky A, Petrova N, Zakharova E, Avakian L, et al. (2013) TNF gene polymorphisms in cystic fibrosis patients: contribution to the disease progression. J Transl Med 11: 19.
34. Jimenez-Morales S, Velazquez-Cruz R, Ramirez-Bello J, Bonilla-Gonzalez E, Romero-Hidalgo S, et al. (2009) Tumor necrosis factor-alpha is a common genetic risk factor for asthma, juvenile rheumatoid arthritis, and systemic lupus erythematosus in a Mexican pediatric population. Hum Immunol 70: 251–256.
35. Vargas-Alarcon G, Ramirez-Bello J, Juarez-Cedillo T, Ramirez-Fuentes S, Carrillo-Sanchez S, et al. (2012) Distribution of the IL-1RN, IL-6, IL-10, INF-gamma, and TNF-alpha Gene Polymorphisms in the Mexican Population. Genet Test Mol Biomarkers 16: 1246–1253.
36. Gomez Flores-Ramos L, Escoto-De Dios A, Puebla-Perez AM, Figuera-Villanueva LE, Ramos-Silva A, et al. (2013) Association of the tumor necrosis factor-alpha −308 G>A polymorphism with breast cancer in Mexican women. Genet Mol Res 12: 5680–5693.
37. Hull J, Thomson AH (1998) Contribution of genetic factors other than CFTR to disease severity in cystic fibrosis. Thorax 53: 1018–1021.
38. Rodriguez-Carreon AA, Zuniga J, Hernandez-Pacheco G, Rodriguez-Perez JM, Perez-Hernandez N, et al. (2005) Tumor necrosis factor-alpha −308 promoter polymorphism contributes independently to HLA alleles in the severity of rheumatoid arthritis in Mexicans. J Autoimmun 24: 63–68.
39. Parra-Rojas I, Ruiz-Madrigal B, Martinez-Lopez E, Panduro A (2006) Influence of the −308 TNF-alpha and −174 IL-6 polymorphisms on lipid profile in Mexican subjects. Hereditas 143: 167–172.
40. Vargas-Alarcon G, Casasola-Vargas J, Rodriguez-Perez JM, Huerta-Sil G, Perez-Hernandez N, et al. (2006) Tumor necrosis factor-alpha promoter polymorphisms in Mexican patients with spondyloarthritis. Hum Immunol 67: 826–832.
41. Castro-Giner F, Kogevinas M, Imboden M, de Cid R, Jarvis D, et al. (2009) Joint effect of obesity and TNFA variability on asthma: two international cohort studies. Eur Respir J 33: 1003–1009.
42. Wu H, Romieu I, Sienra-Monge JJ, del Rio-Navarro BE, Anderson DM, et al. (2007) Parental smoking modifies the relation between genetic variation in tumor necrosis factor-alpha (TNF) and childhood asthma. Environ Health Perspect 115: 616–622.

43. Correa PA, Gomez LM, Anaya JM (2004) [Polymorphism of TNF-alpha in autoimmunity and tuberculosis]. Biomedica 24 Supp 1: 43–51.
44. Correa PA, Gomez LM, Cadena J, Anaya JM (2005) Autoimmunity and tuberculosis. Opposite association with TNF polymorphism. J Rheumatol 32: 219–224.
45. Buranawuti K, Boyle MP, Cheng S, Steiner LL, McDougal K, et al. (2007) Variants in mannose-binding lectin and tumour necrosis factor alpha affect survival in cystic fibrosis. J Med Genet 44: 209–214.
46. Muhlebach MS, MacDonald SL, Button B, Hubbard JJ, Turner ML, et al. (2006) Association between mannan-binding lectin and impaired lung function in cystic fibrosis may be age-dependent. Clin Exp Immunol 145: 302–307.
47. Davies JC, Turner MW, Klein N (2004) Impaired pulmonary status in cystic fibrosis adults with two mutated MBL-2 alleles. Eur Respir J 24: 798–804.
48. Haerynck F, Van Steen K, Cattaert T, Loeys B, Van Daele S, et al. (2012) Polymorphisms in the lectin pathway genes as a possible cause of early chronic Pseudomonas aeruginosa colonization in cystic fibrosis patients. Hum Immunol 73: 1175–1183.
49. Nagy A, Kozma GT, Keszei M, Treszl A, Falus A, et al. (2003) The development of asthma in children infected with Chlamydia pneumoniae is dependent on the modifying effect of mannose-binding lectin. J Allergy Clin Immunol 112: 729–734.
50. Uguz A, Berber Z, Coskun M, Halide Akbas S, Yegin O (2005) Mannose-binding lectin levels in children with asthma. Pediatr Allergy Immunol 16: 231–235.
51. Garred P, Pressler T, Lanng S, Madsen HO, Moser C, et al. (2002) Mannose-binding lectin (MBL) therapy in an MBL-deficient patient with severe cystic fibrosis lung disease. Pediatr Pulmonol 33: 201–207.
52. Summerfield JA (2003) Clinical potential of mannose-binding lectin-replacement therapy. Biochem Soc Trans 31: 770–773.
53. Kilpatrick DC (2003) Introduction to mannan-binding lectin. Biochem Soc Trans 31: 745–747.
54. Hillian AD, Londono D, Dunn JM, Goddard KA, Pace RG, et al. (2008) Modulation of cystic fibrosis lung disease by variants in interleukin-8. Genes Immun 9: 501–508.
55. Heinzmann A, Ahlert I, Kurz T, Berner R, Deichmann KA (2004) Association study suggests opposite effects of polymorphisms within IL8 on bronchial asthma and respiratory syncytial virus bronchiolitis. J Allergy Clin Immunol 114: 671–676.
56. Arinir U, Klein W, Rohde G, Stemmler S, Epplen JT, et al. (2005) Polymorphisms in the interleukin-8 gene in patients with chronic obstructive pulmonary disease. Electrophoresis 26: 2888–2891.
57. Mahadeva R, Stewart S, Bilton D, Lomas DA (1998) Alpha-1 antitrypsin deficiency alleles and severe cystic fibrosis lung disease. Thorax 53: 1022–1024.
58. Mahadeva R, Westerbeek RC, Perry DJ, Lovegrove JU, Whitehouse DB, et al. (1998) Alpha1-antitrypsin deficiency alleles and the Taq-I G–>A allele in cystic fibrosis lung disease. Eur Respir J 11: 873–879.
59. Meyer P, Braun A, Roscher AA (2002) Analysis of the two common alpha-1-antitrypsin deficiency alleles PiMS and PiMZ as modifiers of Pseudomonas aeruginosa susceptibility in cystic fibrosis. Clin Genet 62: 325–327.
60. Frangolias DD, Ruan J, Wilcox PJ, Davidson AG, Wong LT, et al. (2003) Alpha 1-antitrypsin deficiency alleles in cystic fibrosis lung disease. Am J Respir Cell Mol Biol 29: 390–396.
61. Sanchez-Dominguez CN, Buenfil-Lozano JA, Molina-Guajardo CA, Borjas-Almaguer OD, Castillo-Lartigue A, et al. (2008) Frequency of S and Z alleles for alpha-1-antitrypsin and tumor necrosis factor alpha −308 promoter polymorphism in northeastern Mexico. Allergy Asthma Proc 29: 406–410.
62. Kim J, Remick DG (2007) Tumor necrosis factor inhibitors for the treatment of asthma. Curr Allergy Asthma Rep 7: 151–156.

Effect of Different Breathing Aids on Ventilation Distribution in Adults with Cystic Fibrosis

Markus Wettstein[1], Lorenz Radlinger[2], Thomas Riedel[3]*

1 Physiotherapy Institute, Inselspital, Bern University Hospital and University of Bern, Bern, Switzerland, **2** Bern University of Applied Sciences, Health, Bern, Switzerland, **3** Paediatric and Neonatal Intensive Care Medicine, Department of Paediatrics, Inselspital, Bern University Children's Hospital and University of Bern, Bern, Switzerland

Abstract

Background and objectives: We investigated the effect of different breathing aids on ventilation distribution in healthy adults and subjects with cystic fibrosis (CF).

Methods: In 11 healthy adults and 9 adults with CF electrical impedance tomography measurements were performed during spontaneous breathing, continuous positive airway pressure (CPAP) and positive expiratory pressure (PEP) therapy randomly applied in upright and lateral position. Spatial and temporal ventilation distribution was assessed.

Results: The proportion of ventilation directed to the dependent lung significantly increased in lateral position compared to upright in healthy and CF. This effect was enhanced with CPAP but neutralised with PEP, whereas the effect of PEP was larger in the healthy group. Temporal ventilation distribution showed exactly the opposite with homogenisation during CPAP and increased inhomogeneity with PEP.

Conclusions: PEP shows distinct differences to CPAP with respect to its impact on ventilation distribution in healthy adults and CF subjects EIT might be used to individualise respiratory physiotherapy.

Editor: Dominik Hartl, University of Tübingen, Germany

Funding: The authors have no support or funding to report.

Competing Interests: The authors have declared that no competing interests exist.

* Email: thomas.riedel@insel.ch

Introduction

Respiratory Physiotherapy (RPT) is often used for the promotion of lung expansion, minimisation of atelectasis and the airway clearing. RPT contains breathing manoeuvres, positioning, mobilisation/ambulation, exercise therapy and different airway clearance techniques (ACTs) using different devices.

Improved mucus clearance is considered essential in optimising respiratory performance (airway obstruction, atelectasis, ventilation inhomogeneity, increased work of breathing) and might reduce the progression of lung disease in Cystic Fibrosis (CF). [1] Some ACTs have been shown to lead to significantly greater sputum expectoration compared to breathing manoeuvres alone [2].

Probably the most frequently used airway clearance devices are the positive expiratory pressure (PEP) devices. [1] They provide a constant backpressure to the airways during expiration. It has been hypothesised that PEP increases gas pressure behind the mucus via collateral ventilation and maintains airway patency by stabilising the airways during expiration, thereby improving mucus clearance. [3,4] A recent study showed superiority of PEP over high frequency chest wall oscillation as the primary form of airway clearance in CF patients. [5] Ventilation distribution is mainly influenced by factors like gravity (posture), ventilation patterns (tidal volume, flow rate) or breathing manoeuvres (type of respiratory aid) and the quality (age, body weight, genetics) and/or pathology of the lung. [6–11] Hence, to increase their efficacy, ACT's are often combined with positioning and breathing aids such as continuous positive airway pressure (CPAP) or positive expiratory pressure (PEP), in order to benefit from postural drainage effects or changes in ventilation distribution [12,13].

In healthy lungs, most of the tidal volume is directed to the dependent parts of the lung. [11,14] In certain lung diseases and in elderly, children or obese patients these findings may be different, due to early airway closure and lung collapse in the dependent lung during expiration. [15–17] These gravitational effects have been shown to be enhanced with CPAP. [14] PEP devices may homogenise the ventilation distribution and may counteract the early airway closure [3].

To achieve the optimal combination of position and device for each individual patient, it is essential to be aware of the effects of different breathing aids on ventilation distribution in different body positions.

Conventional techniques to assess ventilation distribution such as multiple breath washout (MBW), radio nuclear lung scans or ventilation MRI are either nearly impossible to perform during RPT or give only an overall measure of ventilation distribution without being able to show regional differences. Electrical impedance tomography (EIT) is a imaging technique for bedside monitoring of ventilation distribution. [18] EIT accurately measures tidal volumes and changes in end-expiratory level and describes regional ventilation distribution by measurement of local impedance change and has the advantage of a high temporal resolution [14,19–22].

With the present work, we aimed to compare the effect of different breathing aids on gravity-dependent ventilation distribution in subjects with CF and healthy adults. We hypothesised that the different devices have variable impact on gravity-dependent ventilation distribution in both groups.

Materials and Methods

Ethics Statement

This study was designed as a randomised cross-over study and approved by the ethics committee of the region of Bern, Switzerland. Written informed consent from all subjects was obtained at enrolment.

Subjects

We investigated 11 healthy physiotherapists (5 female), median (range) age 33 (23–45) years and 9 subjects with advanced CF lung disease (2 female), age 31 (19–48) years. All of them were familiar with the use of breathing aids and RPT. Subjects with CF were recruited from outpatient chest clinics at Bern University Hospital, Switzerland. CF subjects showed a forced expiratory volume in the first second (FEV_1) of median (range) 41 (16–63)% predicted, whereas forced vital capacity (FVC) was 48 (20–70)% predicted. FEV_1 and FVC in healthy subjects was 108 (95–118)% predicted and 111 (98–121)% predicted, respectively. In healthy as well as in CF there were no smokers.

Measurements

For each subject, three repetitive recordings of EIT were performed during spontaneous breathing, CPAP (VPAPIII, Resmed AG, Basel, Switzerland) and PEP (PARI-PEP, PARI GmbH, Starnberg, Germany) in upright and right lateral position with the respective commonly used breathing pattern. CPAP pressure were set to 15 mbar in healthy (similar to PEP pressure) and to 10 mbar for CF (according to the hospital guidelines). CPAP was applied by full face mask, PEP was applied by using a mouthpiece and expiratory time was limited to 7 seconds. Body position and the different devices within each body position were applied in a random order. Randomisation was achieved by using sealed envelopes. In between the measurements was a break of at least one minute to check electrodes. Measurements with the new device/position were started after a stabilisation phase of one minute. Based on our own experience this time has shown to lead to stable conditions.

Data acquisition and processing

A Goettingen GoeMF II EIT tomograph (CareFusion, Houten, The Netherlands) was used with a frame rate of 13 Hz and a recording time of 45 seconds in combination with self-adhesive ECG electrodes (Blue Sensor T, Synmedic, Switzerland). EIT scans were generated from the collected potential differences and the known excitation currents with weighted back-projection in a 32×32 pixel matrix using the software provided with the EIT device. The EIT signal was low-pass filtered below the cardiac frequency and a cut-off mask of 20% of the maximum standard deviation of the mean impedance change (912 pixels) was used. [19,23] The proportion of ventilation distributed into the right and left parts of the lung (spatial distribution), relative change in end-expiratory level (EEL), relative change in tidal volume and local filling characteristics (temporal distribution) were calculated adapted to previously-published methods in Matlab R2013a (The MathWorks Inc., Nattick, MA, USA). [14] For the calculation of the temporal distribution the time course of the impedance signal of the region of interest was plotted against the global impedance signal breath by breath. The resulting curve was fitted to the equation $I(g) = a * g^{FI} + c$, where the filling index (FI) describes the shape of the curve. The region of interest is filling faster than the rest of the lung if $FI<1$ and slower if $FI>1$ [24].

Statistics

For spatial distribution EIT results are expressed as the percentage of ventilation directed to the right parts of the lung. For filling characteristics FI-values of the right parts of the lung are reported. Changes in EEL from spontaneous breathing within the same body position were normalised for the impedance change during spontaneous tidal breathing in upright position. Changes in EIT tidal volumes are expressed as percentage change from average EIT tidal volume during spontaneous breathing in the corresponding body position. All data were tested for normal distribution with the Shapiro-Wilk test. The mean value of the three measurements was used for analysis. Descriptive data are presented as means and standard deviation.

Comparison of breathing aids and body positions

Differences in terms of spatial and temporal distribution and change in EEL between spontaneous breathing, CPAP and PEP and between the different body positions within groups were assessed with paired t-tests or two way analysis of variance test with Tukey correction for multiple comparisons where applicable. Comparisons between groups (CF and healthy) were assessed with unpaired t-tests.

A p-value <0.05 was considered significant. All statistics were performed using StatsDirect, version 2.7.9 (StatsDirect Ltd., GB).

Results

Ventilation distribution

In upright position we found no difference in either spatial or temporal ventilation distribution between the right and left lung irrespective of the breathing aid in CF as well as in healthy. In right lateral position there was a significant shift of spatial distribution towards the right lung during spontaneous breathing in CF and healthy. This effect was enhanced by the use of CPAP and neutralised with PEP in both groups. (Figure 1) Temporal distribution showed a lag of the right lung in right lateral position (CF and healthy). This effect was reduced with CPAP and increased with PEP in healthy but no significant difference was noted in CF (Table 1).

Additional results: End-expiratory Level (EEL) and tidal volumes

Compared to spontaneous breathing we found an increase in EEL with CPAP and a decrease in EEL with PEP. This effect was only statistically significant in the healthy group. (Table 2) Tidal volumes during PEP compared to spontaneous breathing increased significantly in upright and right lateral position in both groups. No significant differences in tidal volumes were found between spontaneous breathing and CPAP. Between CPAP and PEP differences were only significant in upright position (Table 3).

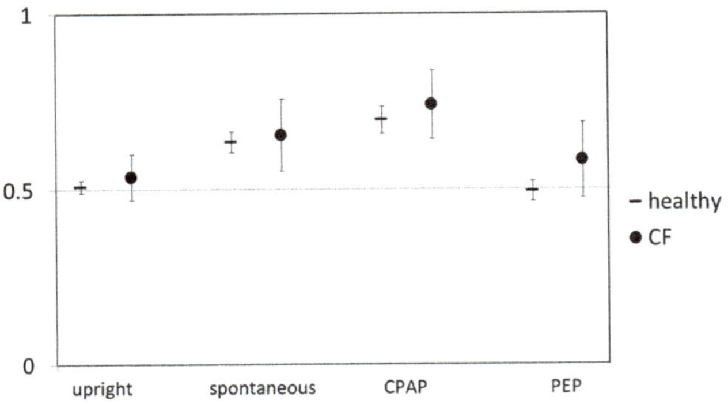

Figure 1. Spatial ventilation distribution with different breathing aids. Mean (95% CI) of the percentage of ventilation directed to the right lung in right lateral position for healthy and CF. For comparison spontaneous breathing in upright position is shown. Values >0.5 indicate more ventilation of the right lung, values <0.5 more ventilation of the left lung.

Discussion

Summary

In healthy adults and subjects with CF gravitational effects on spatial ventilation distribution in both right and left lateral position are enhanced by CPAP but neutralised by PEP. Spatial ventilation inhomogeneity is inversely related to temporal inhomogeneity.

Differences between breathing aids

It is well known that ventilation is increased in the dependent lung during spontaneous breathing and CPAP has been shown previously to enhance gravitational effects in healthy adults, but to our knowledge this is the first study investigating ventilation distribution during PEP therapy. [14] So far the differences between breathing aids have mainly been studied with respect to their clinical effects such as mucus clearance, improvement of gas exchange or improvement of spirometry [25–28].

In our study we compared two devices commonly used during RPT. It has been hypothesised that their effect on mucus clearance is caused by stabilising the airways and by enhancing gravitational effects on ventilation distribution [1,6,29] If it is accepted by the patient and if there are no unwanted side effects, gravity assisted positioning (without any device) as a possibility to enhance mucus clearance is recommended in patients with cystic fibrosis or non-cystic fibrosis-related bronchiectasis [30].

We demonstrated that the investigated devices had a different influence on ventilation distribution in the lateral position, with CPAP enhancing the effect of gravity on spatial distribution whereas PEP appeared to counteract it. Temporal distribution showed the opposite.

We can only speculate on the underlying mechanisms leading to the presented differences between CPAP and the PEP devices. In healthy lungs, the gravity-dependent strain on the independent parts of the lung will lead to a decrease in compliance, corresponding to a shift towards the right, flatter part of the pressure-volume curve. This decrease in compliance will tend to reduce ventilation in these parts of the lung. The application of continuous pressure during inspiration as well as expiration (CPAP) will lead to a further decrease in compliance of the independent parts of the lung and thus decreased local tidal volume. This effect has been described before. [14] As expected from the different breathing patterns used during these therapies end-expiratory level compared to spontaneous breathing was increased with CPAP and decreased with PEP, leading to different lung volumes at the beginning of inspiration. This will influence both spatial and temporal ventilation distribution as shown in healthy adults by Schnidrig et al. [11] With the combination of slightly reduced EEL (healthy −0.38; CF −0.31) and the significantly higher tidal volume (1.8 times normal in both groups) with PEP compared to spontaneous breathing we would expect a shift of ventilation to the right lung in right lateral position. This is not the case in both groups so our results cannot be explained by the change in breathing pattern during PEP therapy alone. PEP is only active during expiration, possibly leading to a homogenisation of the compliance of the lungs at the end of expiration. Similar compliance of the lungs during inspiration will minimise

Table 1. Temporal ventilation distribution: Filling index of the right lung in different body positions.

	spontaneous	CPAP	PEP
upright healthy	0.97 (0.06)	0.96 (0.04)	0.95 (0.06)
		n.s.#	n.s.#
upright CF	0.96 (0.05)	0.95 (0.06)	0.96 (0.04)
		n.s.#	n.s.#
right lateral healthy	1.08 (0.03)	1.01 (0.01)	1.21 (0.11)
	p = 0.006*	p = 0.02*	p<0.001*
	[0.11 (0.07–0.15)]‡	[0.05 (0.03–0.07)]‡	[0.26 (0.19–0.33)]‡
		p = 0.008#	p<0.001#
right lateral CF	1.10 (0.17)	1.05 (0.10)	1.13 (0.24)
	p = 0.021*	p = 0.035*	p = 0.042*
	[0.14 (0.09–0.19)]‡	[0.10 (0.03–0.17)]‡	[0.17 (0.02–0.32)]‡
		n.s.#	n.s.#

Results are given as mean (standard deviation). An index >1 indicating a lag (slower filling than the rest of the lung) and an index <1 a lead (faster filling than the rest of the lung). Mean difference (95% confidence interval) to spontaneous breathing is noted in square brackets‡.
p-values provided for comparison with the upright position* and for comparison with spontaneous breathing within the respective body position#.
n.s. not significant; CF cystic fibrosis; CPAP continuous positive airway pressure; PEP positive end-expiratory pressure.

Table 2. Change in end-expiratory level (EEL) to spontaneous breathing in the corresponding body position expressed as percentage of the average tidal volume during spontaneous breathing in upright position.

	CPAP	PEP
upright healthy	+53 (38–68)%*	−59 (−40−−78)%*
upright CF	+66 (26–106)%	−43 (−10−−76)%
right lateral healthy	+41 (23–59)%*	−38 (−20−−56)%*
right lateral CF	+2 (−16–20)%	−0.31 (−67–5)%

Results are given as mean (95% confidence interval).
All RPT devices showed significant differences in EEL compared to spontaneous breathing in both body positions in healthy (*$p<0.001$) but not CF.
CF cystic fibrosis; CPAP continuous positive airway pressure; PEP positive end-expiratory pressure.

differences of tidal volumes directed to the dependent and independent parts of the lungs.

The much higher inter-subject variability in CF compared to healthy most likely reflects the differences in disease severity. The effect of different devices cannot be predicted by the diagnosis of CF and conventional lung function tests and EIT might help to further individualise RPT in CF.

Strength and weaknesses of the study

To our knowledge this is the first study assessing the influence of different breathing aids on gravity-dependent ventilation distribution in healthy adults and subjects with CF. All participants were familiar with the use of the different devices. EIT itself does not influence the breathing pattern unlike other lung function techniques which use special breathing manoeuvres. With the random order of application of devices/body positions and the consistency of the measured effects we can rule out long lasting effects of one specific device, body position or a potential effect of cardiac oscillations.

Nevertheless, our study has some limitations. First, as the duration of EIT measurements was fixed at 45 seconds for all subjects, the number of breaths analysed was variable. Given the statistical analysis used (intra-subject comparison) and the highly significant differences shown in all subjects this is unlikely to be of any importance. Multiple studies have been performed to evaluate the value of EIT in assessing regional differences of ventilation in animals, infants and adults. EIT has been validated against computer tomography, ventilation scintigraphy and positron emission tomography and a variety of EIT derived indices showed a very good reproducibility. [31–33] In our study we compared ventilation of the right and left lung, which might have led to a certain loss of spatial information. Nevertheless, we were able to show clear differences between breathing aids.

We only investigated young adults. Thus, any conclusions drawn from this study may not apply for elderly people or very young children. This needs to be investigated in different clearly specified disease groups especially since the devices are applied on sick and usually not on healthy lungs.

Pressures for CPAP and PEP were different in CF (10 mbar) and healthy (15 mbar) which might at least partly explain the slightly lower effect of PEP in CF. Nevertheless the distinct differences between devices remain visible even with lower pressures.

Finally, in the present study we did not directly measure tidal volume, which possibly may influence ventilation distribution. We estimated tidal volume using the EIT signal normalised for tidal volume during spontaneous breathing. In right lateral position where we found the biggest differences in spatial and temporal

Table 3. Change in tidal volume expressed as percentage of the average tidal volume during spontaneous breathing in the respective body position.

	CPAP	PEP
upright healthy	11 (−1–43)%	103 (50–156)%
	n.s.*	$p<0.001$*
		$p=0.004$#
upright CF	15 (−2–32)%	97 (51–143)%
	n.s.*	$p<0.001$*
		$p=0.007$#
right lateral healthy	37 (23–51)%	75 (25–125)%
	n.s.*	$p=0.025$
		n.s.#
right lateral CF	28 (−1–57)%	77 (19–135)%
	n.s.*	$p=0.029$*
		n.s.#

Results are given as mean difference (95% confidence interval).
p-values provided for comparison with spontaneous breathing* and for comparison of CPAP and PEP# in the respective body position.

ventilation distribution tidal volumes were only significantly different between spontaneous breathing and PEP.

Clinical relevance

Given the importance of physiotherapy in different pulmonary diseases and the frequent use of breathing aids, it is important to understand the mechanisms of this therapy. We have demonstrated that breathing aids have different effects on ventilation distribution with a very effect size, but the therapeutic effect remains unclear. Whether PEP or CPAP is better for individual subjects needs to be evaluated in an interventional study assessing clinically relevant endpoints. Based on our results one could speculate that for CF PEP combined with lateral position might be superior for mucus clearance and CPAP combined with lateral position might be superior to overcome atelectasis. Nevertheless, EIT might help to find the optimal breathing aid for each patient and to apply individualised, patient-tailored therapy.

Conclusion

Breathing aids show distinct differences in their effects on gravity-dependent ventilation distribution in healthy adults and CF. EIT might be used for individualised RPT in CF. In future studies individualised techniques need to be combined with measures of efficiency such as gas exchange, mucus clearance or other functional outcomes.

Author Contributions

Conceived and designed the experiments: MW LR TR. Performed the experiments: MW. Analyzed the data: MW LR TR. Contributed reagents/materials/analysis tools: TR. Contributed to the writing of the manuscript: MW LR TR.

References

1. Elkins MR, Jones A, van der Schans C (2006) Positive expiratory pressure physiotherapy for airway clearance in people with cystic fibrosis. Cochrane Database Syst Rev: CD003147.
2. Thomas J, Cook DJ, Brooks D (1995) Chest physical therapy management of patients with cystic fibrosis. A meta-analysis. Am J Respir Crit Care Med 151: 846–850.
3. Groth S, Stafanger G, Dirksen H, Andersen JB, Falk M, et al. (1985) Positive expiratory pressure (PEP-mask) physiotherapy improves ventilation and reduces volume of trapped gas in cystic fibrosis. Bull Eur Physiopathol Respir 21: 339–343.
4. Oberwaldner B, Evans JC, Zach MS (1986) Forced expirations against a variable resistance: a new chest physiotherapy method in cystic fibrosis. Pediatr Pulmonol 2: 358–367.
5. McIlwaine MP, Alarie N, Davidson GF, Lands LC, Ratjen F, et al. (2013) Long-term multicentre randomised controlled study of high frequency chest wall oscillation versus positive expiratory pressure mask in cystic fibrosis. Thorax 68: 746–751.
6. Reid WD, Chung F (2004) Clinical Management Notes and Case Histories in Cardiopulmonary Physical Therapy. Thorofare, NJ, USA: SLACK incorporated.
7. Frerichs I, Dudykevych T, Hinz J, Bodenstein M, Hahn G, et al. (2001) Gravity effects on regional lung ventilation determined by functional EIT during parabolic flights. J Appl Physiol 91: 39–50.
8. Tucker B, Jenkins S (1996) The effect of breathing exercises with body positioning on regional lung ventilation. Aust J Physiother 42: 219–227.
9. Tucker B, Jenkins S, Cheong D, Robinson P (1999) Effect of unilateral breathing exercises on regional lung ventilation. Nucl Med Commun 20: 815–821.
10. Crawford AB, Makowska M, Engel LA (1986) Effect of tidal volume on ventilation maldistribution. Respir Physiol 66: 11–25.
11. Schnidrig S, Casaulta C, Schibler A, Riedel T (2013) Influence of end-expiratory level and tidal volume on gravitational ventilation distribution during tidal breathing in healthy adults. Eur J Appl Physiol 113: 591–598.
12. Holland AE, Denehy L, Ntoumenopoulos G, Naughton MT, Wilson JW (2003) Non-invasive ventilation assists chest physiotherapy in adults with acute exacerbations of cystic fibrosis. Thorax 58: 880–884.
13. Placidi G, Cornacchia M, Polese G, Zanolla L, Assael BM, et al. (2006) Chest physiotherapy with positive airway pressure: a pilot study of short-term effects on sputum clearance in patients with cystic fibrosis and severe airway obstruction. Respir Care 51: 1145–1153.
14. Riedel T, Richards T, Schibler A (2005) The value of electrical impedance tomography in assessing the effect of body position and positive airway pressures on regional lung ventilation in spontaneously breathing subjects. Intensive Care Med 31: 1522–1528.
15. Frerichs I, Braun P, Dudykevych T, Hahn G, Genee D, et al. (2004) Distribution of ventilation in young and elderly adults determined by electrical impedance tomography. Respir Physiol Neurobiol 143: 63–75.
16. Davies H, Helms P, Gordon I (1992) Effect of posture on regional ventilation in children. Pediatr Pulmonol 12: 227–232.
17. Hurewitz AN, Susskind H, Harold WH (1985) Obesity alters regional ventilation in lateral decubitus position. J Appl Physiol 59: 774–783.
18. Frerichs I (2000) Electrical impedance tomography (EIT) in applications related to lung and ventilation: a review of experimental and clinical activities. Physiol Meas 21: R1–21.
19. Dunlop S, Hough J, Riedel T, Fraser JF, Dunster K, et al. (2006) Electrical impedance tomography in extremely prematurely born infants and during high frequency oscillatory ventilation analyzed in the frequency domain. Physiol Meas 27: 1151–1165.
20. Frerichs I, Dargaville PA, Dudykevych T, Rimensberger PC (2003) Electrical impedance tomography: a method for monitoring regional lung aeration and tidal volume distribution? Intensive Care Med 29: 2312–2316.
21. Riedel T, Kyburz M, Latzin P, Thamrin C, Frey U (2009) Regional and overall ventilation inhomogeneities in preterm and term-born infants. Intensive Care Med 35: 144–151.
22. Frerichs I, Hahn G, Schiffmann H, Berger C, Hellige G (1999) Monitoring regional lung ventilation by functional electrical impedance tomography during assisted ventilation. Ann N Y Acad Sci 873: 493–505.
23. Pulletz S, van Genderingen HR, Schmitz G, Zick G, Schadler D, et al. (2006) Comparison of different methods to define regions of interest for evaluation of regional lung ventilation by EIT. Physiol Meas 27: S115–127.
24. Grant CA, Fraser JF, Dunster KR, Schibler A (2009) The assessment of regional lung mechanics with electrical impedance tomography: a pilot study during recruitment manoeuvres. Intensive Care Med 35: 166–170.
25. App EM, Kieselmann R, Reinhardt D, Lindemann H, Dasgupta B, et al. (1998) Sputum rheology changes in cystic fibrosis lung disease following two different types of physiotherapy: flutter vs autogenic drainage. Chest 114: 171–177.
26. Gondor M, Nixon PA, Mutich R, Rebovich P, Orenstein DM (1999) Comparison of Flutter device and chest physical therapy in the treatment of cystic fibrosis pulmonary exacerbation. Pediatr Pulmonol 28: 255–260.
27. Bellone A, Lascioli R, Raschi S, Guzzi L, Adone R (2000) Chest physical therapy in patients with acute exacerbation of chronic bronchitis: effectiveness of three methods. Arch Phys Med Rehabil 81: 558–560.
28. Thompson CS, Harrison S, Ashley J, Day K, Smith DL (2002) Randomised crossover study of the Flutter device and the active cycle of breathing technique in non-cystic fibrosis bronchiectasis. Thorax 57: 446–448.
29. Main E, Prasad A, Schans C (2005) Conventional chest physiotherapy compared to other airway clearance techniques for cystic fibrosis. Cochrane Database Syst Rev: CD002011.
30. Bott J, Blumenthal S, Buxton M, Ellum S, Falconer C, et al. (2009) Guidelines for the physiotherapy management of the adult, medical, spontaneously breathing patient. Thorax 64 Suppl 1: i1–51.
31. Victorino JA, Borges JB, Okamoto VN, Matos GF, Tucci MR, et al. (2004) Imbalances in regional lung ventilation: a validation study on electrical impedance tomography. Am J Respir Crit Care Med 169: 791–800.
32. Hinz J, Neumann P, Dudykevych T, Andersson LG, Wrigge H, et al. (2003) Regional ventilation by electrical impedance tomography: a comparison with ventilation scintigraphy in pigs. Chest 124: 314–322.
33. Richard JC, Pouzot C, Gros A, Tourevieille C, Lebars D, et al. (2009) Electrical impedance tomography compared to positron emission tomography for the measurement of regional lung ventilation: an experimental study. Crit Care 13: R82.

7

Plasma sCD14 as a Biomarker to Predict Pulmonary Exacerbations in Cystic Fibrosis

Bradley S. Quon[1,2]*, David A. Ngan[1], Pearce G. Wilcox[1,2], S. F. Paul Man[1,2], Don D. Sin[1,2]

1 Centre for Heart Lung Innovation, St. Paul's Hospital, University of British Columbia, Vancouver, British Columbia, Canada, **2** Division of Respiratory Medicine, St. Paul's Hospital, University of British Columbia, Vancouver, British Columbia, Canada

Abstract

Background: One in four cystic fibrosis (CF) patients diagnosed with a pulmonary exacerbation will not recover their baseline lung function despite standard treatment. This highlights the importance of preventing such events. Clinical decision-making can be improved through a simple blood test that predicts individuals at elevated short-term risk of an exacerbation.

Methods: We obtained plasma samples from 30 stable CF patients from the St. Paul's Hospital Adult CF Clinic (Vancouver, Canada). For 15 patients, an additional plasma sample was obtained during an exacerbation. Soluble CD14 (sCD14) and C-reactive protein (CRP) were quantified using ELISA kits. Myeloperoxidase (MPO), interleukin(IL)-6, IL-1β, monocyte chemoattractant protein-1 (MCP-1), vascular endothelial growth factor (VEGF), and granulocyte colony-stimulating factor (G-CSF) were quantified using Luminex™ immunoassays. Stable state biomarker levels were examined in their ability to predict individuals that would experience a pulmonary exacerbation requiring intravenous (IV) antibiotics within 4 months. Paired stable and exacerbation plasma biomarker levels were also compared.

Results: sCD14 levels were significantly higher in patients that experienced a pulmonary exacerbation requiring IV antibiotics within 4 months ($p = 0.001$). sCD14 cut-off value of 1450 ng/mL was associated with an area under the curve of 0.91 (95% CI 0.83–0.99) for predicting an exacerbation within 4 months of a stable visit, with a sensitivity of 100% and specificity of 82%. Plasma sCD14 levels were significantly higher during exacerbations than during periods of clinical stability ($p = 0.03$).

Conclusions: Plasma sCD14 is a promising biomarker for identifying CF patients who will exacerbate within 4 months of a stable visit but requires further study in larger, independent cohorts.

Editor: Dominik Hartl, University of Tübingen, Germany

Funding: This study was supported by a British Columbia Lung Association Grant-in-Aid (http://www.bc.lung.ca/association_and_services/research.html). The funders had no role in study design, data collection and analysis, decision to publish, or preparation of the manuscript.

Competing Interests: The authors have declared that no competing interests exist.

* E-mail: bradley.quon@hli.ubc.ca

Introduction

Cystic fibrosis (CF) pulmonary exacerbations are clinically important events for CF patients. They are associated with reduced quality of life and survival [1,2,3,4]. Despite aggressive treatment with intravenous (IV) antibiotics targeting airway infection, one in four CF patients diagnosed with an exacerbation will fail to regain their prior baseline lung function post-treatment [5]. This suggests exacerbations may lead to irreversible lung damage, thus highlighting the importance of exacerbation prevention and early diagnosis.

Although CF pulmonary exacerbation definitions vary, they are characterized by a combination of changes in symptoms and lung function (e.g. FEV1% predicted) necessitating an augmentation in treatment [6]. However, because these changes occur downstream from the underlying pathogenic processes, there is invariably a delay of several days (if not weeks) between onset of the exacerbation and diagnosis and treatment of these events. This delay contributes to incomplete recovery of patients' health status and lung function. To prevent these delays, however, clinicians would require a highly sensitive and specific (and inexpensive) test that can accurately risk-stratify these patients for imminent exacerbation even when their symptoms and lung function are stable. Exacerbation outcomes can potentially be improved by identifying patients that are at elevated short-term risk of developing an exacerbation. Such individuals can be selectively targeted for initiation or intensification of maintenance therapies to prevent exacerbations. Exacerbations can potentially be prevented with medications such as mucolytic agents and inhaled antibiotics [7]. These individuals can also be monitored more closely, which may lead to earlier exacerbation detection and treatment. Biomarkers reflective of systemic inflammation have demonstrated promise in monitoring CF lung disease activity, even when patient symptoms are stable [8]. Systemic inflammatory changes likely occur upstream from changes in clinical parameters and thus may enhance exacerbation risk-stratification.

The objectives of this study were to identify systemic inflammatory biomarkers that can be used to: 1) predict CF individuals that are at elevated risk of developing an exacerbation within 4 months of a stable visit; and 2) discriminate between CF individuals that are clinically stable vs. those experiencing an exacerbation.

Methods

Study Population

We enrolled 64 adult patients from the Adult Cystic Fibrosis (CF) Clinic at St. Paul's Hospital (Vancouver, British Columbia, Canada) between April 2009 and June 2010 who were clinically stable at the time of baseline assessment. We included patients with two disease-causing CF transmembrane conductance regulator (CFTR) mutations and at least two sweat chloride measurements of greater than 60 mmol/L. Patients who had experienced an exacerbation within 4 weeks of the initial stable visit or had previously undergone a solid organ transplant were excluded. Patients were not required to have a prior history of exacerbations. Written informed consent was obtained from the research subjects and the University of British Columbia – Providence Health Care Research Ethics Board (UBC-PHC REB) approved the study protocol and consent procedure.

Blood Collection

Venous blood samples were collected in clinic, processed for plasma, and stored at −80°C until thawing for batched analysis. Blood was collected during the initial stable assessment and longitudinally during subsequent stable or exacerbation clinic visits up to August 2010. If an enrolled patient missed a clinic appointment, they were not approached outside of clinic to obtain blood samples. Blood samples were classified as being from a stable clinic visit if the subject did not have a significant change in symptoms warranting escalation in therapy within 4 weeks of the blood draw. Blood samples were classified as being from an exacerbation clinic visit if the subject had the need for additional antibiotic treatment (oral or intravenous) as indicated by a recent change in at least two of the following: change in sputum volume or colour, increased cough, increased malaise, fatigue or lethargy, anorexia or weight loss, increased dyspnea, decrease in pulmonary function by 10% or more, radiographic changes [6,9]. Blood was not collected if the patient was already started on antibiotics prior to the exacerbation clinic visit. CF physicians were not blinded to study participation but were blinded to the blood biomarker results, which were performed several months following the clinic visit.

Clinical Information

Spirometric data were obtained using standard techniques, in accordance with guidelines from the American Thoracic Society [10]. Demographic and other clinical data were extracted through chart review. Exacerbations during the follow-up period were ascertained through chart review (up to 2 years following enrollment) by study personnel blinded to the biomarker results. Because follow-up exacerbations were based on chart review, we could not reliably separate out the use of oral antibiotics for prophylaxis, or extra-pulmonary indications (e.g. sinusitis) versus those used for acute exacerbations. Thus, follow-up exacerbations were defined based on the need for intravenous antibiotic treatment as indicated by a recent change in at least two of the following: change in sputum volume or colour, increased cough, increased malaise, fatigue or lethargy, anorexia or weight loss, increased dyspnea, decrease in pulmonary function by 10% or more, radiographic changes [6,9]. Infection status was defined based on the sputum culture results reported at the time of the CF clinic encounter.

Samples Analyzed

A priori, we decided to analyze plasma samples from 30 out of 64 patients in this pilot study. We selected all 15 (out of 64) patients who had a paired sample collected during clinical stability followed by an exacerbation visit. We then randomly selected an additional 15 patients from the remaining 49 patients. All 15 patients had at least one initial stable sample and 10 of the 15 patients had 2 subsequent stable samples to allow for the analysis of variability in measurements over 3 consecutive stable clinic visits (**Figure 1**).

Biomarker Assays

Circulating proteins from the following inflammatory pathways were selected based on review of the literature and the availability of reliable commercial immunoassays: 1) acute phase proteins; 2) pro-inflammatory cytokines; 3) markers of neutrophilic inflammation; and 4) markers of tissue injury/hypoxia. Acute phase proteins included C-reactive protein (CRP) and soluble cluster of differentiation 14 (sCD14), which were measured using enzyme-linked immunosorbent assay (ELISA) kits (R&D Systems, Minneapolis, MN) with a coefficient of variation of 2.8% and 3.1%, respectively. Cytokines involved in the early phase inflammatory response included interleukin-6 (IL-6), IL-1β, and monocyte chemoattractant protein-1 (MCP-1), which were quantified using high-sensitivity Luminex® bead-based multiplex assays (R&D Systems, Minneapolis, MN) with a coefficient of variation of 3.5%, 6.9%, and 3.3%, respectively. Markers of neutrophilic inflammation included granulocyte colony-stimulating factor (G-CSF) and myeloperoxidase (MPO), and a marker of tissue injury/hypoxia included vascular endothelial growth factor (VEGF). These markers were also quantified using high-sensitivity Luminex® bead-based multiplex assays (R&D Systems, Minneapolis, MN) with a coefficient of variation of 5.3%, 3.9%, and 5.7% respectively. All samples were measured in duplicate and by study personnel who were blinded to patient characteristics and to the study visit number. To mitigate batch effect, baseline and exacerbation paired samples were assayed on the same plates.

Statistical Analysis

Descriptive statistics were presented as medians/interquartile ranges or numbers/proportions. The relationship between stable visit biomarker level and FEV1% predicted was examined using Spearman's rank correlation coefficient. Variability in biomarker measurement, including FEV1% predicted, over three consecutive stable clinic visits was examined using a coefficient of variation (calculated as standard deviation divided by the mean).

Following log transformation to normalize the data, we used the two-group t-test to compare stable visit biomarker levels in patients who did vs. did not develop a pulmonary exacerbation requiring IV antibiotics within 4 months. For biomarkers that were significantly different between the two groups, we performed an area under receiver operating characteristic (ROC) curve analysis to evaluate various biomarker cut-off values to predict exacerbations requiring IV antibiotics within 4 months of the stable visit. We also conducted a post-hoc sub-group analysis to examine area under ROC curve stratified by *Pseudomonas* infection status (positive vs. negative) and median baseline lung function (below median FEV1% predicted vs. equal to or above median FEV1% predicted).

Lastly, biomarker levels when a patient was clinically stable vs. experiencing a pulmonary exacerbation were compared using a paired t-test, following log transformation to normalize the data if

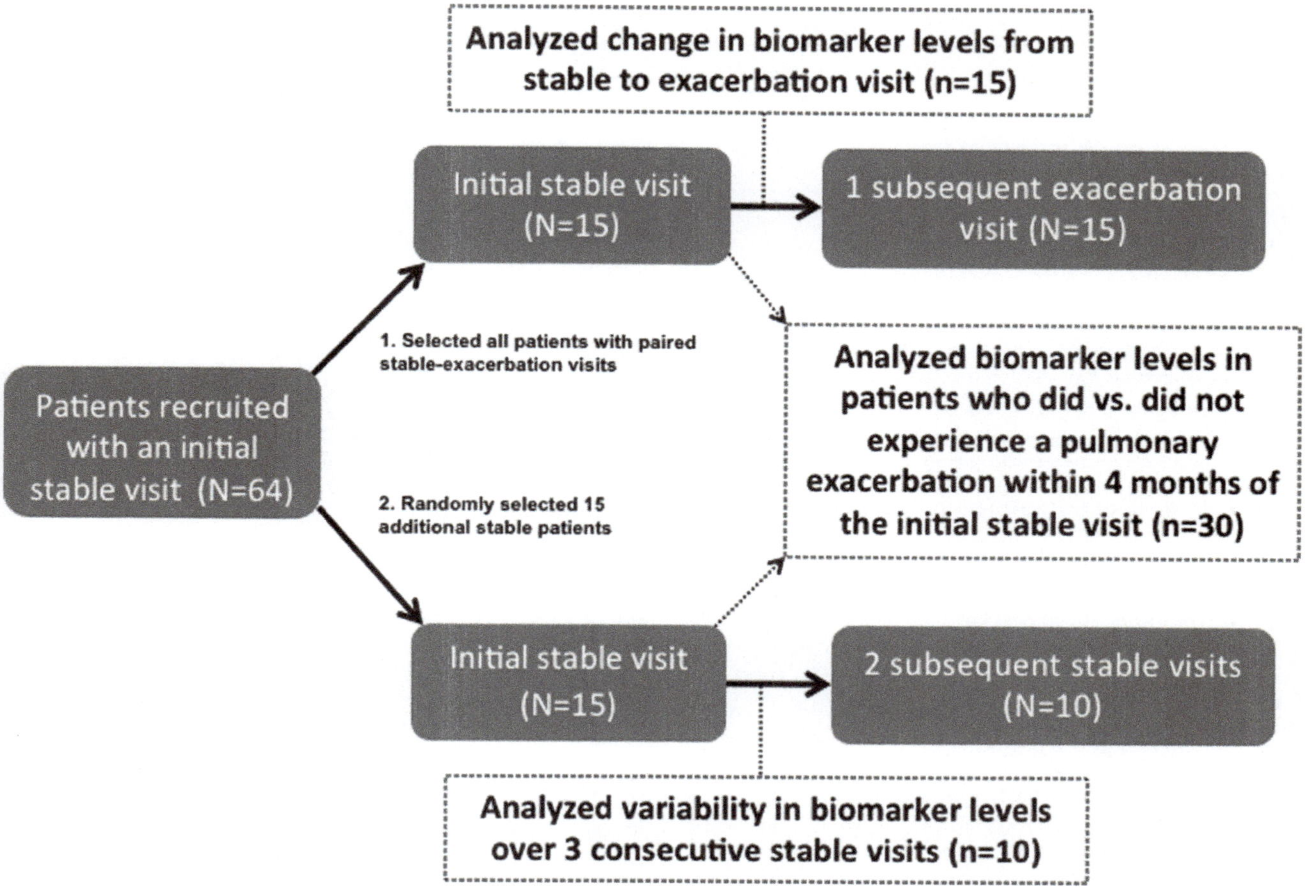

Figure 1. Blood collection schedule and analysis plan.

the paired differences were not normally distributed. P-values of less than 0.05 were considered statistically significant (two-tailed test). All analyses were conducted using STATA 12.1 (College Station, TX) and figures were created using GraphPad PRISM 6 (LaJolla, CA).

Results

Patient Demographics

The study population was generally representative of patients typically followed at an adult CF clinic with a few notable exceptions (**Table 1**). There was a slight over-representation of males and the prevalence of CF-related diabetes was lower than reported in the literature, as it was stringently defined based on the need for insulin therapy. Seven of 30 (23%) patients were diagnosed with an exacerbation requiring IV antibiotics in the year prior to enrolment.

Blood Biomarker Levels and Stable Lung Function

CRP and G-CSF levels inversely correlated with FEV1% predicted at the time of initial assessment, when the patients were deemed clinically stable (**Table 2**). There was also an inverse relationship between MPO level and FEV1% predicted, but did not reach statistical significance ($p = 0.09$). sCD14, IL-6, IL-1β, MCP-1, and VEGF levels were not related with lung function measurements during clinical stability.

Stable Visit Variability in Blood Biomarker Levels

Based on three consecutive stable visit measurements from 10 patients collected longitudinally over a median period of 9.2 (7.1 to 12.4) months, there was wide variability in levels (based on coefficient of variation) of most biomarkers except FEV1% predicted and sCD14 (**Table 3**).

Stable Visit Blood Biomarker Levels in Patients who did vs. did not have an Exacerbation Requiring IV Antibiotics within 4 Months

Eight out of 30 (27%) patients were diagnosed with a pulmonary exacerbation requiring IV antibiotics within 4 months of the stable visit. sCD14 levels measured at the time of stable assessment were significantly higher in patients who went on to develop a pulmonary exacerbation in 4 months, compared to those who did not ($p = 0.001$) (Figure 2). No other biomarker levels were significantly different in patients who did vs. did not exacerbate within 4 months of a stable blood draw (Table 4).

sCD14 Level and the Short-term Risk of Exacerbation Requiring IV Antibiotics

Various sCD14 cut-off values were examined and a cut-off value of 1450 ng/mL resulted in a maximum area under the ROC curve of 0.91 (95% CI 0.83–0.99) (**Figure 3**). This cut-off corresponded to a sensitivity of 100% (8 of 8 patients) and specificity of 82% (18 of 22 patients). In a post-hoc sub-group analysis comparing ROC curves according to baseline *Pseudomonas*

Table 1. Baseline patient characteristics.

Baseline Characteristic*	All Participants (N = 30)	Participants with paired stable-exacerbation visits (N = 15)	Participants with three consecutive stable visits (N = 10)
Age (years)	28 (20–37)	27 (21–33)	27 (22–34)
Male	19 (63%)	11 (73%)	5 (50%)
FEV1% predicted	68 (39–96)	66 (35–92)	78 (59–92)
BMI (kg/m²)	22 (20–26)	22 (21–23)	23 (22–24)
***Pseudomonas* culture (+)**	16 (53%)	10 (67%)	3 (30%)
CF-related diabetes (on insulin)	5 (17%)	1 (7%)	2 (20%)
Use of IV antibiotics in the prior year	7 (23%)	5 (33%)	2 (20%)
Number of exacerbations requiring IV antibiotics in the prior year	0 (0–0)	0 (0–1)	0 (0–0)

*Median (interquartile range) or Number (proportion).
Abbreviations: BMI = body mass index; FEV1 = forced expiratory volume in 1 second; IV = intravenous.

infection status (positive vs. negative) and lung disease severity (below vs. equal to or above median value of 75% predicted), the area under ROC curves were similar across all sub-groups (data not presented).

Paired Stable and Exacerbation Biomarker Measurements

Fifteen out of 30 (50%) patients had paired stable-exacerbation blood samples collected during consecutive CF clinic visits. The median time between paired samples was 3.0 (2.1 to 4.9) months. There was a significant decrease in the geometric mean FEV1% predicted from stable to exacerbation measurement (**Table 5**). Six out of fifteen (40%) exacerbations required treatment with IV antibiotics and the remainder were treated with oral antibiotics. Six out of fifteen (40%) patients had a new bacterium isolated from their exacerbation sputum culture relative to their stable sputum culture (3 *Haemophilus influenza*, 1 *Burkholderia cepacia complex* – genomovar multivorans, 1 *Streptococcus pneumonia*, and 1 *Acinetobacter baumanni*). sCD14 was the only biomarker that changed significantly from paired stable to exacerbation measurements ($p = 0.03$) (**Table 5**). There was a trend toward a significant increase of CRP, MCP-1, and MPO levels from stable to exacerbation measurements (all $p < 0.10$). Subgroup analyses based on potential predictors of more severe systemic inflammation at the time of exacerbation, such as the need for IV antibiotics and growth of new bacteria on sputum culture, did not significantly modify any of the results (data not presented).

Table 2. Correlation between blood biomarker levels and stable (baseline) lung function.

Biomarker	N	Rho (ρ)	P-value†
sCD14	30	−0.15	0.4
CRP	30	−0.42	0.02
IL-6	29*	0.16	0.4
IL-1β	23*	−0.27	0.2
MCP-1	30	0.11	0.6
G-CSF	30	−0.49	0.01
MPO	30	−0.31	0.09
VEGF	26*	0.26	0.2

*Missing individuals had undetectable levels.
†Spearman's rank correlation.
Abbreviations: sCD14 = soluble cluster of differentiation 14; CRP = C-reactive protein; IL = interleukin; MCP-1 = monocyte chemotattractant protein-1; G-CSF = granulocyte colony-stimulating factor; MPO = myeloperoxidase; VEGF = vascular endothelial growth factor.

Discussion

New biomarkers of CF lung disease activity are urgently required to enhance clinical decision-making and improve exacerbation outcomes. Given the adverse impact that exacerbation events have on CF patients, it is a priority to prevent them. A biomarker to identify individuals that are at elevated short-term risk of developing an exacerbation will allow for more selective targeting of preventive therapies (such as mucolytics and inhaled antibiotics) in those most likely to benefit. Discovery of a biomarker that reliably increases early in the course of an exacerbation is also desirable as it may lead to earlier detection

Table 3. Coefficient of variation for blood biomarker levels over 3 consecutive stable visits.

Biomarker	N	Coefficient of Variation†
FEV1 % Predicted	10	4
sCD14	10	7
CRP	10	44
IL-6	7*	43
IL-1β	4*	55
MCP-1	10	25
G-CSF	6*	27
MPO	10	26
VEGF	10	52

*Missing individuals had less than 3 measurements due to undetectable levels
†Standard deviation divided by mean
Abbreviations: sCD14 = soluble cluster of differentiation 14; CRP = C-reactive protein; IL = interleukin; MCP-1 = monocyte chemoattractant protein-1; G-CSF = granulocyte colony-stimulating factor; MPO = myeloperoxidase; VEGF = vascular endothelial growth factor

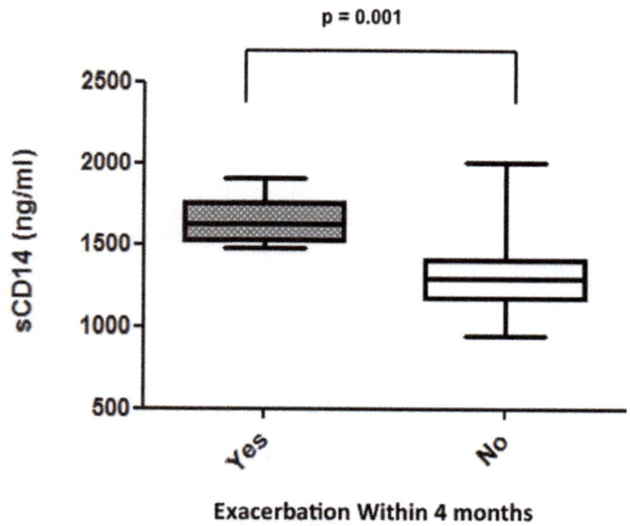

Figure 2. Boxplot of sCD14 levels in patients who did vs. did not experience a pulmonary exacerbation within 4 months.

Table 4. Comparison of blood biomarker levels in patients who did vs. did not experience a pulmonary exacerbation requiring IV antibiotics within 4 months of a stable blood collection.

	Exacerbation within 4 months*		
Biomarker	**Yes (n = 8)**	**No (n = 22)**	**P-value**†
sCD14 (ng/mL)	1645.7 (1.1)	1297.4 (1.2)	0.001
CRP (mg/L)	4.1 (5.3)	2.1 (3.5)	0.2
IL-6 (pg/mL)	2.1 (2.2)	2.8 (3.4)	0.5
IL-1β (pg/mL)	0.5 (2.0)	0.5 (1.8)	0.9
MCP-1 (pg/mL)	95.4 (1.2)	102.3 (1.5)	0.7
G-CSF (pg/mL)	53.0 (3.4)	22.1 (2.8)	0.1
MPO (ng/mL)	454.8 (1.6)	319.6 (1.8)	0.1
VEGF (pg/mL)	53.0 (3.4)	22.1 (2.3)	0.8

*Geometric mean (standard deviation)
†Two-group t-test
Abbreviations: sCD14 = soluble cluster of differentiation 14; CRP = C-reactive protein; IL = interleukin; MCP-1 = monocyte chemoattractant protein-1; G-CSF = granulocyte colony-stimulating factor; MPO = myeloperoxidase; VEGF = vascular endothelial growth factor

and treatment, prior to the establishment of irreversible lung damage.

In this study, we examined several biologically plausible biomarkers of disease activity that could be measured in the systemic circulation. Blood is an attractive biological compartment for biomarker measurement in CF as it can be obtained non-invasively in most clinical laboratories and has the potential for clinical application in patients of all ages and with all stages of lung disease severity. First, we examined whether stable visit biomarker levels were different in patients who were prone to experiencing an exacerbation requiring IV antibiotics within 4 months, compared to those who did not. sCD14 levels were significantly higher in patients who experienced an exacerbation in short-term follow-up. In identifying patients who do vs. do not exacerbate within 4 months of a stable clinic visit, test performance accuracy was optimized using a sCD14 cut-off value of 1450 ng/mL, with an area under ROC curve of 0.91 (95% CI 0.83–0.99). sCD14 possesses other desirable characteristics as a disease activity biomarker as it does not relate to underlying lung disease severity (i.e. FEV1% predicted) and exhibits minimal measurement variability over time when a patient is deemed clinically stable. sCD14 is biologically plausible as a biomarker of disease activity as it is involved in the innate immune response to infection and can mediate phagocytosis by binding to bacterial ligands, such as lipopolyassacharide (LPS), on the surface of gram-negative bacteria [11,12]. It is secreted in a protease-independent manner by monocytes and is cleaved from membrane-bound forms of CD14 on the surface of monocytes and macrophages by proteases such as neutrophil elastase [13]. It is also released as class 2 acute phase proteins from the liver (in response to IL-6), possibly bridging the gap between innate and adaptive immunity [14]. sCD14 has showed promise as a biomarker of pneumonia in children and sepsis in adults [13,15,16].

In our comparison of biomarker levels when a patient was clinically stable vs. experiencing a pulmonary exacerbation, the only biomarker (other than FEV1% predicted) that demonstrated significant change in paired analysis was sCD14. There was also a trend toward a significant increase in CRP, MCP-1, and MPO. For each biomarker, there was substantial overlap observed in stable and exacerbation biomarker levels between patients, which makes the establishment of an absolute cut-off for normal vs. abnormal highly unlikely, which may limit clinical application (**Figure 3**). Moreover, while most patients had an increase in sCD14, CRP, MCP-1 and MPO levels when transitioning from a stable to exacerbation health state, some individual patients had no change or even a slight decrease in biomarker levels (**Figure 4**).

There are several potential limitations to our study. First, this was a pilot study so we selected all 15 patients with paired stable-exacerbation visits and an additional 15 patients of those remaining at random. This aspect of our study design potentially limits the generalizability of our findings but unlikely introduced any systematic bias as this was defined *a priori*. For prediction of exacerbations within 4 months, such events were defined based on IV antibiotic requirement, which allowed for more reliable

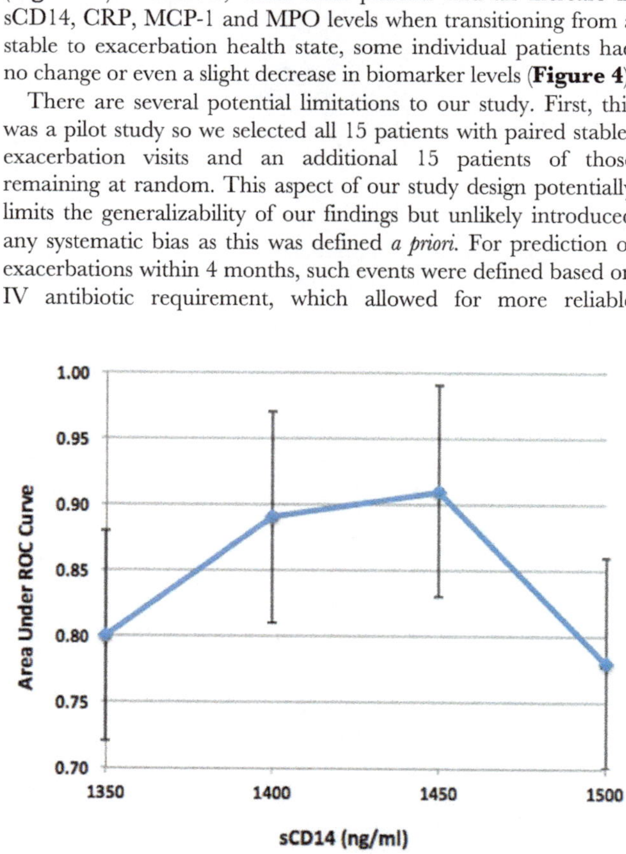

Figure 3. Defining an optimal sCD14 threshold value to predict pulmonary exacerbations requiring IV antibiotics within 4 months.

Table 5. Comparison of paired stable-exacerbation biomarker levels.

Biomarker	N	Stable*	Exacerbation*	P-value†
FEV1 % Predicted	15	64.3 (1.4)	54.6 (1.5)	0.0002
sCD14 (ng/mL)	15	1357.3 (1.2)	1475.0 (1.2)	0.03
CRP (mg/L)	15	4.1 (3.6)	6.7 (3.0)	0.09
IL-6 (pg/mL)	14**	2.2 (2.6)	3.7 (2.3)	0.2
IL-1β (pg/mL)	9**	0.7 (1.8)	0.9 (1.6)	0.8
MCP-1 (pg/mL)	15	95.8 (1.2)	111.7 (1.4)	0.06
G-CSF (pg/mL)	15	46.1 (2.9)	58.4 (3.1)	0.4
MPO (ng/mL)	15	383.2 (1.9)	478.9 (1.8)	0.08
VEGF (pg/mL)	15	10.2 (1.8)	10.0 (1.6)	0.8

*Geometric mean (standard deviation)
**Missing individuals had undetectable levels
†Paired t-test
Abbreviations: sCD14 = soluble cluster of differentiation 14; CRP = C-reactive protein; IL = interleukin; MCP-1 = monocyte chemoattractant protein-1; G-CSF = granulocyte colony-stimulating factor; MPO = myeloperoxidase; VEGF = vascular endothelial growth factor

identification of these events through chart review, as exacerbations requiring oral antibiotics are inconsistently documented in our clinic and are confounded by the fact that almost all patients in the clinic are prophylactically treated with oral macrolides (or a similar antibiotic for those intolerant to macrolides) for exacerbation prevention. This definition resulted in the selection of more severe exacerbations with the likely omission of milder events. Another potential limitation of this definition is that the decision to treat an exacerbation with IV (vs. oral) antibiotics may extend beyond severity of the attack and may relate to the discretion of the treating physician or the preference of the patient. Notwithstanding, it is clinically relevant to focus on the prediction of exacerbations requiring IV antibiotics as they have the greatest impact on patient quality of life and survival and thus should be prioritized for prevention [17,18].

In contrast to the prediction analysis, which exclusively relied on chart review for determining exacerbations, we prospectively collected exacerbation information for the paired analysis. Thus, we could reliably ascertain both mild exacerbations, requiring only oral antibiotics as well as more severe exacerbations requiring IV antibiotic therapy. Indeed, most of the exacerbations determined prospectively were mild events. The enrichment of mild events in the paired analysis may explain the lack of significant change observed in CRP and MPO levels from stable to exacerbation state, both of which have been shown to increase during

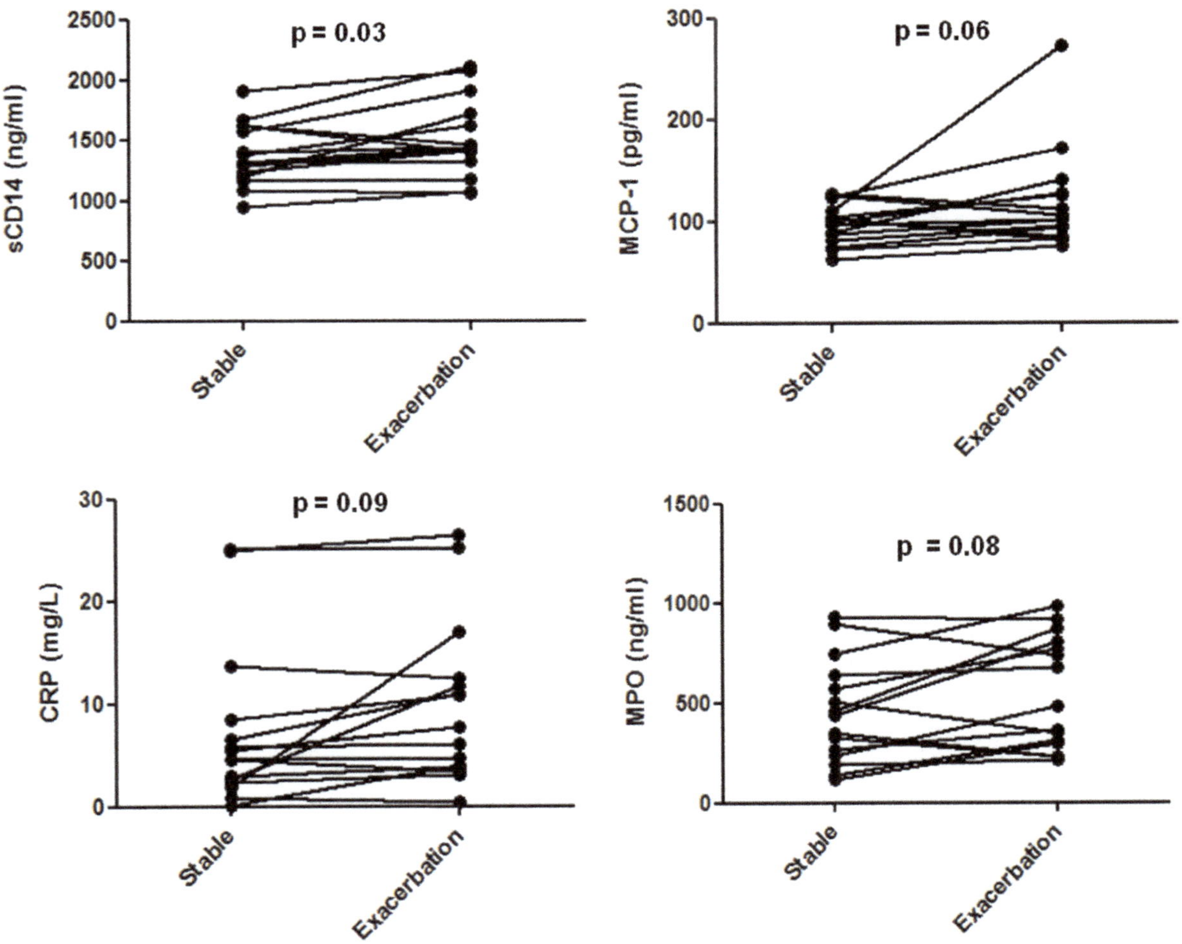

Figure 4. Paired stable-exacerbation biomarker levels for biomarkers with statistically significant (<0.05) or borderline significant change (p<0.10).

exacerbations in prior studies [8,19,20,21,22,23]. We chose four months as the exacerbation prediction interval of interest as most patients are followed-up routinely in the CF clinic every 3 to 4 months and therefore prediction of an event prior to the next clinic visit has the most clinical utility. In a sensitivity analysis, we did not observe a significant difference in the prediction accuracy of sCD14 if the prediction interval was changed to 3 or 6 months (data not presented). Due to our small sample size, we were limited in our ability to combine clinical variables and biomarkers into a multivariate prediction model. However, the high performance accuracy observed for sCD14 alone makes it unlikely that clinical variables would have further improved prognostic accuracy. The small sample size also precluded our ability to identify a high-risk subgroup that is more likely to benefit from blood biomarker analysis.

In conclusion, plasma sCD14 holds promise as a biomarker to identify individuals at elevated short-term risk of a pulmonary exacerbation requiring IV antibiotics but these results must be confirmed in a larger, independent cohort. No plasma biomarkers demonstrated sufficient discriminatory power for the detection of pulmonary exacerbations and therefore new biomarkers of disease activity must be discovered to enhance the early detection of exacerbations.

Author Contributions

Conceived and designed the experiments: BSQ SFPM DDS. Performed the experiments: BSQ DAN. Analyzed the data: BSQ DAN. Contributed reagents/materials/analysis tools: DDS. Wrote the paper: BSQ DAN PGW SFPM DDS.

References

1. Liou TG, Adler FR, Fitzsimmons SC, Cahill BC, Hibbs JR, et al. (2001) Predictive 5-year survivorship model of cystic fibrosis. American journal of epidemiology 153: 345–352.
2. Britto MT, Kotagal UR, Hornung RW, Atherton HD, Tsevat J, et al. (2002) Impact of recent pulmonary exacerbations on quality of life in patients with cystic fibrosis. Chest 121: 64–72.
3. Mayer-Hamblett N, Rosenfeld M, Emerson J, Goss CH, Aitken ML (2002) Developing cystic fibrosis lung transplant referral criteria using predictors of 2-year mortality. American journal of respiratory and critical care medicine 166: 1550–1555.
4. Yi MS, Tsevat J, Wilmott RW, Kotagal UR, Britto MT (2004) The impact of treatment of pulmonary exacerbations on the health-related quality of life of patients with cystic fibrosis: does hospitalization make a difference? The Journal of pediatrics 144: 711–718.
5. Sanders DB, Bittner RC, Rosenfeld M, Hoffman LR, Redding GJ, et al. (2010) Failure to recover to baseline pulmonary function after cystic fibrosis pulmonary exacerbation. American journal of respiratory and critical care medicine 182: 627–632.
6. Bilton D, Canny G, Conway S, Dumcius S, Hjelte L, et al. (2011) Pulmonary exacerbation: towards a definition for use in clinical trials. Report from the EuroCareCF Working Group on outcome parameters in clinical trials. Journal of cystic fibrosis: official journal of the European Cystic Fibrosis Society 10 Suppl 2: S79–81.
7. Flume PA, O'Sullivan BP, Robinson KA, Goss CH, Mogayzel PJ, Jr., et al. (2007) Cystic fibrosis pulmonary guidelines: chronic medications for maintenance of lung health. American journal of respiratory and critical care medicine 176: 957–969.
8. Hakimi Shoki A, Mayer-Hamblett N, Wilcox PG, Sin DD, Quon BS (2013) Systematic Review of Blood Biomarkers in Cystic Fibrosis Pulmonary Exacerbations. Chest.
9. Fuchs HJ, Borowitz DS, Christiansen DH, Morris EM, Nash ML, et al. (1994) Effect of aerosolized recombinant human DNase on exacerbations of respiratory symptoms and on pulmonary function in patients with cystic fibrosis. The Pulmozyme Study Group. The New England journal of medicine 331: 637–642.
10. (1987) Standardization of spirometry–1987 update. Statement of the American Thoracic Society. The American review of respiratory disease 136: 1285–1298.
11. Wright SD (1995) CD14 and innate recognition of bacteria. Journal of immunology 155: 6–8.
12. Wright SD, Ramos RA, Tobias PS, Ulevitch RJ, Mathison JC (1990) CD14, a receptor for complexes of lipopolysaccharide (LPS) and LPS binding protein. Science 249: 1431–1433.
13. Marcos V, Latzin P, Hector A, Sonanini S, Hoffmann F, et al. (2010) Expression, regulation and clinical significance of soluble and membrane CD14 receptors in pediatric inflammatory lung diseases. Respiratory research 11: 32.
14. Bas S, Gauthier BR, Spenato U, Stingelin S, Gabay C (2004) CD14 is an acute-phase protein. Journal of immunology 172: 4470–4479.
15. Landmann R, Zimmerli W, Sansano S, Link S, Hahn A, et al. (1995) Increased circulating soluble CD14 is associated with high mortality in gram-negative septic shock. The Journal of infectious diseases 171: 639–644.
16. Burgmann H, Winkler S, Locker GJ, Presterl E, Laczika K, et al. (1996) Increased serum concentration of soluble CD14 is a prognostic marker in gram-positive sepsis. Clinical immunology and immunopathology 80: 307–310.
17. Hegarty M, Macdonald J, Watter P, Wilson C (2009) Quality of life in young people with cystic fibrosis: effects of hospitalization, age and gender, and differences in parent/child perceptions. Child: care, health and development 35: 462–468.
18. Ellaffi M, Vinsonneau C, Coste J, Hubert D, Burgel PR, et al. (2005) One-year outcome after severe pulmonary exacerbation in adults with cystic fibrosis. American journal of respiratory and critical care medicine 171: 158–164.
19. Eichler I, Nilsson M, Rath R, Enander I, Venge P, et al. (1999) Human neutrophil lipocalin, a highly specific marker for acute exacerbation in cystic fibrosis. The European respiratory journal: official journal of the European Society for Clinical Respiratory Physiology 14: 1145–1149.
20. Rayner RJ, Wiseman MS, Cordon SM, Norman D, Hiller EJ, et al. (1991) Inflammatory markers in cystic fibrosis. Respiratory medicine 85: 139–145.
21. Hendry J, Elborn JS, Nixon L, Shale DJ, Webb AK (1999) Cystic fibrosis: inflammatory response to infection with Burkholderia cepacia and Pseudomonas aeruginosa. The European respiratory journal: official journal of the European Society for Clinical Respiratory Physiology 14: 435–438.
22. Roderfeld M, Rath T, Schulz R, Seeger W, Tschuschner A, et al. (2009) Serum matrix metalloproteinases in adult CF patients: Relation to pulmonary exacerbation. Journal of cystic fibrosis: official journal of the European Cystic Fibrosis Society 8: 338–347.
23. Davidson SJ, Paramothayan S, Hodson ME (2009) Adult cystic fibrosis patients with and without infective exacerbations and their factor XII levels. Blood coagulation & fibrinolysis: an international journal in haemostasis and thrombosis 20: 400–402.

8

Characterization of Defects in Ion Transport and Tissue Development in Cystic Fibrosis Transmembrane Conductance Regulator (CFTR)-Knockout Rats

Katherine L. Tuggle[1,2], Susan E. Birket[1,3], Xiaoxia Cui[4], Jeong Hong[1,5], Joe Warren[4], Lara Reid[4], Andre Chambers[4], Diana Ji[4], Kevin Gamber[4], Kengyeh K. Chu[6,7], Guillermo Tearney[6,8], Li Ping Tang[1], James A. Fortenberry[1], Ming Du[1,9], Joan M. Cadillac[9], David M. Bedwell[1,10], Steven M. Rowe[1,3], Eric J. Sorscher[1,3], Michelle V. Fanucchi[1,2]*

1 Gregory Fleming James Cystic Fibrosis Research Center, University of Alabama at Birmingham, Birmingham, Alabama, United States of America, **2** Department of Environmental Health Sciences, School of Public Health, University of Alabama at Birmingham, Birmingham, Alabama, United States of America, **3** Department of Medicine, University of Alabama at Birmingham, Birmingham, Alabama, United States of America, **4** SAGE Labs, Inc., St. Louis, Missouri, United States of America, **5** Department of Cell, Developmental, and Integrative Biology, University of Alabama at Birmingham, Birmingham, Alabama, United States of America, **6** Wellman Center for Photomedicine, Harvard Medical School, Massachusetts General Hospital, Boston, Massachusetts, United States of America, **7** Department of Dermatology, Massachusetts General Hospital, Boston, Massachusetts, United States of America, **8** Department of Pathology, Massachusetts General Hospital, Boston, Massachusetts, United States of America, **9** Animal Resources Program, Office of the Vice President for Research, University of Alabama at Birmingham, Birmingham, Alabama, United States of America, **10** Department of Microbiology, University of Alabama at Birmingham, Birmingham, Alabama, United States of America

Abstract

Animal models for cystic fibrosis (CF) have contributed significantly to our understanding of disease pathogenesis. Here we describe development and characterization of the first cystic fibrosis rat, in which the cystic fibrosis transmembrane conductance regulator gene (CFTR) was knocked out using a pair of zinc finger endonucleases (ZFN). The disrupted *Cftr* gene carries a 16 base pair deletion in exon 3, resulting in loss of CFTR protein expression. Breeding of heterozygous ($CFTR^{+/-}$) rats resulted in Mendelian distribution of wild-type, heterozygous, and homozygous ($CFTR^{-/-}$) pups. Nasal potential difference and transepithelial short circuit current measurements established a robust CF bioelectric phenotype, similar in many respects to that seen in CF patients. Young $CFTR^{-/-}$ rats exhibited histological abnormalities in the ileum and increased intracellular mucus in the proximal nasal septa. By six weeks of age, $CFTR^{-/-}$ males lacked the vas deferens bilaterally. Airway surface liquid and periciliary liquid depth were reduced, and submucosal gland size was abnormal in $CFTR^{-/-}$ animals. Use of ZFN based gene disruption successfully generated a CF animal model that recapitulates many aspects of human disease, and may be useful for modeling other CF genotypes, including CFTR processing defects, premature truncation alleles, and channel gating abnormalities.

Editor: Prosper N. Boyaka, The Ohio State University, United States of America

Funding: This work was supported by CF Foundation Grant R464-CR07 (www.cff.org) and NIH P30 DK072482 (www.nih.gov) to EJS and R01 HL116213 to SMR. The funders had no role in study design, data collection and analysis, decision to publish, or preparation of the manuscript.

Competing Interests: The authors have read the journal's policy and have the following conflicts: XC, JW, LR, AC, DJ and KG are full-time employees of SAGE Labs, Inc., which sells genetically engineered rats and provides custom model creation services. KKC, EJS, SMR, and GT have filed a patent application related to use of µOCT technology in airways. The application serial number is PCT/US12/52553, entitled "Method for functional investigation of respiratory airways and other ciliated tissues using µOCT," filed August 27, 2012. No financial benefit has yet been derived from this application by any author. SMR receives research support from the NIH, the Cystic Fibrosis Foundation (CFF), the American Lung Association, Synedgen Inc., and Forest Research Institute for basic and translational research. SMR also receives support from CFF Therapeutics (CFFT), Vertex Pharmaceuticals, PTC Therapeutics, N30 Therapeutics, and Novartis to conduct clinical trials related to the treatment and control of cystic fibrosis. SMR receives unrestricted research support for consulting services to Novartis, Kala Pharmaceuticals, Celtaxys Inc., and Bayer Healthcare. SMR receives no personal income from any of the sponsors noted above. GT receives research support from iLumen, Ninepoint Medical, Merck Research Laboratories, Canon, Samsung, and Air Liquide Medical Gases. GT. receives personal income from Ninepoint Medical, Terumo Corporation, and MIT through patent licensing arrangements. GT also receives consulting income from Samsung Advanced Institute of Technology and Ninepoint Medical. EJS receives research support from NIH, CFF, and CFFT. EJS serves as a scientific consultant to Genzyme, Pfizer, and Gilead. He receives consulting income from Gilead. KLT, SEB, JSH, LPT, JAF, MD, JMC, DMB, and MVF have no conflicts of interest to disclose.

* E-mail: fanucchi@uab.edu

Introduction

Cystic fibrosis (CF) is the most common lethal recessive genetic disorder among individuals of European descent, affecting 1 in every 2,500–3,500 newborns each year [1]. The disease is characterized by multi-system pathology, including respiratory complications, intestinal obstruction, exocrine pancreatic disease, hepatoductal blockage, and absence of the vas deferens [2]. The predominant cause of morbidity and mortality in CF results from chronic pulmonary infection and inflammation. CF is caused by mutations in the cystic fibrosis transmembrane conductance regulator (CFTR) gene, encoding an anion channel expressed in epithelial and other tissues.

A variety of CF mice have been generated since the discovery of *Cftr* in 1989 [3,4]. The mouse models, while presenting with CF-related intestinal disease, fail to recapitulate many other manifestations observed in patients. Nonetheless, CF mice have provided a valuable tool for testing pharmaceutical and other interventions, and investigating contributors to pathogenesis, including CF modifier genes [5]. Porcine [6] and ferret [7] CF models exhibit a respiratory phenotype closely resembling that observed in humans, although prolonged gestational period, time to sexual maturation, expense, and specialized care requirements have significantly limited their widespread use.

The development of a CF rat (*Rattus norvegicus*) would provide a number of advantages in comparison with available animal models of CF. First, the rat has a very short gestational period (21–23 days) and time to sexual maturity (8 weeks), allowing rapid colony propagation, breeding studies, and characterization of animals as they mature shortly after birth. Second, there is considerable interest regarding airway glandular function as a mediator of CF respiratory failure [8]. Airway submucosal glands are believed to underlie considerable pathology observed in human CF lungs. Rats are an attractive model in this context because, unlike mice but similar to humans, rats develop extensive submucosal glands throughout the trachea to the level of bronchi [9]. Third, relative to mice, rats are considerably larger in size, even during the early postnatal period, allowing for larger tissue samples to be collected from animals and ease performing surgical procedures [10]. Rats are also a traditional species for pharmacology and toxicology research due to their well-defined pharmacokinetic and biodistribution profiles [11,12]. Previous CF studies have sometimes required transgenic mice for efficacy, with safety studies conducted in rat; however, a CF rat model would facilitate pharmaceutical efficacy and safety studies of potential therapeutic molecules in the same species. Finally, because rats have been well studied in the laboratory for years, there is a large body of literature regarding normal physiology and a vast array of laboratory tools and reagents (i.e. antibodies, siRNA, other genomic probes) readily available for the study of chaperone, binding partner, and other protein based analyses relevant to disease mechanism that would be very difficult to obtain for ferret or pig.

Recent advances in gene manipulation techniques have provided a number of opportunities for developing genetically modified animals other than mouse. Zinc-finger endonuclease (ZFN) technology, for example, allows targeting of user-defined site-specific mutations that generate knockout animals with high efficiency and over a shorter time line than embryonic stem-cell targeting used in many species other than mouse [13,14]. Here, we describe the generation of a CFTR$^{-/-}$ rat by pronuclear microinjection of ZFNs and its characterization. The disease phenotypes observed in young (21–44 days postnatal) CFTR$^{-/-}$ animals, which closely resemble human manifestations, suggest the rat model will be useful for studies of CF pulmonary pathogenesis and drug development.

Materials and Methods

Ethics Statement

This study was carried out in compliance with the Guide for the Care and Use of Laboratory Animals of the National Institutes of Health. Protocols were approved by the SAGE Labs, Inc. or University of Alabama at Birmingham (UAB) Institutional Animal Care and Use Committee (IACUC; SAGE Approval Number 001.02, UAB Approval Number 09479). All surgeries were performed under sodium pentobarbital or ketamine/xylazine/acepromazine anesthesia with all efforts made to minimize animal suffering.

Generation of the Model

ZFN mRNA preparation. *Cftr* specific ZFNs were obtained from the CompoZr product line (Sigma, St. Louis, MO). mRNA was prepared from each construct, linearized with XhoI and modified using MessageMax and Poly(A) polymerase tailing kits (Epicentre Biotechnology). Samples were purified, quantified, and transfected at a 1:1 ratio into rat C6 cells for activity validation.

Animal husbandry. Derivation and breeding of animals was conducted at SAGE Labs (microinjection and founder identification/breeding) operated under approved animal protocols overseen by the SAGE IACUC. Sprague Dawley rats (Ntac:SD) from Taconic Farms (Hudson, New York) were used for microinjection. Animals were bred with housing in standard cages maintained on a 12 h light/dark cycle with *ad libitum* access to food and water. Routine health monitoring of the colony was performed at IDEXX (Columbia, MO) and indicated no evidence of infection with known serious pathogens.

Microinjection. Four to five week-old female donors were injected with 20 units of pregnant mare serum gonadotropin (PMS) followed by injection of 50 units hCG after an additional 48 h, and immediately mated with stud males. Fertilized eggs were harvested a day later. *Cftr* ZFN mRNA was microinjected at 10 ng/ml into the pronucleus of fertilized eggs. Following microinjection, 25–30 eggs were transferred into each pseudo-pregnant female, leading to birth of the founder generation.

Founder identification and breeding. Tail or toe biopsies were used for genomic DNA extraction and analysis as described previously [15]. Primers flanking the target site were forward 5′- AATATCTGGGTGGGCAGTTG and reverse 5′-TTGTTTGCAAGATTGCCCTT. Primers used to detect larger deletions were LD forward 5′-TACGCAATGCCAAGAAGTCA; LD reverse 5′-GAGGATGTTGGGAAGCTTTG. A founder was selected and bred with wild-type to obtain heterozygous animals, and sibling mating of heterozygotes resulted in homozygous SD-$CFTR^{tm1sage}$ rats (termed CFTR$^{-/-}$).

Characterization of the Model

Animals. All animal experiments at UAB were conducted in accordance with UAB IACUC approved protocols. Male and female Sprague-Dawley CFTR$^{+/-}$ rats were paired and housed in HEPA filtered ventilated cages with a 12 hour light/dark cycle and provided sterilized food and water *ad libitum*. Litters remained with lactating dams until weaning. Heterozygous rats were separated from wild-type and CFTR$^{-/-}$ littermates. Heterozygous animals exhibited growth and survival rates similar to wild-type, did not develop intestinal obstruction, and presented with normal dentition and complete male reproductive organs. In preliminary studies, CFTR heterozygotes also exhibited similar bioelectric and other characteristics to wild-type. In order to preclude any subtle confounding variables, CFTR+/− carriers were excluded from data analysis shown in this manuscript. Wild-type and CFTR$^{-/-}$ animals were provided water and standard rodent chow (pellet and ground) with a supplemental diet of DietGel 76A (Clear H_2O). A subset of wild-type and CFTR$^{-/-}$ pups were also provided 1× GoLytely (Braintree Laboratories, Inc) at weaning as a means to reduce gastrointestinal complications.

PCR genotyping. DNA analysis of litters was performed by extracting tail snip genomic DNA prepared in 500 μL lysis buffer (200 mM NaCl, 100 mM Tris-HCl, 5 mM EDTA, 0.25% Tween-20) with 1 mg Proteinase K (Sigma P6556) overnight at room temperature, followed by 60°C incubation to complete tissue lysis. DNA was obtained by standard techniques with 2-propanol, 70% ethanol, and DNA stored TE buffer (10 mM Tris-HCl, 1 mM EDTA) at −20°C. For PCR, 1 μL of DNA was mixed with 8 μL H_20, 10 μL JumpStart Taq ReadyMix (Sigma P2893), and 0.5 μL each primer (forward 5′-GCAGCTCACTGGTC-GATCTT, reverse 5′-GACACTATATTCACAAGGGAGAG). PCR conditions were 95°C for 5 minutes, followed by 35 cycles of 95°C for 30 seconds, 60°C for 30 seconds, and 68°C for 40 seconds, with a fixed cycle at 68°C for 5 minutes. This PCR resulted in amplification of a 172-bp DNA fragment for the wild-type *Cftr* allele and a 156-bp DNA fragment (16-bp deleted) for mutant *Cftr*. PCR products were resolved on a 3.5% agarose gel.

Western blotting. Lung tissue was homogenized in TBS on ice followed by lysis in RIPA buffer (ThermoScientific, Rockford, Il) with Halt protease inhibitor cocktail (ThermoScientific). Protein was quantitated using the BCA assay (ThermoScientific), samples mixed with 4× sample buffer, and incubated at 37°C for 10 minutes. Equal amounts of protein (20 μg) were loaded into each lane, resolved by SDS-PAGE, and blotted onto PVDF membranes. Wild-type Sprague-Dawley rat lung extract (Sc-2396, Santa Cruz Biotechnology, Inc, Dallas, Tx) was used as an additional positive control for CFTR detection. Blocking was with 1% rabbit serum followed by incubation with goat anti-CFTR primary antibody (1:200 Sc-8909) overnight at 4°C, and subsequent rabbit anti-goat HRP conjugated secondary antibody (1:5000 Sc-2768) for 1 hour at room temperature. Labeled proteins were detected using SuperSignal West Femto ECL kit (ThermoScientific).

Histology. Left lung lobes were cannulated and inflation fixed with 1% paraformaldehyde at 30 cm pressure for 30–60 minutes, followed by storage in 10% buffered formalin. Nasal tissue was collected, mandible removed, and nasal passages flushed retrograde with 10% buffered formalin followed by immersion in formalin until processed [16]. Nasal samples were decalcified for 4–5 days in Immunocal (Decal Chemical Corporation, Tallman, NY) solution, and rinsed thoroughly. The nasal cavity was sectioned into four regions at specific anatomic sites as described previously [17,18]. All other tissues were harvested, immersion fixed in 10% buffered formalin or 70% ethanol/formalin and stored at 4°C until processed. Tissues were embedded in paraffin, sectioned, and stained with hematoxylin and eosin (H&E) for evaluation by a board certified veterinary pathologist. Nasal, tracheal, lung, and intestinal tissues were stained with alcian blue periodic acid Schiff (AB-PAS) for identification of mucosubstances. Sections were imaged on an Olympus BX-41 microscope with a digital Q-color 5 camera (Olympus) using Q Capture imaging software (Q Imaging, Surrey, Canada) [19].

Quantitation of intracellular mucus in the nasal septa. The amount of stored mucosubstance in upper respiratory epithelium was estimated by quantifying the area of AB-PAS positive tissue per unit basement membrane. Septa from proximal nasal samples were evaluated at 20×, providing 4–6 fields (entire length of septa) per animal. Images were imported into ImageJ (NIH) and colors separated using the RGB stack feature. Using a green channel, areas of interest were outlined using the polygon tool and maximum threshold set for each image to include all stained intracellular mucus.

Morphometric analysis of tracheal tissue. Tracheas were imaged at 4× and 20× magnification followed by analysis with ImageJ (NIH) using protocols modified from Meyerholz *et al.* [20]. For each animal, three tracheal sections were studied (with a minimum distance of 15 μm between sections) using the following parameters. Lumenal circumference was determined by measuring the apical surface of the epithelium. Cartilage area was quantified by outlining cartilaginous tissue in the tracheal ring, measuring the area, and summing area for all cartilage in each image. Maximal cartilage thickness was evaluated by determining the perpendicular distance between outer boundaries of cartilage rings, with epithelial thickness represented by the distance between the basement membrane (on the serosal surface) and the apical membrane lumenally. Submucosal gland area was determined by circling and measuring both serous and mucus components of the gland structures. Submucosal gland intracellular mucus was assessed by outlining the entire submucosal gland area (same protocol as for quantitation of intracellular mucus in the nasal septa), in order to define the extent of intracellular mucosubstance. The percent of intracellular mucus was determined as the ratio of intracellular mucus/total submucosal gland area.

Bioelectric Measurements

Nasal potential difference. Rats were anesthetized with ketamine (200 mg/kg), acepromazine (0.6 mg/kg), and xylazine (30 mg/kg) by intraperitoneal injection. Potential difference was measured using AgCl electrode and electronic data capture (AD Instruments) as previously described for mouse and human [21,22]. Nasal cavities were perfused sequentially with 1) Ringer solution containing 140 mM NaCl, 5 mM KCl, 1 mM $MgCl_2$, 2 mM $CaCl_2$, 10 mM HEPES, and 100 μM amiloride (pH 7.3); 2) Cl^-free Ringer solution (6 mM Cl^-, pH 7.3) with amiloride; and 3) Cl^-free Ringer solution, amiloride, and forskolin (20 μM). Each condition was studied for 5 to 10 minutes until a stable signal was achieved. Traces were interpreted in a blinded fashion.

Tracheal short-circuit current (I_{SC}). Tracheas were excised, sectioned into 3–4 segments, and opened longitudinally along the dorsal surface. Segments were mounted as flat sheets in modified Ussing chambers (area ~0.031 cm^2) maintained at 37°C and bubbled vigorously with 95% O_2:5% CO_2.

I_{SC} measurements were performed under voltage clamp conductions using MC8 equipment and P2300 Ussing chambers (Physiologic Instruments, San Diego, CA). Tissue segments were equilibrated for 10 minutes in regular Ringer solution that contained (in mM) 120 NaCl, 25 $NaHCO_3$, 3.33 KH_2PO_4, 0.83 K_2HPO_4, 1.2 $CaCl_2$, 1.2 $MgCl_2$, and 10 mannitol to establish a baseline and then tested by one of the following experimental protocols:

1. Administration of amiloride (100 μM) to inhibit the epithelial sodium channel (ENaC), followed by sequential addition of forskolin (10 μM) to activate cAMP-dependent CFTR current, ATP (10 μM) to activate Ca^{2+}- activated chloride channel (CaCC) transport, and bumetanide (100 μM) to block transepithelial Cl^- transport.
2. Administration of $CFTR_{Inh}$-172 (10 μM) to block constitutively active CFTR dependent chloride current, followed by sequential addition of amiloride, ATP, and bumetanide as above.

Changes in I_{SC} attributable to ion transport agonists and inhibitors were calculated following achievement of a stable plateau for several minutes. ATP-sensitive I_{SC} was measured as the highest current value for each sample [21].

Ileal I_{SC} measurements. Tissue segments approximately 8 mm in length sectioned 5 cm above the cecum were stripped of the serosa (visceral peritoneum) and longitudinal/circular muscle layers of the intestinal wall, opened longitudinally along the mesenteric border, and incubated in TTX (Tetrodotoxin, 3.3×10^{-4} μM in PBS) for 10 min to block action potential dependent sodium channels. Segments were mounted as flat sheets onto sliders (area ~0.09 cm^2) and I_{SC} measured under voltage clamp conditions using MC8 equipment and P2300 Ussing chambers (Physiologic Instruments, San Diego, CA) as previously described [23]. Bath solutions were gently stirred and gassed with 95% O_2:5% CO_2.

Regular Ringer solution was utilized for monitoring I_{SC} as above. Low Cl^- Ringer contained (in mM) 1.2 NaCl, 25 $NaHCO_3$, 3.33 KH_2PO_4, 0.83 K_2HPO_4, 1.2 $CaCl_2$, 1.2 $MgCl_2$, 141 Na gluconate, and 10.8 mannitol. Sliders with mounted ileum were equilibrated for 10 minutes in Ringer solution followed by 10 minutes of recording; mucosal side chambers were changed to 1:1 regular Ringer:low Cl^- Ringer. Indomethacin (10 µm) was added to both chambers to block ion transport associated with phospholipase C or A2 activity induced by seromuscular stripping. After 30 minutes of incubation, forskolin (10 µm) and IBMX (3-Isobutyl-1-methylxanthine, 100 µm) were added to both chambers, followed by glybenclamide (200 µM) to block forskolin-activated CFTR short-circuit current.

In all experiments, fully stimulated current was obtained within 3 minutes of forskolin addition. Pulse during voltage clamp measurements was imposed every second after forskolin/IBMX stimulation, and every 20 seconds following other drug treatments.

Micro Optical Coherence Tomography (µOCT)

Tissue preparation. Tracheal tissue was excised, immediately placed on Gelfoam soaked in DMEM/F12 1: 1 media, and incubated under physiologic conditions (37°C, 5% CO_2, and 100% humidity) using an environmentally controlled chamber (Pathology Devices, Westminster, MD). Tracheas were equilibrated for 30 minutes before analysis.

Image acquisition. Measurements of functional microanatomic parameters in tracheal tissue, including measurement of (i) airway surface liquid (ASL) depth, the aqueous layer lining the airway epithelium, (ii) periciliary liquid (PCL) depth, the thin aqueous gel surrounding the cilia, (iii) ciliary beat frequency (CBF), and (iv) velocity of mucociliary transport (MCT) were performed using Micro-Optical Coherence Tomography (µOCT), a high-speed, high-resolution microscopic reflectance imaging modality [24]. µOCT methods for investigation of airway epithelia and quantitative image analysis have been previously described [24,25]. In brief, the µOCT instrument provides cross-sectional images of epithelium with a transverse and axial resolutions of approximately 2 µm and 1 µm, respectively. This resolution is sufficient to directly visualize and quantify parameters including ASL depth, PCL depth, CBF, and MCT rate without using exogenous dyes or particles. Acquisition speed is 20,480 Hz line rate, resulting in 40 frames per second at 512 lines per frame.

Image analysis. Quantitative analysis of ASL and PCL depths were characterized directly by geometric measurement of the respective layers, and images over several frames captured the length of fully extended cilia. CBF was investigated by Fourier analysis of the reflectance due to beating cilia. MCT rate was determined using time elapsed and distance traveled of native particulates in the mucus over multiple frames. Images were acquired at randomly chosen locations on the mucosal surface with the optical beam scanned along the longitudinal axis of the trachea.

Bronchoalveolar lavage fluid cell differentials. Tracheas were cannulated and lungs lavaged with 2.0 mL PBS (7.4 pH). Cells were collected by instilling 2.0 mL phosphate buffered saline (pH 7.2) and the lavage centrifuged onto slides (Cytospin). Slides were stained using Hema 3 stain kit (Fisher Scientific, Kalamazoo, MI) [26]. A minimum of 300 cells were counted per animal.

Complete Blood Counts (CBC) and serum chemistry. Blood (200–500 µL) was collected from the brachial artery into EDTA tubes and processed for CBC by ANATECH Diagnostics (Smyrna, GA). For serum chemistry, whole blood (300–500 µL) was processed in serum separator tubes and allowed to clot at room temperature for 1 hour. Supernatant was obtained by centrifugation at 10,000×*g* for 10 minutes, with serum placed in a fresh tube and frozen at −80°C. Samples were thawed and analyzed on an Abaxis VetScan using a Comprehensive Diagnostic Profile rotor (500–1038, Union City, CA).

Statistical analysis. Data are expressed as mean ± SEM or as individual data points. Statistical significance was determined using unpaired, two-tailed Student's t-test or one-way ANOVA using Prism (GraphPad, LaJolla, CA). For survival analysis, Kaplan-Meier survival curves were plotted and statistical significance determined using the logrank test for trend. P values ≤0.05 were considered significant.

Results

Microinjection and Founder Identification

A pair of ZFNs was confirmed to cleave the target site within exon 3 of *Cftr*, shown in Figure 1A. Following microinjection and embryo transfer, 44 pups were born to six recipients, 18 of which carried at least one mutant allele. The mutations ranged from 9 bp to hundreds of base pairs in length. Seven founders carried the same 9 bp deletion (Figure 1B), presumably due to microhomology within the target site, as discussed previously [15]. One founder was mosaic, harboring wild type *Cftr* allele, an allele with a 16 bp deletion and an allele with a 479 bp deletion. Larger deletions were observed to span the junction of exon 3/intron 3. Heterozygous rats with the 16 bp deletion (a frameshift in the reading frame leading to premature termination in exon 4) (Figure 1C), were used to establish a breeding colony.

Litter Demographics

Four breeding pairs of $CFTR^{+/-}$ rats gave rise to 332 pups from 30 litters with an average litter size of 11 pups. Litters were analyzed by PCR (Figure 2B) and found to have a genotype distribution of 27.1% wild-type, 49.4% heterozygous, and 23.5% $CFTR^{-/-}$, a result similar to the expected 1:2: 1 inheritance pattern. Western blot of whole lung homogenates from wild-type and $CFTR^{-/-}$ animals confirmed that the 16 bp deletion resulted

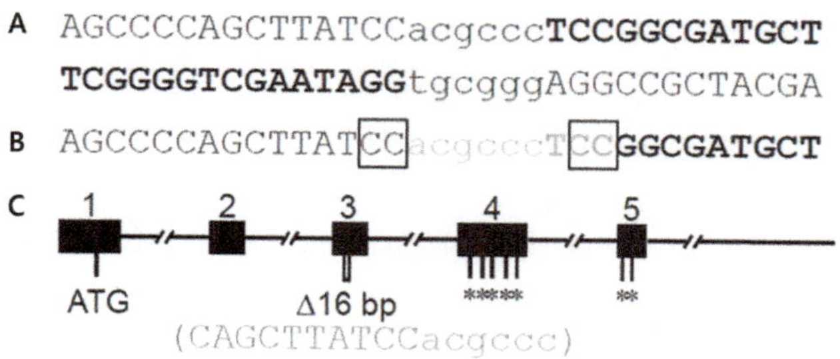

Figure 1. Targeting in exon 3 of *Cftr*. (A) ZFN recognition site sequence. The two ZFN binding sites are in bold uppercase. Cleavage site is in lower case. (B) Nine base pair deletion recovered in multiple founders. The deleted sequence is shown in gray. Microhomology that may have favored this deletion is marked in boxes. (C)Schematic of the gene structure of the first 5 exons of rat *Cftr*. Exons are shown by filled rectangles with exon number above. ATG, position of the translational start codon; Δ16 bp marks the position of 16 bp deletion, with nucleotide sequence below). *indicates premature stop mutations introduced by the 16 bp deletion in exon 3.

in loss of CFTR protein expression (Figure 2C and Figure S3). At birth, body weight and overall body size were similar between wild-type and CFTR$^{-/-}$ animals; however, begining in the second week following birth, CFTR$^{-/-}$ rats gained weight more slowly than wild-type littermates (Figure 2A, 2D). Survival of CFTR$^{-/-}$ rats was similar to wild-type until weaning, but was greatly reduced by 6 weeks (30% vs 99%, p≤0.05; Figure 2E). Mortality was associated with weight loss secondary to gastrointestinal complications (including obstruction, see also below). Addition of GoLytely to water resulted in significantly improved survival rates of CFTR$^{-/-}$ animals at 6 weeks of age (30% vs 64%, p≤0.05; Figure 2E).

Ileal Tissue

CFTR$^{-/-}$ rats developed intestinal obstruction after weaning and exhibited significant weight loss and decreased survival. Histological evaluation of small intestine demonstrated epithelial cell sloughing and crypts dilated with mucus, as well as a qualitative increase in bacterial load (Figure 3A). Ileal tissue was evaluated for CFTR short-circuit current phenotype by Ussing chamber measurements. Wild-type ileal tissue exhibited a strong forskolin-stimulated current (150±49 μA/cm^2), which was absent in CF rats (8±6 μA/cm^2, p<0.0001; Figures 3B, C).

Stored Mucosubstances in Airway Epithelium of the Proximal Septa

The respiratory epithelium of the nasal septum, immediately posterior to the upper incisors, was evaluated and labeled for intracellularly stored mucosubstance. Both wild-type and CFTR$^{-/-}$ animals had normally developed epithelium consisting of a pseudostratified columnar epithelium comprised of both goblet and ciliated epithelial cells. CFTR$^{-/-}$ animals had elevated levels of intracellular mucus that encompassed a significant portion of the airway epithelial cytosol (Figure 4A, Table 1), resulting in cells from CF animals appearing thicker and swollen ("stuffed") compared to wild-type.

Nasal Potential Difference Measurements

To characterize electrophysiology of the upper airway, trans-epithelial potential difference was monitored in response to a series of pharmacologic ion channel regulators. CFTR$^{-/-}$ rats had no evidence of Cl^- dependent secretion upon stimulation of CFTR mediated Cl^- transport by Cl^-free Ringer with forskolin (3.8±0.6 mV), whereas changes were robust in wild-type littermates (−9.3±2.7 mV, p≤0.01; Figure 4B, C). There were no differences between CF and non-CF following perfusion with amiloride. These measurements indicate a bioelectric phenotype consistent with absence of CFTR in the nasal airways, but without concomitant increase in amiloride sensitive voltage, the conventional ion transport pathway associated with sodium reabsorption.

Morphometric Analysis of Tracheal Rings

Tracheal morphology in young CF animals appeared grossly similar between wild-type and CFTR$^{-/-}$ genotypes (Figure 5); however, morphometric analysis revealed important differences attributable to absent CFTR (Table 1). While lumenal circumference was not significantly different between wild-type and CFTR$^{-/-}$ rats at 3–6 weeks after birth, cartilage area was significantly diminished in CF animals. CF rats also exhibited reduced tracheal gland area (~50% compared to wild-type) even after normalization for tracheal lumen circumference. Additionally, at all time points during the 3–6 week growth period, alcian blue positive (AB+) staining of submucosal glandular cells was

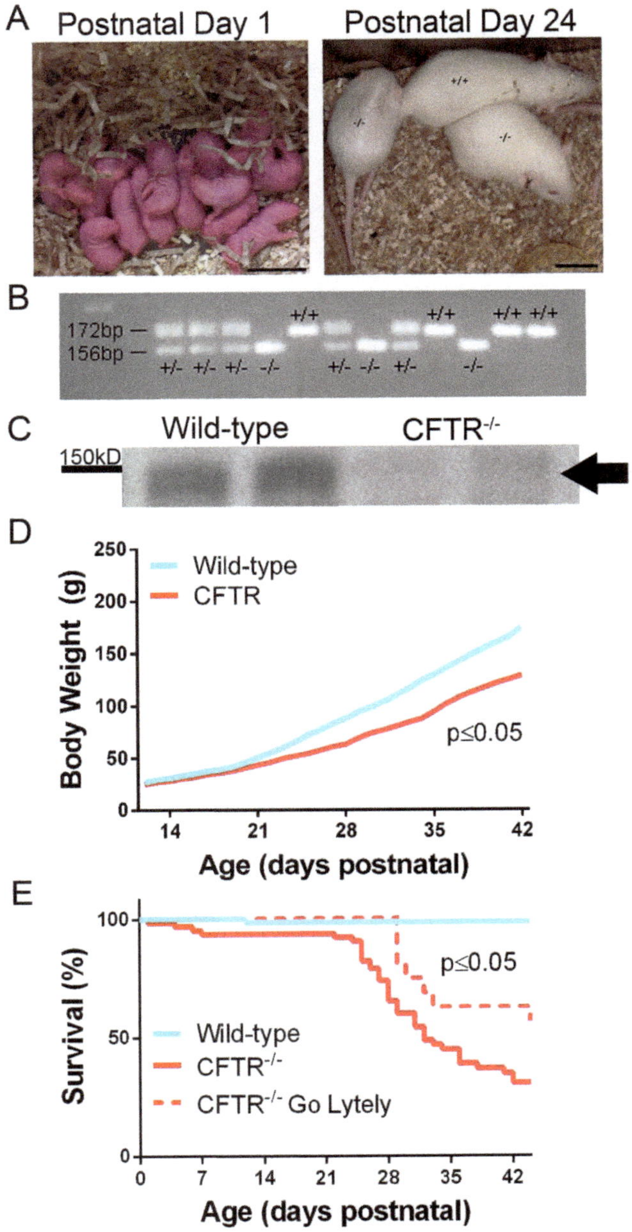

Figure 2. Generation of CFTR$^{-/-}$ rats. (A) Animals at days 1 and 24 postnatal. (B) Results of PCR genotyping from a representative litter. (C) Western blot indicating expression of CFTR in wild-type rats and absence of CFTR protein from lungs of CFTR$^{-/-}$ animals. Arrow - CFTR. (D) Body weight values (mean ± SD) from wild-type and CFTR$^{-/-}$ rats from 12 to 44 days postnatal. (E) Survival curve for CFTR$^{-/-}$ rats from postnatal day 1 to 44 (p<0.05 for all groups, n = 12–67 animals/group).

decreased in CF versus wild-type rats, suggesting that glandular maturation in the CF animals was delayed in comparison to age-matched controls.

Tracheal I_{SC} Measurements

Baseline I_{SC} of freshly excised trachea was significantly lower in CFTR$^{-/-}$ animals compared to wild-type (Figure 5B), a finding predominantly attributable to $CFTR_{Inh}$-172 sensitive current. To determine the contribution of Na^+ transport to basal currents,

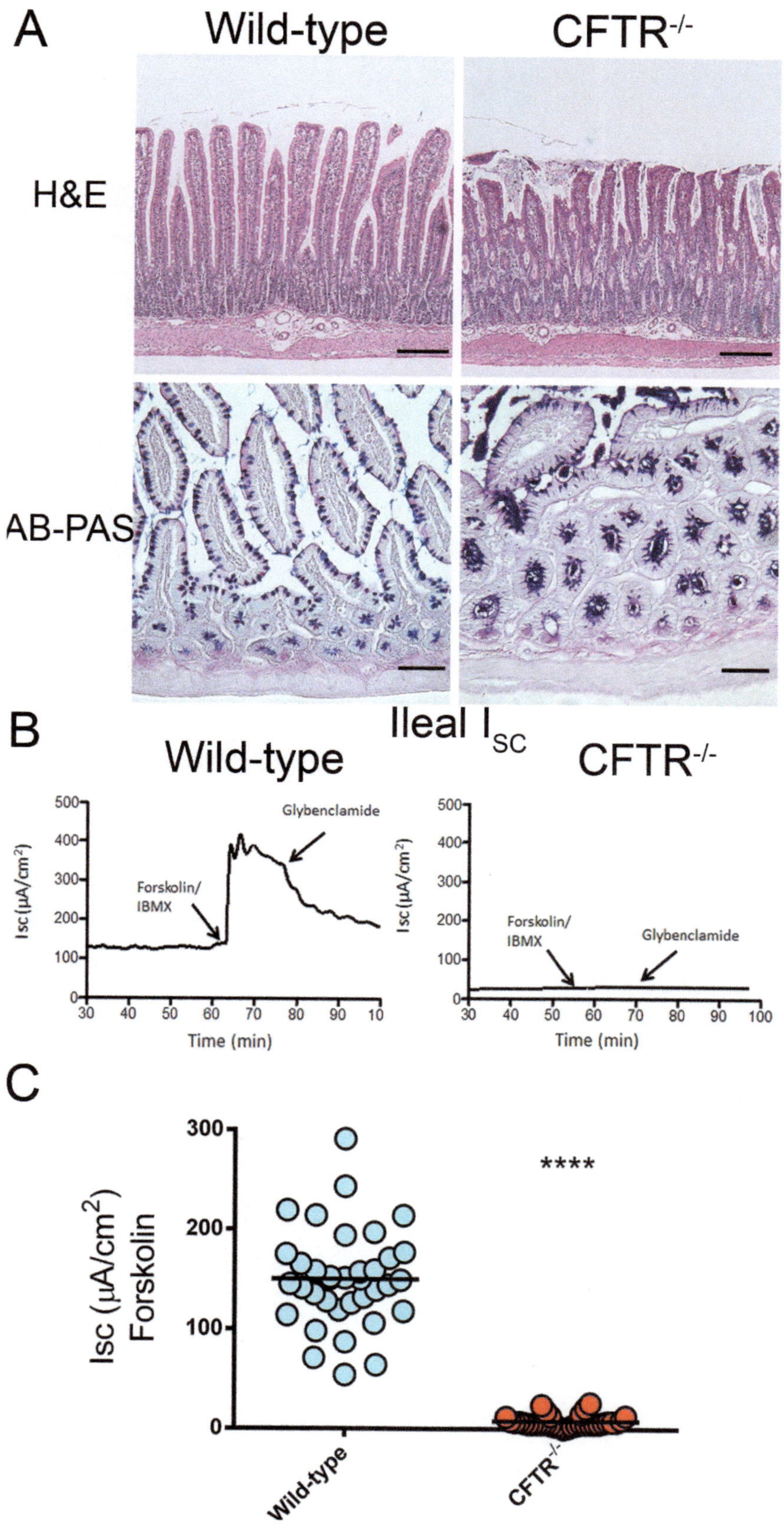

Figure 3. Histology and short-circuit current measurements from small intestines of wild-type and CFTR$^{-/-}$ rats. H&E (bar = 200 μm) and AB-PAS (bar = 100 μm) stained sections of the small intestines from wild-type and CFTR$^{-/-}$ rats. (n = 3–5 animals/group) (B) I_{SC} tracings from wild-type and CFTR$^{-/-}$ rat ileum. (C) Summary of forskolin stimulated current measurements from ileal sections. (n = 5 animals/group) ****$p \leq 0.0001$.

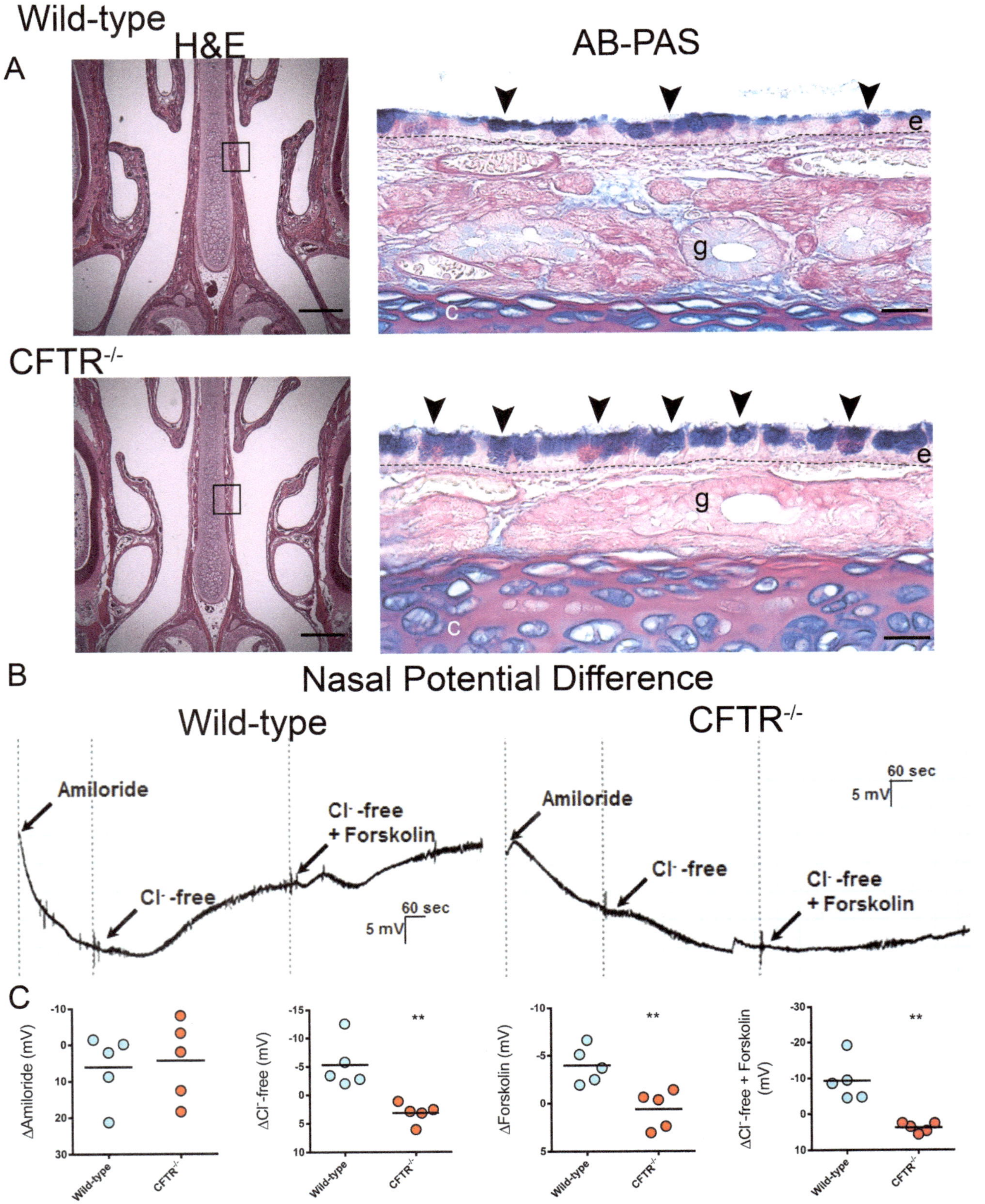

Figure 4. Proximal nasal histology and nasal potential difference measurements. (A) Low power magnification (4×) H&E stained sections from the proximal nasal passages bar = 500 μm. 20× images of ABPAS stained nasal septa from boxed areas bar = 25 μm. Arrowheads, cells swollen with intracellular mucus; e, respiratory epithelium; g, submucosal gland; dashed line (–), basement membrane (n = 4 animals/group) (B) NPD tracings from wild-type and $CFTR^{-/-}$ rats. (C) Summary data from NPD measurements for Δamiloride, ΔCl^--free Ringers, Δforksolin, and $\Delta Cl^{-/-}$free Ringers+ forskolin. (n = 5 animals/group) $^{**}p \leq 0.01$.

Table 1. Morphometric analysis of respiratory tissue from 3–6 week old wild-type and CFTR$^{-/-}$ rats.

	Wild-type	CFTR$^{-/-}$
Nasal Septa		
Intracellular mucus/basement membrane (μm²/μm)	3.5±0.9	7.5±0.9*
Trachea		
Lumen circumference (mm)	5.5±0.3	5.1±0.2
Cartilage area (mm²)	0.63±0.06	0.42±0.03**
Cartilage area/lumenal circumference (mm²/mm)	0.11±0.01	0.08±0.01*
Maximum cartilage thickness (mm)	0.20±0.01	0.17±0.01
Epithelial thickness (μm)	11.5±0.7	9.9±1.09
Submucosal gland area (mm²)	0.057±0.005	0.032±0.006*
Submucosal gland area/lumenal circumference (mm²/mm)	0.016±0.001	0.006±0.001*
Submucosal gland intracellular mucus (μm²)	7409±1481	2877±752*
% intracellular mucus	12±2	8.4±2

Values shown as mean ± SEM (n = 4–6 animals/group).
*p≤0.05, **p≤0.001 (Student's t-test).

amiloride was added apically (Figure 5B, left panel). The reduction in I_{SC} was similar for both wild-type and CFTR$^{-/-}$ rats (49±11 μA/cm^2 and 64±21 μA/cm^2, respectively; Figure 5C) indicating comparable levels of sodium transport irrespective of CFTR expression (Figure 5B, left panel; a finding similar to the nasal ion transport phenotype, Figure 4). Subsequent addition of forskolin did not confer substantial I_{SC} activation in either group, suggesting CFTR may be constitutively active in wild-type sections, diminishing the additional activation otherwise expected from forskolin. In contrast, ATP stimulated current was much greater for CFTR$^{-/-}$ animals (although maximal Cl^- currents for both genotypes were comparable and inhibited by addition of bumetanide), suggesting a compensatory increase of ATP-dependent Cl^- transport in the absence of functional CFTR, as also seen in humans [27]. To confirm that CFTR was constitutively active in wild-type animals, an alternative protocol was developed to test this interpretation (Figure 5B, right panel). Using the modified assay, wild-type rats demonstrated a baseline current of 547±102 μA, while current was far less (61±17 μA) in CFTR$^{-/-}$ animals. Addition of CFTR$_{Inh}$-172 reduced the current in wild-type by 304±63 μA, demonstrating high level basal CFTR activity, whereas CFTR$_{Inh}$-172 had minimal effect on constitutive current in CFTR$^{-/-}$ rats (9±7 μA, $p \le 0.001$). ATP sensitive currents were strongly inhibited by the addition of bumetanide.

Measurement of Functional Airway Microanatomy

We used μOCT to visualize and quantify the functional microanatomy of the airway surface (Figure 6). Excised tracheas from wild-type animals had significantly greater ASL depth compared to CFTR$^{-/-}$ rats ($p \le 0.05$; Figure 6). In addition, PCL thickness was reduced in CFTR$^{-/-}$ animals ($p \le 0.05$). Ciliary beat frequency and mucociliary transport were not different between wild-type and CFTR$^{-/-}$ groups.

CFTR$^{-/-}$ Male Rats Exhibit Bilateral Absence of the Vas Deferens

Evaluation of gross genitourinary anatomy revealed absence of the vas deferens in 6 week old CFTR$^{-/-}$ male rats (Figure 7). When sections from 6 month old males were evaluated histologically, only connective tissue and vasculature were observed with no evidence of the vas identified (data not shown).

CF rats have Abnormal Dentition

Incisors of wild-type rats presented with yellow-brown enamel while CFTR$^{-/-}$ rats exhibited white incisors (Figure 8A). Wild-type rats maintained normally filed teeth while CF animals exhibited grossly malformed dentition, possibly due to defective physiological trimming. Without intervention, incisors of CF rats developed dental malformations, including curvature of the incisors and penetration of the hard palate (Figure 8B).

Lung and Major Exocrine Tissues from CFTR$^{-/-}$ Rats are without Pathology or Inflammatory Cell Infiltrates During Early Life

Pulmonary sections from wild-type and CFTR$^{-/-}$ rats appear to develop normally from days 22 to 42 (Figure S1). In addition, BAL profiles were not different between genotypic groups, indicating the absence of overt pulmonary inflammation. Pancreas and liver from young animals were also histologically normal (Figure S2).

Hematology and Serum Chemistry

Hypoalbuminemia, decreased total protein, and increased blood urea nitrogen (Table S1) were observed in CFTR$^{-/-}$ rats. Because many animals experienced substantial weight loss prior to euthanasia, these findings may be attributable in part to malnourishment and poor hydration. Serum electrolytes (Ca^{2+}, Na^+, K^+) were not different between wild-type and CFTR$^{-/-}$ groups (Table S1). A trend towards increased blood glucose levels was observed in CF animals with very high values in a subset (data not shown) which is currently under investigation.

Red blood cells, hemoglobin, and hematocrit were all within normal range for young animals. Total white blood cell counts were not different between groups, although the differential was influenced by genotype (Wild-type: 21±4% neutrophils and 76±4% circulating lymphocytes, CFTR$^{-/-}$ animals: 52±5% neutrophils and 44±6% circulating lymphocytes), likely attributable to gastrointestinal or other stress-related complications observed in CFTR$^{-/-}$ animals.

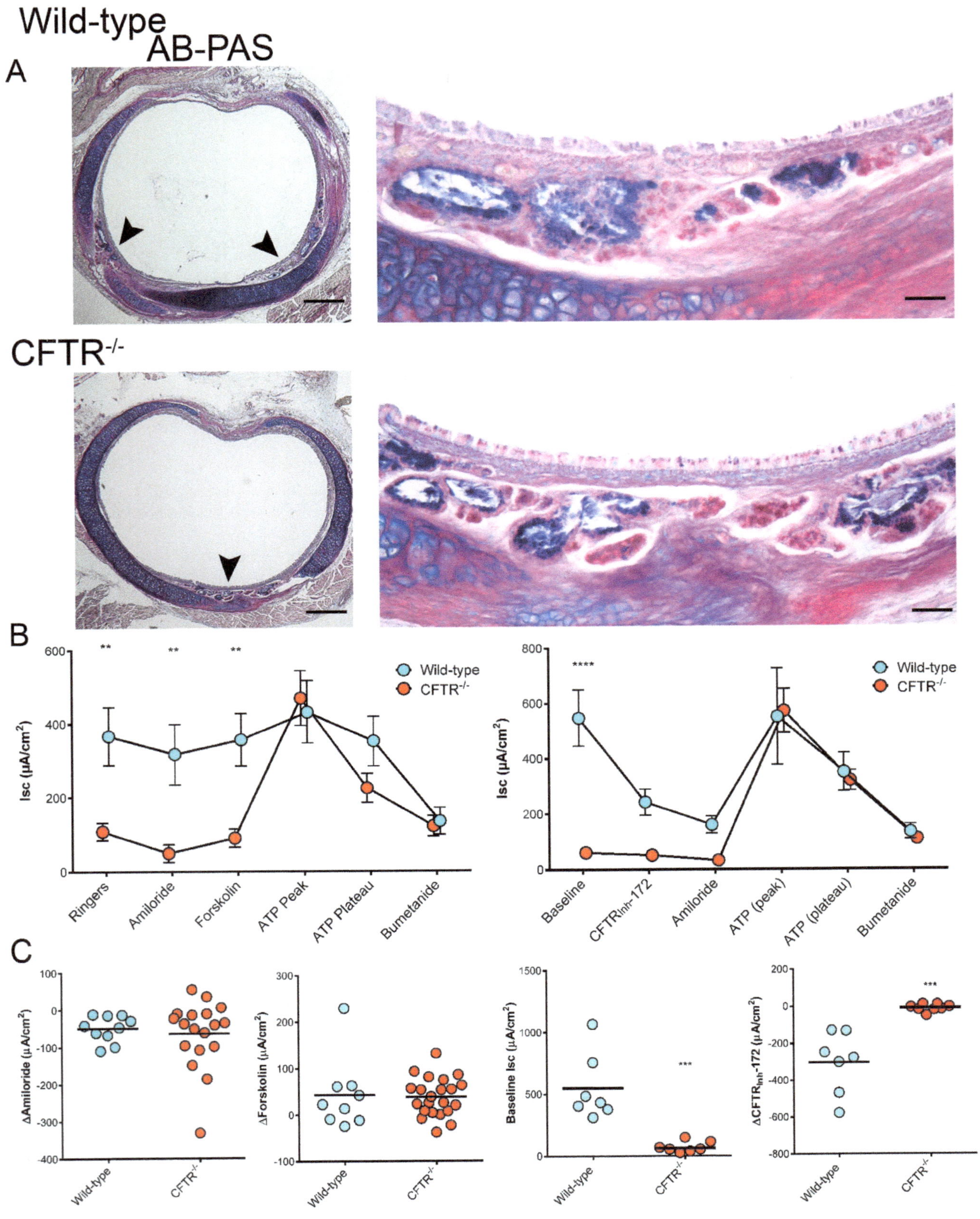

Figure 5. Tracheal histology and short circuit current measurements. (A) AB-PAS stained tracheal sections from 6 week old rats. Submucosal glandular tissue indicated by arrowheads. Low magnification bar = 500 μm, high magnification bar = 50 μm (B & C) Summary data from Ussing chamber short circuit current measurements. Panels on right depict a modified protocol designed to specifically detect baseline (constitutive) CFTR function. (n = 3–6 animals/group) $^{**}p \leq 0.01$, $^{***}p \leq 0.001$, $^{****}p \leq 0.0001$.

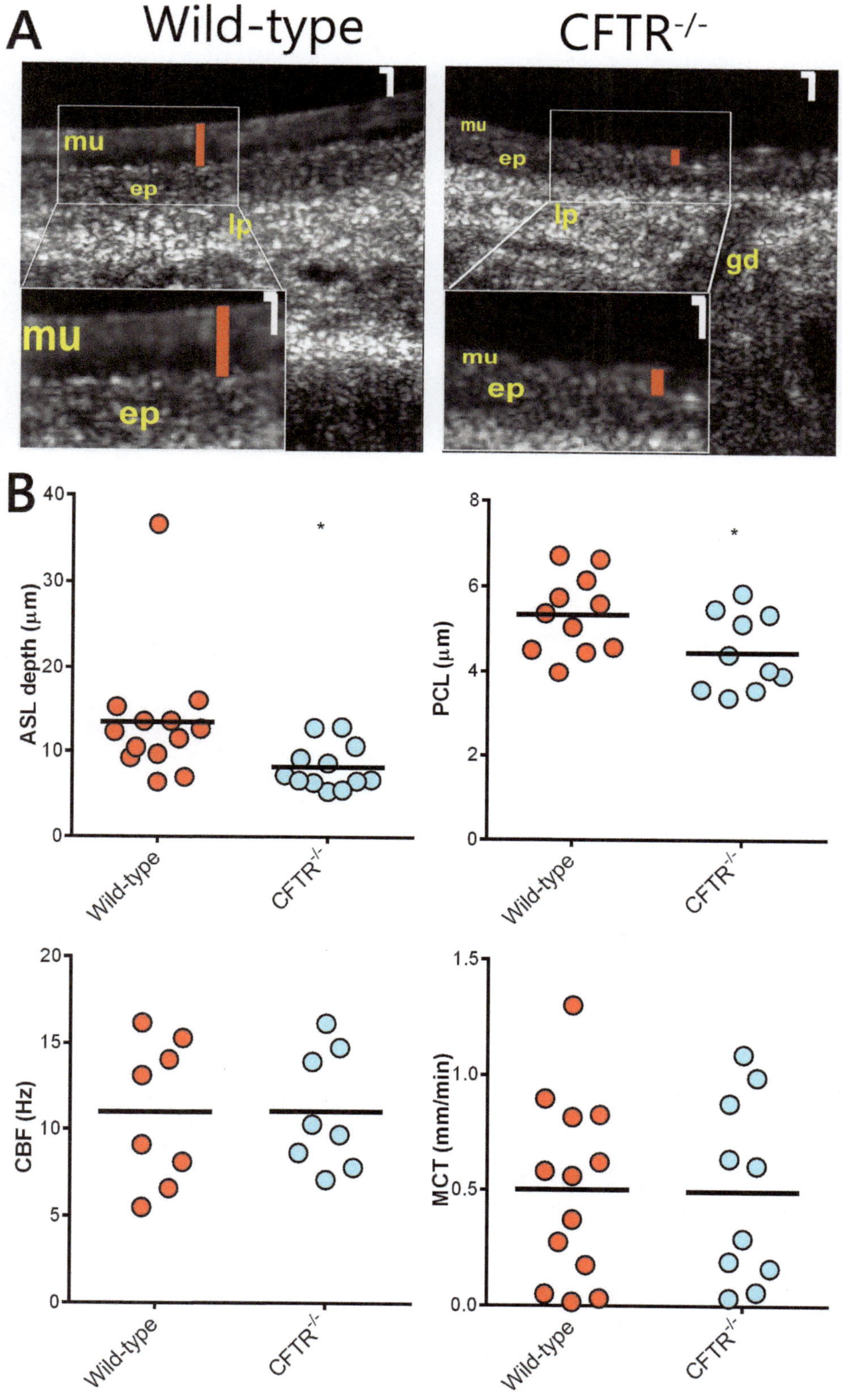

Figure 6. Functional anatomy of rat trachea. (A) Representative time-averaged µOCT images of wild-type and $CFTR^{-/-}$ tracheas. Higher magnification insets (bottom left corner) show differences in ASL height between wild-type and $CFTR^{-/-}$ animals. White magnification bar = 10 µm. Red bars indicate ASL height. Mucus layer (mu), epithelium (ep), lamina propria (lp), and gland duct (gd) are also visualized. (B) Summary data for airway surface liquid depth (ASL), periciliary liquid depth (PCL), ciliary beat frequency (CBF), and mucociliary transport (MCT). (n = 8–13 animals/group) $^{*}p \leq 0.05$.

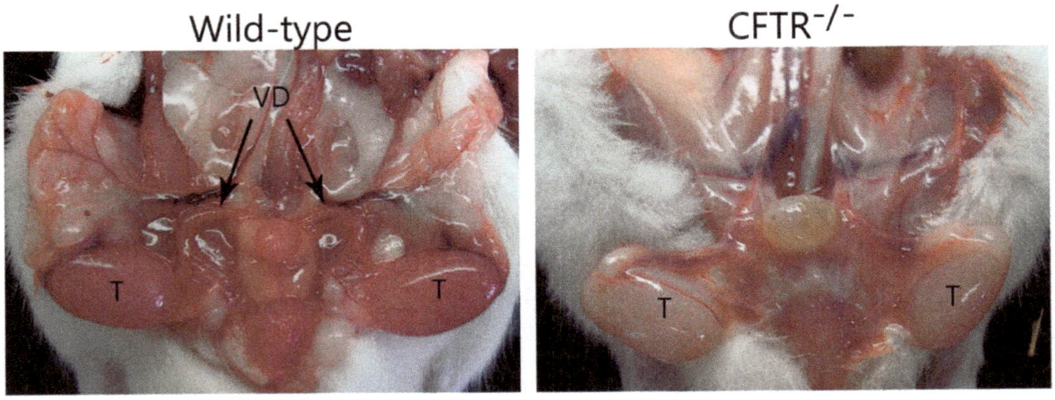

Figure 7. Male CFTR$^{-/-}$ rats have bilateral absence of the vas deferens by 6 weeks of age. Wild-type males (left) have an intact reproductive tract. CFTR$^{-/-}$ males (right) develop other reproductive organs, but exhibit absent vas at 6 weeks. T, testis; VD, vas deferens. (n = 3 animals/group).

Discussion

We present here a novel cystic fibrosis rat with a number of phenotypic characteristics that resemble the human disease. The CF rat furnishes a new opportunity to investigate (i) developmental processes that affect disease progression and severity, (ii) the impact of CFTR and other ion channels with regard to ASL depth in CF airways, (iii) contributions of ASL and PCL abnormalities to manifestations of CF respiratory pathology, and (iv) the role of CFTR in mucus synthesis and release.

Developmental defects attributable to absent CFTR have received considerable recent attention, including abnormal airway remodeling and tracheal formation [20], deficient levels of growth hormone [28], absent vas deferens [7,29], and problems with enamel deposition in teeth [30–33]. Similar to CF pig [20] and human subjects [20,34], we observed reduced tracheal circumference and a loss of submucosal gland area in the CF rat model (Figure 2), supporting the notion that CFTR may play a critical role during normal lung development [20]. The CF rat offers an ideal opportunity to monitor phenotypes such as these more longitudinally than has been practical in the past (e.g. from intrauterine tissue formation to adulthood).

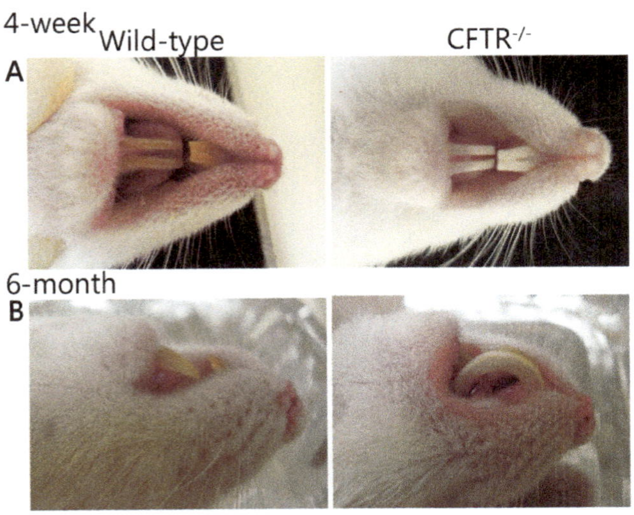

Figure 8. CF rats have abnormal dentition. (A) Wild-type rats (left) have yellowish-brown enamel while CFTR$^{-/-}$ rats (right) exhibit bright white incisors. (B) Incisors from CF rats exhibit uncontrolled growth and penetrate the hard palate. (n = 3 animals/group).

The rat model will also serve as a valuable resource for investigating developmental events that lead to abnormalities of the male reproductive tract. The majority (~99%) of men with CF are sterile due to degeneration or complete absence of the vas deferens [35]. In both the CF pig and ferret, the vas deferens is poorly formed or absent at birth [7,29]. The most commonly utilized CF animal model, the mouse, does not exhibit this feature. CF rats have lost the vas deferens by 6 weeks of age. The role of chloride secretion versus intracellular or other CFTR functions with regard to vas deferens involution are not well understood, but can be more readily characterized *in vitro* and *in vivo* using this new animal model. The rat may also facilitate experiments intended to determine the extent to which vas tissue destruction can be ameliorated by early (e.g. prenatal) therapeutic intervention.

Another area of increasing interest is the development of dental complications in CF subjects. Similar to observations in mice [33], CFTR$^{-/-}$ rats exhibit white incisors compared to yellow dentition of wild-type littermates (Figure 8A). Moreover, by three months of age CF rats demonstrate grossly malformed upper and lower incisors, characterized by curved dentition and penetration of the hard palate (Figure 8B). Additional studies are in progress to determine whether this phenotype is the result of (i) dysregulated growth and/or (ii) reduced wearing of the teeth, and the extent to which hypomineralization or other defects in enamel contribute to the findings [30,31,33,36]. Human data indicate that many CF patients have diminished mineralization of enamel [37–40] which may predispose to development of caries. The rat represents an ideal means of further investigating this feature of clinical CF.

The relationship of ASL depth to pathogenesis of cystic fibrosis lung disease has engendered considerable controversy. Previous studies have concluded that depleted ASL is primarily responsible for cystic fibrosis pulmonary damage, and associated with defects in ciliary extension [41]. The present results in CFTR$^{-/-}$ animals indicate ASL depletion in lower airways (Figure 6) that is qualitatively and quantitatively very similar to that noted in human subjects [42], but without evidence of overt respiratory pathology (Figure S1). Our findings establish that defective ASL hydration can occur for several weeks without resulting in manifestations of a CF pulmonary phenotype. While spontaneous lung disease is absent in very young CF rats, it is important to note that the animals described here have been housed in HEPA

Table 2. Summary of phenotypes across numerous CF species.

	Human	Mouse	Pig	Ferret	Rat
Increased Stored Nasal Mucus	NR	Yes [52]	Yes [51]	NR	Yes
Airway Surface Hydration	NR	Depleted [55]	Not Depleted [47]	NR	Depleted
Sodium Hyperabsorption	Yes [41,56], No [57]	Yes [58], No [59]	No [47]	No [48]	No
Hypoplastic Tracheal Submucosal Glands	Inconclusive [20,34]	NR	Hypoplastic at birth [20]	NR	Hypoplastic 21–42 DPN
Intestinal Obstruction	13–17% MI, 7–8% DIOS in childhood [60]	0–95% OB at weaning [4][a]	100% MI [61]	50–100% MI [7]	~70% OB between weaning and 42 DPN
Vas deferens	~99% CBAVD [35]	Normal	Degenerate or absent vas at birth [29]	Degenerate or absent vas at birth [7]	Vas absent before 42 DPN
Dentition	Abnormal [37–39]	Abnormal [33]	Abnormal [31]	NR	Abnormal

CBAVD – congenital bilateral absence of the vas deferens, DIOS – distal intestinal obstruction syndrome, DPN – Days postnatal, NR – Not reported, MI – meconium ileus, OB – Obstruction.
[a]Background strain and/or CFTR genotype dependent.

filtered ventilated cages. Future studies will determine whether older animals maintained under more natural housing conditions develop evidence of lower respiratory involvement. If such experiments fail to elicit a CF phenotype, the findings would indicate that defects in ASL and PCL hydration by themselves do not represent a proximate cause of CF pathology. The rat model will therefore furnish a valuable means to address unanswered questions regarding airway surface hydration and cystic fibrosis pathogenesis.

Decreased ASL depth has classically been attributed to Na^+ hyperabsorption as a consequence of absent CFTR [43–46]. Similar to what has recently been reported in CF pig [47] and ferret [48], the cystic fibrosis rat does not exhibit sodium hyperabsorption in either nasal or lower airways. Although amiloride-sensitive sodium transport is not significantly different between wild-type and $CFTR^{-/-}$ rats, ASL depth is markedly diminished (Figures 4 and 5). The abrogation of constitutively active CFTR fluid secretion may provide part of the explanation for ASL depletion in CF animals (as opposed normal levels of ASL observed in the CF porcine model) [47]. Our findings therefore suggest that CFTR (rather than ENaC) serves as the dominant regulator of ASL depth in the rat airway *in vivo*.

It has recently been argued that mucus in cystic fibrosis lungs is excessively viscous due to loss of CFTR dependent bicarbonate secretion, and that the newly formed mucus gel fails to properly expand [49]. We observed markedly increased mucus stores (i.e. cells appear 'stuffed' with mucins; Figure 4) in epithelial cells from the proximal nasal septa of CF compared to non-CF rats. Histological findings such as these are compatible with an intrinsic defect in mucus secretion/release [50]. CF pigs develop mucous cell hyperplasia [51] qualitatively similar to that observed in our young $CFTR^{-/-}$ animals, and CF mice have also been reported to exhibit a phenotype characterized by measurably increased numbers of mucous cells [52]. Based on findings shown in Figure 4 and Table 1, the rat model should be useful for investigating CFTR-dependent airway mucin synthesis, expansion, and release.

The generation of the first $CFTR^{-/-}$ rat using zinc finger nuclease technology suggests a clear path to other CF animal models with specific mutations relevant to therapeutic development, including animals that express F508del or CFTR premature truncations alleles. The advantages of a rat model for CF drug development include robust and multi-organ bioelectric and histological findings, ease of breeding, short gestation, manageable expense, availability of antibodies and other reagents for mechanistic studies, and standard use for pharmacokinetic and drug toxicity analysis.

In summary, the $CFTR^{-/-}$ rat exhibits many features of the CF phenotype found in human subjects and CF animal models (summarized in Table 2), including defects in airway mucus production (Figure 4), tracheal development (Table 1), airway surface and periciliary fluid depth (Figure 6), nasal mucus (Figure 4), dentition (Figure 8), and involution of the vas deferens (Figure 7). Bioelectric findings in rat are also informative and demonstrate significantly diminished periciliary fluid without evidence of ENaC hyperactivity. Moreover, unlike the CF ferret or pig, the $CFTR^{-/-}$ rat does not present with meconium ileus at birth. Only after weaning do large numbers of animals develop intestinal blockage, which appears similar to the distal intestinal obstruction syndrome observed in children and adults with cystic fibrosis [53]. Complications due to intestinal obstruction can be managed by use of dietary modification (Figure 2). The new CF rat model will provide a very useful resource for longitudinal studies of tissue development, electrophysiology, and other endpoints relevant to disease mechanism in the future.

Supporting Information

Figure S1 Analysis of lung tissue from CF rats. (A) Lung histology of wild-type and $CFTR^{-/-}$ animals. Magnification bar = 200 μm (n = 7–11 animals/group) (B) Total cell counts and cell differential of BAL in wild-type and CF rats (n = 4 animals/group).

Figure S2 Histology of pancreas and liver from CF rats. H&E stained paraffin sections of (A) pancreas and (B) liver from 22–44 day old wild-type and $CFTR^{-/-}$ rats. Magnification bar = 100 μm (n = 3–5 animals/group).

Figure S3 Expanded western blot (see Figure 2). Western indicating absence of CFTR protein from lungs of $CFTR^{-/-}$ animals and expression of CFTR in wild-type samples. Arrow - rat CFTR (~150 kD as previously reported [54]); *indicates likely CFTR degradation product commonly observed in CFTR preparations. This experiment has been repeated three times in separate animals with similar results.

Table S1 CBC and serum chemistry for wild-type and CFTR−/− rats.

Acknowledgments

We thank the UAB Comparative Pathology and CMBD Core Laboratories for processing samples. We also thank the UAB Animal Resource Program staff, who have assisted with breeding and rat husbandry. The authors also thank Dr. Trenton Schoeb for his review and analysis of tissue sections.

Author Contributions

Conceived and designed the experiments: KLT SEB XC DMB SMR EJS MVF. Performed the experiments: KLT SEB JH JW LR AC DJ LPT JF MD MVF. Analyzed the data: KLT SEB KKC GT MD DMB SMR EJS MVF. Contributed reagents/materials/analysis tools: KKC GT. Wrote the paper: KLT SEB XC MD EJS MVF. Coordinated Collaboration: KG. Provided veterinary care and assisted with animal husbandry: JMC.

References

1. Grosse SD, Boyle CA, Botkin JR, Comeau AM, Kharrazi M, et al. (2004) Newborn screening for cystic fibrosis: evaluation of benefits and risks and recommendations for state newborn screening programs. MMWR Recomm Rep 53: 1–36.
2. Derichs N (2013) Targeting a genetic defect: cystic fibrosis transmembrane conductance regulator modulators in cystic fibrosis. Eur Respir Rev 22: 58–65.
3. Riordan JR, Rommens JM, Kerem B, Alon N, Rozmahel R, et al. (1989) Identification of the cystic fibrosis gene: cloning and characterization of complementary DNA. Science 245: 1066–1073.
4. Guilbault C, Saeed Z, Downey GP, Radzioch D (2007) Cystic fibrosis mouse models. Am J Respir Cell Mol Biol 36: 1–7.
5. Carvalho-Oliveira I, Scholte BJ, Penque D (2007) What have we learned from mouse models for cystic fibrosis? Expert Rev Mol Diagn 7: 407–417.
6. Rogers CS, Hao Y, Rokhlina T, Samuel M, Stoltz DA, et al. (2008) Production of CFTR-null and CFTR-DeltaF508 heterozygous pigs by adeno-associated virus-mediated gene targeting and somatic cell nuclear transfer. J Clin Invest 118: 1571–1577.
7. Sun X, Sui H, Fisher JT, Yan Z, Liu X, et al. (2010) Disease phenotype of a ferret CFTR-knockout model of cystic fibrosis. J Clin Invest 120: 3149–3160.
8. Pilewski JM, Frizzell RA (1999) Role of CFTR in airway disease. Physiol Rev 79: S215–255.
9. Smolich JJ, Stratford BF, Maloney JE, Ritchie BC (1978) New features in the development of the submucosal gland of the respiratory tract. J Anat 127: 223–238.
10. Mashimo T, Serikawa T (2009) Rat resources in biomedical research. Curr Pharm Biotechnol 10: 214–220.
11. Aitman TJ, Critser JK, Cuppen E, Dominiczak A, Fernandez-Suarez XM, et al. (2008) Progress and prospects in rat genetics: a community view. Nat Genet 40: 516–522.
12. Jacob HJ (1999) Functional genomics and rat models. Genome Res 9: 1013–1016.
13. Urnov FD, Rebar EJ, Holmes MC, Zhang HS, Gregory PD (2010) Genome editing with engineered zinc finger nucleases. Nat Rev Genet 11: 636–646.
14. Cui X, Ji D, Fisher DA, Wu Y, Briner DM, et al. (2011) Targeted integration in rat and mouse embryos with zinc-finger nucleases. Nat Biotechnol 29: 64–67.
15. Carbery ID, Ji D, Harrington A, Brown V, Weinstein EJ, et al. (2010) Targeted genome modification in mice using zinc-finger nucleases. Genetics 186: 451–459.
16. Fanucchi MV, Hotchkiss JA, Harkema JR (1998) Endotoxin potentiates ozone-induced mucous cell metaplasia in rat nasal epithelium. Toxicology and Applied Pharmacology 152: 1–9.
17. Young JT (1981) Histopathologic examination of the rat nasal cavity. Fundam Appl Toxicol 1: 309–312.
18. Harkema JR, Hotchkiss JA, Harmsen AG, Henderson RF (1988) In vivo effects of transient neutrophil influx on nasal respiratory epithelial mucosubstances. Quantitative histochemistry. Am J Pathol 130: 605–615.
19. Fanucchi MV, Bracher A, Doran SF, Squadrito GL, Fernandez S, et al. (2012) Post-exposure antioxidant treatment in rats decreases airway hyperplasia and hyperreactivity due to chlorine inhalation. Am J Respir Cell Mol Biol 46: 599–606.
20. Meyerholz DK, Stoltz DA, Namati E, Ramachandran S, Pezzulo AA, et al. (2010) Loss of cystic fibrosis transmembrane conductance regulator function produces abnormalities in tracheal development in neonatal pigs and young children. Am J Respir Crit Care Med 182: 1251–1261.
21. Solomon GM, Konstan MW, Wilschanski M, Billings J, Sermet-Gaudelus I, et al. (2010) An international randomized multicenter comparison of nasal potential difference techniques. Chest 138: 919–928.
22. Pyle LC, Fulton JC, Sloane PA, Backer K, Mazur M, et al. (2010) Activation of the cystic fibrosis transmembrane conductance regulator by the flavonoid quercetin: potential use as a biomarker of ΔF508 cystic fibrosis transmembrane conductance regulator rescue. Am J Respir Cell Mol Biol 43: 607–616.
23. Dawson DC (1977) Na and Cl transport across the isolated turtle colon: parallel pathways for transmural ion movement. J Membr Biol 37: 213–233.
24. Liu L, Chu KK, Houser GH, Diephuis BJ, Li Y, et al. (2013) Method for quantitative study of airway functional microanatomy using micro-optical coherence tomography. PLoS One 8: e54473.
25. Rutland J, Cole PJ (1981) Nasal mucociliary clearance and ciliary beat frequency in cystic fibrosis compared with sinusitis and bronchiectasis. Thorax 36: 654–658.
26. Brand JD, Ballinger CA, Tuggle KL, Fanucchi MV, Schwiebert LM, et al. (2012) Site-specific dynamics of CD11b+ and CD103+ dendritic cell accumulations following ozone exposure. Am J Physiol Lung Cell Mol Physiol 303: L1079–1086.
27. Clarke LL, Boucher RC (1992) Chloride secretory response to extracellular ATP in human normal and cystic fibrosis nasal epithelia. Am J Physiol 263: C348–356.
28. Rosenberg LA, Schluchter MD, Parlow AF, Drumm ML (2006) Mouse as a model of growth retardation in cystic fibrosis. Pediatr Res 59: 191–195.
29. Pierucci-Alves F, Akoyev V, Stewart JC, Wang LH, Janardhan KS, et al. (2011) Swine models of cystic fibrosis reveal male reproductive tract phenotype at birth. Biol Reprod 85: 442–451.
30. Arquitt CK, Boyd C, Wright JT (2002) Cystic fibrosis transmembrane regulator gene (CFTR) is associated with abnormal enamel formation. J Dent Res 81: 492–496.
31. Chang EH, Lacruz RS, Bromage TG, Bringas P, Welsh MJ, et al. (2011) Enamel pathology resulting from loss of function in the cystic fibrosis transmembrane conductance regulator in a porcine animal model. Cells Tissues Organs 194: 249–254.
32. Dabrowska E, Błahuszewska K, Minarowska A, Kaczmarski M, Niedźwiecka-Andrzejewicz I, et al. (2006) Assessment of dental status and oral hygiene in the study population of cystic fibrosis patients in the Podlasie province. Adv Med Sci 51 Suppl 1: 100–103.
33. Wright JT, Kiefer CL, Hall KI, Grubb BR (1996) Abnormal enamel development in a cystic fibrosis transgenic mouse model. J Dent Res 75: 966–973.
34. Sturgess J, Imrie J (1982) Quantitative evaluation of the development of tracheal submucosal glands in infants with cystic fibrosis and control infants. Am J Pathol 106: 303–311.
35. Jarzabek K, Zbucka M, Pepiński W, Szamatowicz J, Domitrz J, et al. (2004) Cystic fibrosis as a cause of infertility. Reprod Biol 4: 119–129.
36. Wright JT, Hall KI, Grubb BR (1996) Enamel mineral composition of normal and cystic fibrosis transgenic mice. Adv Dent Res 10: 270–274; discussion 275.
37. Azevedo TD, Feijó GC, Bezerra AC (2006) Presence of developmental defects of enamel in cystic fibrosis patients. J Dent Child (Chic) 73: 159–163.
38. Ferrazzano GF, Sangianantoni G, Cantile T, Amato I, Orlando S, et al. (2012) Dental enamel defects in Italian children with cystic fibrosis: an observational study. Community Dent Health 29: 106–109.
39. Primosch RE (1980) Tetracycline discoloration, enamel defects, and dental caries in patients with cystic fibrosis. Oral Surg Oral Med Oral Pathol 50: 301–308.
40. Jagels AE, Sweeney EA (1976) Oral health of patients with cystic fibrosis and their siblings. J Dent Res 55: 991–996.
41. Boucher RC (2007) Evidence for airway surface dehydration as the initiating event in CF airway disease. J Intern Med 261: 5–16.
42. Song Y, Namkung W, Nielson DW, Lee JW, Finkbeiner WE, et al. (2009) Airway surface liquid depth measured in ex vivo fragments of pig and human trachea: dependence on Na+ and Cl- channel function. Am J Physiol Lung Cell Mol Physiol 297: L1131–1140.
43. Chinet TC, Fullton JM, Yankaskas JR, Boucher RC, Stutts MJ (1994) Mechanism of sodium hyperabsorption in cultured cystic fibrosis nasal epithelium: a patch-clamp study. Am J Physiol 266: C1061–1068.
44. Boucher RC, Stutts MJ, Knowles MR, Cantley L, Gatzy JT (1986) Na+ transport in cystic fibrosis respiratory epithelia. Abnormal basal rate and response to adenylate cyclase activation. J Clin Invest 78: 1245–1252.
45. Boucher RC, Cotton CU, Gatzy JT, Knowles MR, Yankaskas JR (1988) Evidence for reduced Cl- and increased Na+ permeability in cystic fibrosis human primary cell cultures. J Physiol 405: 77–103.
46. Cotton CU, Stutts MJ, Knowles MR, Gatzy JT, Boucher RC (1987) Abnormal apical cell membrane in cystic fibrosis respiratory epithelium. An in vitro electrophysiologic analysis. J Clin Invest 79: 80–85.
47. Chen JH, Stoltz DA, Karp PH, Ernst SE, Pezzulo AA, et al. (2010) Loss of anion transport without increased sodium absorption characterizes newborn porcine cystic fibrosis airway epithelia. Cell 143: 911–923.

48. Fisher JT, Tyler SR, Zhang Y, Lee BJ, Liu X, et al. (2013) Bioelectric Characterization of Epithelia from Neonatal CFTR Knockout Ferrets. Am J Respir Cell Mol Biol 49: 837–844.
49. Chen EY, Yang N, Quinton PM, Chin WC (2010) A new role for bicarbonate in mucus formation. Am J Physiol Lung Cell Mol Physiol 299: L542–549.
50. Garcia MA, Yang N, Quinton PM (2009) Normal mouse intestinal mucus release requires cystic fibrosis transmembrane regulator-dependent bicarbonate secretion. J Clin Invest 119: 2613–2622.
51. Chang EH, Pezzulo AA, Meyerholz DK, Potash AE, Wallen TJ, et al. (2012) Sinus hypoplasia precedes sinus infection in a porcine model of cystic fibrosis. Laryngoscope 122: 1898–1905.
52. Tarran R, Grubb BR, Parsons D, Picher M, Hirsh AJ, et al. (2001) The CF salt controversy: in vivo observations and therapeutic approaches. Mol Cell 8: 149–158.
53. Houwen RH, van der Doef HP, Sermet I, Munck A, Hauser B, et al. (2010) Defining DIOS and constipation in cystic fibrosis with a multicentre study on the incidence, characteristics, and treatment of DIOS. J Pediatr Gastroenterol Nutr 50: 38–42.
54. Collaco A, Marathe J, Kohnke H, Kravstov D, Ameen N (2010) Syntaxin 3 is necessary for cAMP- and cGMP-regulated exocytosis of CFTR: implications for enterotoxigenic diarrhea. Am J Physiol Cell Physiol 299: C1450–1460.
55. Jayaraman S, Song Y, Vetrivel L, Shankar L, Verkman AS (2001) Noninvasive in vivo fluorescence measurement of airway-surface liquid depth, salt concentration, and pH. J Clin Invest 107: 317–324.
56. Boucher RC (2004) New concepts of the pathogenesis of cystic fibrosis lung disease. Eur Respir J 23: 146–158.
57. Itani OA, Chen JH, Karp PH, Ernst S, Keshavjee S, et al. (2011) Human cystic fibrosis airway epithelia have reduced Cl- conductance but not increased Na+ conductance. Proc Natl Acad Sci U S A 108: 10260–10265.
58. Grubb BR, Vick RN, Boucher RC (1994) Hyperabsorption of Na+ and raised Ca(2+)-mediated Cl- secretion in nasal epithelia of CF mice. Am J Physiol 266: C1478–1483.
59. Livraghi-Butrico A, Kelly EJ, Wilkinson KJ, Rogers TD, Gilmore RC, et al. (2013) Loss of Cftr function exacerbates the phenotype of Na(+) hyperabsorption in murine airways. Am J Physiol Lung Cell Mol Physiol 304: L469–480.
60. van der Doef HP, Kokke FT, van der Ent CK, Houwen RH (2011) Intestinal obstruction syndromes in cystic fibrosis: meconium ileus, distal intestinal obstruction syndrome, and constipation. Curr Gastroenterol Rep 13: 265–270.
61. Rogers CS, Stoltz DA, Meyerholz DK, Ostedgaard LS, Rokhlina T, et al. (2008) Disruption of the CFTR gene produces a model of cystic fibrosis in newborn pigs. Science 321: 1837–1841.

9

Stationary Phase-Specific Virulence Factor Overproduction by a *lasR* Mutant of *Pseudomonas aeruginosa*

Matthew T. Cabeen*

Department of Molecular and Cellular Biology, Harvard University, Cambridge, Massachusetts, United States of America

Abstract

Secreted virulence factors of the human pathogen *Pseudomonas aeruginosa* are often under quorum sensing control. Cells lacking the quorum-sensing regulator LasR show reduced virulence factor production under typical laboratory conditions and are hypo-virulent in short-term animal infection models, yet *lasR* mutants are frequently associated with long-term infection in cystic fibrosis patients. Here, I show that in stationary-phase or slow-growth conditions, *lasR* cells continuously and strongly produce the important virulence factor pyocyanin while wild-type cells do not. Pyocyanin overproduction by *lasR* cells is permitted by loss of repression by RsaL, a LasR-dependent negative regulator. *lasR* cells also contribute pyocyanin in mixed cultures, even under "cheating" conditions where they depend on their wild-type neighbors for nutrients. Finally, some clinical *P. aeruginosa* isolates with *lasR* mutations can overproduce pyocyanin in the laboratory. These results imply that slow-growing clinical populations of *lasR* cells in chronic infections may contribute to virulence by producing pyocyanin under conditions where *lasR*$^+$ cells do not.

Editor: Tom Coenye, Ghent University, Belgium

Funding: This work was funded by the BASF (www.basf.com) Advanced Research Initiative at Harvard University, Grant 5366005-01. The funders had no role in study design, data collection and analysis, decision to publish, or preparation of the manuscript.

Competing Interests: This work was funded by the BASF (www.basf.com) Advanced Research Initiative at Harvard University, Grant 5366005-01.

* E-mail: cabeen@fas.harvard.edu.

Introduction

Pseudomonas aeruginosa is a common opportunistic bacterial pathogen that causes human infections in a variety of clinical situations [1] but is especially important in cystic fibrosis lung infections [2]. Many of the numerous virulence factors produced by *P. aeruginosa* are under the control of quorum sensing, which uses diffusible autoinducer molecules as a way to monitor cell density [3]. Specific genes are thus activated when bacterial cell population density, and hence autoinducer concentration, exceeds a threshold. *P. aeruginosa* has at least three quorum-sensing systems, with distinct autoinducer molecules and partially overlapping regulons, that are hierarchically arranged. The Las system is the first to become activated, and it in turn stimulates additional systems known as Rhl and PQS, which additionally regulate each other (Fig. 1) [3]. Finally, pyocyanin, a phenazine small molecule and virulence factor, acts as a terminal signaling factor in the quorum-sensing cascade [4]. Consistent with this hierarchy, inactivation of LasR, the regulatory protein of the Las quorum-sensing system, has been reported to severely attenuate quorum sensing, the production of quorum-regulated factors, and virulence in typical laboratory culture and in short-term animal models [5,6,7,8,9,10,11].

Decreased quorum sensing can permit *lasR* mutants to become social cheaters that gain a growth advantage by utilizing quorum-regulated "public goods" (including virulence factors) produced by nearby wild-type cells rather than producing their own [12,13]. Cheating was thus proposed as one reason [13] why *lasR* mutants are detected in highly chronic human infections such as those occurring in cystic fibrosis patients [14]. Consistent with this idea, *lasR* mutant cells outcompeted co-infected wild-type cells and lowered overall virulence in a murine burn-infection model, consistent with their being non-producing cheaters [11]. However, recent work has revealed that cells lacking LasR function can in fact accomplish quorum sensing by employing the Rhl and PQS systems [15,16]. Without activation by LasR, the quorum response is substantially delayed, but it appears to resemble the wild-type response in terms of gene expression and virulence factor synthesis [15]. Such LasR-independent virulence factor production is another potential explanation for why *lasR* mutants may not reduce overall virulence in long-term cystic fibrosis infections. In accord with this idea, the presence of *lasR* mutant cells has been correlated with disease progression and declining lung function in cystic fibrosis patients [17].

Pyocyanin is one of the most important quorum-regulated virulence factors of *P. aeruginosa*. It has numerous toxic effects on host tissues at such infection sites as the respiratory epithelium, where its toxicity is thought to be related to the generation of reactive oxygen species when pyocyanin is oxidized [18]. Pyocyanin is under the control of the Rhl and PQS systems and can accordingly be produced even in the absence of LasR after a delay [15]. As with the presence of *lasR* mutants, high levels of sputum pyocyanin have been associated with advanced infection in cystic fibrosis patients [19]. Pyocyanin also serves as an antibiotic thanks to its redox activity, can act as a terminal electron

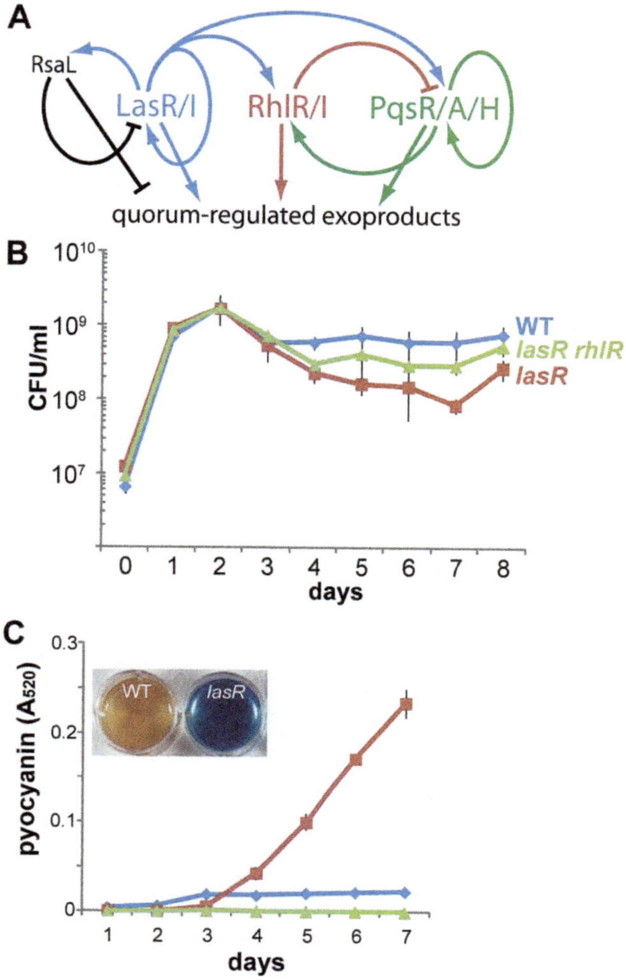

Figure 1. A *lasR* mutant overproduces pyocyanin under stationary-phase culture conditions. A. A simplified diagram showing some of the regulatory pathways linking the three quorum-sensing systems of *P. aeruginosa* and exoproduct synthesis. Each system and its regulatory pathways is color coded. B. Plot of the number of live cells (colony-forming units) in static cultures of strains with wild-type (WT) PA14 (MTC772), PA14 *lasR* (MTC774), and PA14 *lasR rhlR* (MTC797) backgrounds in LB at 25°C. C. Pyocyanin quantification in static cultures of wild-type (WT) PA14 (MTC1), PA14 *lasR* (MTC390), and PA14 *lasR rhlR* (MTC626) in LB at 25°C. The inset image shows the appearance of the cultures in a 12-well plate after 7 d. All plots show the mean ± standard deviation of 3 biological replicates.

acceptor for *P. aeruginosa*, and is a terminal signaling molecule in the quorum-sensing cascade [4]. It is therefore useful for monitoring quorum-sensing activity in *P. aeruginosa*, especially given its bright blue color when oxidized.

Most previous laboratory studies of *P. aeruginosa* quorum sensing have observed bacteria exponentially growing in shaking culture. Under such conditions, wild-type quorum-sensing behaviors begin during late exponential phase and continue into stationary phase, while LasR-independent behaviors do not begin to appear until the onset of stationary phase, between 8 and 24 h [15]. However, most bacterial cells in nature are not growing in optimal laboratory-like conditions. Instead, pathogens often form biofilms during infection [20]. The physiology of slowly growing bacteria resembles that of bacteria growing in biofilms [21], and *P. aeruginosa* expresses the stationary-phase sigma factor RpoS both in clinical sputum samples [22] and in continuously fed biofilms in vitro [23]. Indeed, one reason for the treatment resistance of cells growing in biofilms is their relatively slow growth [24]. Therefore, I reasoned that slow-growing or stationary-phase cells maintained in longer-term culture might manifest phenotypes that reflect their behavior in a more physiologically relevant state. Here, I report that wild-type and *lasR* cells exhibit clearly distinct yet complementary stationary-phase phenotypes. Moreover, wild-type/*lasR* mixtures can collaborate to enact behaviors inaccessible to the individual strains.

Materials and Methods

Routine bacterial culture

Pseudomonas aeruginosa and *Escherichia coli* strains were routinely cultured on LB Lennox solid (1.5% agar) and liquid media at 37°C. Culture stocks were stored in 25% glycerol at -80°C, and fresh plates were grown for each experiment. The following antibiotics were used for selection/maintenance for *P. aeruginosa*; the maintenance concentration was used for *E. coli* culture: gentamycin (75/15 μg/ml) and tetracycline (75/25 μg/ml). Irgasan (25 μg/ml) was used as an *E. coli*-specific selective agent. *P. aeruginosa* strains are listed in Table 1. *E. coli* strains are listed in Table S1 in File S1, plasmids are listed in Table S2 in File S1, and primer sequences are listed in Table S3 in File S1.

Specialized media

M63 medium contained 100 μM (13.6 g/L) KH_2PO_4, 15.14 mM (2 g/L) $(NH_4)_2SO_4$, and 0.36 μM (0.1 mg/L) $FeSO_4 \cdot H_2O$. A 5X salts stock was adjusted to pH 7.0 with KOH before autoclaving. To make the final medium, the 5X stock was mixed with 0.2% casamino acids and 0.5% glycerol from 20% and 50% sterile stocks, respectively, and adjusted to 1X with sterile H_2O.

M9 medium was based on a salt solution of 12.8 g/L $NaHPO_4 \cdot 7H_2O$, 3 g/L KH_2PO_4, 0.5 g/L NaCl, 1 g/L NH_4Cl. A 5X salts stock was prepared and autoclaved. To make the final medium, the 5X stock was mixed with 2 mM $MgSO_4$ and 0.1 mM $CaCl_2$ from sterile 1M stocks, the appropriate carbon sources (sodium caseinate was added from a 10% autoclaved stock), and was adjusted to 1X with sterile H_2O.

SCFM medium was made as described by Palmer *et al.* [25] and was prepared and used freshly, as it displayed a short shelf life.

Specialized culture conditions

Static cultures of *P. aeruginosa* were grown in 4-ml volumes in 12-well microtiter plates, in 2-ml volumes in 24-well plates, or in 200-μl volumes in 96-well plates. A 1% volume of stationary-phase LB starter culture (OD_{600}~2-3), adjusted to OD_{600} = 1.0, was used for inoculation (hence, the starting OD_{600} was equivalent to 0.01). Pure autoinducer molecules (3OC12-HSL, C4-HSL, and PQS; Sigma) were added from 100 mM stocks in DMSO, and equivalent volumes of DMSO were used for controls.

Reporter assays

Luminescent *lux* reporter strains were grown in static 200-μL LB cultures in 96-well microtiter plates. The cultures were inoculated at an initial OD_{600} of 0.01 (from starter cultures diluted to OD_{600} = 1.0) and grown at 25°C and 40% relative humidity. At daily time points, the luminescence values of the plate were read with a BioTek Synergy 2 plate reader. Data were collected using BioTek Gen5 software. At the same time points, static cultures with isogenic backgrounds, bearing an empty reporter and prepared identically, were taken, vortexed to disperse cells

Table 1. Strains used in this study.

Strain	Alias	Relevant genotype or description	Source or reference
P. aeruginosa			
MTC1		PA14	
MTC63		PA14 Δ*phz*	[4]
MTC390		PA14 Δ*lasR*	This study
MTC498		PA14 Δ*rsaL*	This study
MTC500		PA14 Δ*rsaL* Δ*lasI*	This study
MTC537		PA14 Δ*pqsA*	This study
MTC556		PA14 Δ*rhlI* Δ*pqsA*	This study
MTC625		PA14 Δ*lasR* Δ*rhlI*	This study
MTC626		PA14 Δ*lasR* Δ*rhlR*	This study
MTC628		PA14 Δ*lasR* Δ*pqsA*	This study
MTC637		PA14 Δ*lasR attB::CTX-1-aacC1* (Gent^R)	This study
MTC723		PA14 *attB::CTX-1-*P_{lasB}*-lux*	This study
MTC725		PA14 *attB::CTX-1-*P_{phzA1}*-lux*	This study
MTC733		PA14 *attB::CTX-1-*P_{hcnA}*-lux*	This study
MTC735		PA14 *attB::CTX-1-*P_{rhlA}*-lux*	This study
MTC737		PA14 *attB::CTX-1-*P_{rsaL}*-lux*	This study
MTC745		PA14 Δ*lasR attB::CTX-1-*P_{lasB}*-lux*	This study
MTC747		PA14 Δ*lasR attB::CTX-1-*P_{phzA1}*-lux*	This study
MTC755		PA14 Δ*lasR attB::CTX-1-*P_{hcnA}*-lux*	This study
MTC757		PA14 Δ*lasR attB::CTX-1-*P_{rhlA}*-lux*	This study
MTC759		PA14 Δ*lasR attB::CTX-1-*P_{rsaL}*-lux*	This study
MTC772		PA14 *attB::CTX-1-lux*	This study
MTC774		PA14 Δ*lasR attB::CTX-1-lux*	This study
MTC789		PA14 Δ*lasR* Δ*rhlR attB::CTX-1-*P_{lasB}*-lux*	This study
MTC790		PA14 Δ*lasR* Δ*rhlR attB::CTX-1-*P_{phzA1}*-lux*	This study
MTC794		PA14 Δ*lasR* Δ*rhlR attB::CTX-1-*P_{hcnA}*-lux*	This study
MTC795		PA14 Δ*lasR* Δ*rhlR attB::CTX-1-*P_{rhlA}*-lux*	This study
MTC797		PA14 Δ*lasR* Δ*rhlR attB::CTX-1-lux*	This study
MTC838		PA14 Δ*lasR* Δ*ambB*	This study
MTC842		PA14 Δ*lasR* Δ*phoB*	This study
MTC949		PA14 Δ*lasR* Δ*rhlI* Δ*pqsA*	This study
0007-2	CF1	*lasR* wild type (confirmed by sequencing)	[17]
0022-1	CF2	$lasR_{179C>T}$ (W60STOP identified by sequencing)	[17]
0024-5	CF3	*lasR* wild-type (identified by sequencing)	[17]
0029-1	CF4	$lasR_{557T>G}$ (Q186P identified by sequencing)	[17]
0053-2	CF5	$lasR_{520G>A}$ (P174S identified by sequencing)	[17]
0063-6	CF6	$lasR\Delta_{350-362}$ (deletion and frameshift identified by sequencing)	[17]

(effective dispersion was verified by phase-contrast microscopy) and serially diluted to obtain colony-forming unit (CFU) counts. The resulting CFU counts were then used to normalize the luminescence values of their respective reporter strains.

Pyocyanin extraction and quantification

Pyocyanin was extracted from the supernatants of liquid cultures by adding an equal volume of chloroform ($CHCl_3$) and vigorously vortexing. The lower, pyocyanin-containing organic layer was then taken and vortexed with an equal volume of 0.2 M HCl. The pink pyocyanin-containing aqueous layer was taken, and its absorbance at 520 nm (A_{520}) was read in a BioTek Synergy 2 plate reader.

For some experiments, pyocyanin was quantified directly in culture supernatants by reading the absorbance at 691 nm as previously described [19]. Sterile medium was used as a blank.

Cheating experiments

For cheating experiments, PA14 cells or mixtures of PA14 or PA14 *phz* cells with *lasR* cells were grown in liquid M9 medium (6 mL) containing 1% casein at 25°C in a tube roller. Pyocyanin was quantified as described above. The fraction of *lasR* cells within a mixture was determined using a *lasR* strain chromosomally marked with gentamycin resistance (MTC637). Cultures were serially diluted in 1X M9 salts and plated on LB or LB containing 5 µg/ml gentamycin to obtain CFU counts.

Statistical analysis

Comparisons between samples were analyzed using unpaired equal-variance two-tailed Student's t-tests. The threshold for significance was set as $p<0.01$.

Results

Pyocyanin is overproduced by *lasR* cells in extended stationary-phase culture

To observe the behavior of stationary-phase cells over a time period of days rather than hours, as in traditional laboratory studies, I examined static liquid LB cultures of PA14 and a *lasR* mutant derivative growing at 25°C. Under these conditions, cells grow to a high density that then very gradually falls over the course of several days (Fig. 1B) but do not exhibit the "death phase" that typically precedes long-term adaptation to stationary phase [26]. In shaking culture, wild-type cells produce noticeable pyocyanin beginning in late exponential phase [4], while *lasR* cells begin to produce it by 24 h of culture [15]. After 3–4 days in static culture, I unexpectedly observed strong and continuing production of pyocyanin by stationary-phase *lasR* cells that turned the cultures dark blue, while wild-type cells produced virtually no visible pyocyanin at any time during the experiment (Fig. 1C). This effect was strongest in LB at 25°C, but the same trend appeared in static cultures of minimal M63 medium and in a nutritional mimic of cystic fibrosis sputum [25] at both 25°C and 37°C (Fig. S1 in File S1). Therefore, the wild type and *lasR* mutant display distinct stationary-phase phenotypes in that *lasR* cells continually produce pyocyanin while wild-type cells barely produce any pyocyanin. The phenotype of the *lasR* mutant was not due to additional mutations accumulated during the experiment, as cells from 6-day-old blue cultures displayed the same time course of pyocyanin production when inoculated into liquid LB, grown overnight at 37°C, and re-inoculated into static LB (Fig. S2 in File S1).

Stationary-phase wild-type and *lasR* cells express distinct quorum-regulated virulence genes

Because stationary-phase wild-type and *lasR* cells displayed distinct phenotypes with respect to pyocyanin production, I analyzed the expression of additional quorum-regulated genes with roles in virulence factor production. Two distinct expression patterns were apparent. The first, typified most strongly by *lasB* but also seen for *rhlA* (encoding the LasB elastase and a rhamnolipid biosynthesis protein, respectively), showed strong early expression in the wild-type but only weak expression in *lasR* cells (Fig. 2). The second, seen most strongly for *phzA1* but also for *hcnA* (involved in phenazine and hydrogen cyanide synthesis, respectively), showed delayed but stronger expression by *lasR* mutant cells but weaker expression by the wild type (Fig. 2). These results revealed that wild-type cells were successfully performing quorum sensing, as they very strongly expressed *lasB* and also expressed *rhlA*. However, *phzA1* was notable for being largely turned off in the wild-type. The *lasR* mutant displayed the opposite phenotype, most strongly expressing genes that were weakly expressed by the wild type. Among the sampled quorum-regulated virulence genes, the wild-type and *lasR* strains thus showed distinct but complementary expression profiles, and the *lasR* profile was characterized by strong *phzA1* expression and pyocyanin production.

LasR-independent expression requires the Rhl and PQS quorum-sensing systems

Previously reported LasR-independent quorum sensing in shaking culture required the Rhl quorum sensing system [15], in accord with its position in the quorum-sensing network (Fig. 1A). I thus tested whether the Rhl and PQS systems were also required for quorum expression in stationary-phase *lasR* cells. Indeed, additional deletion of *rhlR*, encoding the RhlR regulator, in a *lasR* background abolished the expression of all tested genes (Fig. 2). Similarly, pyocyanin production did not occur in *lasR rhlI* or *lasR pqsA* double mutants, which are unable to produce the Rhl autoinducer *N*-butyryl-L-homoserine lactone (C4-HSL) or 2-heptyl-4-quinolone (HHQ) and 2-heptyl-3-hydroxy-4-quinolone (PQS), respectively (Fig. 3A). Each of these double mutants could be complemented for pyocyanin production by exogenous addition of the appropriate autoinducer (C4-HSL or PQS), with stronger induction at 100 µM than at 10 µM (Fig. 3A). Consistent with these results, a triple *lasR rhlI pqsA* mutant required the addition of both autoinducers to restore pyocyanin production (Fig. 3A). Moreover, exogenous addition of PQS alone or in combination with C4-HSL to the *lasR* mutant accelerated pyocyanin production, while C4-HSL alone did not (Fig. 3B). This result is consistent with the idea that cellular RhlR levels are a limiting factor for LasR-independent pyocyanin production, as PQS signaling can stimulate *rhlR* transcription [27] and addition of constitutively expressed plasmid-borne *rhlR* greatly accelerated and increased pyocyanin production in a *lasR* mutant in shaking culture [15].

A *lasR pqsH* double mutant, which is unable to convert HHQ to PQS [28,29], was able to produce pyocyanin (Fig. 3C), suggesting that HHQ is itself a signaling molecule that can functionally substitute for PQS to induce pyocyanin production under stationary-phase conditions. This result contrasts with a previous report [29], but the difference may be due to the different strain background, culture media and conditions used in this work.

It has been suggested that LasR-independent quorum sensing and pyocyanin production may occur through the PhoB-mediated phosphate starvation pathway [27] or use the newly discovered signaling molecule IQS, whose synthesis requires the AmbB protein [30]. To test whether pyocyanin production by stationary-phase *lasR* cells required either of these proteins in addition to Rhl and PQS quorum signaling, I constructed *lasR phoB* and *lasR ambB* double mutants and assayed them for pyocyanin production in static culture. Each of the double mutants produced pyocyanin indistinguishably from the *lasR* mutant (Fig. S3 in File S1), showing that neither of these pathways is required for LasR-independent overproduction of pyocyanin in stationary-phase culture.

Repression by RsaL explains the different quorum profiles of wild-type and *lasR* cells

The weak expression by wild-type cells of genes that were strongly expressed by the *lasR* mutant suggested that they might be under negative regulation. Notably, *phzA1* and *hcnA*, which displayed the strongest LasR-independent expression and the weakest expression by the wild type, are direct targets of negative regulation by RsaL, a repressor whose primary role is to provide negative homeostatic feedback to Las quorum sensing [31]. Meanwhile, *lasB* and *rhlA*, which are not under RsaL repression [31], were strongly expressed in the wild type. Because expression of *rsaL* is under LasR control [32], RsaL was an excellent candidate for a negative repressor that would be present in the wild type but absent in a *lasR* mutant. Indeed, stationary-phase *rsaL* expression in static culture was very strong in wild-type cells

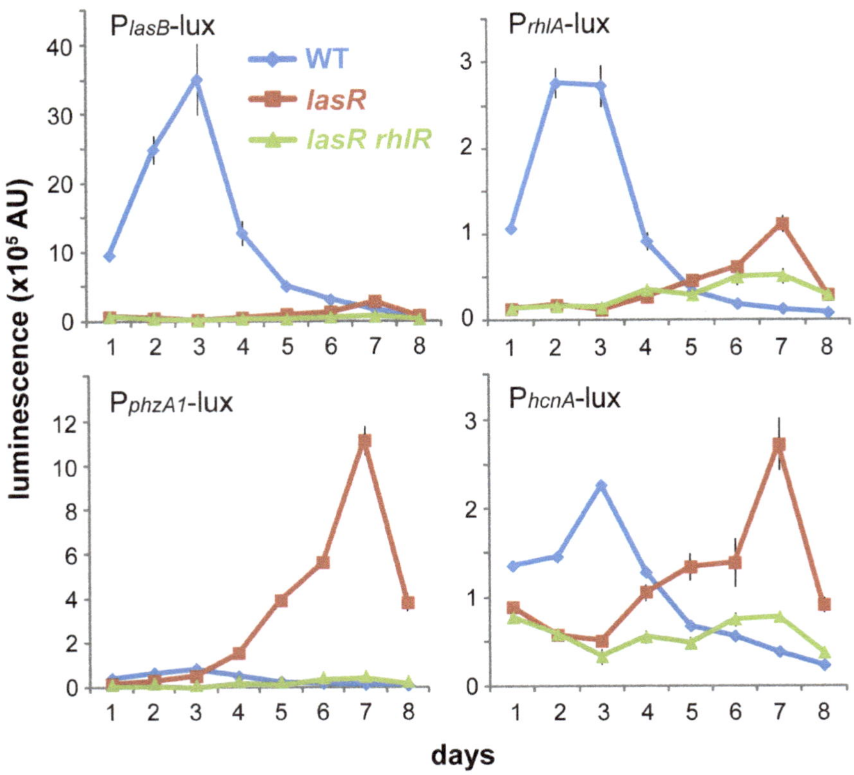

Figure 2. Wild-type and *lasR* mutant cells display distinct virulence gene expression patterns in stationary-phase culture. Gene expression was measured using chromosomally integrated *lux* reporters in the listed strain backgrounds. Plots show the mean ± standard deviation of 3 biological replicates each composed of 3 technical replicates.

but quite weak in *lasR* cells (Fig. 4A). Presumably, the RsaL protein produced during the initial peak of expression in wild-type cells continues to stably bind its target DNA sequences [33], such as *phzA1*, in subsequent days, ensuring their continued repression.

If RsaL were responsible for repressing genes such as *phzA1* in otherwise quorum-active wild-type cells in stationary phase, inactivation of *rsaL* in a wild-type background would relieve this repression. Consistent with this hypothesis, an *rsaL* mutant in static culture displayed copious pyocyanin production that began significantly earlier than in a *lasR* mutant (Fig. 4B), suggesting that RsaL normally blocks pyocyanin production by the wild type. Deletion of *rsaL* also disrupts Las homeostasis, resulting in overabundance (25 μM, compared to 2 μM in the wild type) of the Las autoinducer *N*-3-oxo-dodecanoyl-L-homoserine lactone (3OC12-HSL) [31]. It was thus possible that high concentrations of 3OC12-HSL abetted the early production of pyocyanin. To correct for any such effect, I constructed an *rsaL lasI* double mutant unable to produce 3OC12-HSL and exogenously added a low (100 nM) concentration of 3OC12-HSL at the time of inoculation. The double mutant displayed 3OC12-HSL-dependent early pyocyanin production that was even stronger than that of the *rsaL* mutant (Fig. 4B), confirming that stationary-phase wild-type cells are capable of pyocyanin production but that it is repressed by the presence of the RsaL repressor. Therefore, expression of a specific set of quorum-regulated genes (including *phzA1* and *hcnA*) in *lasR* cells is caused by LasR-independent Rhl and PQS quorum-sensing activity in combination with deactivation of RsaL-mediated repression.

lasR cells contribute pyocyanin in mixed culture even under conditions that permit cheating

A *lasR* mutant is a well-known example of a "cheater". Typical cheating experiments use defined medium containing casein as the sole carbon source [12,13,34]. Because casein utilization requires quorum-regulated extracellular proteases such LasB, whose production in early phases of growth is induced by the Las system [35], a *lasR* mutant fails to grow on casein medium (Fig. S4 in File S1). When a wild-type strain is grown together with a *lasR* mutant, the *lasR* mutant benefits from the casein proteolysis performed by wild-type-derived LasB without the associated costs of producing quorum-regulated factors and thereby gains an advantage [12,13]. In light of the distinct quorum-sensing profiles of stationary-phase wild-type and *lasR* cells, I hypothesized that *lasR* cells might be able to contribute quorum-regulated factors such as pyocyanin even while "cheating" with respect to nutrition. To test this hypothesis, I cultivated wild-type and *lasR* cells alone and in a 1:4 mutant-to-wild-type mixture for several days in shaking liquid M9 medium with 1% casein, a typical cheating medium. As expected, the *lasR* mutant alone did not grow in this medium (Fig. S4 in File S1), while the wild-type grew (Fig. S4 in File S1) and produced some pyocyanin (Fig. 5A), indicating quorum sensing. The mixture of the two strains, however, produced much more pyocyanin than the wild-type alone (Fig. 5A), suggesting that the *lasR* mutant was contributing to pyocyanin production. To test this idea, I grew 1:4 *lasR*-to-*phz* mixtures in which only the *lasR* mutant could contribute pyocyanin. Such mixtures produced only slightly less pyocyanin than mixtures with the wild-type and substantially more pyocyanin than the wild-type alone (Fig. 5A), confirming that the *lasR* mutant contributed the majority of pyocyanin in

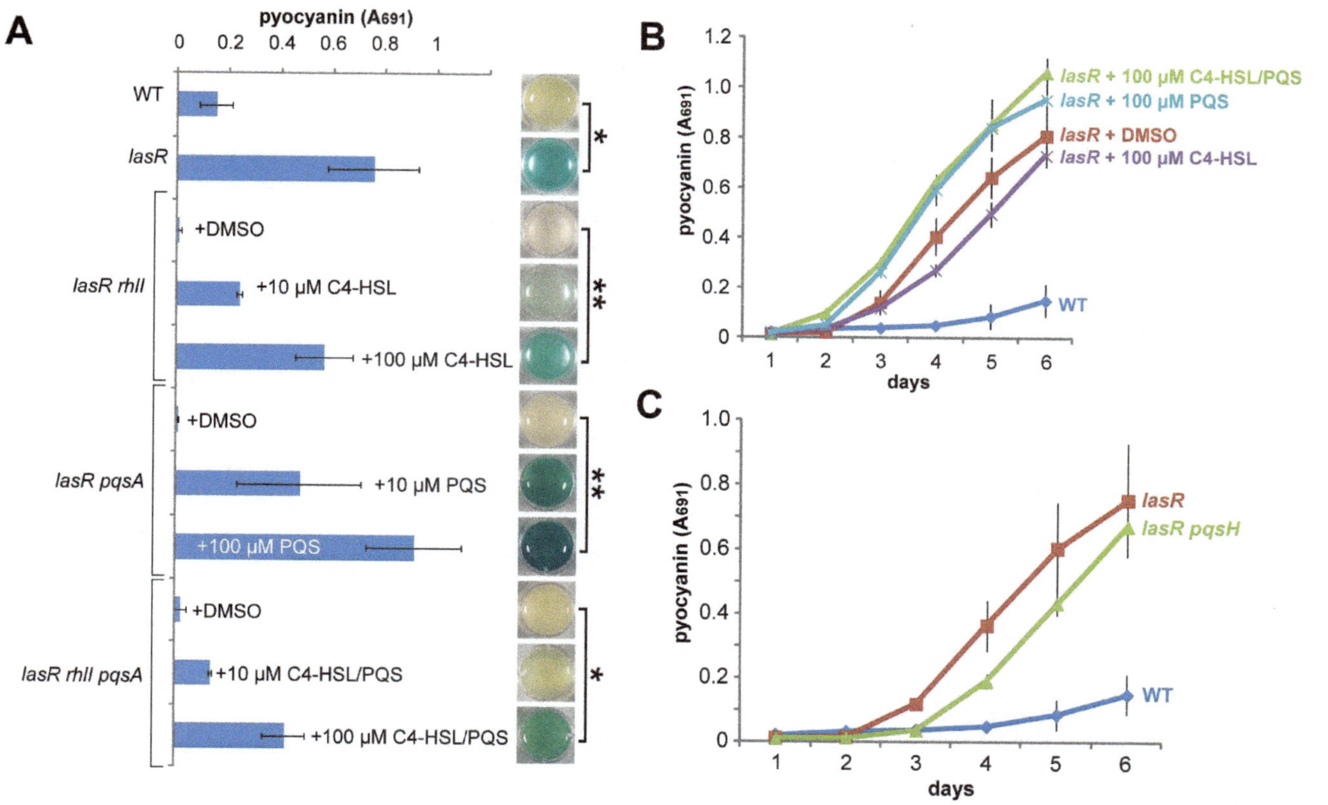

Figure 3. Pyocyanin production by stationary-phase *lasR* mutant cells requires Rhl and quinolone signaling. A. Pyocyanin quantification in the listed strains with or without the listed signaling molecules after 6 days of LB static culture at 25°C. The images to the right of the bar graph show the appearance of representative cultures. *, $p<0.005$; **, $p<0.001$. The differences between *lasR* and the 100 µM-complemented autoinducer-negative samples were not significant ($0.04<p<0.33$). B. Pyocyanin quantification in static LB cultures of the listed strains and conditions at 25°C. C. Pyocyanin quantification in static LB cultures of the listed strains at 25°C. All plots show the mean ± standard deviation of 3 biological replicates.

mixtures. In such mixtures, the relative *lasR* population increased from its initial 20% level to 30–40% after 7 days of culture (Fig. 5B), suggestive of a slight advantage gained by nutritional cheating. These results demonstrated that the *lasR* mutant cooperated with respect to pyocyanin production even under conditions (casein medium) that forced it to cheat with respect to LasB. Notably, pyocyanin production by the *lasR* cells was not detected until the third day of culture (Fig. 5A), explaining why this *lasR* phenotype is not seen in cheating assays when cultures are diluted every 1–2 days [12,13].

Clinical *lasR* isolates can overproduce pyocyanin

The overproduction of pyocyanin by stationary-phase *lasR* cells in monoculture and in mixtures with wild-type cells raised the interesting possibility that *lasR* cells may overproduce pyocyanin in clinical infections, thereby increasing virulence. A relationship between the presence of *lasR* cells and high pyocyanin is at least suggested by separate studies associating high sputum pyocyanin [19] and *lasR* cell presence [17] with *P. aeruginosa* disease progression in cystic fibrosis patients. Assessing the relative contributions of *lasR*$^+$ and *lasR* cells to pyocyanin or virulence factor production in actual chronic human infections is very difficult, due to the spatial and genetic complexity of human lung infections. However, as a simple test of principle, I subjected a small set of clinical cystic fibrosis isolates that were wild type or mutant for *lasR* (Fig. 6A) to a static culture assay and looked for pyocyanin production. The *lasR*$^+$ strains exhibited minimal pyocyanin production, whereas *lasR* mutant strains showed widely varied production ranging from minimal to very strong (Fig. 6B). This variability may reflect differences in the severity of the different *lasR* mutant alleles (Fig. 6A) and other mutations in the genetic backgrounds of these strains that modulate pyocyanin production. Nonetheless, these results demonstrate that some clinical *lasR* mutant strains have the ability to overproduce pyocyanin under stationary-phase conditions where *lasR*$^+$ isolates cannot.

Discussion

This work shows that the quorum response by *lasR* mutants in slow-growth or stationary-phase conditions is distinct from the wild-type response and is characterized by strong expression of virulence factor genes that are repressed in wild-type cells by RsaL. For example, the pattern of low pyocyanin production by wild-type and high production by *lasR* cells in static stationary-phase culture is a reversal of the pattern seen for cells growing exponentially in shaking culture, showing that "typical" lab conditions uncover only part of the full range of cell behaviors. Experiments conducted in shaking culture for 24 hours showed that *lasR* cells could manifest a quorum response [15], but did not reveal the distinctions between the wild-type and *lasR* stationary-phase phenotypes that develop after longer-term culture under slow-growth conditions.

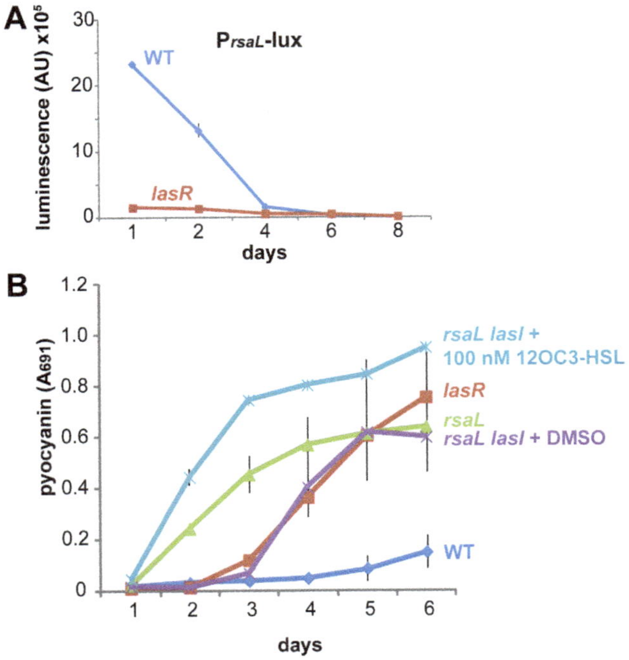

Figure 4. RsaL prevents pyocyanin production by stationary-phase *lasR*[+] cells. A. Transcription from the *rsaL* promoter in wild-type (PA14) and *lasR* mutant cells in static 25°C LB culture. B. Pyocyanin quantification in static LB cultures of the listed strains and conditions at 25°C. All plots show the mean ± standard deviation of 3 biological replicates.

Stationary-phase phenotypes are highly relevant for bacterial physiology in natural settings, including within infective biofilms [20,21,22]. The relative metabolic inactivity of some biofilm-embedded cells is one mechanism of resistance against killing by host defenses or by antibiotics [24]. Moreover, host environments like the cystic fibrosis lung contain hypoxic niches that slow bacterial growth [36,37]. It is therefore likely that many *P. aeruginosa* cells in long-term infections are enacting stationary-phase behaviors. In such conditions, the presence of *lasR* mutants within the *P. aeruginosa* population may permit the expression of important virulence factors such as pyocyanin that are repressed by RsaL in *lasR*[+] cells, thus expanding the range of phenotypes available to the total population. In this way, niches containing *lasR* cells could make a key contribution to virulence.

If repression by RsaL prevents *lasR*[+] cells from producing important virulence factors, why are mutations in *rsaL* not commonly isolated in clinical samples from chronic infections? One likely reason is because of the homeostatic function of RsaL in the normal quorum response. Cells lacking RsaL function display constitutive overproduction of quorum-regulated factors [38], perhaps making an *rsaL* cell population less competitive than wild-type cells under faster-growth conditions in the same way that wild-type cells can be cheated on by *lasR* cells. In contrast, a *lasR* mutant can be competitive under fast-growth conditions (as illustrated by its well-known cheating behavior) before overproducing a more narrowly defined set of quorum-regulated factors specifically during stationary phase. This fine tuning is made possible by a combination of three features of the quorum-sensing regulatory circuit: first, RsaL is under LasR control and thus is not produced in a *lasR* mutant [32]; second, RsaL has many other targets in addition to its homeostatic regulation of *lasI* [31]; and

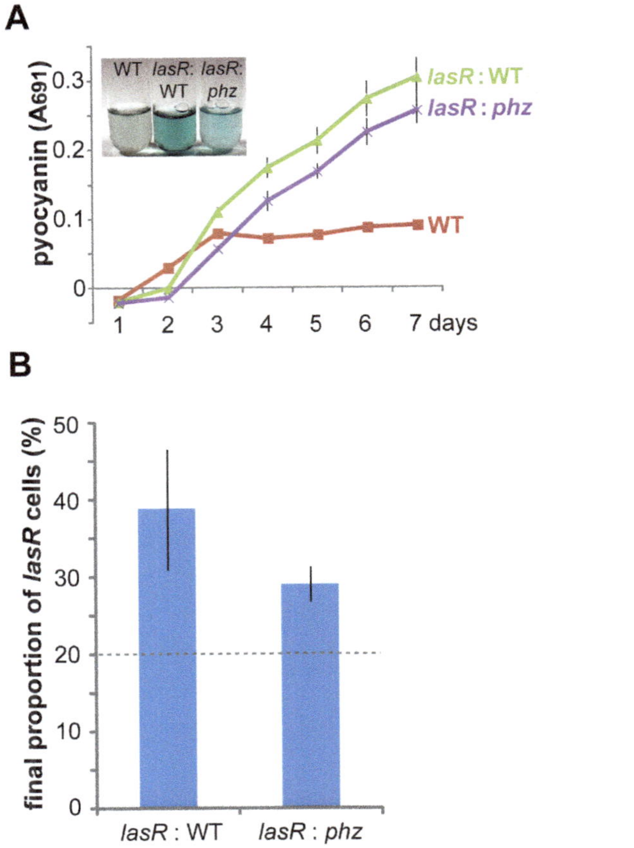

Figure 5. A *lasR* mutant contributes pyocyanin in a cheating mixture. Starting mixtures were 1:4 *lasR* mutant to PA14 or PA14 *phz*. All plots show the mean ± standard deviation of 3 biological replicates. A. Pyocyanin quantification in shaking M9-casein medium at 25°C. Inset shows appearance of cultures after 7 days of incubation. B. Relative proportions of *lasR* mutant cells in the indicated mixtures after 7 days of incubation. The difference between the two mixtures was not significant ($p = 0.12$).

third, the Rhl and PQS systems, which are normally activated by LasR, can also self-activate in a *lasR* mutant [15,16].

The distinct contributions of *lasR*[+] and *lasR* cells in a mixture allows them to collaborate to produce otherwise inaccessible phenotypes. This is seen most clearly in casein medium, where the *lasR*[+] cells secrete LasB to break down casein and feed the *lasR* cells, and the *lasR* cells in turn produce high levels of pyocyanin. It is conceivable that such a division of labor, where *lasR* cells overproduce pyocyanin and other virulence factors, may have a role in host infection. In this scenario, slow-growing or stationary-phase *lasR* cells within an infecting population might continually produce pyocyanin under conditions where *lasR*[+] cells do not. Overproduction of pyocyanin by some clinical *lasR* isolates under stationary-phase laboratory conditions suggests that they may do likewise in an infection setting, in accord with the findings that *lasR* strains [17] and high sputum pyocyanin [19] are both correlated with disease progression in cystic fibrosis patients. One corollary of this idea is that treatment strategies based on strong pharmacological inhibition of LasR (thus making cells functionally null for LasR) may in fact increase pyocyanin production by *lasR*[+] cells in stationary phase.

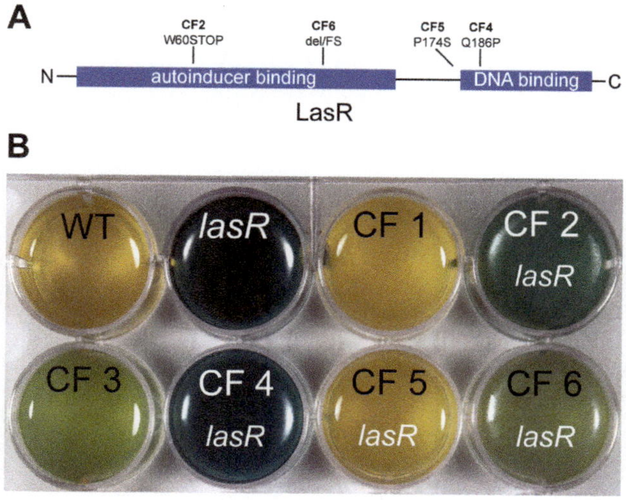

Figure 6. Clinical *lasR* isolates can overproduce pyocyanin. A. Locations of mutations in the LasR protein detected by sequencing. The mutations are in clinical isolates from Ref. 17. B. Appearance of static LB cultures of PA14 and *lasR* laboratory strains and of clinical isolates (CF1-6) [17] with and without *lasR* mutations. The cultures were grown for 12 days at 25°C to allow weaker phenotypes to develop.

Supporting Information

File S1 This file contains Tables S1–S3 and Figure S1–S4. Table S1, *Escherichia coli* strains used in this study. Table S2, Plasmids used in this study. Table S3, Primer sequences used in this study. Figure S1, Pyocyanin production in static culture. Figure S2, Pyocyanin production by *lasR* cells after overnight regrowth. Figure S3, LasR-independent pyocyanin production does not depend on AmbB or PhoB. Figure S4, Growth of wild-type PA14 or lasR cells in M9 medium with added casamino acids or casein.

Acknowledgments

I gratefully acknowledge my postdoctoral advisor Richard Losick, in whose laboratory this work was performed, for invaluable advice about the experiments in this study and during the preparation of the manuscript and for giving me the opportunity to publish on my own. I also thank Stephen Lory and Debbie Yoder-Himes for valuable advice and for supplying strains and vectors. I received clinical isolates from Jane Burns. Thanks to Marvin Whiteley, Karine Gibbs and Christine Jacobs-Wagner for comments on an earlier version of the paper and to Roberto Kolter, Quincey Justman, Peter Girguis and Thomas Norman for helpful discussions. M.T.C. is a Merck Fellow of the Jane Coffin Childs Foundation for Medical Research.

Author Contributions

Conceived and designed the experiments: MTC. Performed the experiments: MTC. Analyzed the data: MTC. Contributed reagents/materials/analysis tools: MTC. Wrote the paper: MTC.

References

1. Driscoll JA, Brody SL, Kollef MH (2007) The epidemiology, pathogenesis and treatment of *Pseudomonas aeruginosa* infections. Drugs 67: 351–368.
2. Lyczak JB, Cannon CL, Pier GB (2002) Lung infections associated with cystic fibrosis. Clin Microbiol Rev 15: 194–222.
3. Rutherford ST, Bassler BL (2012) Bacterial quorum sensing: its role in virulence and possibilities for its control. Cold Spring Harb Perspect Med 2.
4. Dietrich LE, Price-Whelan A, Petersen A, Whiteley M, Newman DK (2006) The phenazine pyocyanin is a terminal signalling factor in the quorum sensing network of *Pseudomonas aeruginosa*. Mol Microbiol 61: 1308–1321.
5. D'Argenio DA, Wu M, Hoffman LR, Kulasekara HD, Deziel E, et al. (2007) Growth phenotypes of *Pseudomonas aeruginosa* lasR mutants adapted to the airways of cystic fibrosis patients. Mol Microbiol 64: 512–533.
6. Hentzer M, Wu H, Andersen JB, Riedel K, Rasmussen TB, et al. (2003) Attenuation of *Pseudomonas aeruginosa* virulence by quorum sensing inhibitors. EMBO J 22: 3803–3815.
7. Pesci EC, Pearson JP, Seed PC, Iglewski BH (1997) Regulation of *las* and *rhl* quorum sensing in *Pseudomonas aeruginosa*. J Bacteriol 179: 3127–3132.
8. Schuster M, Lostroh CP, Ogi T, Greenberg EP (2003) Identification, timing, and signal specificity of *Pseudomonas aeruginosa* quorum-controlled genes: a transcriptome analysis. J Bacteriol 185: 2066–2079.
9. Smith RS, Iglewski BH (2003) *P. aeruginosa* quorum-sensing systems and virulence. Curr Opin Microbiol 6: 56–60.
10. Wagner VE, Bushnell D, Passador L, Brooks AI, Iglewski BH (2003) Microarray analysis of *Pseudomonas aeruginosa* quorum-sensing regulons: effects of growth phase and environment. J Bacteriol 185: 2080–2095.
11. Rumbaugh KP, Diggle SP, Watters CM, Ross-Gillespie A, Griffin AS, et al. (2009) Quorum sensing and the social evolution of bacterial virulence. Curr Biol 19: 341–345.
12. Diggle SP, Griffin AS, Campbell GS, West SA (2007) Cooperation and conflict in quorum-sensing bacterial populations. Nature 450: 411–414.
13. Sandoz KM, Mitzimberg SM, Schuster M (2007) Social cheating in *Pseudomonas aeruginosa* quorum sensing. Proc Natl Acad Sci U S A 104: 15876–15881.
14. Smith EE, Buckley DG, Wu Z, Saenphimmachak C, Hoffman LR, et al. (2006) Genetic adaptation by *Pseudomonas aeruginosa* to the airways of cystic fibrosis patients. Proc Natl Acad Sci U S A 103: 8487–8492.
15. Dekimpe V, Deziel E (2009) Revisiting the quorum-sensing hierarchy in *Pseudomonas aeruginosa*: the transcriptional regulator RhlR regulates LasR-specific factors. Microbiology 155: 712–723.
16. Diggle SP, Winzer K, Chhabra SR, Worrall KE, Camara M, et al. (2003) The *Pseudomonas aeruginosa* quinolone signal molecule overcomes the cell density-dependency of the quorum sensing hierarchy, regulates rhl-dependent genes at the onset of stationary phase and can be produced in the absence of LasR. Mol Microbiol 50: 29–43.
17. Hoffman LR, Kulasekara HD, Emerson J, Houston LS, Burns JL, et al. (2009) *Pseudomonas aeruginosa lasR* mutants are associated with cystic fibrosis lung disease progression. J Cyst Fibros 8: 66–70.
18. Rada B, Leto TL (2013) Pyocyanin effects on respiratory epithelium: relevance in *Pseudomonas aeruginosa* airway infections. Trends Microbiol 21: 73–81.
19. Hunter RC, Klepac-Ceraj V, Lorenzi MM, Grotzinger H, Martin TR, et al. (2012) Phenazine content in the cystic fibrosis respiratory tract negatively correlates with lung function and microbial complexity. Am J Respir Cell Mol Biol 47: 738–745.
20. Bjarnsholt T, Alhede M, Alhede M, Eickhardt-Sørensen SR, Moser C, et al. (2013) The in vivo biofilm. Trends in microbiology 21: 466–474.
21. Fux CA, Costerton JW, Stewart PS, Stoodley P (2005) Survival strategies of infectious biofilms. Trends Microbiol 13: 34–40.
22. Foley I, Marsh P, Wellington EM, Smith AW, Brown MR (1999) General stress response master regulator *rpoS* is expressed in human infection: a possible role in chronicity. J Antimicrob Chemother 43: 164–165.
23. Xu KD, Franklin MJ, Park CH, McFeters GA, Stewart PS (2001) Gene expression and protein levels of the stationary phase sigma factor, RpoS, in continuously-fed *Pseudomonas aeruginosa* biofilms. FEMS Microbiol Lett 199: 67–71.
24. Mah TF, O'Toole GA (2001) Mechanisms of biofilm resistance to antimicrobial agents. Trends Microbiol 9: 34–39.
25. Palmer KL, Aye LM, Whiteley M (2007) Nutritional cues control *Pseudomonas aeruginosa* multicellular behavior in cystic fibrosis sputum. J Bacteriol 189: 8079–8087.
26. Navarro Llorens JM, Tormo A, Martinez-Garcia E (2010) Stationary phase in gram-negative bacteria. FEMS Microbiol Rev 34: 476–495.
27. Jensen V, Lons D, Zaoui C, Bredenbruch F, Meissner A, et al. (2006) RhlR expression in *Pseudomonas aeruginosa* is modulated by the *Pseudomonas* quinolone signal via PhoB-dependent and -independent pathways. J Bacteriol 188: 8601–8606.
28. Deziel E, Lepine F, Milot S, He J, Mindrinos MN, et al. (2004) Analysis of *Pseudomonas aeruginosa* 4-hydroxy-2-alkylquinolines (HAQs) reveals a role for 4-hydroxy-2-heptylquinoline in cell-to-cell communication. Proc Natl Acad Sci U S A 101: 1339–1344.
29. Gallagher LA, McKnight SL, Kuznetsova MS, Pesci EC, Manoil C (2002) Functions required for extracellular quinolone signaling by *Pseudomonas aeruginosa*. J Bacteriol 184: 6472–6480.

30. Lee J, Wu J, Deng Y, Wang J, Wang C, et al. (2013) A cell-cell communication signal integrates quorum sensing and stress response. Nat Chem Biol.
31. Rampioni G, Schuster M, Greenberg EP, Bertani I, Grasso M, et al. (2007) RsaL provides quorum sensing homeostasis and functions as a global regulator of gene expression in *Pseudomonas aeruginosa*. Mol Microbiol 66: 1557–1565.
32. de Kievit T, Seed PC, Nezezon J, Passador L, Iglewski BH (1999) RsaL, a novel repressor of virulence gene expression in *Pseudomonas aeruginosa*. J Bacteriol 181: 2175–2184.
33. Rampioni G, Polticelli F, Bertani I, Righetti K, Venturi V, et al. (2007) The *Pseudomonas* quorum-sensing regulator RsaL belongs to the tetrahelical superclass of H-T-H proteins. J Bacteriol 189: 1922–1930.
34. Dandekar AA, Chugani S, Greenberg EP (2012) Bacterial quorum sensing and metabolic incentives to cooperate. Science 338: 264–266.
35. Van Delden C, Pesci EC, Pearson JP, Iglewski BH (1998) Starvation selection restores elastase and rhamnolipid production in a *Pseudomonas aeruginosa* quorum-sensing mutant. Infect Immun 66: 4499–4502.
36. Alvarez-Ortega C, Harwood CS (2007) Responses of *Pseudomonas aeruginosa* to low oxygen indicate that growth in the cystic fibrosis lung is by aerobic respiration. Mol Microbiol 65: 153–165.
37. Worlitzsch D, Tarran R, Ulrich M, Schwab U, Cekici A, et al. (2002) Effects of reduced mucus oxygen concentration in airway *Pseudomonas* infections of cystic fibrosis patients. J Clin Invest 109: 317–325.
38. Rampioni G, Schuster M, Greenberg EP, Zennaro E, Leoni L (2009) Contribution of the RsaL global regulator to *Pseudomonas aeruginosa* virulence and biofilm formation. FEMS Microbiol Lett 301: 210–217.

Voice Disorder in Cystic Fibrosis Patients

Bruna Mendes Lourenço[1,2], Kauê Machado Costa[1¤a¤b], Manoel da Silva Filho[1*]

1 Institute of Biological Sciences, Federal University of Pará, Belém, Pará, Brazil, 2 João de Barros Barreto University Hospital, Federal University of Pará, Belém, Pará, Brazil

Abstract

Cystic fibrosis is a common autosomal recessive disorder with drastic respiratory symptoms, including shortness of breath and chronic cough. While most of cystic fibrosis treatment is dedicated to mitigating the effects of respiratory dysfunction, the potential effects of this disease on vocal parameters have not been systematically studied. We hypothesized that cystic fibrosis patients, given their characteristic respiratory disorders, would also present dysphonic symptoms. Given that voice disorders can severely impair quality of life, the identification of a potential cystic fibrosis-related dysphonia could be of great value for the clinical evaluation and treatment of this disease. We tested our hypothesis by measuring vocal parameters, using both objective physical measures and the GRBAS subjective evaluation method, in male and female cystic fibrosis patients undergoing conventional treatment and compared them to age and sex matched controls. We found that cystic fibrosis patients had a significantly lower vocal intensity and harmonic to noise ratio, as well as increased levels of jitter and shimmer. In addition, cystic fibrosis patients also showed higher scores of roughness, breathiness and asthenia, as well as a significantly altered general grade of dysphonia. When we segregated the results according to sex, we observed that, as a group, only female cystic fibrosis patients had significantly lower values of harmonic to noise ratio and an abnormal general grade of dysphonia in relation to matched controls, suggesting that cystic fibrosis exerts a more pronounced effect on vocal parameters of women in relation to men. Overall, the dysphonic characteristics of CF patients can be explained by dysfunctions in vocal fold movement and partial upper airway obstruction, potentially caused by the accumulation of mucus and chronic cough characteristic of CF symptomatology. Our results show that CF patients exhibit significant dysphonia and suggest they may potentially benefit from voice therapy as a parallel treatment strategy.

Editor: Donald A. Robin, University of Texas Health Science Center at San Antonio, Research Imaging Institute, United States of America

Funding: This study was supported by the Federal University of Pará and the João de Barros Barreto University Hospital. MSF is a research fellow of the National Council for Research and Development (CNPQ). The funders had no role in study design, data collection and analysis, decision to publish, or preparation of the manuscript. Funder's websites: http://www.ufpa.br/, http://www.barrosbarreto.ufpa.br/, http://www.cnpq.br/.

Competing Interests: The authors have declared that no competing interests exist.

* E-mail: manoel@ufpa.br

¤a Current address: International Max Planck Research School for Neural Circuits, Max Planck Institute for Brain Research, Frankfurt am Main, Germany
¤b Current address: Institute for Neurophysiology, Johann Wolfgang Goethe University Frankfurt, Frankfurt am Main, Germany

Introduction

Voice disorders, or dysphonias, can be caused by neurological, structural or functional problems affecting breathing, phonation, articulation, resonance and prosody or the production of sounds at the level of the larynx [1]. A variety of respiratory tract disorders, including chronic cough and laryngeal tension, can lead to reduced voice quality [2]. Dysphonias can cause severe drawbacks in communication and significantly impair quality of life [3,4]. Given the importance of vocal communication to human interaction, subjects with abnormal voice patterns are at high risk for anxiety disorders and depression [5]. Patients with voice disorders score significantly lower on all health status subscales, as measured by the SF-36 form, a highly validated questionnaire assessing quality of life [4].

Cystic fibrosis (CF) is a common autosomal recessive disorder, with a prevalence of approximately 1:2500 live births in people of European descent [6]. This disease is caused by mutations in the cystic fibrosis transmembrane regulator gene, which encodes an epithelial chloride channel. Dysfunctions in this ion channel lead to abnormal transport of chloride and sodium across epithelial membranes and result in the production of thick, viscous secretions in various organs, including the respiratory tract [6,7]. Respiratory dysfunctions, such as shortness of breath and chronic cough, are a hallmark of CF and a major cause of morbidity in CF patients. Therefore, in current medical practice a large part of CF treatment is dedicated to mitigating the effects of respiratory dysfunction [7,8]. However, the potential effects of CF respiratory complications on the vocal capacity of CF patients have not been studied in detail.

We hypothesized that CF patients, given their characteristic respiratory disorders, would also present intrinsic voice alterations. If this is true, CF patients could potentially benefit from voice therapy as a way to improve their quality of life. We tested our hypothesis by measuring vocal parameters, using both objective and subjective clinical evaluation methods, in male and female CF patients undergoing conventional treatment and compared them to age and sex matched controls.

Methods

Subject selection and Ethics Statement

Subjects aged between 10 and 30 years were divided into four groups: a male control group ($n = 25$), a female control group ($n = 16$), male patients with CF ($n = 15$) and female patients with CF ($n = 8$). For some analyses, CF patients ($n = 23$) and control subjects ($n = 41$) were pooled independently of their sex. CF patients were diagnosed based on the standard sweat test, family

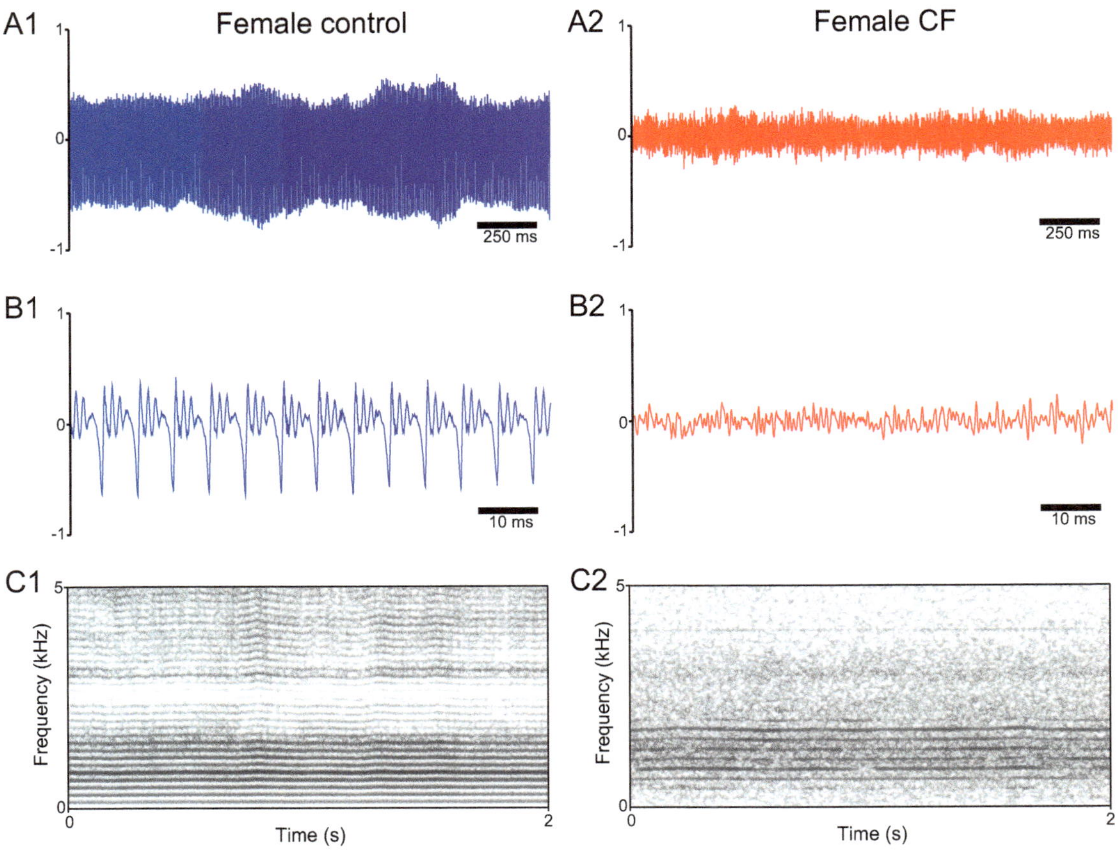

Figure 1. Representative voice recordings and spectrograms of female patients with CF (red) and healthy controls (blue). A: Sound recordings of/a/vowel phonations from a female control subject (A1) and a female patient with CF (A2); note the markedly reduced amplitude range of the signal from the CF patient in relation to the control. B: Amplified views of the recordings presented in A1 and A2; note the irregularity of the voice signal from the CF patient in relation to the control. C: Spectrogram (frequency domain) representations of the recordings presented in A1 and A2; note the higher level of background noise and low formant segregation in the CF patient in relation to the healthy control.

history and the presence of chronic pulmonary disease and pancreatic insufficiency. Previous laryngoscopic examination (conducted prophylactically as part of the patients' clinical monitoring) confirmed that the selected CF patients had no drastic vocal cord dysfunctions or laryngeal diseases, such as vocal cord polyps, laryngeal carcinoma or laryngeal paralysis. CF patients and control subjects had never received voice therapy.

Patients with CF were receiving, individually, regular treatment accompanied by physician, dietician, physiotherapist and psychologist. At the time of the study, none of the CF patients had signs of infection and were not being medicated with inhalatory antibiotics or hypertonic saline. Further information on the clinical status of the subjects can be found in Tables S1–S4, including body mass index (BMI) and FEV1 (a common measure of lung function defined as the volume of air that is exhaled in the first second of forced expiration and normalized by the mean values for the population). The low number of CF patients of each sex is a limitation of this study and was due to the limited pool of willing CF patients which fitted the necessary criteria. This study was approved by the research ethics committee of the João de Barros Barreto University Hospital (#112/09) and all subjects or their legal caretakers signed an informed consent form.

Vocal recordings

Subjects were asked to produce a sustained/a/vowel phonation in their usual intensity for a maximum voicing time. Voice recordings were conducted using a hand-held microphone (PG42-LC, Shure) always positioned six centimeters from the subject's mouth and at a 45° angle to ensure comparable intensity measurements. The initial second of the recording was always excluded from the analysis and parameters were measured over the three second time window that followed this period. Signals were recorded with a sampling rate of 44.1 kHz and analyzed with the Praat 5.1.36 software.

Objective vocal analysis

We measured the following quantitative vocal parameters: fundamental frequency (F_0), intensity, jitter (index of F_0 variability), shimmer (index of intensity variability) and the harmonics to noise ratio (HNR; index of glottal turbulence noise and hoarseness). These parameters have been extensively validated as quantitative, objective measures of vocal quality and are routinely used by voice care professionals as diagnostic tools [9]. Low values of vocal intensity and HNR, high values of jitter and shimmer and altered F_0 are all potential signs of dysphonia.

Subjective vocal analysis

In addition to these objective acoustic variables, we also conducted a perceptual assessment of voice quality in CF and control subjects using the GRBAS (Grade, Roughness, Breathiness, Asthenia, Strain) scale [10]. This vocal assessment method evaluates a patient's general grade of dysphonia (represented by

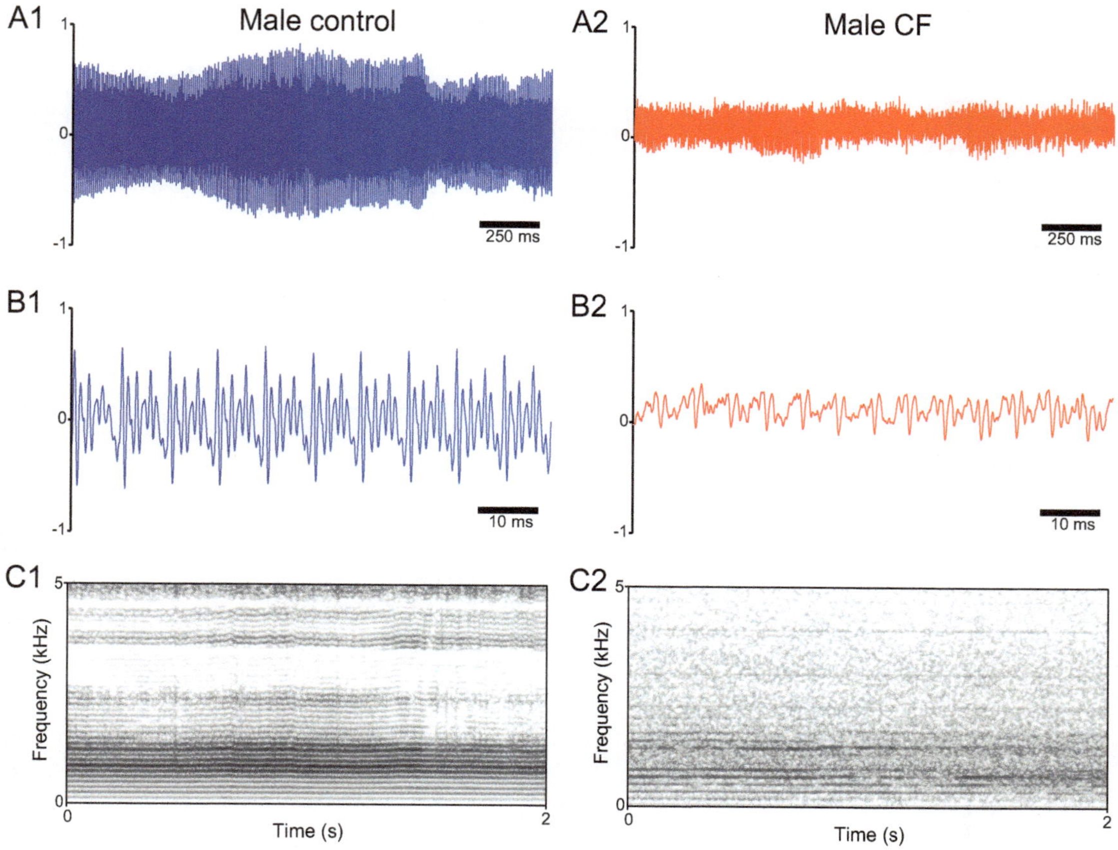

Figure 2. Representative voice recordings and spectrograms of male patients with CF (red) and healthy controls (blue). A: Sound recordings of/a/vowel phonations from a male control subject (A1) and a male patient with CF (A2); note the markedly reduced amplitude range of the signal from the CF patient in relation to the control. B: Amplified views of the recordings presented in A1 and A2; note the irregularity of the voice signal from the CF patient in relation to the control. C: Spectrogram (frequency domain) representations of the recordings presented in A1 and A2; note the higher level of background noise and low formant segregation in the CF patient in relation to the healthy control.

the letter G) through four subjective parameters: roughness (R), breathiness (B), asthenia (A), and strain (S). These variables are determined by a voice care professional, who quantifies his perception of the patients voice as zero (normal), one (mild alteration), two (moderate alteration) or three (severe alteration) on each of the abovementioned factors. The reliability of this method has been extensively validated [10–13]. In order to avoid any confirmation bias in our analyses, we asked an independent practicing clinical voice therapist, with no ties to the research project, to perform the GRBAS evaluation of all our recordings. The evaluator received the recordings in a pseudo-randomized order and was completely blind to the structure of the experimental protocol, the project's objective and the identification and diagnosis of each subject. The evaluator had 9 years of professional experience in voice therapy and GRBAS analysis methods and was instructed to analyze our recordings exactly as it would be performed in clinical practice.

Data analysis and statistics

Differences in objective and subjective vocal parameters were evaluated with the Mann-Whitney test. Data distribution was non-Gaussian for many variables, as defined by the Shapiro-Wilk normality test (Table S5), and therefore data are represented as median values or median and interquartile range (IQR). Statistical significance level was initially set at $P<0.05$; to account for multiple comparisons within the objective and subjective categories of vocal parameters, the Bonferroni correction method was applied. This procedure adjusted the significance level to $P<0.01$ for all analyses.

Results

Representative recordings

Voice signal recordings and spectrograms of representative individuals from all studied groups are shown in Figures 1 and 2. In the control group, recordings show clear features of a euphonic voice [14], such as high periodicity and wide amplitude ranges (Figures 1-B1 and 2-B1). In contrast, signals from subjects in the CF group showed remarkable aperiodicity and reduced amplitude (Figures 1-B2 and 2-B2). The spectrograms of CF patients also showed high noise levels and the loss of high frequency harmonics in relation to the controls (Figures 1-C2 and 2-C2).

CF-related changes in vocal parameters

Analysis of objective voice parameters revealed that CF patients presented a significant decrease in intensity (Figure 3-B; $P<0.0001$), an increase in jitter (Figure 3-C: $P<0.0001$) and shimmer (Figure 3-D; $P<0.0001$) and a much lower HNR (Figure 3-E; $P<0.0001$) in relation to controls. No differences were observed in F_0 (Figure 3-A; $P>0.01$) between the two groups.

The perceptual assessment of voice quality on the GRBAS scale also revealed clear signs of dysphonia in CF patients. In relation to

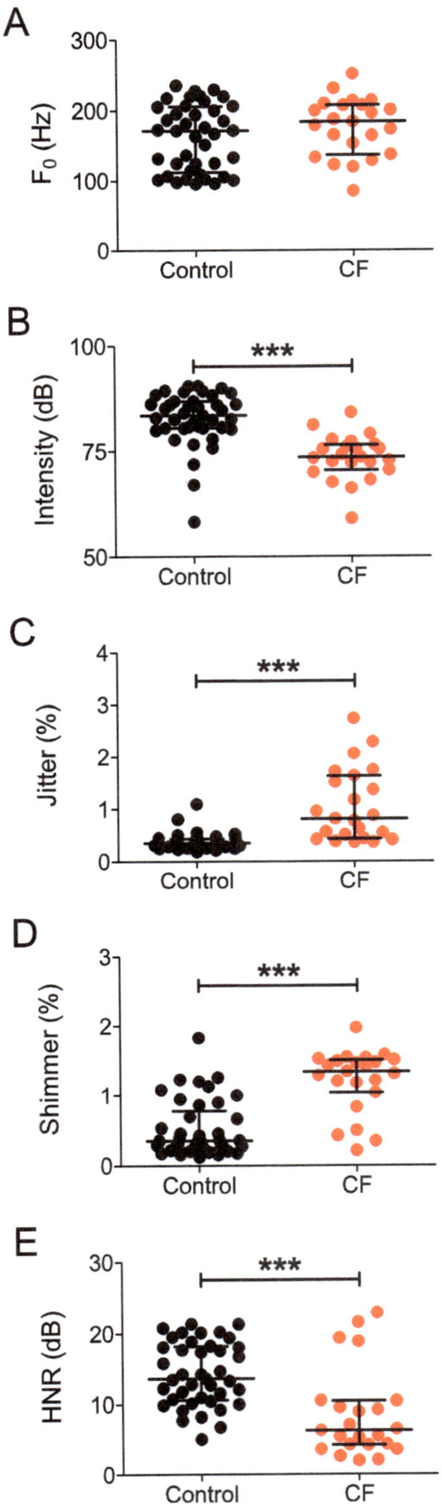

Figure 3. Objective measurements of vocal parameters of control subjects and CF patients. Horizontal lines and error bars represent median±IQR for all variables. Subjects were pooled independently of their sex. **A:** Values of F_0 for each group. **B:** Values of intensity for each group; note the significant reduction in intensity in the CF group. **C:** Values of jitter for each group; note the significant increase in jitter in the CF group. **D:** Values of shimmer for each group; note the significant increase in shimmer in the CF group. **E:** Values of HNR for each group; note the significant reduction in this variable in the CF group. *** $= P < 0.0001$.

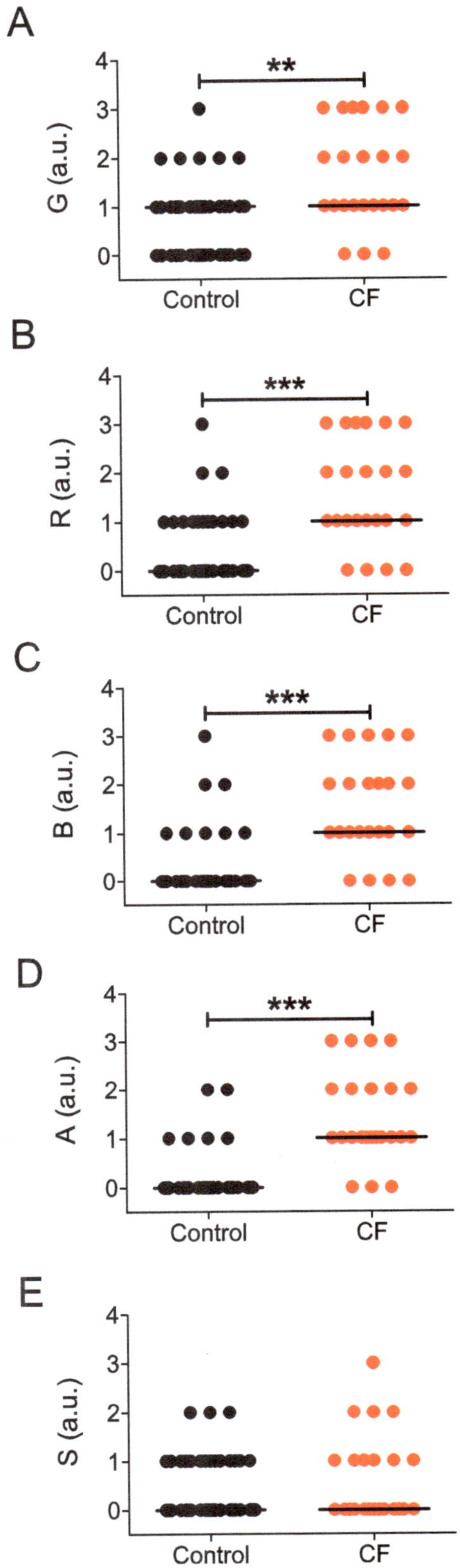

Figure 4. Subjective measurements of vocal parameters of male and female control subjects and CF patients. Horizontal lines and error bars represent the median value of each group. Subjects were pooled independently of their sex. **A:** Values of G for each group; note the significant increase in G in the CF group. **B:** Values of R for each group; note the significant increase in R in the CF group. **C:** Values

of B for each group; note the significant increase in B in the CF group. **D:** Values of A for each group; note the significant increase in A in the CF group. **E:** Values of S for each group. ** $= P<0.001$; *** $= P<0.0001$.

the control group, patients with CF presented an overall increase in R (Figure 4-B; $P<0.0001$), B (Figure 4-C; $P<0.0001$) and A (Figure 4-D; $P<0.0001$). In addition, CF patients showed an increase in G in relation to controls (Figure 4-A; $P=0.0012$). Interestingly, no difference was observed in the S score between CF patients and healthy controls (Figure 4-E; $P>0.01$). All median values and IQRs for the studied variables and statistical comparisons between groups are summarized in Table S6.

It is important to note that it is highly unlikely that the CF-related changes in vocal parameters are related to the age or lung function of the subjects, as none of the objective variables that were affected in CF patients had any significant correlation with age or FEV1 (Figures S1 and S2; $r2<0.2$ and $P<0.01$ for correlations of age or FEV1 with intensity, jitter, shimmer and HNR).

Influence of sex in CF-related dysphonia

We also analyzed our data segregating the control and CF groups according to sex, in order to reveal any possible influence of sex in CF-related dysphonia. These analyses revealed that both male and female CF patients, in relation to their matched controls, presented a significant decrease in intensity (Figure 5-B1 and 5-B2; $P<0.0001$ for both males and females) and an increase in jitter (Figure 5-C1 and 5-C2; for males: $P=0.001$ for females and $P<0.0001$ for males) and shimmer (Figure 5-D1 and 5-D2; $P=0.0001$ for females and $P=0.0038$ for males). Interestingly, while female CF patients showed drastically lower values of HNR (Figure 5-E1; $P=0.0002$) in relation to the control group, this feature was not observed in male CF patients (Figure 5-E2; $P>0.01$) compared to their respective controls. No differences between CF patients and control subjects were observed in F_0 for both sexes (Figure 5-A1 and 5-A2; $P>0.01$ for both comparisons).

In relation to the subjective vocal parameters analyzed on the GRBAS scale, both male and female patients with CF presented an overall increase in R (Figure 6-B1 and 6-B2; $P=0.0019$ for females and $P=0.0025$ for males), B (Figure 6-C1 and 6-C2; $P=0.0003$ for females and $P=0.0004$ for males) and A (Figure 6-D1 and 6-D2; $P=0.0003$ for females and $P<0.0001$ for males) compared to matched controls. However, only female CF patients showed an increase in G in relation to controls (Figure 6-A1; $P=0.0081$), which was not observed in male subjects (Figure 6-A2; $P=0.0293$). No difference was observed in the S score between CF patients and healthy controls of both sexes (Figure 6-E1 and 6-E2; $P>0.01$ for both comparisons). All median values and IQRs for the studied variables and statistical comparisons between CF patients and control subjects segregated by sex are summarized in Table S7.

Discussion

Our results show that subjects with CF present significantly altered vocal parameters, both objectively and subjectively. To our knowledge, this is the first systematic investigation of voice dysfunction in CF. Our findings suggest that dysphonia is a relevant manifestation of CF pathology.

Objective vocal parameters affected by CF were intensity, jitter, shimmer and HNR. Changes in vocal intensity can be observed in cases of vocal microtrauma, neurological dysfunction and obstructive respiratory diseases [15]. Vocal intensity depends

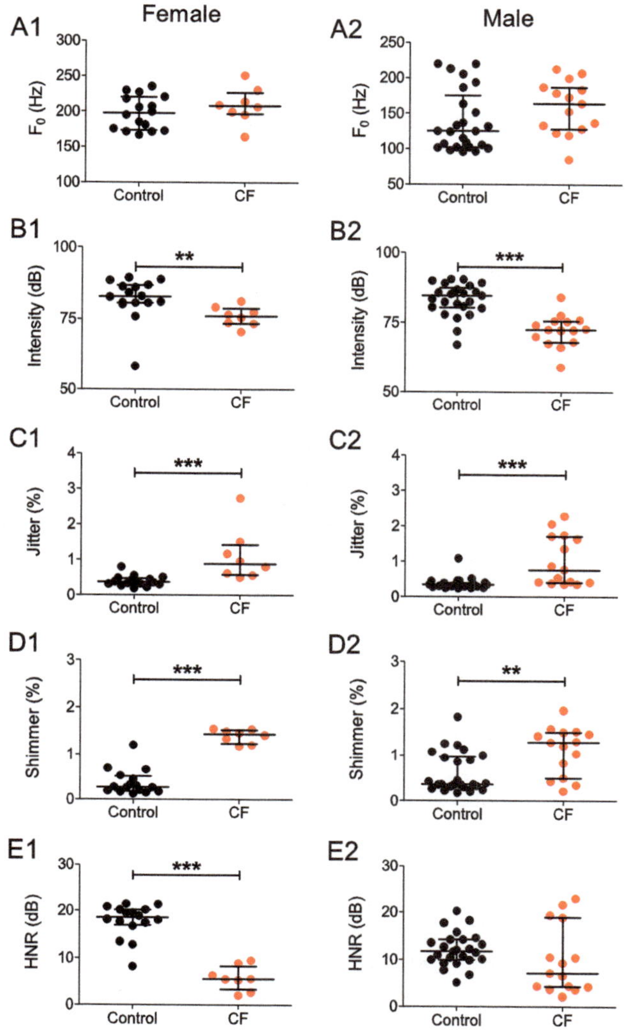

Figure 5. Objective measurements of vocal parameters of male and female control subjects and CF patients. Horizontal lines and error bars represent median±IQR for all variables. **A:** Values of F_0 for female (A1) and male (A2) subject groups. **B:** Values of intensity for female (A1) and male (A2) subject groups. **C:** Values of jitter for female (A1) and male (A2) subject groups. **D:** Values of shimmer for female (A1) and male (A2) subject groups. **E:** Values of HNR for female (A1) and male (A2) subject groups; note that only female CF patients have a lower HNR in relation to the matched controls. ** $= P<0.001$; *** $= P<0.0001$.

fundamentally of subglottal air pressure, upper airway airflow and glottal resistance [16]. The observed decrease in intensity in CF patients could thus be explained by the inefficient lung function and partial upper airway obstruction characteristic of CF physiopathology [6,8]. Chronic cough, a major symptom of CF, could also contribute to this effect [2,6,7,15].

Changes in jitter and shimmer are typically related to irregularities in vocal fold vibration, and are also usually related to vocal harshness and the presence of noise in the vocal signal [9,17,18]. The differences in these variables observed in our dataset can be due to the presence of thick mucous secretions in the vocal folds of CF patients, which can potentially interfere in the oscillatory motion of the vocal folds [19,20]. In addition, chronic cough is also known to cause dysfunction of vocal fold movement [2].

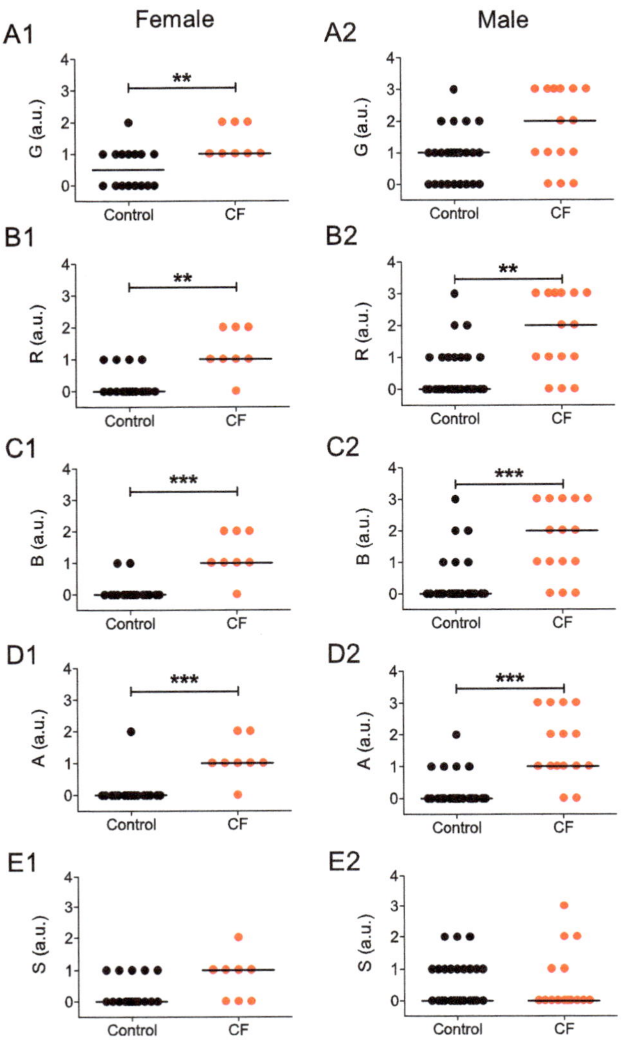

Figure 6. Subjective measurements of vocal parameters of male and female control subjects and CF patients. Horizontal lines and error bars represent the median value of each group. **A:** Values of G for female (A1) and male (A2) subject groups; note that only female patients have a significant change in G in relation to the matched controls. **B:** Values of R for female (A1) and male (A2) subject groups. **C:** Values of B for female (A1) and male (A2) subject groups. **D:** Values of A for female (A1) and male (A2) subject groups. **E:** Values of S for female (A1) and male (A2) subject groups. ** $=P<0.001$; *** $=P<0.0001$.

Decreases in HNR are caused by increases in the variation of vocal amplitude and frequency and in upper airway turbulence. This produces distortions in the vocal signal, emphasizing the sub-harmonic components and vocal breaks and, consequently, reducing the relative contribution of harmonic components to the overall vocal signal [21]. More importantly, it has been reported that high vocal noise (low HNR) is the most characteristic sign of dysphonia [13]. CF patients showed drastically low HNR values, which can be considered pathologically hoarse and highly detrimental to a normal voice production [15,22]. This decrease in HNR could have the same physiological underpinning as the changes in jitter and shimmer, namely the accumulation of mucus and chronic cough.

The changes in objective vocal parameters in CF patients were confirmed in the subjective evaluation of vocal quality using the GRBAS scale. CF patients showed significant differences in most perceptual vocal parameters, with the exception of S [23]. Previous studies have shown that increases in R and B are strongly related with increases in shimmer [23], which is in agreement with our finding that all three variables are higher in CF patients in relation to the controls. Increases in A are caused by decreases in airflow rate in the upper airways, a common feature of many respiratory diseases [24]. In these cases, subglottal pressure does not rise to the appropriate levels during voice production, causing asthenia and hoarseness. In our dataset of CF patients, this feature can be related to the observed decrease in intensity.

Differences in G represent the general degree of vocal disorder, i.e. a subjective summation of all other perceptual parameters [11,12]. This makes G the most important index within the GRBAS scale [10]. The significantly higher values of G in CF patients indicated that the individual changes in R, B and A combine to produce a noticeable condition of dysphonia.

A notable finding of our study is that female CF patients appear to have more vocal alterations in relation to the controls than male CF patients. When data from each sex was analyzed separately, only female CF patients presented significant lower values of HNR, and higher values of G compared to matched controls. This difference between sexes may be due to the intrinsic differences in the structure of the vocal apparatus observed between men and women. On average, men have thicker vocal folds, larger glottal area and airflow, and lower laryngeal airway resistance than women [25–28]. Our data show that CF vocal pathology is probably due to disorders in vocal fold oscillation and obstruction of the upper airways, and these dysfunctions can be exacerbated when associated to thinner vocal folds and higher airway resistance, respectively. Taken together, these gender-related structural differences are likely to be a major factor in making female patients more susceptible to CF-related dysphonia.

In addition, several other studies have reported that healthy males have voices with significantly lower HNR than healthy females across different languages and age ranges [29–32]. This is also the case in our dataset, as recordings from male control subjects had significantly lower HNRs than female control subjects (Figure 5-E1 and 5-E2; $P=0.0001$ between female and male controls). This intrinsic difference might be explained both by the already mentioned gender related differences in the structure of the vocal apparatus and by social influences, as some authors speculate that women have better vocal training than men, as they use their voices more frequently [29]. Because the perception of what is a normal or appropriate voice depends on what is expected from a person's gender, age and social group, deviations in vocal parameters must be compared with matched controls. Indeed, because healthy women might be expected to have higher HNRs than men, it is fair to predict that the significantly larger decrease in HNR observed in female CF patients might have a highly deleterious impact in their quality of life.

Our data suggests that, as a group, only female patients have their voices affected by the pathophysiology of CF to a degree in which the general perception of their voice, and presumably its communication function, is significantly affected. Nevertheless, it is important to point out that 6 out of 15 subjects in the male CF patient group also presented very low values of HNR (under 5dB), even though the median values of the group were not significantly different from the control. In addition, 6 male CF subjects also presented levels of G above 2, while no such values were observed in the male control group. This would mean that, even though female CF patients might be more susceptible to the deleterious effects of CF on vocal capacity (and thus present more dysphonic symptoms than males), some individual male CF patients might also develop significant changes in HNR and G.

Our results open the possibility that CF patients may benefit from voice therapy as a clinical intervention strategy to reduce dysphonia and increase life quality. Voice therapy consists of a series of techniques applied to the mitigation of voice disorders, which include enhancing the patient's awareness of his or her dysphonia, application of vocal health guidelines, hearing training, muscle relaxation and psychodynamic vocal training [33,34]. This form of therapy has been shown to be an effective treatment in reducing dysphonic symptoms in several diseases, including respiratory disorders, and is capable of at least partially restoring quality of life to affected patients [35–37].

The dysphonic characteristics observed in CF patients can be potentially attributed to dysfunctions in vocal fold movement and partial upper airway obstruction, both of which can be caused by the accumulation of mucus and chronic cough, which are standard symptoms of CF respiratory pathology. While there is no available data on which therapy would be adequate for CF patients, therapy for vocal disorders with hyperfunctional origins have been shown to be effective in patients with chronic cough [2]. Given that chronic cough is a major manifestation of CF pathology, this strategy could potentially be applied to CF patients. This type of intervention is usually based on voice education and vocal hygiene as strategies for cough suppression and also applies exercises that improve dysfunctional vocal fold vibration [2], which according to our data are probably the major features of CF-related dysphonia. Of course, further studies must be conducted to confirm the efficacy of this form of treatment, as well as any other form of voice therapy, for patients with CF.

Conclusion

We showed that patients with CF exhibit symptoms of dysphonia, with changes in both objective and subjective vocal parameters. This may be a relevant feature of CF pathology and morbidity. Voice alterations were more pronounced in female patients, which exhibited a marked reduction in both HNR and overall subjective voice quality. Our results suggest that CF patients might potentially benefit from voice therapy.

Supporting Information

Figure S1 Linear correlation analyses between age and objective vocal parameters for the control and CF groups. *P* values indicate if the slope of the linear regression line is significantly different from zero. **A:** Linear correlation between age and F_0 for each group; note that there is a relatively high inverse correlation (r^2 around 0.2) between these two variables in both the control and CF groups. **B:** Linear correlation between age and intensity for each group. **C:** Linear correlation between age and jitter for each group. **D:** Linear correlation between age and shimmer for each group. **E:** Linear correlation between age and HNR for each group. ** = $P<0.001$.

Figure S2 Linear correlation analyses between FEV1 and objective vocal parameters in the CF group. FEV1 is a common measure of lung function, defined as the volume of air that is exhaled in the first second of forced expiration and normalized to the mean values for the population. *P* values indicate if the slope of the linear regression line is significantly different from zero. Note that only very small correlations were found between FEV1 and each objective vocal parameter. **A:** Linear correlation between FEV1 and F_0 for each group. **B:** Linear correlation between FEV1 and intensity. **C:** Linear correlation between FEV1 and jitter. **D:** Linear correlation between FEV1 and shimmer. **E:** Linear correlation between FEV1 and HNR.

Table S1 Age and body mass index (BMI) for all subjects of the female control group.

Table S2 Age and body mass index (BMI) for all subjects of the male control group.

Table S3 Age, body mass index (BMI), FEV1 and medical status of the female cystic fibrosis group.

Table S4 Age, body mass index (BMI), FEV1 and medical status of the male cystic fibrosis group.

Table S5 Summary of mean ± standard error values and normality test results for all studied groups.

Table S6 Summary of median and IQR values for pooled data of CF and control subjects, with statistical comparison including values for the Mann-Whitney U (U), Z-score (Z), effect size (r) and P.

Table S7 Summary of median and IQR values for data of CF and control subjects segregated according to sex, with statistical comparison including values for the Mann-Whitney U (U), Z-score (Z), effect size (r) and P.

Acknowledgments

We thank Dr. Francisco Palheta Neto for his assistance in diagnosing and selecting the subjects. We also thank Milena Freitas for performing the blind GRBAS evaluation of our acoustic data. We are grateful to Ivaylo Borislavov Iotchev and Dr. Felipe Camargo Munhoz for critically reviewing the manuscript and providing important suggestions.

Author Contributions

Conceived and designed the experiments: BML MSF. Performed the experiments: BML. Analyzed the data: BML KMC. Contributed reagents/materials/analysis tools: BML KMC MSF. Wrote the paper: KMC BML MSF.

References

1. Cohen SM, Elackattu A, Noordzij JP, Walsh MJ, Langmore SE (2009) Palliative Treatment of Dysphonia and Dysarthria. Otolaryngol Clin North Am 42: 107–121. doi:10.1016/j.otc.2008.09.010.
2. Gibson PG, Vertigan AE (2009) Speech pathology for chronic cough: a new approach. Pulm Pharmacol Ther 22: 159–162. doi:10.1016/j.pupt.2008.11.005.
3. Murry T, Medrado R, Hogikyan ND, Aviv JE (2004) The relationship between ratings of voice quality and quality of life measures. J Voice 18: 183–192. doi:10.1016/j.jvoice.2003.11.003.
4. Wilson JA, Deary IJ, Millar A, Mackenzie K (2002) The quality of life impact of dysphonia. Clin Otolaryngol Allied Sci 27: 179–182.
5. Deary IJ, Scott S, Wilson IM, White A, MacKenzie K, et al. (1997) Personality and psychological distress in dysphonia. Br J Health Psychol 2: 333–341. doi:10.1111/j.2044-8287.1997.tb00547.x.
6. Ratjen F, Döring G (2003) Cystic fibrosis. The Lancet 361: 681–689. doi:10.1016/S0140-6736(03)12567-6.

7. Yankaskas JR, Marshall BC, Sufian B, Simon RH, Rodman D (2004) Cystic fibrosis adult care: consensus conference report. Chest 125: 1S–39S.
8. Zemanick ET, Harris JK, Conway S, Konstan MW, Marshall B, et al. (2010) Measuring and improving respiratory outcomes in cystic fibrosis lung disease: opportunities and challenges to therapy. J Cyst Fibros Off J Eur Cyst Fibros Soc 9: 1–16. doi:10.1016/j.jcf.2009.09.003.
9. Baken RJ, Orlikoff RF (2000) Clinical Measurement of Speech and Voice. Cengage Learning. 628 p.
10. Hirano M (1981) Clinical examination of voice. Springer London, Limited. 124 p.
11. Nemr K, Simões-Zenari M, Cordeiro GF, Tsuji D, Ogawa AI, et al. (2012) GRBAS and Cape-V scales: high reliability and consensus when applied at different times. J Voice 26: 812.e17–22. doi:10.1016/j.jvoice.2012.03.005.
12. De Bodt MS, Wuyts FL, Van de Heyning PH, Croux C (1997) Test-retest study of the GRBAS scale: Influence of experience and professional background on perceptual rating of voice quality. J Voice 11: 74–80. doi:10.1016/S0892-1997(97)80026-4.
13. Bhuta T, Patrick L, Garnett JD (2004) Perceptual evaluation of voice quality and its correlation with acoustic measurements. J Voice Off J Voice Found 18: 299–304. doi:10.1016/j.jvoice.2003.12.004.
14. Kosztyła-Hojna B, Andrzejewska A, Moskal D, Rogowski M, Falkowski D, et al. (2011) Morphological aspects of the euphonic voice. Folia Histochem Cytobiol Pol Acad Sci Pol Histochem Cytochem Soc 49: 72–79.
15. Pontes PAL, Vieira VP, Gonçalves MIR, Pontes AAL (2002) Characteristics of hoarse, rough and normal voices: acoustic spectrographic comparative analysis. Rev Bras Otorrinolaringol 68: 182–188. doi:10.1590/S0034-72992002000200005.
16. Hodge FS, Colton RH, Kelley RT (2001) Vocal intensity characteristics in normal and elderly speakers. J Voice 15: 503–511. doi:10.1016/S0892-1997(01)00050-9.
17. Yelken K, Gultekin E, Guven M, Eyibilen A, Aladag I (2010) Impairment of voice quality in paradoxical vocal fold motion dysfunction. J Voice 24: 724–727. doi:10.1016/j.jvoice.2009.05.004.
18. Maryn Y, Corthals P, De Bodt M, Van Cauwenberge P, Deliyski D (2009) Perturbation measures of voice: a comparative study between Multi-Dimensional Voice Program and Praat. Folia Phoniatr Logop Off Organ Int Assoc Logop Phoniatr IALP 61: 217–226. doi:10.1159/000227999.
19. Grini-Grandval MN, Bingenheimer S, Maunsell R, Ouaknine M, Giovanni A (2002) Phonatory threshold pressure in a healthy population before and after aerosol treatment, a preliminary study. Rev Laryngol - Otol - Rhinol 123: 311–314.
20. Verdonck-de Leeuw IM, Festen JM, Mahieu HF (2001) Deviant vocal fold vibration as observed during videokymography: the effect on voice quality. J Voice Off J Voice Found 15: 313–322. doi:10.1016/S0892-1997(01)00033-9.
21. Franca MC (2012) Acoustic comparison of vowel sounds among adult females. J Voice 26: 671.e9–17. doi:10.1016/j.jvoice.2011.11.010.
22. Yumoto E, Gould WJ, Baer T (1982) Harmonics-to-noise ratio as an index of the degree of hoarseness. J Acoust Soc Am 71: 1544–1549.
23. Lopes LW, Barbosa Lima IL, Alves Almeida LN, Cavalcante DP, de Almeida AAF (2012) Severity of voice disorders in children: correlations between perceptual and acoustic data. J Voice 26: 819.e7–12. doi:10.1016/j.jvoice.2012.05.008.
24. Omori K (2011) Diagnosis of Voice Disorders. JMAJ 54: 248–253.
25. Hollien H (1962) Vocal fold thickness and fundamental frequency of phonation. J Speech Hear Res 5: 237–243.
26. Holmes LC, Leeper HA, Nicholson IR (1994) Laryngeal Airway Resistance of Older Men and Women as a Function of Vocal Sound Pressure Level. J Speech Hear Res 37: 789–799.
27. Lucero JC, Koenig LL (2005) Simulations of temporal patterns of oral airflow in men and women using a two-mass model of the vocal folds under dynamic control. J Acoust Soc Am 117: 1362–1372. doi:10.1121/1.1853235.
28. Holmberg EB, Hillman RE, Perkell JS (1988) Glottal airflow and transglottal air pressure measurements for male and female speakers in soft, normal, and loud voice. J Acoust Soc Am 84: 511–529. doi:10.1121/1.396829.
29. Dehqan A, Ansari H, Bakhtiar M (2010) Objective voice analysis of Iranian speakers with normal voices. J Voice Off J Voice Found 24: 161–167. doi:10.1016/j.jvoice.2008.07.005.
30. Naufel de Felippe AC, Grillo MHMM, Grechi TH (2006) Standardization of acoustic measures for normal voice patterns. Braz J Otorhinolaryngol 72: 659–664.
31. Ferrand CT (2000) Harmonics-to-noise ratios in normally speaking prepubescent girls and boys. J Voice Off J Voice Found 14: 17–21.
32. Toran KC, Lal BK (2009) Objective analysis of voice in normal young adults. Kathmandu Univ Med J KUMJ 7: 374–377.
33. Holmberg EB, Hillman RE, Hammarberg B, Södersten M, Doyle P (2001) Efficacy of a behaviorally based voice therapy protocol for vocal nodules. J Voice 15: 395–412. doi:10.1016/S0892-1997(01)00041-8.
34. Schindler A, Mozzanica F, Maruzzi P, Atac M, De Cristofaro V, et al. (2013) Multidimensional assessment of vocal changes in benign vocal fold lesions after voice therapy. Auris Nasus Larynx 40: 291–297. doi:10.1016/j.anl.2012.08.003.
35. Gartner-Schmidt JL, Roth DF, Zullo TG, Rosen CA (2013) Quantifying Component Parts of Indirect and Direct Voice Therapy Related to Different Voice Disorders. J Voice 27: 210–216. doi:10.1016/j.jvoice.2012.11.007.
36. Speyer R (2008) Effects of Voice Therapy: A Systematic Review. J Voice 22: 565–580. doi:10.1016/j.jvoice.2006.10.005.
37. Mueller PB, Larson GW (1992) Voice therapy practices and techniques: A survey of voice clinicians. J Commun Disord 25: 251–260. doi:10.1016/0021-9924(92)90019-S.

11

Poor Survival in Rheumatoid Arthritis Associated with Bronchiectasis: A Family-Based Cohort Study

Xavier Puéchal[1,2]*, Emmanuelle Génin[3], Thierry Bienvenu[4], Claire Le Jeunne[1], Daniel J. Dusser[5]

1 National Referral Center for Rare Systemic Autoimmune Diseases, Department of Internal Medicine, Hôpital Cochin, Assistance Publique-Hôpitaux de Paris, Université Paris Descartes, Paris, France, **2** INSERM U1016, CNRS UMR 8104, Institut Cochin, Paris, France, **3** INSERM UMR-1078, Centre Hospitalier Universitaire, Brest, France, **4** Biochemistry and Molecular Biology Laboratory, Hôpital Cochin, Assistance Publique-Hôpitaux de Paris, Université Paris Descartes, Paris, France, **5** Department of Respiratory Diseases, Hôpital Cochin, Assistance Publique-Hôpitaux de Paris, Université Paris Descartes, Paris, France

Abstract

Background: Diffuse bronchiectasis (DB) may occur in rheumatoid arthritis (RA). *CFTR* (cystic fibrosis transmembrane conductance regulator) mutations predispose RA patients to DB, but the prognosis of RA-associated DB (RA-DB) is unclear.

Methods: We report long-term mortality data from a nationwide family-based association study of patients with RA only, DB only or RA-DB. We assessed mortality as a function of clinical characteristics and CF/*CFTR*-RD (*CFTR*-related disorders) mutations in 137 subjects from 24 kindreds. Potential risk factors were investigated by Cox proportional-hazard analysis with shared Gaussian random effects to account for within-family correlations.

Results: During a median follow-up of 11 years after inclusion, 18 patients died, mostly from cardiorespiratory causes. Survival was significantly lower for RA-DB patients than for unaffected relatives and for patients with RA or DB only. RA patients with DB had also a poorer prognosis in terms of survival after RA diagnosis (HR, 8.6; 95% CI, 1.5–48.2; $P = 0.014$) and from birth (HR, 9.6; 95% CI, 1.1–81.7; $P = 0.039$). Early onset of DB (HR, 15.4; 95% CI, 2.1–113.2; $P = 0.007$) and CF/*CFTR*-RD mutation (HR, 7.2; 95% CI, 1.4–37.1; $P = 0.018$) were associated with poorer survival in patients with RA-DB. Thus, CF/*CFTR*-RD mutations in RA patients with early-onset DB defined a subgroup of high-risk patients with higher mortality rates (log-rank test $P = 1.28 \times 10^{-5}$).

Conclusion: DB is associated with poorer survival in patients with RA. Early-onset DB and *CFTR* mutations are two markers that identify RA patients at a high risk of death, for whom future therapeutic interventions should be designed and evaluated.

Editor: Dominique Heymann, Faculté de médecine de Nantes, France

Funding: This work was supported by grants from the Assistance Publique-Hôpitaux de Paris (Contrat de Recherche et d'Innovation Clinique CRC98046) (to XP) and the Société Française de Rhumatologie (to XP). The funders had no role in study design, data collection and analysis, decision to publish, or preparation of the manuscript.

Competing Interests: The authors have declared that no competing interests exist.

* Email: xavier.puechal@cch.aphp.fr

Introduction

Rheumatoid arthritis (RA) is a systemic autoimmune disease, of unknown origin, that affects 0.5–1.0% of the adult population worldwide [1]. It primarily involves the joints, but extra-articular manifestations, such as lung involvement, have been observed and may increase the burden of this frequently disabling disease. Most studies in RA patients have reported higher mortality rates than for the general population and have shown that extra-articular manifestations contribute to premature death [2,3].

There is a well-established association between RA and diffuse bronchiectasis (DB). In prospective blind studies based on high-resolution computed tomography (HRCT) in patients with RA, the prevalence of diffuse bronchiectasis has been reported to range from 5.6% to 30% [4–9]. Conversely, RA is found in 2.7% to 5.2% of patients with DB referred to respiratory medicine departments for investigation [10,11]. In cases of symptomatic DB in RA patients, respiratory symptoms precede the onset of RA in more than 90% of cases, with a mean interval of more than 30 years between the onset of the two diseases (early-onset, mostly childhood DB) [10,12–16]. In less than 10% of patients, respiratory symptoms of DB occur concomitantly with the onset of arthritis (late-onset and adulthood DB) [17]. The prognosis of these two subtypes of DB in RA patients remains unclear. Recent data have suggested that the lung may be an early site of autoimmune-related injury in RA patients and a potential site involved in RA-related autoimmunity [18,19]. Further analyses of the link between RA and DB are, therefore, required.

Cystic fibrosis transmembrane conductance regulator (*CFTR*) gene mutations have been identified as the cause of cystic fibrosis (CF) [20], a disease associated with DB and impaired survival due to respiratory insufficiency in most cases [21]. Beside CF, some DB may be classified as *CFTR*-related diseases (*CFTR*-RD), defined as a clinical entity associated with CFTR dysfunction not fulfilling the diagnostic criteria for CF [22].

We previously reported a higher prevalence of CF/*CFTR*-RD mutations in patients suffering from RA-associated DB (RA-DB) than in the general population [16]. We found a strong association and linkage between mutations in the CF/*CFTR*-RD gene and RA-DB phenotypes in a French nationwide family-based association study [23]. CF/*CFTR*-RD mutations were five times more frequent in RA-DB patients than in patients with RA only (no DB) and cosegregated with RA-DB in the families. Furthermore, RA-DB patients carrying at least one abnormal *CFTR* allele but not fulfilling the diagnostic criteria for CF more frequently had chronic sinusitis, a trend toward more severe pulmonary involvement, and CFTR protein dysfunction, as demonstrated by the lower nasal potential difference of these patients than of patients with both RA and DB but without CF/*CFTR*-RD mutations [16]. These data suggest that CF/*CFTR*-RD mutations may predispose patients with RA to DB, but the vital prognosis of the RA-DB association has not been investigated in detail, and the influence of the clinical onset of DB and the presence of CF/*CFTR*-RD mutations on survival has not been studied.

We therefore investigated long-term mortality and variables predictive of the risk of death in a well characterized, prospectively followed family-based cohort of patients with a diagnosis of RA only, DB only, or RA-DB.

Methods

The study protocol was reviewed and approved by the institutional review board for clinical research of *Assistance Publique-Hôpitaux de Paris* and the ethics committee of the Medical Faculty of Paris Descartes University. Written informed consent was obtained from all participants.

Study population

The study was performed in a prospectively followed family-based cohort recruited between September 1999 and February 2002, which has been described elsewhere [23]. Briefly, for inclusion in the study, each family had to include at least one proband with both RA and symptomatic DB and one affected first-degree relative with RA and/or DB. Once a family was deemed eligible for inclusion, all affected subjects and unaffected relatives were interviewed and blood samples were taken for *CFTR* genotyping.

Interview and clinical assessment at inclusion

At inclusion, pedigree analysis was carried out and each family member underwent face-to-face semi-structured interviews and clinical assessment. Given the known association of RA and DB and the possibility of asymptomatic or paucisymptomatic DB, all RA patients underwent HRCT of the lungs. An HRCT scan of the lungs was also conducted for other participants presenting respiratory symptoms. All cases of DB were confirmed by two independent observers finding evidence of diffuse (more than one lobe) bronchiectasis on HRCT scan, without knowledge of the *CFTR* mutational status of the individual concerned. In patients with both RA and DB, DB was defined as early-onset DB if respiratory symptoms preceded RA by more than 10 years (mostly childhood DB) and as late-onset DB for patients whose respiratory symptoms occurred at the same time or less than 10 years before RA onset (adulthood DB). Participants were classified into four categories: RA-DB, RA without DB (RA only), DB only and unaffected.

CFTR genotyping

We checked the entire coding region and exon/intron junctions of *CFTR* for CF/*CFTR*-RD mutations, which were subsequently confirmed by direct DNA sequencing, as previously described [23]. Nucleotide substitutions were classified according to their known or predicted functional consequences [23] and groups of mutations were considered collectively in the analyses.

Survival

The primary outcome measure was survival between November 2011 and December 2012. Data were censored on December 31st, 2012. Vital status was recorded in this family-based cohort, with a new questionnaire that was sent to each participant and a follow-up interview carried out for all families. Information about the cause of death was collected retrospectively from a family questionnaire and medical reports. Survival from inclusion was determined for all participants and survival from birth and from RA diagnosis was also analyzed.

Statistical analysis

The characteristics of the patients (sex ratio, age at inclusion, age at diagnosis, median follow-up) were compared between the groups in chi-squared tests, Fisher's exact tests or Kruskal-Wallis tests, as appropriate.

Survival analysis was performed with the R package "survival" [24]. Kaplan-Meier survival curves were plotted with the "plot.survfit" function and the log-rank test, implemented in the "survdiff" function, was used to compare survival between groups.

We adjusted for the effect of covariates and estimated hazard ratios (HR) while accounting for family correlations, by fitting Cox models with Gaussian random effects models to the data with the R package "coxme" [25]. Each individual was assumed to have a random genetic risk, but risks were correlated between individuals according to the strength of their pedigree relationship, as assessed by their kinship coefficient. We report HR and 95% confidence intervals (95% CI) and the *P*-value of the *z* test.

We compared survival from inclusion, adjusted for age at inclusion, between the individuals included in the study, as a function of their disease status. We then focused on RA patients and compared their survival from birth and from RA diagnosis as a function of whether or not they had DB (comparison of RA-DB with RA only). Finally, we focused on patients with both RA and DB and investigated the factors potentially influencing their survival from birth or from RA diagnosis.

All analyses were conducted with R version 2.15.1 [26].

Results

Patients' characteristics

The family-based cohort comprised 137 subjects from 24 kindreds, including 30 patients with RA-DB, 25 patients with RA only and eight patients with DB only; the remaining participants constituted the unaffected relatives.

The main demographic features of the participants enrolled in the family-based cohort are shown in Table 1. The median follow-up time after inclusion was 10, 11, 11, and 12 years for patients with RA-DB, RA only, DB only, and unaffected relatives, respectively.

Survival in different groups of individuals

At the time of analysis, vital status was known for all subjects. Eighteen patients and 11 unaffected relatives from the study cohort had died (Table 1). In patients with RA-DB, the reported cause of death was identified in 12 of the 14 patients who died, and

Table 1. Characteristics and outcome of the 137 participants in the family-based cohort study.

Characteristics	RA-DB	RA only	DB only	Unaffected relatives	*P* value
	(*N* = 30)	(*N* = 25)	(*N* = 8)	(*N* = 74)	
Sex ratio (F/M)	25/5	17/8	5/3	37/37	0.011[a]
Median (mean) age at RA onset – yr	45 (45.1)	39 (42.0)	-	-	0.35[b]
Median (mean) age at inclusion – yr	64.0 (60.1)	51.0 (51.1)	45.5 (50.1)	52.0 (54.7)	0.08[b]
Symptoms at inclusion					
Dyspnea – no. (%)	24 (80%)		7 (86%)		1[a]
Cough and sputum – no. (%)	24 (80%)		7 (86%)		1[a]
>1 respiratory infection/year – no. (%)	19 (63%)		6 (71%)		0.69[a]
Sinus involvement – no. (%)	14 (47%)		5 (63)%		0.69[a]
Hemoptysis – no. (%)	7 (23%)		3 (38%)		0.41[a]
Subjects with at least one *CFTR* mutation – no. (%)	18 (60%)	5 (20%)	6 (75%)	16 (22%)	5.5×10^{-5} [a]
Age when last seen – yr					0.15[b]
Median	70.5	62	56	65.5	
Mean±SD	69.57±9.74	62.80±12.70	61.00±17.74	67.07±14.45	
Median (mean) follow-up time – yr	10 (9.5)	11 (11.7)	11 (10.9)	12 (12.4)	0.06[b]
Deaths – no. (%)	14 (46.7%)	2 (8.0%)	2 (25.0%)	11 (14.9%)	0.0015[a]
Cause of death – no.					
cardiorespiratory	8	1		1	
others	4*	1[†]	1[‡]	5[¥]	
unknown	2		1	5	

RA: rheumatoid arthritis; DB: diffuse bronchiectasis. *CFTR*: cystic fibrosis transmembrane conductance regulator gene.
Plus-minus values are means+SD.
[a] *P*-values of Fisher exact tests.
[b] *P*-values of Kruskal-Wallis tests.
* Causes of death included CVA, Hodgkin lymphoma, cancer, and refractory RA, in one patient each.
[†] Cause of death was CVA.
[‡] Cause of death was cancer.
[¥] Causes of death included cancer in 4 patients and degenerative neurological disease in one patient.

cardiorespiratory disease was the principal cause of death reported for eight of these patients.

There were more deaths after inclusion among the patients with RA-DB than among the other groups (RA only, DB only, unaffected relatives) (Table 1), even after adjustment for age at inclusion (Fig. 1A). RA-DB patients tended to be older at inclusion than patients with RA only or DB only (Table 1). We therefore also compared survival from birth between the different groups (Fig. S1A). For patients with RA or DB only, survival after inclusion or since birth was not significantly different from the survival of unaffected relatives (log-rank test $P = 0.71$ and $P = 0.21$, respectively). By contrast, survival was a mean of 8.6 years shorter for RA-DB patients than for unaffected relatives (log-rank test $P = 6.2\times10^{-5}$) (Fig. 1A and Fig. S1A). In mixed effect Cox models, with unaffected relatives as the reference group, the HR for death was significant only for patients with RA-DB, whether we took inclusion in the study (HR, 7.61; 95% CI, 2.68–21.59; *z*-test $P = 0.00014$) (Fig. 1B) or birth as the starting points (Fig. S1B).

Survival in rheumatoid arthritis patients with and without bronchiectasis

The survival of RA-DB patients after RA diagnosis was significantly lower than that of patients with RA only, even after adjusting for age of diagnosis (Fig. 2). Kaplan-Meier estimates of the probability of survival 15 years after RA diagnosis were 82.8% (95% CI, 70.2% to 97.8%) for RA-DB patients and 95.2% (95% CI, 86.6% to 100%) for patients with RA only ($P = 0.022$). In the mixed effect Cox model adjusted for age at RA diagnosis, the HR for death associated with the presence of DB was 8.6 (95% CI, 1.5 to 48.2; *z*-test $P = 0.014$) (Fig. 2B). We obtained similar results if we considered survival from birth, with a HR for death associated with the presence of DB of 9.6 (95% CI, 1.1 to 81.7; *z*-test $P = 0.039$).

Factors influencing survival in patients with both rheumatoid arthritis and bronchiectasis

We found that 18 of the 30 patients with RA-DB (60%) had early-onset DB, whereas the other 12 patients with RA-DB (40%) had late-onset DB. Individuals with early-onset DB tended to be diagnosed with RA at younger ages than those with late-onset DB. We therefore studied survival from birth in RA-DB patients.

In univariate analyses of survival from birth, early-onset DB, CF/*CFTR*-RD mutations and being male were associated with poorer survival (Table 2).

Multivariate analysis of survival from birth showed that, in patients with RA-DB, an early onset of DB (HR, 15.4; 95% CI, 2.1 to 113.2; $P = 0.0072$) and CF/*CFTR*-RD mutations (HR, 7.2; 95% CI, 1.4 to 37.1; $P = 0.018$) were the two major determinants associated with poorer survival (Table 2). Eight of the 14 RA-DB

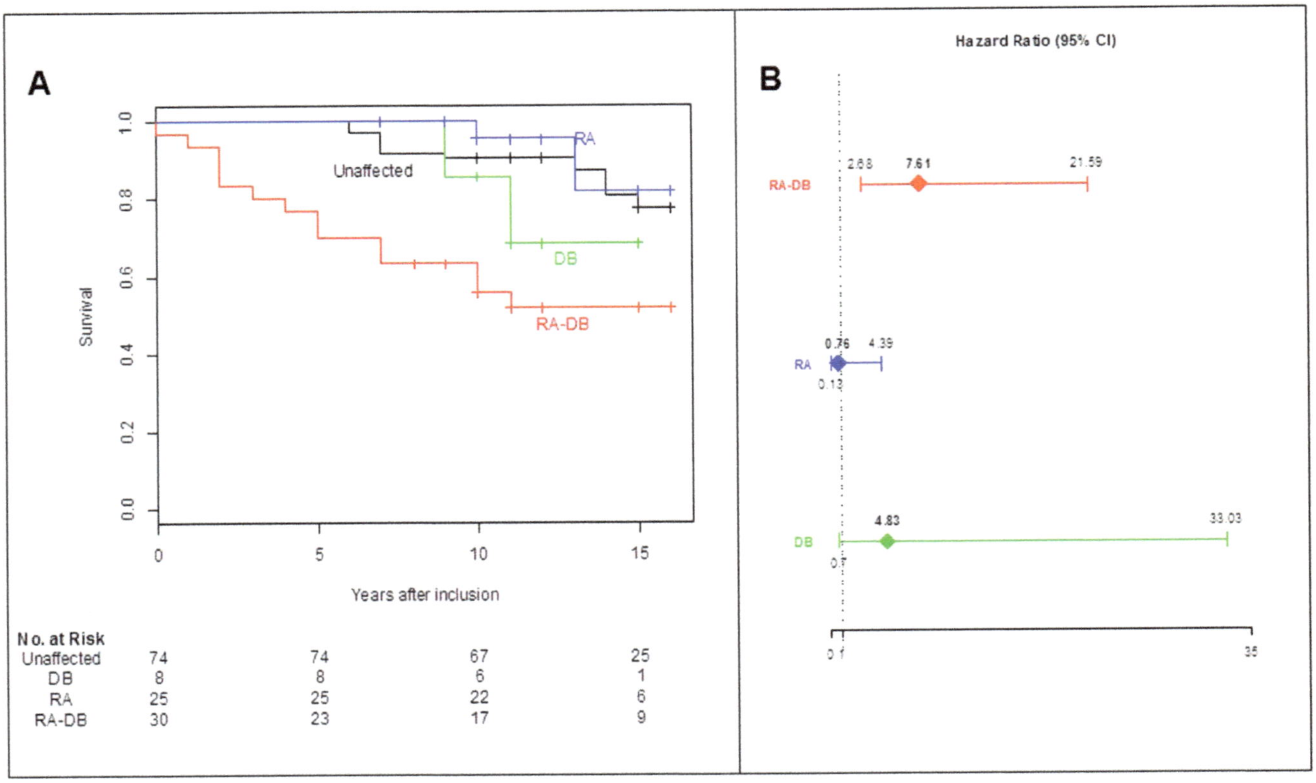

Panel A. Kaplan-Meier survival curves from inclusion in the study for the various groups of individuals.
Panel B. Hazard ratios (95% CI) of death after inclusion for the various disease groups, compared with unaffected relatives as the reference group.
A mixed effect Cox model was fitted, taking inclusion as the starting point and adjusting for age at inclusion. Individual random effects were assumed to be correlated as a function of the corresponding kinship coefficients. The variance of the random effect was 1.48.
RA: rheumatoid arthritis; DB: diffuse bronchiectasis.

Figure 1. Kaplan-Meier probability of survival from inclusion of the various participants in the study cohort, according to their phenotype. Panel A. Kaplan-Meier survival curves from inclusion in the study for the various groups of individuals. **Panel B.** Hazard ratios (95% CI) of death after inclusion for the various disease groups, compared with unaffected relatives as the reference group. A mixed effect Cox model was fitted, taking inclusion as the starting point and adjusting for age at inclusion. Individual random effects were assumed to be correlated as a function of the corresponding kinship coefficients. The variance of the random effect was 1.48. RA: rheumatoid arthritis; DB: diffuse bronchiectasis.

patients who died (57.1%) carried CF/*CFTR*-RD mutations and 10 (71.4%) had early-onset DB. The corresponding figures were six of 16 (37.5%) and 8 of 16 (50%) for the surviving RA-DB patients. The analysis classified RA patients with DB into categories of low or high risk of death. CF/*CFTR*-RD mutations in RA patients with early-onset DB defined a subgroup of high-risk patients with higher mortality rates (log-rank test $P = 1.28 \times 10^{-5}$). Only RA patients with both an early onset of DB and CF/*CFTR*-RD mutations were found to have significantly poorer survival and these patients tended to develop RA at a younger age than the other RA-DB patients. Survival from birth did not differ significantly between patients with late-onset DB and no mutation, patients with late-onset DB and CF/*CFTR*-RD mutations and patients with early-onset DB and no mutation (log-rank test = 2.8; 2 df; $P = 0.251$). Survival in RA-DB patients is shown according to risk of death categories in Figure 3.

Discussion

In this prospective cohort study, DB was associated with poorer survival in RA patients. This analysis further identified early-onset DB and CF/*CFTR*-RD mutation as factors associated with a poorer survival in RA-DB patients.

This study provides the first evidence of long-term poor survival in patients with DB-associated RA, who were found to have an eight times higher probability of death after RA diagnosis than family members with RA only. Cardiorespiratory causes were the most frequently reported causes of death in this population. These results are similar to those of a previous controlled study, in which the five-year probability of mortality in patients with RA-DB was found to be five times that of a matched control group of patients with RA alone and 2.4 times that of a group of patients with DB alone [14]. Most of the deaths of patients with RA-DB (60%) in this previous study were attributed to respiratory infection, whereas the severity of RA, as assessed by HAQ, grip strength, nodules and steroid treatment, was not significantly associated with poorer survival [14].

In patients with RA, childhood-onset DB is much more prevalent than late-onset DB [10,12-16]. Most (60%) of the 30 patients from our cohort with both RA and DB had early-onset DB, beginning more than 10 years before the onset of RA. These data are consistent with the hypothesis that the lung may be an early target of systemic RA autoimmunity or a site at which RA-related autoimmunity is initiated, with an initial autoimmune response in the lung [18,19]. We found that RA-DB patients with early-onset DB had a poorer prognosis than those with late-onset

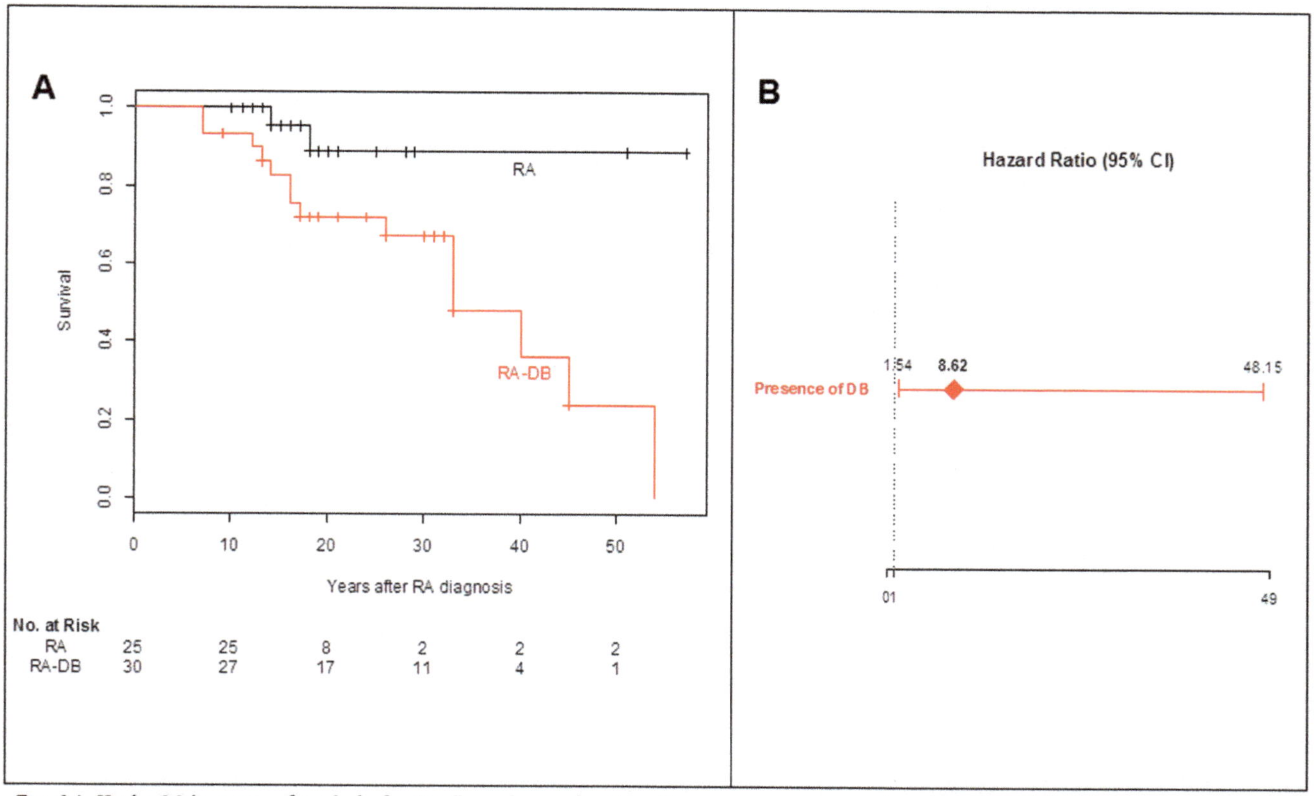

Panel A. Kaplan-Meier curves of survival after RA diagnosis, as a function of the presence or absence of associated DB.
Panel B. Hazard ratios (95% CI) for death after RA diagnosis associated with the presence of DB.
A mixed effect Cox model was fitted, taking RA diagnosis as the starting point. Individual random effects were assumed to be correlated as a function of the corresponding kinship coefficients. The variance of the random effect was 4 10^{-4}.
RA: rheumatoid arthritis; DB: diffuse bronchiectasis.

Figure 2. Kaplan-Meier probability of survival after RA diagnosis in patients, as a function of the presence or absence of associated DB. Panel A. Kaplan-Meier curves of survival after RA diagnosis, as a function of the presence or absence of associated DB. **Panel B.** Hazard ratios (95% CI) for death after RA diagnosis associated with the presence of DB. A mixed effect Cox model was fitted, taking RA diagnosis as the starting point. Individual random effects were assumed to be correlated as a function of the corresponding kinship coefficients. The variance of the random effect was 4 10^{-4}. RA: rheumatoid arthritis; DB: diffuse bronchiectasis.

DB, and early-onset DB was identified as a major determinant of survival in RA patients in multivariate analysis. The role of CF/*CFTR*-RD mutation in the association between RA and DB has been described before [23] and such mutations were found in 50% of the RA-DB patients with early-onset DB and 42% of those with late-onset DB. Not only do CF/*CFTR*-RD mutations predispose RA patients to DB, they are also associated with poorer survival. The prognostic implications of *CFTR* gene mutations have been considered to date only for in patients with CF. Our results demonstrate that RA patients with both early-onset DB and CF/*CFTR*-RD mutations should be considered at high risk of death and should receive more aggressive treatment, including smoking cessation and physiotherapy. Most of our patients were enrolled before the widespread use of biological agents likely to modify

Table 2. Analysis of survival from birth of 30 patients with both RA and DB.

	Univariate analysis	Multivariate analysis	
	P value	Hazard ratio [95% CI]	*P* value
Early-onset DB	0.009	15.4 [2.1; 113.2]	0.0072
***CFTR* mutations**	0.073	7.2 [1.4; 37.1]	0.018
Male versus female	0.06	1.1 [0.2; 5.6]	0.92

RA: rheumatoid arthritis; DB: diffuse bronchiectasis.
Early-onset DB: respiratory symptoms preceding RA by >10 years (mostly childhood DB).
CFTR: cystic fibrosis transmembrane conductance regulator gene.
A mixed effect Cox model was used, with shared random effects, depending on the kinship coefficient of individuals.
The variance of the random effect was 4×10^{-4}.

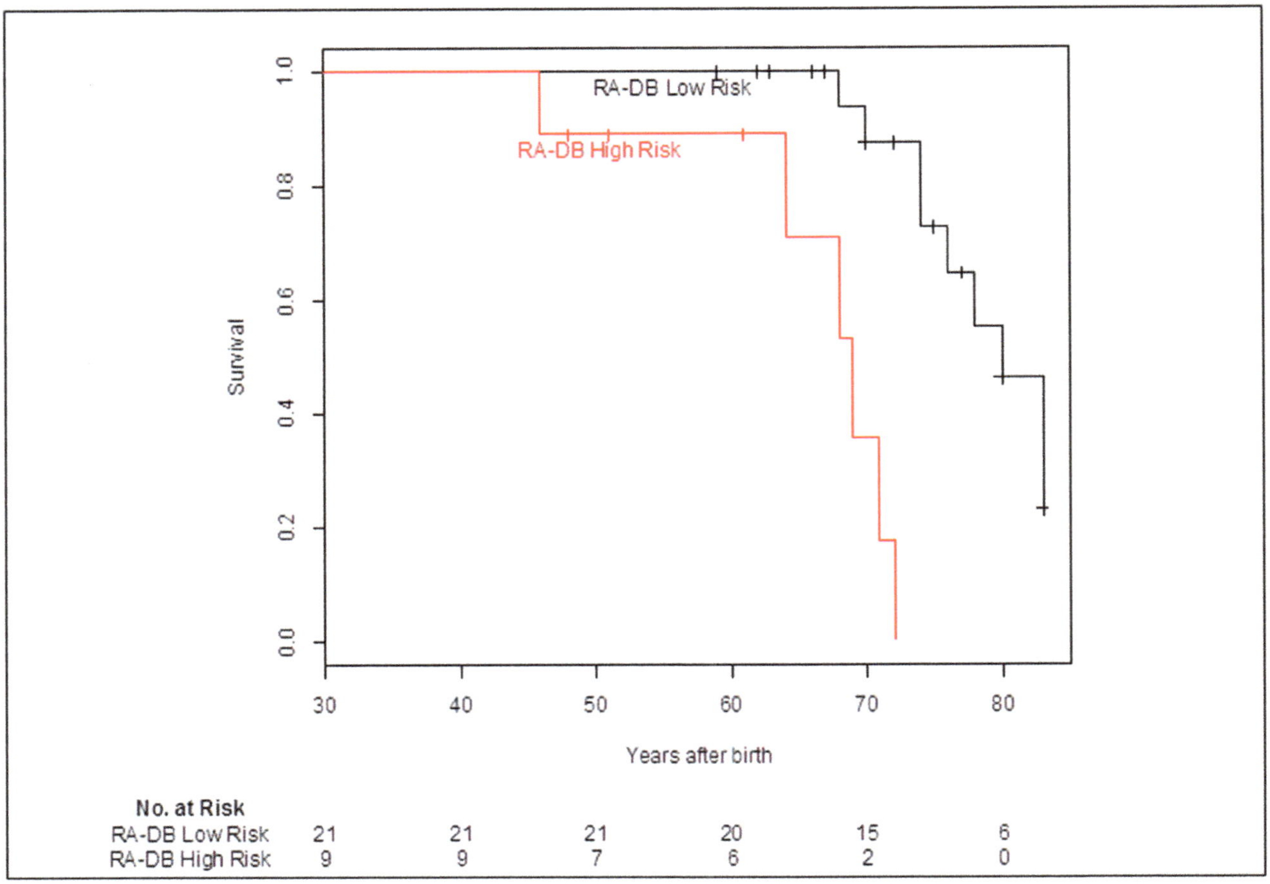

The analysis classified RA patients with DB into categories of low or high risk of death.
Patients with early onset of DB and CF/*CFTR*-related disorders mutations were classified in the high group as compared with the other patients with both RA and DB who were classified into the low risk (log-rank test, P=1.28 x 10^{-5}).
RA: rheumatoid arthritis; DB: diffuse bronchiectasis.
Early-onset DB: respiratory symptoms preceding RA by > 10 years (mostly childhood DB).
Late-onset DB: respiratory symptoms occurring at the same time or < 10 years before RA onset (adulthood DB).
Mutations: cystic fibrosis (CF) and cystic fibrosis transmembrane conductance regulator (*CFTR*)-related disorder mutations.
See Methods for additional information.

Figure 3. Kaplan-Meier probability of survival from birth of patients with both RA and DB according to risk of death categories. The analysis classified RA patients with DB into categories of low or high risk of death. Patients with early onset of DB and CF/*CFTR*-related disorders mutations were classified in the high group as compared with the other patients with both RA and DB who were classified into the low risk. RA: rheumatoid arthritis; DB: diffuse bronchiectasis. Early-onset DB: respiratory symptoms preceding RA by >10 years (mostly childhood DB). Late-onset DB: respiratory symptoms occurring at the same time or <10 years before RA onset (adulthood DB). Mutations: cystic fibrosis (CF) and cystic fibrosis transmembrane conductance regulator (*CFTR*)-related disorder mutations. See Patients and Methods for additional information.

mortality [27], but frequent pulmonary superinfections may constitute a contraindication for such treatments in these patients [15]. These high-risk patients should be eligible in priority in protocols evaluating new treatment interventions such as long-term macrolide therapy which may be beneficial in patients with non-CF bronchiectasis [28–33] and significantly improve the signs and symptoms of RA [34,35]. It remains unclear which patients should receive antibiotic treatment [36], but we suggest that RA patients with early-onset DB carrying CF/*CFTR*-RD mutations should be among those treated and evaluated for long-term azithromycin therapy.

Our study has several strengths. It is a family-based study, which made it possible to gather long-term data for all the individuals included. Such a family-based design limits research bias, by providing appropriate controls and follow-up. Furthermore, phenotypic characterization was carried out and mutational *CFTR* status was determined for all individuals. We systematically checked for DB on HRCT scans for all RA patients and for all individuals with respiratory symptoms. These scans were assessed by two investigators blind to the results of genetic tests.

Several limitations of this study merit further comment. The predictors of mortality in RA include severe extra-articular manifestations [2,37–41]. One of the limitations of this nationwide study is the lack of information regarding other risk factors for mortality in RA patients. These confounding factors may influence the outcome, but the strongest predictor of mortality has been shown to be extra-articular manifestations of the disease [2,40] and the leading cause of death of our RA-DB patients was cardiorespiratory complications. Sample size is another potential limitation of this study. The limited number of patients in each subgroup restricts the power of this study to detect differences. However, this series of patients with RA-DB is one of the largest ever studied, and differences in age at onset of DB and genetic background appear to have a significant, independent, and strong effect on mortality. In addition, our patients were selected from families with a history of RA or DB. It therefore remains unclear to what extent these results can be extrapolated to patients with no such family history. Another limitation of this study is the possible overestimation of the survival of patients with RA and late-onset DB with respect to that of patients with RA and early-onset DB. Indeed, for recruitment in the study, a family had to include at least one patient with RA and DB. Thus, if this patient had late-onset DB, there is the possibility of a survival advantage because he or she must have lived long enough after the onset of RA to develop DB meeting the late-onset criterion. However, this should not have biased the results concerning the deleterious effects of CF/*CFTR*-RD mutations on survival in patients with early-onset DB, in whom the presence of a mutation was found to lead to a mean decrease in survival of 7.1 years on average (log rank test = 6.3; 1 df; $P = 0.012$).

Conclusions

In this prospective family cohort, DB in RA patients was associated with lower overall survival. CF/*CFTR*-RD mutations predispose RA patients with early-onset DB to more severe disease, associated with a shorter lifespan. The identification of early-onset DB and the genotyping of such patients may make it possible to define high-risk patients for whom new treatments should be developed and evaluated specifically.

Supporting Information

Figure S1 Kaplan-Meier probability of survival from birth of the various participants in the study cohort as a function of their phenotype. Panel A. Kaplan-Meier survival curves from birth for the various groups of individuals. **Panel B.** Hazard ratios (95% CI) for death since birth for the various disease groups, compared with unaffected relatives as the reference group. A mixed effect Cox model was fitted, taking birth as the starting point and age as the scale. Individual random effects were assumed to be correlated as a function of the corresponding kinship coefficient. The variance of the random effect was 1.35. RA: rheumatoid arthritis; DB: diffuse bronchiectasis.

Acknowledgments

We thank the patients and their families for their participation. We thank Paul Legmann for HRCT scan analysis. We thank Eglantine Rouanet for assistance with data management, and the French Society of Rheumatology and the French National Society of Internal Medicine. We thank Philippe Saint Pierre for his helpful comments and advice on the analysis of correlated survival data.

Author Contributions

Conceived and designed the experiments: XP EG TB DD. Performed the experiments: EG TB. Analyzed the data: XP EG TB CLJ DD. Contributed reagents/materials/analysis tools: EG TB. Wrote the paper: XP EG TB CLJ DD.

References

1. Firestein GS (2003) Evolving concepts of rheumatoid arthritis. Nature 423: 356–361.
2. Turesson C, O'Fallon WM, Crowson CS, Gabriel SE, Matteson EL (2002) Occurrence of extraarticular disease manifestations is associated with excess mortality in a community based cohort of patients with rheumatoid arthritis. J Rheumatol 29: 62–67.
3. Aviña-Zubieta JA, Choi HK, Sadatsafavi M, Etminan M, Esdaile JM, et al. (2008) Risk of cardiovascular mortality in patients with rheumatoid arthritis: a meta-analysis of observational studies. Arthritis Rheum 59: 1690–1697.
4. Fewins HE, McGowan I, Whitehouse GH, Williams J, Mallya R (1991) High definition computed tomography in rheumatoid arthritis associated pulmonary disease. Br J Rheumatol 30: 214–216.
5. McDonagh J, Greaves M, Wright AR, Heycock C, Owen JP, et al. (1994) High resolution computed tomography of the lungs in patients with rheumatoid arthritis and interstitial lung disease. Br J Rheumatol 33: 118–122.
6. Hassan WU, Keaney NP, Holland CD, Kelly CA (1995) High resolution computed tomography of the lung in lifelong non-smoking patients with rheumatoid arthritis. Ann Rheum Dis 54: 308–310.
7. Vergnenègre A, Pugnere N, Antonini MT, Arnaud M, Melloni B, et al. (1997) Airway obstruction and rheumatoid arthritis. Eur Respir J 10: 1072–1078.
8. Perez T, Remy-Jardin M, Cortet B (1998) Airways involvement in rheumatoid arthritis: clinical, functional, and HRCT findings. Am J Respir Crit Care Med 157: 1658–1665.
9. Zrour SH, Touzi M, Bejia I, Golli M, Rouatbi N, et al. (2005) Correlations between high-resolution computed tomography of the chest and clinical function in patients with rheumatoid arthritis: prospective study in 75 patients. Joint Bone Spine 72: 41–47.
10. Solanki T, Neville E (1992) Bronchiectasis and rheumatoid disease: is there an association? Br J Rheumatol 31: 691–693.
11. Pasteur MC, Helliwell SM, Houghton SJ, Webb SC, Foweraker JE, et al. (2000) An investigation into causative factors in patients with bronchiectasis. Am J Respir Crit Care Med 162: 1277–1284.
12. Mathieu JP, Stack BH, Dick WC, Buchanan WW (1978) Pulmonary infection and rheumatoid arthritis. Br J Dis Chest 72: 57–61.
13. McMahon MJ, Swinson DR, Shettar S, Wolstenholme R, Chattopadhyay C, et al. (1993) Bronchiectasis and rheumatoid arthritis: a clinical study. Ann Rheum Dis 52: 776–779.
14. Swinson DR, Symmons D, Suresh U, Jones M, Booth J (1997) Decreased survival in patients with co-existent rheumatoid arthritis and bronchiectasis. Br J Rheumatol 36: 689–691.
15. Puéchal X (1998) Bronchiectasis in rheumatoid arthritis. Rev Rhum Engl Ed 65: 447–450.
16. Puéchal X, Fajac I, Bienvenu T, Desmazes-Dufeu N, Hubert D, et al. (1999) Increased frequency of cystic fibrosis deltaF508 mutation in bronchiectasis associated with rheumatoid arthritis. Eur Respir J 13: 1281–1287.
17. Shadick NA, Fanta CH, Weinblatt ME, O'Donnell W, Coblyn JS (1994) Bronchiectasis. A late feature of severe rheumatoid arthritis. Medicine (Baltimore) 73: 161–170.
18. Demoruelle MK, Weisman MH, Simonian PL, Lynch DA, Sachs PB, et al. (2012) Airways abnormalities and rheumatoid arthritis-related autoantibodies in subjects without arthritis: early injury or initiating site of autoimmunity? Arthritis Rheum 64: 1756–1761.
19. Reynisdottir G, Karimi R, Joshua V, Olsen H, Hensvold AH, et al. (2014) Structural changes and antibody enrichment in the lungs are early features of anti-citrullinated protein antibody-positive rheumatoid arthritis. Arthritis Rheumatol 66: 31–39.
20. Knowles MR, Durie PR (2002) What is cystic fibrosis? N Engl J Med 347: 439–442.
21. McKone EF, Emerson SS, Edwards KL, Aitken ML (2003) Effect of genotype on phenotype and mortality in cystic fibrosis: a retrospective cohort study. Lancet 361: 1671–1676.
22. Bombieri C, Claustres M, De Boeck K, Derichs N, Dodge J, et al. (2011) Recommendations for the classification of diseases as CFTR-related disorders. J Cyst Fibros 10 Suppl 2: S86–S102.
23. Puéchal X, Bienvenu T, Génin E, Berthelot JM, Sibilia J, et al. (2011) Mutations of the cystic fibrosis gene in patients with bronchiectasis associated with rheumatoid arthritis. Ann Rheum Dis 70: 653–659.
24. Therneau T (2013) A package for survival analysis in S. R package version 2.37–4. Available: http://CRAN.R-project.org/package=survival. Accessed 2014 Sep 19.
25. Therneau T (2012) Coxme: Mixed Effects Cox Models. R package version 2.2–3. Available: http://CRAN.R-project.org/package=coxme. Accessed 2014 Sep 19.
26. R Core Team (2012) R: A language and environment for statistical computing. R Foundation for Statistical Computing, Vienna, Austria. ISBN 3-900051-07-0. Available: http://www.R-project.org/. Accessed 2014 Sep 19.
27. Jacobsson LT, Turesson C, Nilsson JA, Petersson IF, Lindqvist E, et al. (2007) Treatment with TNF blockers and mortality risk in patients with rheumatoid arthritis. Ann Rheum Dis 66: 670–675.
28. Koh YY, Lee MH, Sun YH, Sung KW, Chae JH (1997) Effect of roxithromycin on airway responsiveness in children with bronchiectasis: a double-blind, placebo-controlled study. Eur Respir J 10: 994-999.
29. Tsang KW, Ho PI, Chan KN, Ip MS, Lam WK, et al. (1999) A pilot study of low-dose erythromycin in bronchiectasis. Eur Respir J 13: 361–364.

30. Wong C, Jayaram L, Karalus N, Eaton T, Tong C, et al. (2012) Azithromycin for prevention of exacerbations in non-cystic fibrosis bronchiectasis (EMBRACE): a randomised, double-blind, placebo-controlled trial. Lancet 380: 660–667.
31. Altenburg J, de Graaff CS, Stienstra Y, Sloos JH, van Haren EH, et al. (2013) Effect of azithromycin maintenance treatment on infectious exacerbations among patients with non-cystic fibrosis bronchiectasis: the BAT randomized controlled trial. JAMA 309: 1251–1259.
32. Serisier DJ, Martin ML, McGuckin MA (2013) Effect of long-term, low-dose erythromycin on pulmonary exacerbations among patients with non-cystic fibrosis bronchiectasis: the BLESS randomized controlled trial. JAMA 309: 1260–1267.
33. Elborn JS, Tunney MM (2013) Macrolides and bronchiectasis: clinical benefit with a resistance price. JAMA 309: 1295–1296.
34. Ogrendik M, Karagoz N (2011) Treatment of rheumatoid arthritis with roxithromycin: a randomized trial. Postgrad Med 123: 220–227.
35. Ogrendik M (2007) Effects of clarithromycin in patients with active rheumatoid arthritis. Curr Med Res Opin 23: 515–522.
36. Wilson R, Wells AU (2012) Azithromycin in bronchiectasis: when should it be used? Lancet 380: 627–629.
37. Foster CS, Forstot SL, Wilson LA (1984) Mortality rate in rheumatoid arthritis patients developing necrotizing scleritis or peripheral ulcerative keratitis. Effects of systemic immunosuppression. Ophthalmology 91: 1253–1263.
38. Erhardt CC, Mumford PA, Venables PJ, Maini RN (1989) Factors predicting a poor life prognosis in rheumatoid arthritis: an eight year prospective study. Ann Rheum Dis 48: 7–13.
39. Turesson C, Jacobsson L, Bergström U (1999) Extra-articular rheumatoid arthritis: prevalence and mortality. Rheumatology (Oxford) 38: 668–674.
40. Gabriel SE, Crowson CS, Kremers HM, Doran MF, Turesson C, et al (2003) Survival in rheumatoid arthritis: a population-based analysis of trends over 40 years. Arthritis Rheum 48: 54–58.
41. Turesson C, McClelland RL, Christianson TJ, Matteson EL (2007) Severe extra-articular disease manifestations are associated with an increased risk of first ever cardiovascular events in patients with rheumatoid arthritis. Ann Rheum Dis 66: 70–75.

12

A Little CFTR Goes a Long Way: CFTR-Dependent Sweat Secretion from G551D and R117H-5T Cystic Fibrosis Subjects Taking Ivacaftor

Jessica E. Char[1], Marlene H. Wolfe[1], Hyung-ju Cho[1], Il-Ho Park[1], Jin Hyeok Jeong[1], Eric Frisbee[1], Colleen Dunn[2], Zoe Davies[2], Carlos Milla[2], Richard B. Moss[2], Ewart A. C. Thomas[3], Jeffrey J. Wine[1,2,3]*

1 Cystic Fibrosis Research Laboratory, Stanford University, Stanford, California, United States of America, **2** Department of Pediatrics, Stanford University School of Medicine, Stanford, California, United States of America, **3** Department of Psychology, Stanford University, Stanford, California, United States of America

Abstract

To determine if oral dosing with the CFTR-potentiator ivacaftor (VX-770, Kalydeco) improves CFTR-dependent sweating in CF subjects carrying G551D or R117H-5T mutations, we optically measured sweat secretion from 32–143 individually identified glands in each of 8 CF subjects; 6 F508del/G551D, one G551D/R117H-5T, and one I507del/R117H-5T. Two subjects were tested only (−) ivacaftor, 3 only (+) ivacaftor and 3 (+/−) ivacaftor (1–5 tests per condition). The total number of gland measurements was 852 (−) ivacaftor and 906 (+) ivacaftor. A healthy control was tested 4 times (51 glands). For each gland we measured both CFTR-independent (M-sweat) and CFTR-dependent (C-sweat); C-sweat was stimulated with a β-adrenergic cocktail that elevated $[cAMP]_i$ while blocking muscarinic receptors. Absent ivacaftor, almost all CF glands produced M-sweat on all tests, but only 1/593 glands produced C-sweat (10 tests, 5 subjects). By contrast, 6/6 subjects (113/342 glands) produced C-sweat in the (+) ivacaftor condition, but with large inter-subject differences; 3–74% of glands responded with C/M sweat ratios 0.04%–2.57% of the average WT ratio of 0.265. Sweat volume losses cause proportionally larger underestimates of CFTR function at lower sweat rates. The losses were reduced by measuring C/M ratios in 12 glands from each subject that had the highest M-sweat rates. Remaining losses were estimated from single channel data and used to correct the C/M ratios, giving estimates of CFTR function (+) ivacaftor = 1.6%–7.7% of the WT average. These estimates are in accord with single channel data and transcript analysis, and suggest that significant clinical benefit can be produced by low levels of CFTR function.

Editor: Giuseppe Novelli, Tor Vergata University of Rome, Italy

Funding: This work was supported by Cystic Fibrosis Foundation Therapeutics, Grant WINE08A0 to JJW. http://www.cff.org/research/cfft/. The funders had no role in study design, data collection and analysis, decision to publish, or preparation of the manuscript.

Competing Interests: The authors have declared that no competing interests exist.

* E-mail: wine@stanford.edu

Introduction

Genetic mutations that reduce CFTR-mediated anion conductance ($G_{anion} = nP_O\gamma$) cause cystic fibrosis (CF). Over 1,000 mutations are known or predicted to reduce CFTR channel number (n), open probability (P_O), and/or conductance (γ), and 127 of these have been identified as disease-causing mutations [1]. A complex set of interacting pathophysiological consequences follows large reductions in CFTR function, most resulting from defective ion and fluid transport. The most efficient way to stop this cascade is to correct the defective gene or protein. Ivacaftor (VX-770, Kalydeco) increases P_O in a wide variety of CFTR mutations as well as WT CFTR [2]. VX-770 was shown to improve the function of G551D in cultured cells [3], and patients having at least one G551D mutation treated with oral ivacaftor showed marked clinical improvement [4,5], leading to FDA approval of ivacaftor for use in G551D patients. Recently, ivacaftor was shown to improve CFTR-dependent ion transport in human airway epithelial cells carrying an R117H mutation [6], and trials are now underway to determine if ivacaftor will be clinically beneficial for patients with R117H-5T mutations.

Most CFTR mutations are rare, and marked phenotypic differences can occur in patients having the same mutations [7,8,9]. Therefore, n-of-1 studies are informative. With that in mind, a bioassay was developed that compares the volume of CFTR-independent and CFTR-dependent sweat secretion gland-by-gland for ~50 individually identified glands within each subject [10]. On the premise that the therapeutics of interest will act directly on CFTR, we treated individual glands as the units of analysis, providing sufficient statistical power to determine efficacy for individual subjects in n-of-1 studies.

The assay takes advantage of two parallel pathways for sweat secretion: a CFTR-independent, cholinergic pathway stimulated with methacholine ('M-sweat') and a β-adrenergic pathway that is CFTR-dependent ('C-sweat') [10]. When C-sweating is expressed as a function of M-sweating, the assay gives a near-linear readout of CFTR function over a wide range: i.e. the C-sweat/M-sweat ratio for carriers of one CFTR mutation is 50% that of non-CF controls, while the ratio for CF subjects is zero. However, at very low levels of CFTR function the C-sweat assay departs from linearity and becomes less sensitive: at present it doesn't detect C-sweating in most pancreatic sufficient (PS) CF subjects, who are

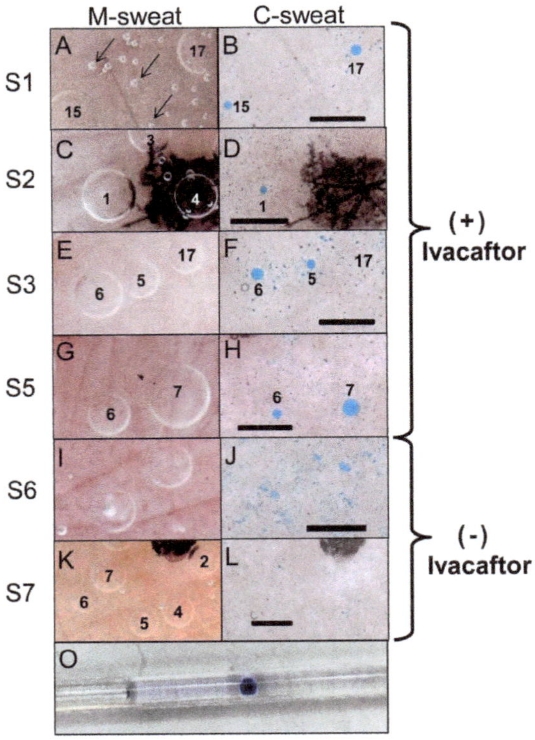

Figure 1. CFTR independent (M-sweat) and CFTR dependent (C-sweat) secretion in G551D CF subjects. Each image shows a small region (~1.5 mm^2) of the stimulated field of sweat glands (full imaged field is 0.63 cm^2) for each subject. Images for S1-3 and S5 were (+) ivacaftor and S6, 7 (−) ivacaftor. A portion of each field was selected to show glands that responded (or not) to the β-adrenergic cocktail (right column). (A-B). S1, male. Arrows in (A) point to air bubbles in the oil. (C-D) S2, female. (D) Shows the single sweat gland that responded to the β-adrenergic stimulus in this experiment. The dark stain is an ink spot on the freckle used for image registration. (E-F) S3, female. This subject had high background staining. (G-H) S5, male. (I-J) S6, female, (-) ivacaftor. This subject showed the most background staining of any subject in this series. (K-L) S7, female, (−) ivacaftor. (O) C-sweat collected in 2 µl constant bore capillary from S1 (+) ivacaftor. Calibration bars = 0.5 mm.

known to have some residual CFTR function [10]. The sweat volume bioassay is thus complementary to the sweat chloride test, which does discriminate between CF patients based on their pancreatic status, but which can't discriminate CF heterozygotes from WT subjects [10]. Both tests benefit by using an organ that is unaffected by the progressive, destructive changes that occur in many other CFTR-expressing organs [11].

Given the assay's present inability to discriminate between PI and PS subjects, it was important to determine if it could detect functional efficacy of ivacaftor in CF subjects carrying the G551D mutation, where its clinical efficacy has already been demonstrated [4,5]. Therefore, in the present study we measured the efficacy of ivacaftor in 4 individuals of G551D/F508del genotype. In addition, we wanted to use the assay with patients having mutations for which clinical efficacy of ivacaftor is presently unknown. Therefore, we also used the assay to measure the efficacy of ivacaftor in two CF subjects with R117H-5T mutations.

Materials and Methods

Subjects

The study was approved by the Institutional Review Board of Stanford University. After written informed consent, six adults with genotypes G551D/F508del, one with G551D/R117H-5T and one with I507del/R117H-5T were enrolled, along with a healthy control. All CF subjects were classified as having cystic fibrosis by the Stanford Cystic Fibrosis Center on the basis of elevated sweat chloride levels, CFTR mutations, and clinical indications. The healthy control subject was genotyped by the Molecular Pathology Laboratory, Stanford University Medical Center and was free of any CFTR mutations and had (TG)12-7T and (TG)10-9T.

Two subjects were tested only off drug, three only on drug, and two were tested both off and on. There were no adverse events. Seven subjects had been enrolled in multi-center studies of ivacaftor and were studied either during the open label period, during the month prior to the start of open label, or both. One G551D subject who was not enrolled in an ivacaftor trial was studied off drug prior to FDA approval and then on-drug after starting ivacaftor as prescribed by his physician.

Ratiometric measurement of sweat secretion from identified individual glands

We used the single gland, ratiometric, optical assay for CFTR secretory function as described by Wine *et al.* [10]. In brief, a specific region of skin on the volar forearm was sequentially injected intradermally with methacholine to stimulate CFTR-independent sweating (M-sweat) and then with a cocktail of agents that blocked M-sweating and produced CFTR-dependent sweating (C-sweat). Bubbles of sweat from single glands were captured in an oil layer, visualized by oblique lighting or dye-partioning, and digitally imaged at 30 sec intervals. The individual glands were identified by location as follows: a region of interest (ROI) was defined by counting bubbles of M-sweat starting at the center of the field and spiraling outward until ~50 individual glands were numbered. For each identified gland the increases in M- and C-sweat volumes over time were measured. Plots of volume vs. time were made at 5-6 min intervals for selected glands to latencies and rates of volume increase. Plots correlating M- and C-sweat volumes were based on M-sweat volumes at the end of 15 min, and C-sweat volumes/2 at the end of 30 min. In the plots of M- and C-sweat correlations, each point represents the average volume for a single identified gland based on all trials where the gland was measured.

To provide a common, meaningful basis of comparison among the CF subjects, we obtained a mean C/M ratio of 0.2651 from testing six healthy controls subjects [10], set that value = 100%, and expressed the responses of the CF subjects with reference to it. Proportionality between CFTR-dependent and CFTR-independent secretory function, i.e., the constancy of the C/M ratio across glands, is compromised by sweat volume losses via ductal absorption and physical capacitance [10], as well as by finite losses into the oil from very small bubbles in spite of extensive water saturation of the oil (P.M. Quinton, personal communication). Indeed, the C/M values showed a positive relation to
M-sweat rates, consistent with proportionally less sweat volume loss in the faster secreting glands. To take advantage of this relationship for each subject, we plotted the C/M ratio for the 12 highest M-sweat secreting glands, in which sweat loss is much reduced and the C/M ratio is expected to be relatively constant. A further correction factor was obtained by using single channel

Table 1. G551D/F508del subjects.

			Gland numbers			Gland volumes/rates				Ratios			
ID	**G**	**TestDate**	**MCh glands (n)**	**Cktl glands (n)**	**C/M n glands (%)**	**MCh Avg. Final Vol. (nl/gland)**	**MCh Rate Estimate nl/gl/min**	**Cktl Avg Final Vol (pl/gl)**	**Cktl Rate (pl/gl/min)**	**C mean/ M mean**	**% WT**	**% WT (Highest 12 M-sweat)**	**% WT (Hi-12, Loss-Corrected)**
S1 G551D/F508del (−) ivacaftor													
S1	M	10/20/2011	71	0	0%	75.83	5.06	0	0	0.00%	0.00%	-	—
S1	M	1/13/2012	85	0	0%	64.58	4.31	0	0	0.00%	0.00%	-	—
S1	M	2/4/2012	75	0	0%	71.34	4.76	0	0	0.00%	0.00%	-	—
S1 (−) Averages			**77**	**0**	**0%**	**70.58**	**4.71**	**0**	**0**	**0.00%**	**0.00%**	**0.00%**	**0.00%**
S1 G551D/F508del (+) ivacaftor													
S1	M	3/23/2012	82	13	16%	70.99	4.73	152	5.06	0.11%	0.42%	-	—
S1	M	4/10/2012	71	15	21%	91.91	6.13	105	3.52	0.06%	0.22%	-	—
S1	M	4/17/2012	66	11	17%	97.02	6.47	110	3.66	0.06%	0.22%	-	—
S1 (+) A xverages			**73**	**13**	**18%**	**86.64**	**5.78**	**122**	**4.08**	**0.07%**	**0.29%**	**0.64%**	**1.59%**
S2 G551D/F508del (−) ivacaftor													
S2	F	2/2/2012	99	0	0%	28.61	1.91	0	0	0.00%	0.00%	-	—
S2	F	3/20/2012	100	0	0%	29.16	1.94	0	0	0.00%	0.00%	-	—
S2 (−) Averages			**99.5**	**0**	**0%**	**28.88**	**1.93**	**0**	**0**	**0.00%**	**0.00%**	**0.00%**	**0.00%**
S2 G551D/F508del (+) ivacaftor													
S2	F	5/8/2012	82	4	5%	35.55	2.37	11	0.37	0.02%	0.06%	-	—
S2	F	5/15/2012	90	1	1%	29.16	1.94	2	0.07	0.00%	0.01%	-	—
S2 (+) Averages			**86**	**2.5**	**3%**	**32.36**	**2.16**	**7**	0.22	**0.01%**	**0.04%**	**0.13%**	**2.75%**
S3 G551D/F508del (+) ivacaftor													
S3	**F**	**7/24/2012**	**90**	**21**	**23%**	**45.03**	**3.00**	**95**	**3.18**	**0.11%**	**0.41%**	**0.58%**	**2.27%**
S5 G551D/F508del (+) ivacaftor data													
S5	**M**	**11/2/2012**	**58**	**29**	**50%**	**78.94**	**5.26**	**703**	**23.42**	**0.45%**	**1.74%**	**3.07%**	**4.11%**
S6 G551D/F508del (−) ivacaftor data													
S6	**F**	**2/2/2012**	**143**	**0**	**0%**	**14.37**	**0.96**	**0**	**0**	**0.00%**	**0.00%**	**0.00%**	**0.00%**
S7 G551D/F508del (−) ivacaftor data													
S7	**F**	**2/13/2012**	**123**	**0**	**0%**	**32.16**	**2.14**	**0**	**0**	**0.00%**	**0.00%**	**0.00%**	**0.00%**
Summary (−) ivacaftor: 4 G551D subjects													
Sums or Averages			**852**	**0**	**0%**	**36.50**	**2.43**	**0**	**0**	**0.00%**	**0.00%**	**0.00%**	**0.00%**
Summary (+) ivacaftor 4 G551D subjects													
Sums or Averages			**906**	**317**	**29%**	**42.93**	**2.84**	**267**	**6.80**	**0.29%**	**1.15%**	**1.84%**	**4.07%**

Summary of results for CF subjects with G551D mutations. Six adult G551D CF subjects were tested. Table is arranged by subject and condition, each row shows the results for a single test or means/sums when multiple tests were performed. Subjects had been taking ivacaftor for at least 3 weeks prior to (+) ivacaftor testing. Columns labeled 'gland numbers' show the number of glands that secreted to an intradermal injection of MCh, then to the β-adrenergic cocktail at the same site (C-sweat), and the ratio of the two expressed as a percentage. Columns labeled 'gland volumes/rates' show the average final M-sweat or C-sweat volumes per gland expressed as nanoliters for a 15 min period (M-sweat) or 30 min period (C-sweat) followed by average rates (per min, per gland). The 4 columns labeled 'ratios' show: 1) the mean C-sweat rate as a percent of the mean M-sweat rate; 2) the C/M ratios as a percentage of the average C/M ratio of 0.2651 obtained for 6 control subjects [10]; 3) that value for the 12 glands having the highest M-sweat rates; and 4) the value for the 12 highest glands after correcting for sweat volume loss.

measures of P_O and γ for R117H [12] and mRNA transcript measurements of n [13] to provide an independent estimate of unpotentiated R117H-5T channel function. We then subtracted the C/M measure from the predicted single channel value to obtain an estimate of the amount of fluid loss, and added this back for a final, best estimate of CFTR function (see discussion). For G551D, our corrected C/M values were compared with single channel measures made (±) ivacaftor [14,15].

The small volumes of C-sweat observed for the CF subjects made us alert to possible artifacts. In addition to other criteria [10], we also used pipets to collect C-sweat from three CF subjects after optically recording secretion in the presence of ivacaftor. The small amounts collected were in accord with the optical measurements. We tried but failed to collect any C-sweat from CF subjects (−) ivacaftor. Skin staining seen in some experiments (−) ivacaftor (e.g. **Fig. 1L**) had no detectable volume and could not be dislodged by the collecting pipet. Such staining was seen variably in 6 experiments done prior to 2/13/2012 when it was eliminated by a rinse procedure between the M-sweat and C-sweat trials. All (+) ivacaftor trials were done with minimized background

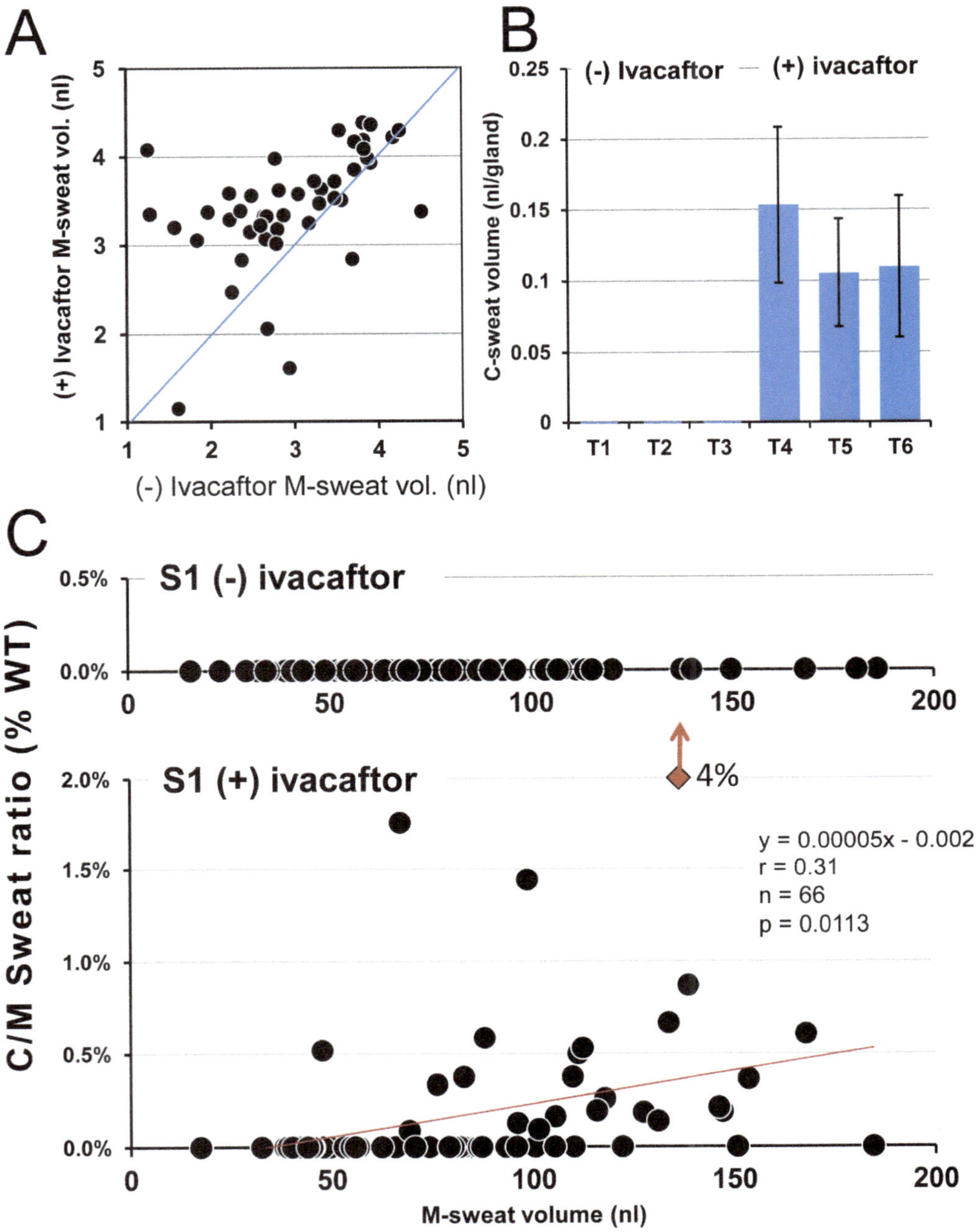

Figure 2. M- and C-sweat secretion (±) ivacaftor for CF subject 1: male, F508del/G551D. (A) Larger M-sweat responses (+) ivacaftor were seen (uniquely) in this subject. Scatter plot shows gland-by-gland volumes measured 7.5 min post MCh injection before any appreciable mergers for 46 glands. Each point is the average of 2–3 measures (2.93 measures per gland per condition), log transformed. Value (−) ivacaftor are on the x-axis and (+) ivacaftor on the y axis. Mean volume at the 7.5 min time point was 28.7±20 vs. 38.35±20 nl^{-gland}, $p = 0.004$, paired t-test on log transformed data. Diagonal line shows equivalence. (B) Bar graphs showing mean C-sweat volumes ± ivacaftor; 3 tests in each condition; zero C-sweat seen (−) ivacaftor. (C) Gland-by-gland sweat secretion (±) ivacaftor. Each point in these graphs is jointly determined by the mean of M-sweat responses (x axis) and C-sweat/M-sweat ratios expressed as a% of the mean WT C/M ratio (y axis). Top graph with truncated y axis shows measurements (−) ivacaftor. Each point is mean ratio measured in 1–3 tests (mean 2.1 tests) for each of 94 identified glands. C-sweating and hence ratio was zero for all glands. Bottom graph, (+) ivacaftor. 25/66 glands produced C-sweat on 1–3 trials (average 1.56 trials). The dark outlined red diamond and arrow show an outlier gland (G19) which secreted ~10 times more than the mean of all responding glands on each of 3 (+) ivacaftor trials. Red line is linear fit.

and hence had reduced chances of false positives, but extremely low levels of secretion might have been missed in 3 (−) ivacaftor tests done before the rinse procedure.

Statistical Analysis

Single, identified sweat glands were the units of analysis for the within-subject comparisons in our "n-of-1" analyses [10]. Paired t-tests on log transformed data, Pearson r, ANOVA, and mixed

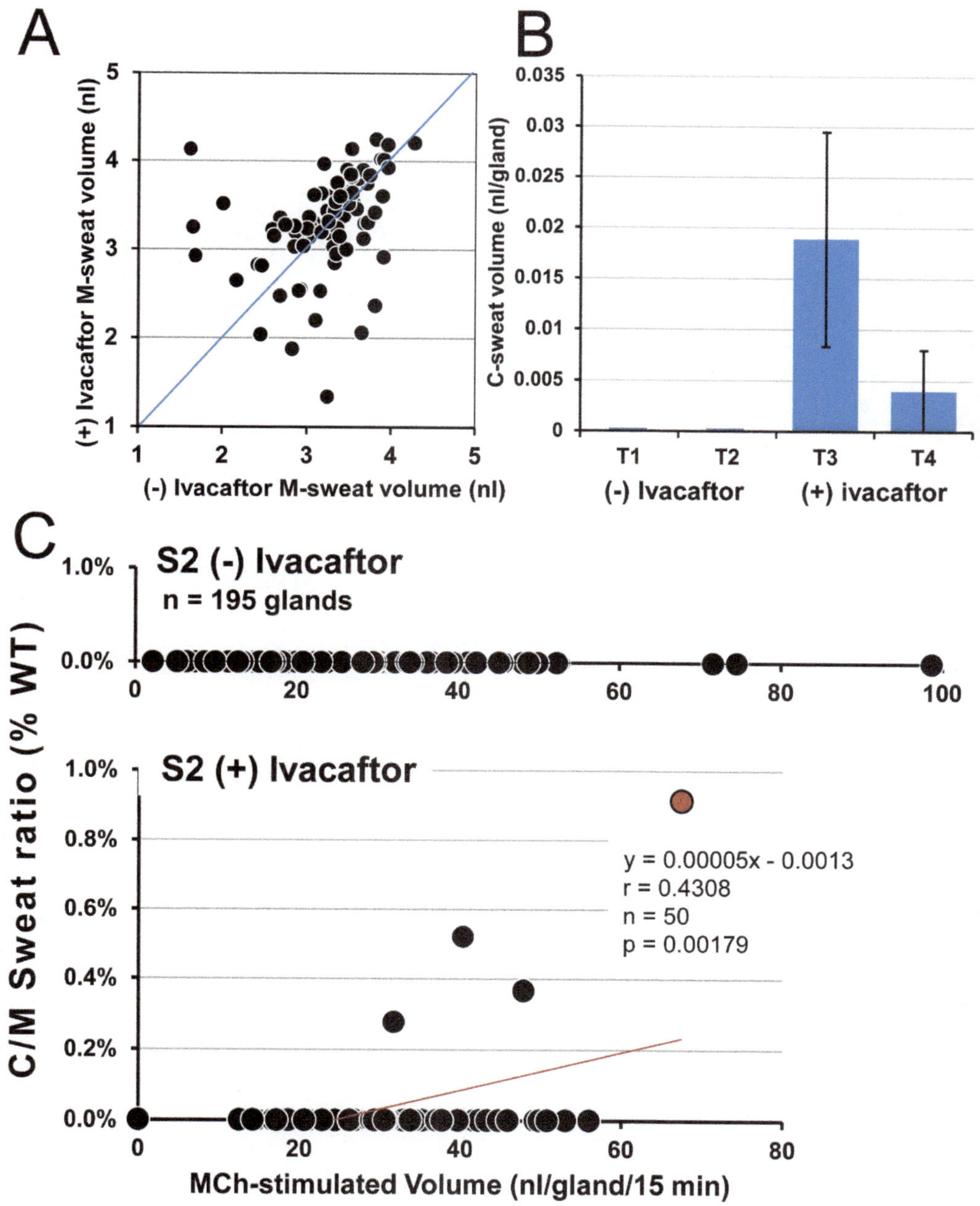

Figure 3. M- and C-sweat secretion (±) ivacaftor for CF subject 2: female, F508del/G551D. (A) M-sweat responses were unchanged by ivacaftor in this subject. Each point is log transformed values for a single pre-test and mean of 2 post-test measures for each of 87 glands. Mean volumes were 28.2±12.5 vs. 31.9±14.6 nl^{-gland}, pre and post, n=87 glands $p=0.12$, paired t-test on log transformed data, plotted as in Fig. 2A. (B) Bar graphs show C-sweat volumes (mean ± SEM) for (±) ivacaftor conditions; 2 tests in each condition. One (−) ivacaftor test was at a different site. (The means are based on glands 1–50). (C) Gland-by-gland C-sweat secretion ± ivacaftor. Each symbol shows correlations for each gland between mean M-sweat volumes (x axis) vs. C-sweat/M-sweat ratio expressed as a% of mean WT value (y axis). (Top graph, truncated y axis) shows measurements (−) ivacaftor. Each point is M-sweat volume for a single test for 195 identified glands at two sites; C-sweat was zero. (Bottom graph) shows measurements (+) ivacaftor (mean of 2 tests). Four of 87 glands produced C-sweat, only one gland secreted on both tests (red symbol). Red line is linear fit. This was the smallest response observed for any subject (+) ivacaftor.

models regression with lmer() from the lme4 package in R (see methods, ref [10]) were used as appropriate.

The ratio of the average rates of M- and C-sweat produced per gland (averaged over 15 min for M-sweat and 30 min for C-sweat) is the main index of sweat production, and we use it here to estimate the proportion of CFTR function in various conditions relative to a sample of healthy controls. However, for CF subjects, virtually no glands produced C-sweat in the (-) ivacaftor condition, and the majority still failed to produce measurable C-sweat (+) ivacaftor. We assume that glands sometimes secrete amounts of sweat that fail to exceed the threshold resulting from subtractive processes [10]. To assess this assumption, we dichotomized the C-sweat response as 0, if there is no observed secretion, and 1, otherwise. With this recoding, the average recoded C-sweat response is simply the *probability* that a gland produces C-sweat on

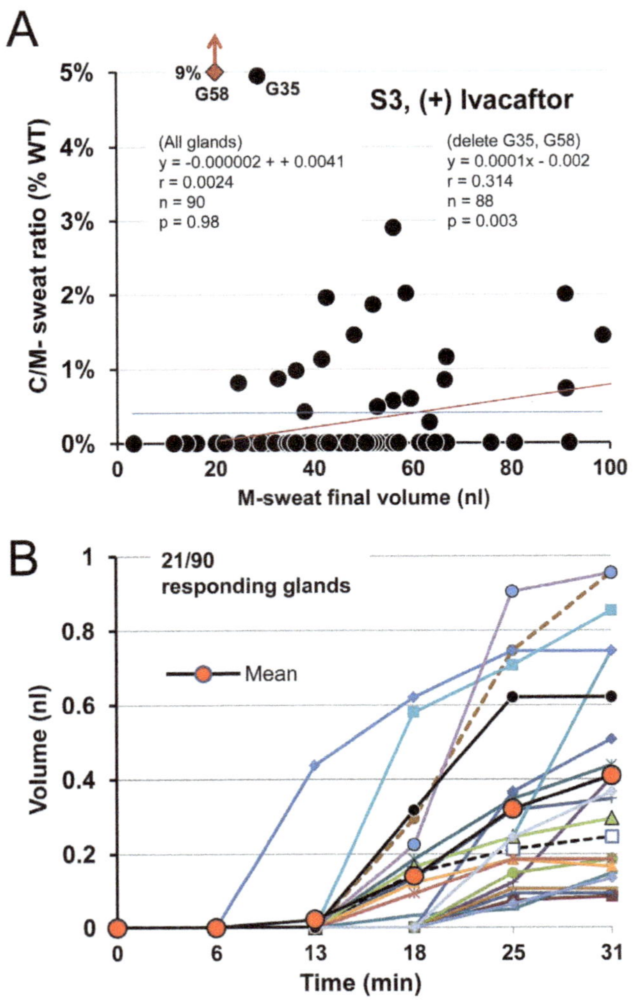

Figure 4. C-sweat secretion (+) ivacaftor in CF subject 3: female, F508del/G551D. S4 was tested only once, (+) ivacaftor. (A) Gland-by-gland correlations of M- and C-sweating using the same conventions as above. M-sweat was measured for 90 glands of which 21 also produced C-sweat with C/M ratios of 0.3% to 5% of the mean WT ratio. (B) Volume vs. time plots for C-sweating of each responding gland. β-adrenergic cocktail injected at time 0, and no observations were made during the first 3 min when atropine was taking effect and when the site was rinsed and dried before reapplying oil. Note slow time course of response.

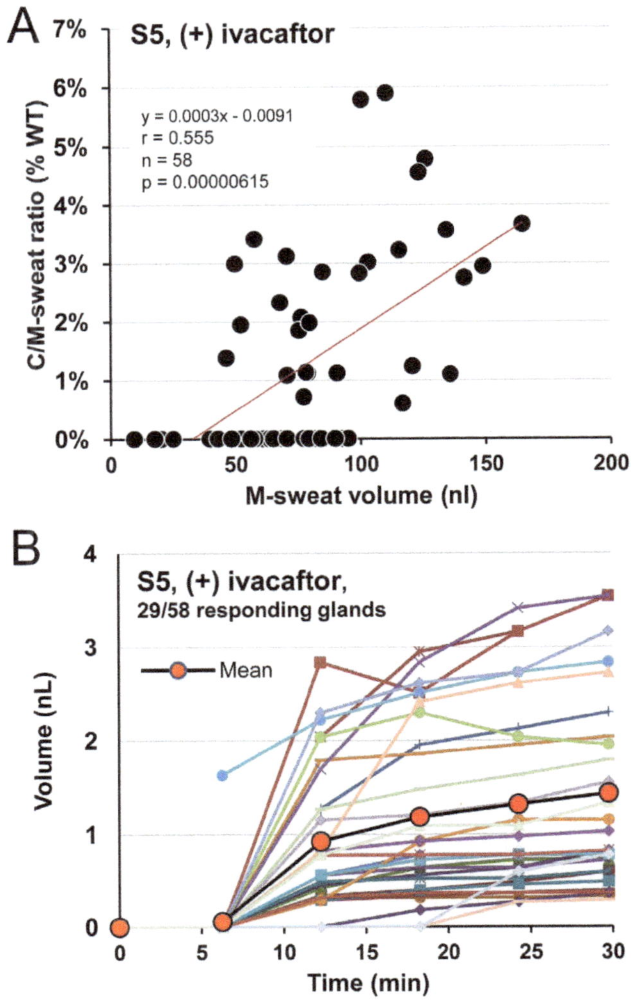

Figure 5. C-sweat secretion (+) ivacaftor in CF subject 5: male, F508del/G551D. S5 was tested only once, (+) ivacaftor. (A) Gland-by-gland correlations of M- and C-sweating using the same conventions as previously. M-sweating was measured in 58 glands. Of these, 29 (50%) also produced C-sweat, with C/M ratios of 0.6% to 5.9% of the mean WT ratio. (B) Volume vs. time plots for β-stimulated, C-sweating. β-adrenergic cocktail injected at time 0.

a test, and we use this probability as an alternative index of C-sweat production (see **Appendix S1**).

Note that this method is useful for testing statistical significance when many glands do not respond, the situation with CF subjects (−) ivacaftor, but becomes insensitive as the response rate increases and P(C-sweat) approaches 1. For example, WT and HZ both have P(C-sweat) ≈ 1, but C/M ratios of 1 and 0.5 respectively. The upper limit for the utility of this method is a function of CFTR functional levels and gland secretory capacity (M-sweat rate) and remains to be determined.

Results

For six CF subjects each carrying one G551D mutation, CFTR-independent M-sweating was imaged for 15 minutes, allowing us to identify 58–143 sweat glands per subject and measure the M-sweat rates for each gland. The same glands were then stimulated with the β-adrenergic cocktail to stimulate CFTR-dependent
C-sweating, which was imaged for 30 min. Two subjects were tested (+/−) ivacaftor, two only (+) ivacaftor and two only (−) ivacaftor (**Table 1**). Images of M-sweat and C-sweat bubbles are shown for each G551D CF subject in **Fig. 1**.

G551D subjects: within-subject comparisons (−) and (+) ivacaftor

Subject 1 (**S1**, male, F508del/G551D) was tested 3 times in each condition. (This is the preferred paradigm for testing, but it could not be used with all subjects because of limited subject availability.) M-sweat is considered to be CFTR-independent [16,17], but unexpectedly, S1's M-sweat rates were significantly larger (+) ivacaftor (78.0 versus 58.5 nl^{-gland}, p<.01; see **Fig. 2A**). Glands differed significantly in their typical M-sweat rates (p<.0001), but not in their sensitivity to ivacaftor (p>.38). Indeed,

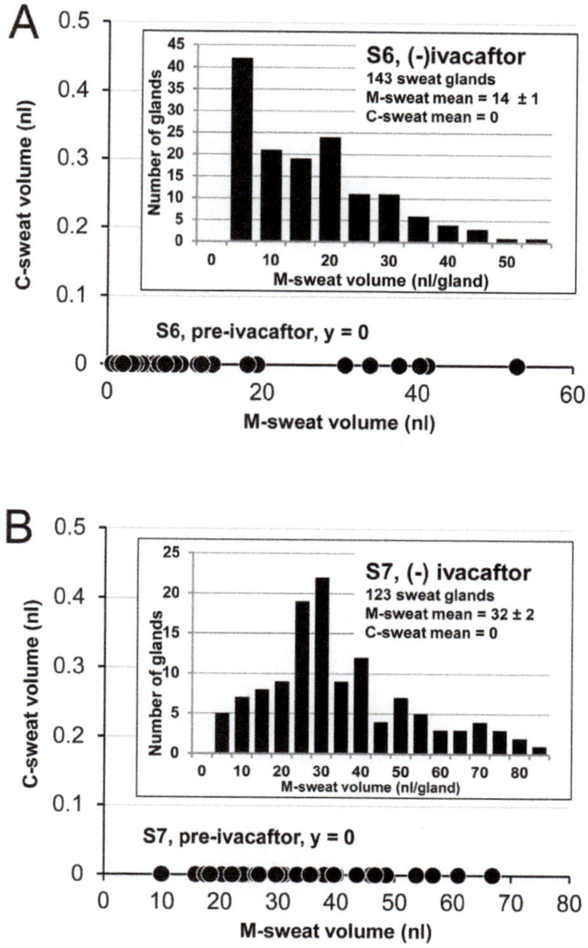

Figure 6. Absence of C-sweat secretion (−) ivacaftor in two G551D CF subjects. (A) S6: female, F508del/G551D. Each symbol in the main graph shows M-sweat volumes produced by a single sweat gland (x-axis) and C-sweat (truncated y axis, all C-sweat values were zero). The distribution of M-sweat volumes is shown in the inset. (B) S7: female, F508del/G551D. Same format as for S6.

M-sweating, presumably reflecting gland size, varied ~10 fold, as previously observed [10]. There was also significant variation in average M-sweat rates across weeks ($p<.05$); but in this subject the 6 tests were spread out across a 6 month period.

Ivacaftor caused a qualitative difference in C-sweating. No gland produced C-sweat in any of 3 tests (−) ivacaftor, but (+) ivacaftor 16–21% of the glands responded (**Table 1**) and produced an average of 0.1–0.15 nl^{-gland} on each of 3 tests (**Fig. 2B**). (Glands with zero C-sweat were included in the averages). As noted in **Appendix S1**, we dichotomized the C-sweat response, and then replaced by '1' one of the '0's (i.e., non-secretions) in the (−) ivacaftor condition. A logistic mixed model analysis of the minimally perturbed responses showed the effect of ivacaftor was significant [P(C-sweat) was estimated to be.1035 and.0009 in the (+) and (−) ivacaftor conditions, respectively, $p<.0005$]. Here too, glands ($p<.0001$), but not weeks ($p>.99$), differed significantly in the probability of a C-sweat response.

Fig. 2C presents data for S1 on a gland-by-gland basis, in which each point represents the joint mean values for C-sweat and M-sweat for a single gland. The top, truncated graph of **Fig. 2C** shows that no glands produced C-sweat in the absence of ivacaftor across the full range of M-sweat responses (0/231 = 0% response rate based on a mean of 2.35 measurements for each of 98 glands), hence all points are arrayed along the x axis according to their M-sweat responses. The bottom graph of **Fig. 2C** shows the results (+) ivacaftor. C-sweat responses were observed for 24 glands on at least one test with an overall response rate of 17.9% and C/M ratios 0%–4% of the average WT ratio. **Fig. 2C** also shows that the C/M ratio was not constant across the glands, but increased significantly as a function of the M-sweat rate ($r = 0.31$, $p<0.02$), see also [10]. The positive relationship between C/M and M, which was significant for all but one subject, was used to arrive at better estimates of the% of CFTR function restored by ivacaftor (see discussion).

As an additional means to estimate the level and significance of CFTR function that is restored by ivacaftor, we developed a prediction equation based on the gland's M-sweat response (+) ivacaftor, as discussed in **Appendix S1**. If the significant differences in P(C-sweat) across glands is due mainly to factors, e.g., gland size, that are reflected in the M-sweat response (+) ivacaftor, then one would expect that, when M-sweat response is included as a predictor, 'gland' would no longer be significant as a random effect. Similarly, to the extent that differences among weeks are reflected in the M-sweat response, 'week' would no longer be significant as a random effect. A logistic mixed model analysis showed that M-sweat response (on a log scale) was a significant predictor of P(C-sweat) ($b = 2.43$, $p<.0001$) in the (+) ivacaftor condition. Further, neither 'gland' ($p>.17$) nor 'week' ($p\approx1$) was significant, suggesting that differences in CFTR function (i.e., in the CFTR-dependent C-sweat response) across glands and weeks can be adequately accounted for, or 'explained', by differences in the CFTR-independent M-sweat responses of the glands. On the log scale, M-sweat levels vary from 0 to 5.527, and the corresponding probabilities of a C-sweat response are.00006 and.23

Subject S2 (**S2**, female, F508del/G551D) was tested twice in each condition. Unlike S1, S2's M-sweat values did not differ between (+) and (−) ivacaftor (26.5 versus 25.3 nl^{-gland}, $p>.9$; see **Fig. 3A**). C-sweating for S2 was evaluated in the same way as for S1. **Fig. 3B** shows that no C-sweat volume was produced (−) ivacaftor, and only a tiny average volume (<20 pl^{-gland}) was produced (+) ivacaftor because only 1–4 out of 90 glands responded (**Fig. 3C, D**). A logistic mixed model analysis of the minimally perturbed responses showed a non-significant effect of ivacaftor ($p>.13$). Here too glands ($p<.0001$), but not weeks ($p>.99$), differed significantly in the probability of a C-sweat response. In predicting P(C-sweat) from M-sweat response (+) ivacaftor, a logistic mixed model analysis yielded unreliable estimates of the variances of the random effects for gland and week, most likely because less than 3% of glands yielded observable levels of

C-sweat. A simple logistic regression without random effects did show that M-sweat response (on a log scale) was a significant predictor of P(C-sweat) ($b = 3.88$, $p<.05$) (see discussion).

Two additional G551D subjects tested only (+) ivacaftor

Subject 3 (**S3**, female, F508del/G551D) was tested only once. M-sweating was measured for 90 glands, of which 21 (23%) produced measureable C-sweat with C/M ratios 0.3%–9% of the mean WT ratio (**Fig. 4A**). The average C/M for all glands was 0.41% WT. **Fig. 4B** plots volumes vs. time for C-sweat from each of the 21 responding glands. Most responding glands had long post-injection latencies, and many continued to increase throughout the 30 min period. This subject (or test) was unusual in that

Table 2. Summary of results for R117H-5T CF subjects and the healthy control.

			Gland numbers			Gland volumes/rates				Ratios			
ID	**G**	**Test Date**	**MCh glands (n)**	**Cktl glands (n)**	**C/M n glands (%)**	**MCh Avg. Final Vol. (nl/gland)**	**MCh Rate Estimate nl/gl/min**	**Cktl Avg Final Vol (pl/gl)**	**Cktl Rate (pl/gl/min)**	**C mean/ M mean**	**% WT**	**% WT (Highest 12 M-sweat)**	**% WT (Hi-12, Loss-Corrected)**
S4 G551D/R117H-5T (+) ivacaftor data													
S4	F	8/22/ 2012	37	8	22%	16.05	1.07	100	3.33	0.31%	1.22%	-	—
S4	F	11/6/ 2012	32	6	19%	10.66	0.69	30	1.00	0.14%	0.55%	-	—
S4	F	4/30/ 2013	37	11	30%	13.57	0.57	150	5.00	0.55%	2.16%	-	—
S4 (+) Averages			**35.33**	**8.33**	**23%**	**13.43**	**0.78**	**93**	**3.11**	**0.35%**	**1.31%**	**2.13%**	**7.83%**
S8 R117H/I508del (−) ivacaftor													
S8	M	1/31/ 2013	52	1	2%	46.76	3.12	6	0.19	0.01%	0.02%	—	—
S8	M	2/8/2013	54	1	2%	49.88	3.33	12	0.39	0.01%	0.04%	—	—
S8	M	2/15/ 2013	50	1	2%	59.51	3.97	4	0.14	0.00%	0.01%	—	—
S8 (−) Averages			**52**	**1**	**0%**	**52**	**3**	**7**	**0.24**	**0.01%**	**0.03%**	**0.06%**	**1.50%**
S8 R117H/I508del (+) ivacaftor													
S8	M	3/15/ 2013	53	28	53%	41.40	2.76	531	17.70	0.64%	2.42%	—	—
S8	M	3/22/ 2013	53	45	84%	54.35	3.62	766	25.55	0.71%	2.66%	—	—
S8	M	3/29/ 2013	49	42	86%	53.88	3.59	1146	38.20	1.06%	4.01%	—	—
S8	M	6/17/ 2013	53	43	81%	57.84	3.86	645	21.49	0.56%	2.10%	—	—
S8	M	6/24/ 2013	53	40	75%	53.85	3.59	474	15.80	0.44%	1.66%	—	—
S8 (+) Averages			**52.2**	**39.6**	**76%**	**52.26**	**3.48**	**712**	**23.75**	**0.68%**	**2.57%**	**4.51%**	**5.89%**
Healthy Control													
WT	F	3/14/ 2013	51	50	98%	35.94	2.40	9687	323	13%	51%	—	—
WT	F	3/25/ 2013	51	51	100%	36.98	2.47	9371	312	13%	48%	—	—
WT	F	3/28/ 2013	51	51	100%	28.81	1.92	11519	384	20%	75%	—	—
WT	F	5/2/2013	51	50	98%	36.48	2.43	10540	351	14%	54%	—	—
WT Averages			**51**	**50.5**	**99%**	**34.55**	**2.30**	**10279**	**343**	**15%**	**57%**	**60.65%**	**62.97%**

Table is arranged using same format as Table 1 and shows data for S8, S4 and the healthy control.

two glands with low M-sweat rates had high C-sweat rates, leading to unusually high C/M ratios and resulting in a non-significant association between C/M ratio and M-sweat rate ($r = 0.002$, $p = 0.98$). Excluding those two glands gave $r = 0.314$, $p = 0.003$).

Subject 5 (**S5**, male, F508del/G551D), was tested only once (+) ivacaftor. M-sweating was measured in 58 glands, of which 29 (50%) produced C-sweat, giving C/M ratios of 0.6% to 5.9% of the mean WT ratio (**Fig. 5A**). The time course of increases in C-sweat bubble volumes in this subject was similar to S4 (**Fig. 5B**). (Time courses of responding glands from S1 and S2 were similar to S3 and S5, data not shown). The C/M ratio increased significantly as a function of the M-sweat rate ($r = 0.555$, $p = 0.000006$).

In predicting P(C-sweat) from M-sweat response (+) ivacaftor, a logistic mixed model analysis showed that M-sweat response (on a log scale) was a significant predictor of P(C-sweat) (S3: $b = 1.43$, $p < .05$; S5: $b = 3.73$, $p < .01$).

Two additional G551D subjects tested only (−) ivacaftor

Two female G551D CF subjects, **S6** and **S7**, were each tested once only (−) ivacaftor. They did not return for repeat pre-testing or since starting ivacaftor. Each subject had abundant sweat glands, none of which responded to the β-adrenergic cocktail with any measureable C-sweat (0/266 glands, main graphs of **Fig. 6A, B**). The insets show the distribution of M-sweat volumes for these two subjects; note the prevalence of low-secreting glands for S6.

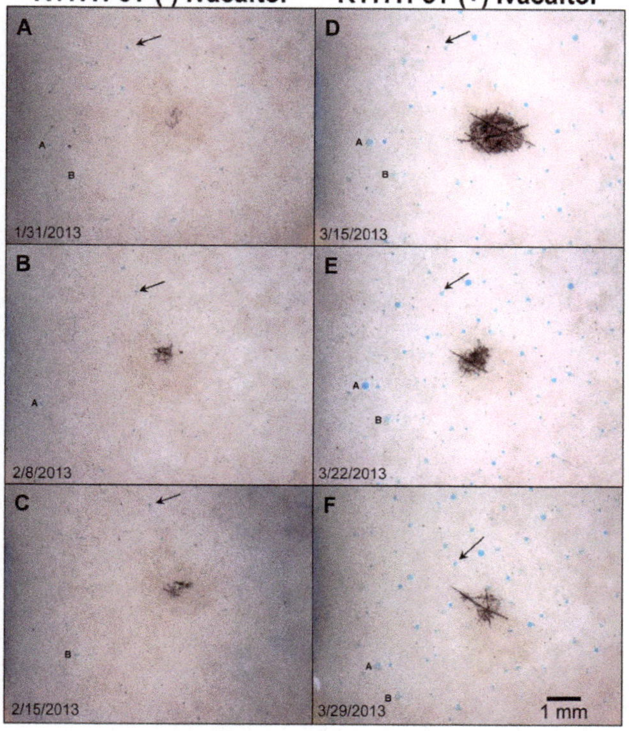

Figure 7. Images of C-sweat responses for CF subject 8: male, I507del/R117H-5T (±) ivacaftor (N of 1 trial). S8 was tested 3 times (−) ivacaftor and 5 times (+) ivacaftor. Only the first 3 (+) ivacaftor tests are shown. (A-C) (−) ivacaftor; (D-F) (+) ivacaftor. Each image shows the field 30 min after the cocktail injection. A light freckle served as the landmark, with an ink spot on the freckle to improve registration and focusing. For image (F) the ink spot was too high causing the field to shift down. In this pancreatic sufficient subject, a few glands marked as A, B, or arrows) produced small amounts of C-sweat (−) ivacaftor.

Within-subject study of an R117H-5T subject (−) and (+) ivacaftor

Subject 8 has genotype I507del/R117H-5T. The I507del mutation does not traffic [18,19] and so is predicted to be unresponsive to ivacaftor, allowing us to assess the *in vivo* effect of ivacaftor on the R117H-5T mutation in isolation. S8 was tested 3 times (−) ivacaftor and 5 times (+) ivacaftor **(Table 2)**. In the (−) ivacaftor condition, the C-sweat response to the β-adrenergic cocktail was not completely absent for this pancreatic sufficient subject. One gland (G43, arrows in **Fig. 7**) in the region of interest (ROI) and two glands outside the ROI (glands A, B in **Fig. 7A-C**) responded to cocktail in the (−) ivacaftor condition on all 3 tests. Using just the glands in the ROI gave a response rate of 3/153 (1.9%).

C-sweating increased unequivocally in the (+) ivacaftor condition (**Figs. 7, 8**). After starting ivacaftor, 53–85% of the glands responded on each test, with an average response rate of 75±15% (SD) across the 5 tests. **Fig. 8A** shows the mean final volumes of C-sweat for each of 8 tests. C-sweat volume (−) ivacaftor could be measured in only one gland so the average was almost undetectable (0.007 nl^{-gland} accumulated over the 30 min observation period), but in the presence of ivacaftor 53 glands produced an average of 0.71±0.04 nl^{-gland} during the 30 min period. The C/M-sweat ratio expressed as a% of the WT mean was 0.01% (−) ivacaftor and was 2.2±0.6% (SD) (+) ivacaftor (**Fig. 9B**). Mean responses for each of the 53 glands (±) ivacaftor are shown in **Fig. 9C, D** where each point is the mean of 5 M-sweat responses (x axis) and 5 C/M ratios as a% of the mean WT value (y axis). The response rate for 10 selected glands is shown in **Fig. 8E**.

As we did for S1 and S2, we performed an additional analysis by dichotomizing the C-sweat response before conducting a logistic mixed model analysis of the raw responses. The effect of ivacaftor was significant [P(C-sweat) was estimated to be.8065 and.0085 in the (+) and (−) ivacaftor conditions, respectively, p<.0001]. Like S2 but unlike S1, S8's M-sweat values did not differ between (+) and (−) ivacaftor (46.1 versus 46.0 nl^{-gland}, p>.9; see **Fig. 8F**). Consistent with the other subjects tested in this way, glands differed significantly from one another in their typical M-sweat rates (p<.0001), but not in their sensitivity to ivacaftor (p>.45). In predicting P(C-sweat) from M-sweat response (+) ivacaftor, M-sweat (on a log scale) was a significant predictor of P(C-sweat) (b = 2.00, p<.0001), with M-sweat levels varying from −0.064 to 4.998, and P(C-sweat) levels from 0.0013 to 0.9711 (**Appendix S1**).

Study of a CF subject with two responsive mutations: G551D/R117H-5T

Subject 4 (**S4**, female, G551D/R117H-5T) has two mutations that are each expected to respond to ivacaftor. This led us to expect a greater response, but she also had the fewest glands and lowest M-sweat rate of any subject, which predicted a smaller C-sweat response as noted above. S4 was tested 3 times (+) ivacaftor (**Table 2**). We identified 40 glands; 2 are shown in (**Fig. 9A, B**). M-sweating was measured from 32–37 of these gland on each trial (the lowest number for any subject). Of these, 13 (40%) also produced C-sweat on at least one of the three tests. On average, 22% of glands (range 15–30%) in a given trial produced C-sweat. The C/M ratios for responding glands ranged from 0.7% to 11.4% of the mean C/M ratio for WT subjects (**Fig. 9C**); the average ratio for all glands was 1.31% WT. The response time course (**Fig. 9D**) was similar to other subjects, presumably reflecting the offsetting factors of a larger response to ivacaftor and a smaller M-sweat rate. The C/M ratio increased significantly as a function of the M-sweat rate (r = 0.61, p = 0.00003). M-sweat response (on a log scale) was a significant predictor of P(C-sweat) (b = 2.03, p<.0001), with M-sweat levels varying from −0.60 to 3.78, and the P(C-sweat) levels from 0.0005 to 0.7876 (**Appendix S1**).

Responses of a control subject

As stated in methods, the comparison C/M ratio for the CF subjects in this study was the mean C/M ratio of 0.2651 obtained from 6 healthy control subjects in our initial report of the bioassay [10]. As an additional, contemporaneous control, we tested a female healthy control 4 times using an identical protocol. Summary results are shown in **Fig. 10** and **Table 2**). For this subject the ROI contained 51 identified glands. The mean M-sweat final volume for the 15 min test period was 33.9± 1.8 nl^{-gland} (51 glands, 4 tests); means for individual tests were: 35.9±2.0, 37.0±2.1, 28.8±1.8 and 36.5±3.2 $nl^{-gland-30\ min}$ (**Fig. 10A**, open columns). C-sweating was observed for all but one gland in one test. The mean final volume of C-sweat for the 30 min observation period was 10.24±0.77 nl^{-gland}; mean values for each of the four trials were: 9.7±0.7, 9.4±0.7 11.5±1.0 and 10.5±0.9 (**Fig 10A**, blue columns). The mean C/M ratio was 0.143±0.005; ratios for each test were: 0.129±0.006, 0.124±0.004, 0.203±0.015 and 0.178±0.016 (**Fig. 10B**). **Fig. 10C** plots the gland-by-gland comparison of C-sweating (as C/M ratio as a percent of the previously determined WT mean)

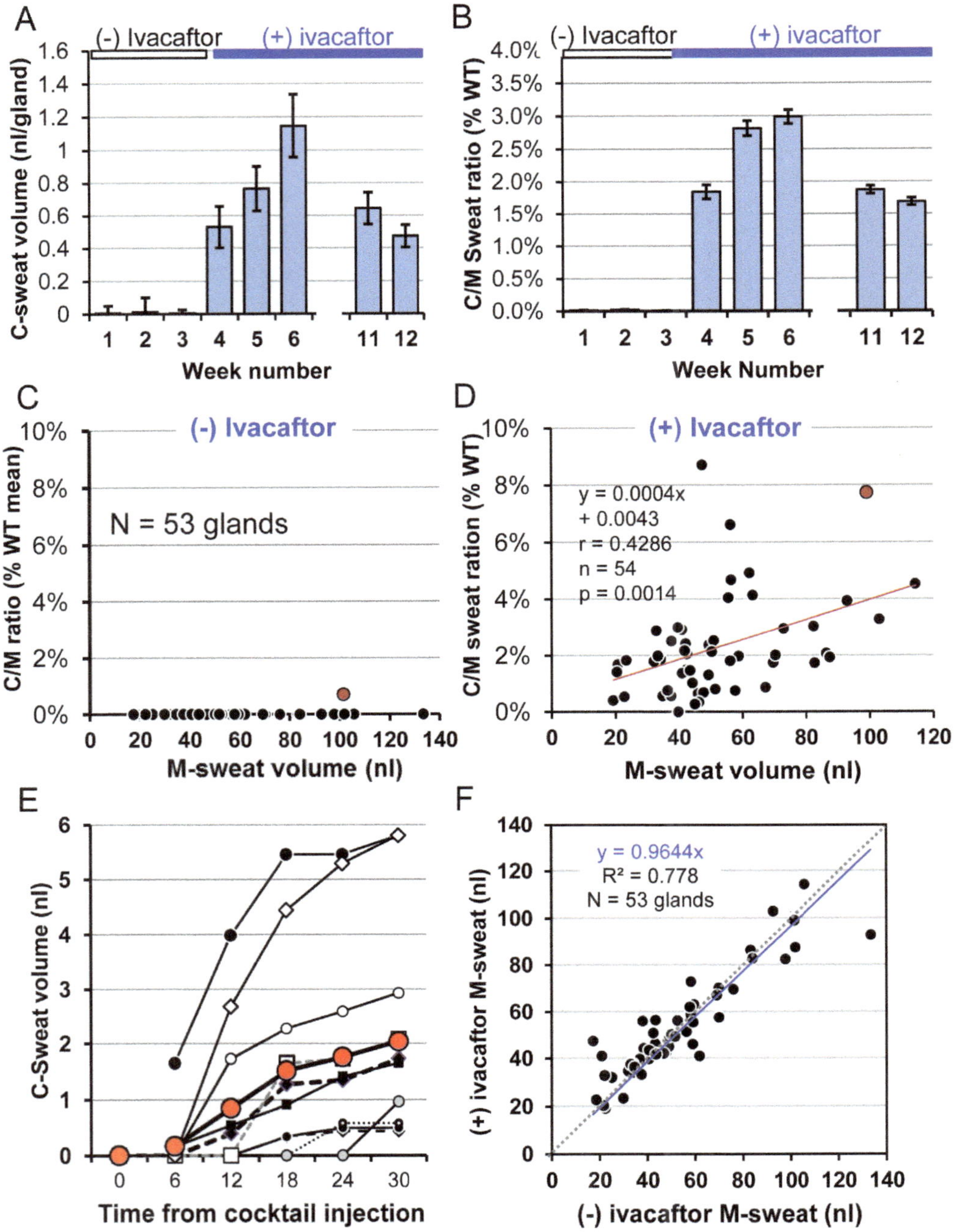

Figure 8. Summary data for S8, R117H-5T, (±) ivacaftor. (**A**) Mean ± SEM for the final (30 min) volume of C-sweat secretion per gland (50–53 glands measured for each test) (±) ivacaftor. (B) C-sweat/M-sweat ratios expressed as percent of the WT mean. Results are means ± SEM for 49–53 glands per test. (C-D) Gland-by-gland correlations of M-sweat and C-sweat responses in the absence (C), and presence (D) of ivacaftor. Each symbol represents a single gland and shows its average C/M ratio expressed as a% of the WT average (y-axis) vs. its mean M-sweat volume (x-axis). A single gland (G43) in the original ROI produced C-sweat (−) ivacaftor (red symbol); this gland had the second highest C/M ratio in the (+) ivacaftor condition (red symbol). In the (+) ivacaftor condition, 92% of the glands in the ROI produced C-sweat on at least one of the 3 trials, at C/M ratios 0.3%–8.7% of the mean WT C/M ratio. (E) C-sweat volume vs. time for 10 responding glands selected to represent the range of responses for S8 (+) ivacaftor. β-adrenergic cocktail injected at time 0. (F) Absence of ivacaftor effect on M-sweating in this subject. Each point represents a single identified sweat gland, and shows the average M-sweat volumes from 3 tests (−) ivacaftor (x-axis) and 5 tests (+) ivacaftor (y-axis). Dashed 45 degree line indicates equivalence; linear fit does not differ significantly from it.

vs. M-sweat. The overall C/M ratio for this control subject was 54±0.02% of the WT average, which is at the lower end of the range for the WT subjects (range: 52–142%). A significantly positive trend between the C/M ratio and M-sweat volumes was also observed in this WT subject; $r = 0.55$, $p = 0.00002$. The response time course for C-sweating of 11 selected glands from one test is shown in **Fig. 10D**; unlike the CF subjects, all glands had produced measureable C-sweat volumes by 12 min post-injection.

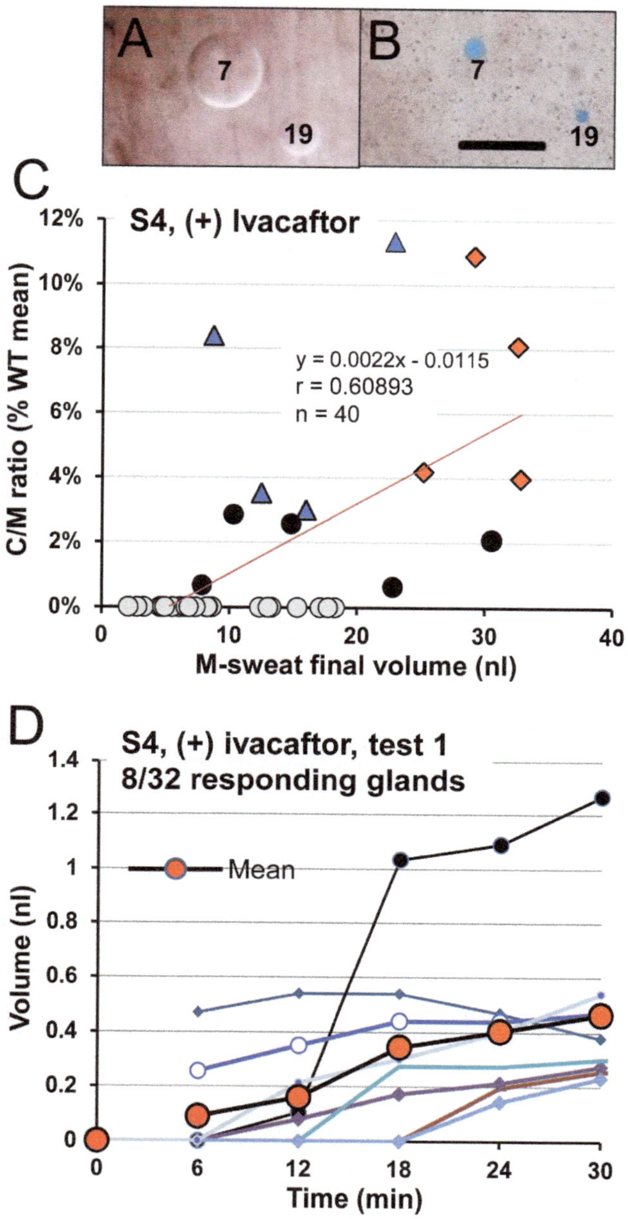

Figure 9. Summary data for S4, a female CF subject having two potentially responsive mutations: G551D & R117H-5T who was tested 3 times (+) ivacaftor. (A) Examples of M-sweat. (B) Examples of C-sweat. Calibration = 0.5 mm. (C) Gland-by-gland correlations of M- and C-sweating using same conventions as previous figures. Symbols: Filled circles, C-sweat on 1/3 trials, blue triangles, 2/3 trials and red diamonds, 3/3 trials. (D) Volume vs. time plots for C-sweating from a single experiment (test 1). β-adrenergic cocktail injected at time 0.

Individual differences across subjects and sensitivity of the C/M ratio to sweat gland secretory capacity

Table 1 shows summary results for all 6 G551D CF subjects; **Table 2** has the summary results for the other subjects.

Fig. 11 provides summary data and analyses for all 6 CF subjects tested (+) ivacaftor. **Fig. 11A** plots the mean C/M ratios (left axis, blue columns) and M-sweat rates (right axis, red symbols that also indicate the subject's gender). Mean single gland M-sweat rates (probably determined mainly by gland size) varied widely and were larger for males. (The number [density] of glands also varies widely among individuals, but because we use individual glands as the units of analysis, this factor was not confounded with secretion rate, as it is in most sweat assays.) **Fig. 11B** plots the percentage of identified glands from each subject that produced measurable volumes of C-sweat. The G551D subjects differed significantly from one another in the proportion of glands that produced measureable C-sweat (ANOVA, $F = 54.8$, $p = 0.001$). **Fig. 11C** plots the C/M ratios after equating M-sweat rates. Because C-sweating is jointly dependent on M-sweating and CFTR function, we isolated CFTR's contribution by selecting a subset of glands from each subject such that the average M-sweat rates for the samples were nearly equivalent (**Fig. 11C**, right axis, red squares). The corresponding C/M ratios for these matched samples of glands (**Fig. 11C**, left axis, blue columns,) show that G551D subjects still differ widely: e.g. S5's ratio is ~7-fold >S1's. Even so, the differences within G551D subjects are overshadowed by the much higher C/M ratio seen in R117H-5T subject 8, and in S4, who, with two responsive mutations, had the highest C/M ratio after partially correcting for M-sweat rate.

A consistent result of this study is that the C/M ratio in subjects with low C-sweat rates is positively correlated with M-sweat rates (**Figs. 2C, 3C, 4A, 5A, 8D** and **9C** and **10A**). This relationship is summarized for all subjects in **Fig. 12A**. It was previously hypothesized that the positive correlation resulted from at least two subtractive processes: physical capacitance (filling of gland lumen before sweat emerges) and absorption of sweat volume in the duct [10]. These have negligible consequences at high sweat rates, but become progressively evident at lower sweat rates. If this hypothesis is correct, it follows that the larger values for each subject, rather than the average for all glands, should more accurately quantify CFTR function. Accordingly, **Fig. 13** (blue columns, left axis) plots for each subject the mean C/M (% WT) of the 12 glands having the highest M-sweat rates, which yielded C/M ratios from <1%–4.5% of the mean WT ratio. The red columns in **Fig. 13** are based on an additional correction that incorporates data from single channel measurements (see discussion).

Discussion

Our first goal in this study was to determine if this bioassay could detect improved CFTR function in CF subjects with G551D or R117H-5T mutations who were taking ivacaftor. We knew before starting that ivacaftor increases G551D CFTR function sufficiently to benefit health [4,5]. Therefore, the positive results with these subjects validate the assay rather than the compound. But no clinical data were available on ivacaftor treated R117H-5T subjects, so our finding of a strong ivacaftor effect for subjects with this compound allele provides *in vivo* support for the prediction that ivacaftor will be therapeutic in such patients [2].

A second goal was to determine if the assay could detect individual differences among the subjects. In fact, we observed large (~6-fold), inter-subject differences in C-sweat responses among the four G551D subjects taking ivacaftor, after correcting for M-sweat rates (**Fig. 11C**). Individual differences could arise from different G551D-CFTR expression levels, differences in transport processes affecting CFTR-dependent sweat secretion, drug pharmacokinetics/tissue distribution, different responses of the in trans F508del allele, and compliance. Such differences are expected to have clinical implications. We were blinded to results from clinical studies of these subjects, but it will be possible to compare the two data sets in the future.

A third goal was to determine if the assay could quantify the extent to which ivacaftor restored function to G551D and

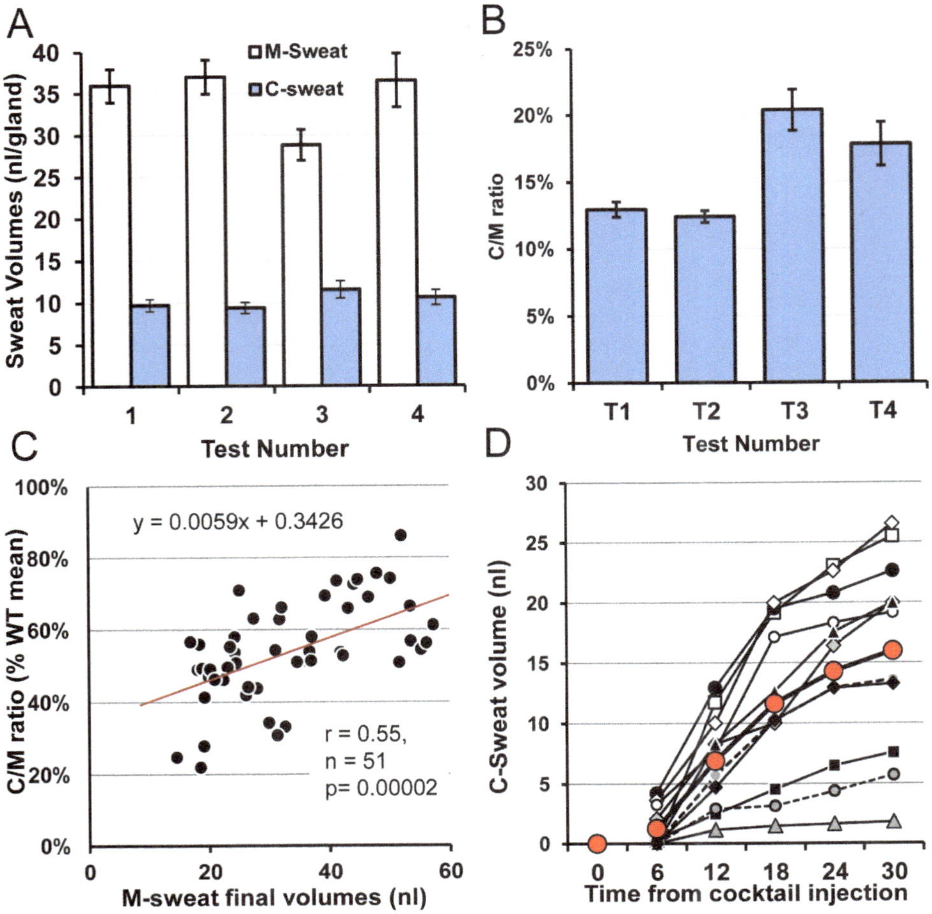

Figure 10. M- and C-sweating in a female, healthy control subject. (A) M-sweat and C-sweat responses for each of 4 tests (Mean ± SEM, n = 51 glands). Each open bar is the average final M-sweat volume in response to 15 min stimulation with MCh; each blue bar is the average final C-sweat volume in response to 30 min of β-adrenergic cocktail. (B) C-sweat/M-sweat ratios for each test. (C) Gland-by-gland correlation of mean C/M sweat ratios, expressed as a% of the WT average, vs. the mean M-sweat response. Each symbol represents mean values for a single gland based on ~4 tests. Responses for this subject were at the low end of the control range. (D) Time course of C-sweating in 11 responsive glands selected to cover the range of C-sweat secretion rates.

R117H-5T CFTR. We hypothesized that primary C-sweat (as elaborated in the secretory coil) provides an accurate readout of CFTR function [10], and that some primary secretion was occurring in most treated glands. However, because subtractive processes reduce the volume of primary C-sweat, uncorrected C-sweating underestimates CFTR function. Therefore, we used independent evidence about channel number and P_O to correct for the losses.

CF is caused by reductions in apical membrane conductance mediated by CFTR, which in turn is a function of channel number, open probability, and single channel conductance: $G_{CFTR} = nP_O\gamma$. The P_O of WT CFTR is ~0.4, e.g. ref. [2]. When considering channel number (n), it is necessary to take account of wide variations arising especially from the length of a polythymidine tract in intron 8 [13]. This tract is found as 3 variable repeat alleles of 9T, 7T or 5T, which in the non-CF population exist in proportions of ~9%, 80% and 11% respectively [20]. The tract length influences splicing of exon 9 such that as tract length shortens, exon 9 skipping increases, resulting in less functional CFTR [13]. With the 5T allele, only ~10% of full-length, functional CFTR is produced, *vs.* 50–100% with 7T and >95% with 9T [13]. Furthermore, a variable TG repeat also affects the number of functional CFTR transcripts [21]. Thus, healthy controls have a wide range of CFTR (n) and hence CFTR function. Importantly, this variation is seldom considered when assessing the operation of most organs with *in vivo* assays, because CFTR function is logarithmically related to most outputs (e.g. sweat chloride, **Fig. 14**) and hence is not rate limiting until it approaches zero (which is why CF is a recessive disease). However, CFTR *is* rate-limiting for C-sweating, which accounts for its linear output [10,22] and (**Fig. 14**). Thus, variation in CFTR (n) is expected to be expressed quantitatively in the C/M sweat ratio. Indeed, the C/M ratio varied 3-fold among 6 healthy controls tested with this method [10] and varied 4-fold among 19 controls in the original study of C/M ratios using a different method [22]. In both studies CF heterozygotes showed a similar dispersion around a mean C/M value half that of the healthy controls [10,22]. On average, healthy control subjects have 70% full length transcripts [13], which we used to set the average WT value for n in the following estimates of CFTR function, i.e. we assume that ~70% transcripts gave the mean C/M ratio of 0.265 for healthy controls [10]. With this background, we first consider results for the R117H-5T subject.

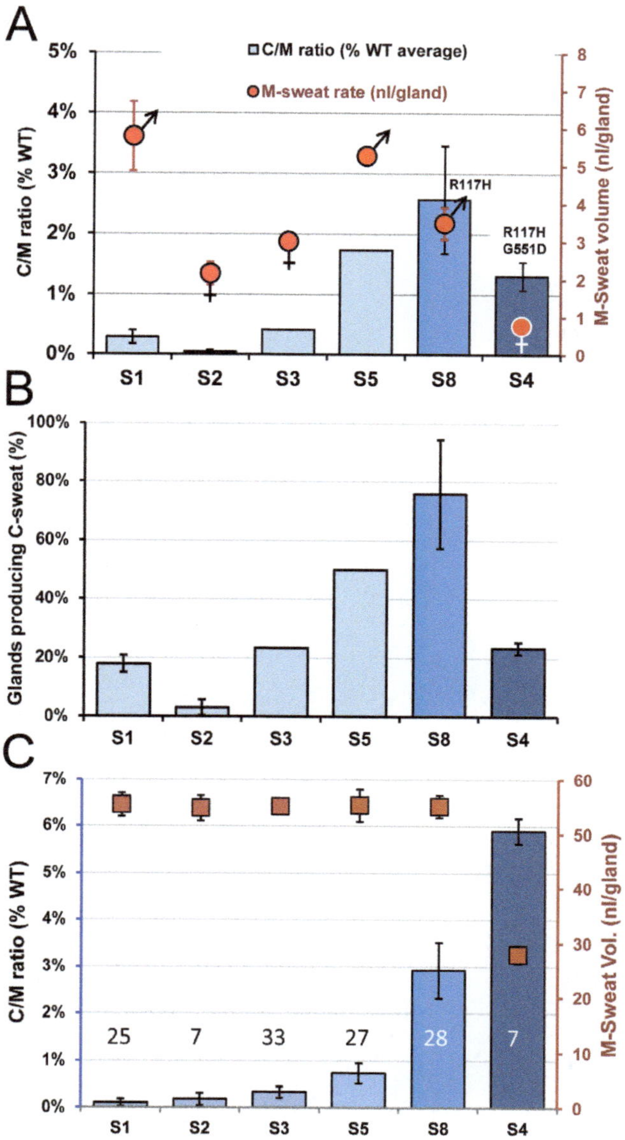

Figure 11. Summary of CFTR-dependent sweat secretion for six CF subjects (+) ivacaftor. (A) Columns (left axis) show C-sweat/M-sweat ratios (mean ± SEM) for each subject, expressed as% of mean WT value. Filled red gender signs (right axis) show M-sweat rates for each subject in the presence of ivacaftor (Mean ± SD). Error bars for S1, S4 and S8 are based on 3 tests, S2 on 2 tests. S1-S3 and S5 each has one G551D mutation, S8 has R117H-5T, and S4 has both. (B) Percentage of glands producing C-sweat in each subject (Mean ± S.D). For healthy control and CF heterozygote (carrier) subjects this value is 97–99±3% [10]. (C) C/M ratios (+) ivacaftor at equivalent M-sweat rates. Filled red squares (right axis) show M-sweat rates (mean ± S.D) for a sample of 7–33 glands from each subject chosen to give a mean M-sweat volume of ~55 nl^{-gland} (= 3.67 $nl^{-min-gland}$). Columns (left axis) show C/M ratios (mean ± SEM), expressed as% of mean WT value for the same sample of glands. Numbers indicate sample size for each subject. S4 had the fewest glands and the lowest M-sweat rates, which prevented matching her sample to the others.

Quantifying R117H-5T CFTR function in vivo and in vitro

R117H-5T CFTR retains partial function and confers pancreatic sufficiency when *trans* to a severe allele. Studies of heterologously expressed CFTR channels by Sheppard and colleagues [12] found that the whole-cell Cl^- conductance of R117H was reduced to 15% of WT, while single channel analysis found that both P_O and γ were reduced predicting ~24% WT CFTR channel function. In a male and a female each having R117H/R117H on a 7T/7T background, all clinical indices were normal except for CBAVD in the male, electrophysiological measurements of nasal and intestinal epithelia were also normal, and sweat chloride values were 34 mM for the male and 42 mM for the female [23]. However, when R117H-CFTR is in *cis* with a 5T allele, n = 0.1/0.7 = 14% WT, reducing R117H-5T function to 2.1–3.7% of WT function. If the other allele is nonfunctional, as it is in S8, the expected residual function will be 1.1%–1.85% of WT (average 1.5%). Remarkably then, <2% of CFTR function, if also found in the pancreas, appears to be sufficient to confer pancreatic sufficiency and to reduce sweat chloride levels from 100 to ~80 mM [24].

To estimate the amount of primary sweat in S8 that was lost in the (−) ivacaftor condition, we assigned a CFTR functional level = 1.5% WT to S8, based on the above analysis of R117H-5T function [12,13]. For S8's 12 glands with highest M-sweat rates, the predicted rate of C-sweating, if he were a WT subject, would be 1.59 $nl^{-min-gland}$, and 1.5% of that value = 0.024 $nl^{-min-gland}$. However, we observed only 0.001 $nl^{-min-gland}$, leading to a loss estimate of 0.023 $nl^{-min-gland}$. If ivacaftor restored normal P_O to R117H and left n and γ unchanged, it would increase R117H-5T CFTR function equivalent to 5T function on 1 allele, or 7% of WT. The C/M ratio for the top 12 glands of S8 (+) ivacaftor was 4.51% of WT (left axis, blue column, **Fig. 12B**). Correcting for the loss estimate increased the C/M ratio to 6.1% of WT (right axis, red column, **Fig. 12B**). Thus, in this R117H-5T subject, functional estimates based on patch-clamp [12] and mRNA transcript analysis [13] converged with those of based on C/M-sweat bubble analysis.

Quantifying G551D CFTR function in vivo and in vitro

The G551D mutation severely decreases P_O to near zero (~0.004) without a known effect on n or γ [15]. The calculations used above predict that this level of function is invisible to the sweat bubble test, consistent with the lack of any observed sweating in the 4 G551D subjects tested (−) ivacaftor. The P_O of G551D-CFTR (+)-ivacaftor has been measured as 0.04 [14] and 0.12 [2] or 10–30% of the WT value of 0.4. Subjects S1–S3 and S5 each have one G551D and one (nonfunctional) F508del allele, so their ivacaftor-potentiated CFTR function should have been half of those values or 5–15% of WT. C/M ratios from the top 12 M-sweat rate glands (**Fig. 12A, B**) gave values of 0.24% to 2.77%, and correcting for the loss estimate of 0.023 $nl^{-min-gland}$ gave 1.56% for S1 to 4.08% for S5. The highest value is similar to the estimate of ~5% CFTR function predicted from the ivacaftor-potentiated P_O value of 0.04 [**14**]. Based on all the data and on comparisons with the ivacaftor-treated R117H subject, we estimate ivacaftor-potentiated CFTR function in G551D/F508del subjects to be <5% WT.

Subject S4 has mutations R117H-5T and G551D. In the (+) ivacaftor condition, the data from patch clamp and transcript analysis predicts CFTR function of 2.6–5% function for R117H-5T, and up to 5% for G551D, or up to 10% function for the combination. The corrected C/M value for this subject was 7.7%, the highest value observed, consistent with an additive effect of ivacaftor acting on both mutations.

Does ivacaftor increase M-sweating?

The present experiments do not answer that question. Two of 3 subjects where M-sweating was tested (+/−) ivacaftor did not show a change. The increased M-sweating seen in S1 (+) ivacaftor occurred in tests that were run over a 6 month period, and two

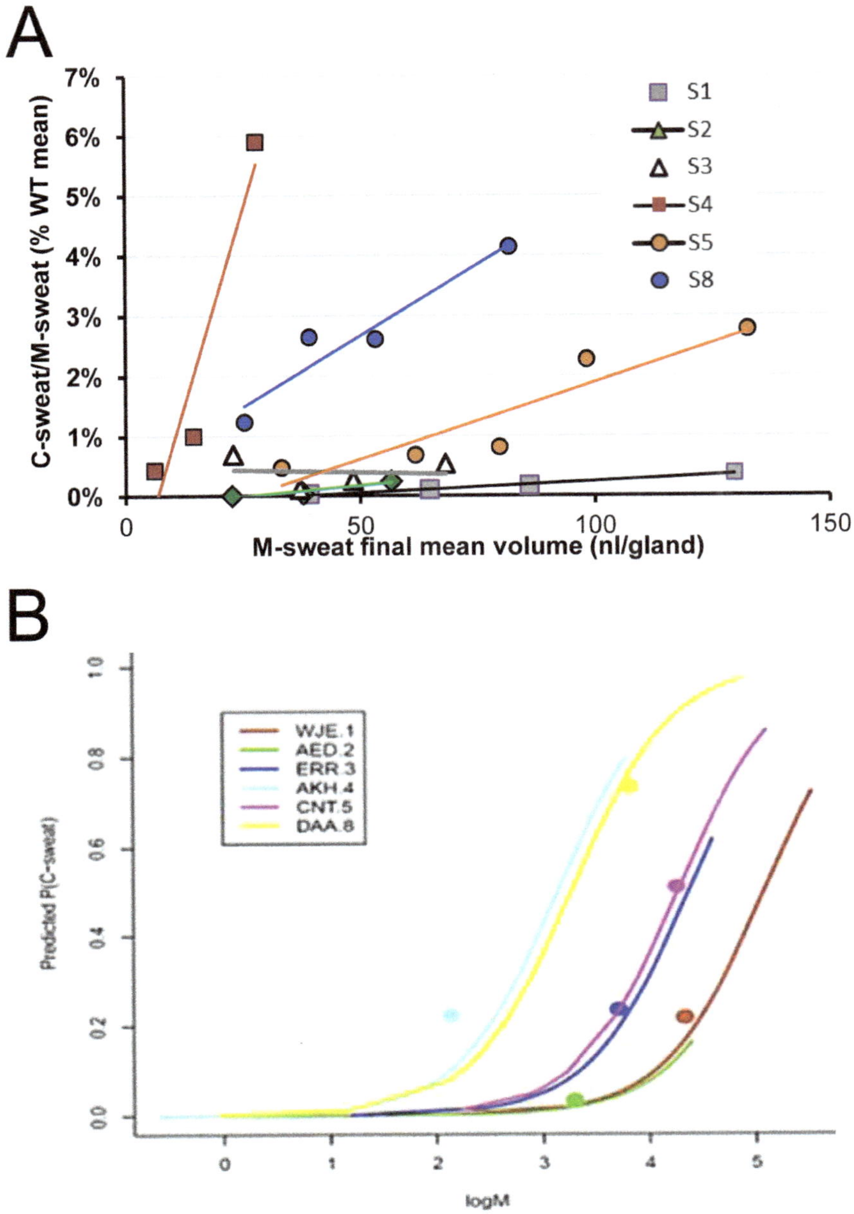

Figure 12. C-sweat values as a function of M-sweat rates. (A) Summary data showing dependence of C/M ratios to M-sweat rates for all 6 subjects tested (+) ivacaftor. For clarity, each subject's glands, glands were rank ordered according to their M-sweat rates and then divided into 3–5 bins according to their M-sweat rates (mean of 16.6 glands per bin). Each point plots the average M-sweat response on the x-axis and the average C/M ratio as a% of the WT mean on the y-axis for each bin; lines are linear fits. Each gland was measured 1–3 times, and the average number of glands included in each bin was 16.6 (range 5–26 glands). C/M vs. M-sweat correlations were significant for all subjects except S3. (B) C-sweat response is coded as 1, if some C-sweat is observed on a test, and 0, otherwise; and P(C-sweat) denotes the probability that C-sweat is observed. Then P(C-sweat) is also the average of the recoded 0/1 C-sweat response. We predicted P(C-sweat) as a function of log M-sweat using the combined data from all 6 CF subjects tested (+) ivacaftor. A logistic mixed model analysis showed that CF patients differed in their overall P(C-sweat) levels, but not in the within-patient effect of M-sweat response on P(C-sweat) across glands ($p>.57$), and that the average across patients of the within-patient effect of M-sweat was significantly positive ($b=2.14$, $p<.0001$). The predicted P(C-sweat) levels are plotted for each patient. See methods and Appendix S1.

(−) ivacaftor tests in winter months gave lower values than any other tests. There was no opportunity to test again off-drug. M-sweating has been considered to be CFTR-independent because of its persistence in CF subjects [16,17], but CFTR contributes to cholinergically-mediated fluid secretion in several tissues and species [25,26,27,28,29,30,31]. Stimulation of M3 muscarinic receptors strongly activates CFTR when both are expressed in BHK cells [32], and apical UTP activates CFTR in primary human airway cells [33]. It is possible that CFTR is activated during M-sweating, but its contribution may be masked by a high apical conductance conferred by CaCC channels.

Limitations

Four limitations specific to the present study are that it was done open label, with a small number of subjects, the results could not be correlated with clinical or sweat chloride data because of

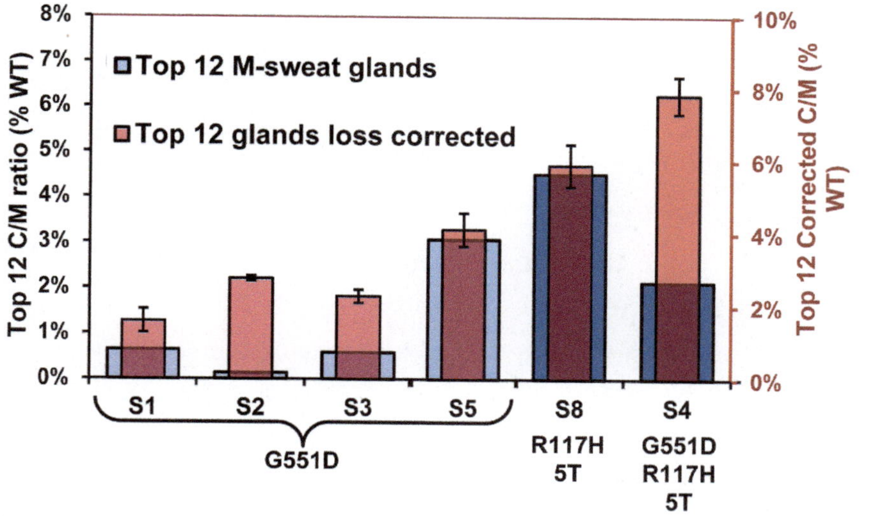

Figure 13. Loss-reduced and loss-corrected estimates of CFTR function in CF subjects (+) ivacaftor. Each blue column (left axis) shows mean C/M ratios (mean ± SEM) for the 12 glands with the highest M-sweat rates for each subject; higher sweat rates reduce C-sweat losses. Each transparent red column (right axis) shows the corrected C/M ratios (mean ± SEM) for the 12 fastest M-secreting glands, obtained by adding 0.029 $nl^{-min-gland}$ to the observed C-sweat secretion rates (see text).

ongoing studies, and only two subjects were tested with triplicate (±) ivacaftor tests. The inaccessibility of subjects for repeated (±) testing was our main concern, because the assay is well suited for n-of-1 studies where each subject (and each gland) serves as its own control [34,35,36,37]. It will be important to carry out more n-of-1 studies with ivacaftor in which this assay is one component of the assessment, and to establish the assay in other laboratories. Because of large and consistent individual differences in measurements of healthy controls, it will be important to expand the number control subjects and to correlate their results with genotype, sweat chloride, and CFTR transcript analysis.

Conclusions

Multiple measures of C-sweating and M-sweating from individual glands revealed that oral dosing with ivacaftor improved β-adrenergic cocktail-stimulated, CFTR-dependent sweating (C-sweating) in CF subjects with G551D or R117H-5T mutations. The C/M ratio across all measured glands was smaller than predicted based on patch clamp/transcript analyses. We hypothesize that this resulted from a proportionally larger loss of sweat volume via ductal absorption and gland capacitance at lower sweat rates. After correcting for these losses, estimated CFTR

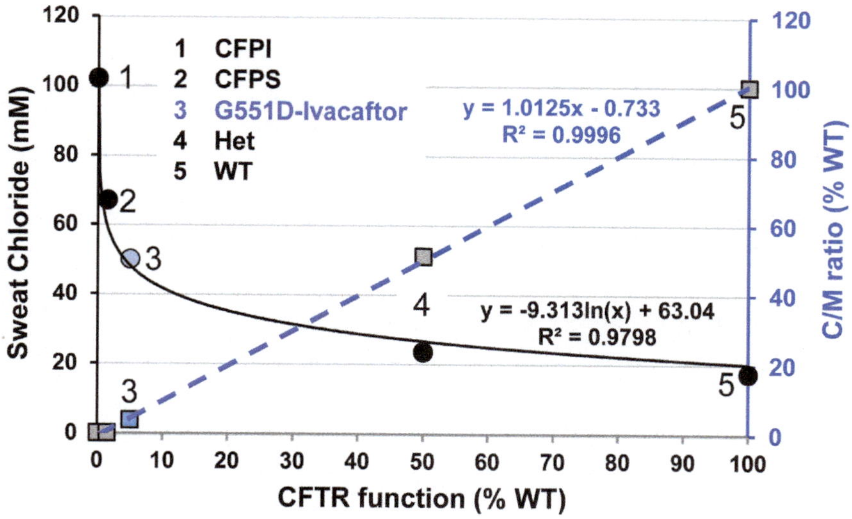

Figure 14. Two measures of CFTR function in the sweat gland. The sweat chloride concentration (left y axis,) is plotted (solid line) against CFTR function as a% of average WT values, plotted on the x axis. Sweat chloride is an inverse logarithmic function of CFTR function (n P_O γ) and hence is most sensitive at the lowest levels of CFTR function. The C-sweat/M-sweat ratio as% WT (right axis), is plotted (dashed line) against CFTR function as a% of average WT values, plotted on the x axis. The C/M ratio provides a direct readout of CFTR function and is linear over most of the range; the loss-reduced and loss-corrected values extend the linear range close to zero CFTR function. Sweat chloride point 3 is from ref. [5], the rest are from ref. [38]. C/M point 3 is from present paper, other points are from ref. [10]. CFTR values 0, 50 and 100 are defined, 1.5% and 5% function assigned by patch clamp and mRNA measures.

function was 2.66±1.06% of WT for the 4 G551D subjects, 6.1% for the R117H-5T subject, and 7.7% for the subject with both mutations. The finding that CFTR-dependent sweat secretion was greater in R117H-5T than in G551D subjects supports prior work suggesting that ivacaftor will be clinically useful for subjects with the R117H-5T mutation [6]. In sum, the corrected *in vivo* estimates of restored CFTR function overlap estimates based on patch clamp data, and suggest that excellent clinical responses can be expected by restoring less than 10% of CFTR function.

Supporting Information

Appendix S1

Acknowledgments

We are grateful to the subjects who participated in these trials and in previous trials required to develop this assay. We thank Dr. Iris Schrijver, Stanford Medical Center for genotyping the healthy control, and Jonathan Chen, Julie Desch, Nam Soo Joo, Franklin B. Krasne, Mauri Krouse, Sara E. Modlin, Olivia Peeps, Barkha Tiwana, and members of the Cystic Fibrosis Foundation Therapeutics Sweat Consortium for valuable assistance and discussions.

Author Contributions

Conceived and designed the experiments: JJW. Performed the experiments: JEC MHW HJC IHP JHJ JJW. Analyzed the data: JEC JJW MHW EACT. Contributed reagents/materials/analysis tools: EF EACT. Wrote the paper: JJW EACT RBM JEC. Recruited subjects: CD ZD CM. Supplied relevant clinical data: CD ZD CM. Discussed interpretations: CD ZD CM.

References

1. Sosnay PR, Siklosi KR, Van Goor F, Kaniecki K, Yu H, et al. (2013) Defining the disease liability of variants in the cystic fibrosis transmembrane conductance regulator gene. Nat Genet.
2. Yu H, Burton B, Huang CJ, Worley J, Cao D, et al. (2012) Ivacaftor potentiation of multiple CFTR channels with gating mutations. Journal of cystic fibrosis: official journal of the European Cystic Fibrosis Society 11: 237–245.
3. Van Goor F, Hadida S, Grootenhuis PD, Burton B, Cao D, et al. (2009) Rescue of CF airway epithelial cell function in vitro by a CFTR potentiator, VX-770. Proc Natl Acad Sci U S A 106: 18825–18830.
4. Accurso FJ, Rowe SM, Clancy JP, Boyle MP, Dunitz JM, et al. (2010) Effect of VX-770 in persons with cystic fibrosis and the G551D-CFTR mutation. N Engl J Med 363: 1991–2003.
5. Ramsey BW, Davies J, McElvaney NG, Tullis E, Bell SC, et al. (2011) A CFTR potentiator in patients with cystic fibrosis and the G551D mutation. The New England journal of medicine 365: 1663–1672.
6. Van Goor F, Yu H, Burton B, Huang C, Hoffman B (2012) Ivacaftor potentiates multiple mutant cystic fibrosis transconductance regulator (CFTR) forms. Pediatr Pulmonol 47: 233.
7. Drumm ML, Konstan MW, Schluchter MD, Handler A, Pace R, et al. (2005) Genetic modifiers of lung disease in cystic fibrosis. N Engl J Med 353: 1443–1453.
8. Guo X, Pace RG, Stonebraker JR, Commander CW, Dang AT, et al. (2011) Mucin variable number tandem repeat polymorphisms and severity of cystic fibrosis lung disease: significant association with MUC5AC. PLoS One 6: e25452.
9. Veeze HJ, Halley DJ, Bijman J, de Jongste JC, de Jonge HR, et al. (1994) Determinants of mild clinical symptoms in cystic fibrosis patients. Residual chloride secretion measured in rectal biopsies in relation to the genotype. The Journal of clinical investigation 93: 461–466.
10. Wine JJ, Char JE, Chen J, Cho HJ, Dunn C, et al. (2013) In Vivo Readout of CFTR Function: Ratiometric Measurement of CFTR-Dependent Secretion by Individual, Identifiable Human Sweat Glands. PLoS One 8: e77114.
11. Farber S (1945) Some organic digestive disturbances in early life. J Mich Med Soc 44: 587.
12. Sheppard DN, Rich DP, Ostedgaard LS, Gregory RJ, Smith AE, et al. (1993) Mutations in CFTR associated with mild-disease-form Cl- channels with altered pore properties. Nature 362: 160–164.
13. Chu CS, Trapnell BC, Curristin S, Cutting GR, Crystal RG (1993) Genetic basis of variable exon 9 skipping in cystic fibrosis transmembrane conductance regulator mRNA. Nat Genet 3: 151–156.
14. Jih KY, Hwang TC (2013) Vx-770 potentiates CFTR function by promoting decoupling between the gating cycle and ATP hydrolysis cycle. Proc Natl Acad Sci U S A 110: 4404–4409.
15. Bompadre SG, Sohma Y, Li M, Hwang TC (2007) G551D and G1349D, two CF-associated mutations in the signature sequences of CFTR, exhibit distinct gating defects. J Gen Physiol 129: 285–298.
16. Cooke RE, Gochberg SH (1956) Physiology of the sweat gland in cystic fibrosis of the pancreas. Pediatrics 18: 701–715.
17. Bijman J, Quinton PM (1984) Influence of abnormal Cl- impermeability on sweating in cystic fibrosis. Am J Physiol 247: C3–9.
18. Cheng SH, Gregory RJ, Marshall J, Paul S, Souza DW, et al. (1990) Defective intracellular transport and processing of CFTR is the molecular basis of most cystic fibrosis. Cell 63: 827–834.
19. Champigny G, Imler JL, Puchelle E, Dalemans W, Gribkoff V, et al. (1995) A change in gating mode leading to increased intrinsic Cl- channel activity compensates for defective processing in a cystic fibrosis mutant corresponding to a mild form of the disease. EMBO J 14: 2417–2423.
20. Friedman KJ, Heim RA, Knowles MR, Silverman LM (1997) Rapid characterization of the variable length polythymidine tract in the cystic fibrosis (CFTR) gene: association of the 5T allele with selected CFTR mutations and its incidence in atypical sinopulmonary disease. Hum Mutat 10: 108–115.
21. Cuppens H, Lin W, Jaspers M, Costes B, Teng H, et al. (1998) Polyvariant mutant cystic fibrosis transmembrane conductance regulator genes. The polymorphic (Tg)m locus explains the partial penetrance of the T5 polymorphism as a disease mutation. J Clin Invest 101: 487–496.
22. Behm JK, Hagiwara G, Lewiston NJ, Quinton PM, Wine JJ (1987) Hyposecretion of beta-adrenergically induced sweating in cystic fibrosis heterozygotes. Pediatr Res 22: 271–276.
23. de Nooijer RA, Nobel JM, Arets HG, Bot AG, van Berkhout FT, et al. (2011) Assessment of CFTR function in homozygous R117H-7T subjects. J Cyst Fibros 10: 326–332.
24. Wilschanski M, Zielenski J, Markiewicz D, Tsui LC, Corey M, et al. (1995) Correlation of sweat chloride concentration with classes of the cystic fibrosis transmembrane conductance regulator gene mutations. J Pediatr 127: 705–710.
25. Taylor CJ, Baxter PS, Hardcastle J, Hardcastle PT (1988) Failure to induce secretion in jejunal biopsies from children with cystic fibrosis. Gut 29: 957–962.
26. Berschneider HM, Knowles MR, Azizkhan RG, Boucher RC, Tobey NA, et al. (1988) Altered intestinal chloride transport in cystic fibrosis. Faseb J 2: 2625–2629.
27. Bijman J, Veeze H, Kansen M, Tilly B, Scholte B, et al. (1991) Chloride transport in the cystic fibrosis enterocyte. Adv Exp Med Biol 290: 287–294; discussion 294–286.
28. Salinas D, Haggie PM, Thiagarajah JR, Song Y, Rosbe K, et al. (2005) Submucosal gland dysfunction as a primary defect in cystic fibrosis. Faseb J 19: 431–433.
29. Joo NS, Cho HJ, Khansaheb M, Wine JJ (2010) Hyposecretion of fluid from tracheal submucosal glands of CFTR-deficient pigs. J Clin Invest 120: 3161–3166.
30. Cho HJ, Joo NS, Wine JJ (2011) Defective fluid secretion from submucosal glands of nasal turbinates from CFTR−/− and CFTR (DeltaF508/DeltaF508) pigs. PloS one 6: e24424.
31. Sun X, Sui H, Fisher JT, Yan Z, Liu X, et al. (2010) Disease phenotype of a ferret CFTR-knockout model of cystic fibrosis. J Clin Invest 120: 3149–3160.
32. Billet A, Luo Y, Balghi H, Hanrahan JW (2013) Role of tyrosine phosphorylation in the muscarinic activation of the Cystic Fibrosis Transmembrane conductance Regulator (CFTR). J Biol Chem.
33. Namkung W, Finkbeiner WE, Verkman AS (2010) CFTR-adenylyl cyclase I association responsible for UTP activation of CFTR in well-differentiated primary human bronchial cell cultures. Mol Biol Cell 21: 2639–2648.
34. Rochon J (1990) A statistical model for the "N-of-1" study. Journal of clinical epidemiology 43: 499–508.
35. Spiegelhalter DJ (1988) Statistical issues in studies of individual response. Scandinavian journal of gastroenterology Supplement 147: 40–45.
36. Barlow DH, Hersen M (1984) Single Case Experimental Designs MA, USA: Allyn and Bacon.
37. Kazdin AE (1982) Single-Case Research Designs: Methods for Clinical and Applied Settings. New York, USA: Oxford University Press.
38. Gonska T, Choi P, Stephenson A, Ellis L, Martin S, et al. (2012) Role of Cystic Fibrosis Transmembrane Conductance Regulator (CFTR) in patients with chronic sinopulmonary disease. Chest 142: 996–1004.

13

Reduced Blood Pressure of CFTR-F508del Carriers Correlates with Diminished Arterial Reactivity Rather than Circulating Blood Volume in Mice

Veronica A. Peotta, Prasad Bhandary, Ugochi Ogu, Kenneth A. Volk, Robert D. Roghair*

Department of Pediatrics, University of Iowa Carver College of Medicine, Iowa City, Iowa, United States of America

Abstract

The F508del mutation of the cystic fibrosis transmembrane conductance regulator (CFTR) is the most common cause of cystic fibrosis (CF). Both CF patients and F508del carriers have decreased blood pressure. While this has been attributed to salt depletion, recent studies have shown F508del expression interferes with smooth muscle cell calcium mobilization. We tested the hypothesis that carriers of the F508del mutation have lower adult blood pressures and reduced aortic contractility without a reduction in circulating blood volume. By radiotelemetry, F508del heterozygous mice had significantly lower arterial pressures than wild-type C57BL/6 controls, with the greatest effect seen at the time of dark-to-light cycle transition (mean difference of 10 mmHg). To replicate the vascular effects of sympathetic arousal, isoproterenol and epinephrine were co-infused, and F508del mice again had significantly reduced arterial pressures. Aortas isolated from F508del heterozygous mice had significantly decreased constriction to noradrenaline (0.9 ± 0.2 versus 2.9 ± 0.7 mN). Inhibition of wild-type CFTR or the inositol triphosphate receptor replicated the phenotype of F508del aortas. CFTR carrier status did not alter circulating blood volume. We conclude the CFTR-F508del mutation decreases aortic contractility and lowers arterial pressures. As a cAMP-activated chloride channel that facilitates calcium mobilization, we speculate wild-type CFTR co-activation during adrenergic receptor stimulation buffers the vasodilatory response to catecholamines, and loss of this compensatory vasoconstrictor tone may contribute to the lower arterial pressures seen in heterozygote carriers of a CFTR-F508del mutation.

Editor: Jörn Karhausen, Duke University Medical Center, United States of America

Funding: Funding was provided by the National Institutes of Health (HL102659 to RDR) and the Children's Miracle Network (RDR). The funders had no role in study design, data collection and analysis, decision to publish, or preparation of the manuscript.

Competing Interests: The authors have declared that no competing interests exist.

* E-mail: robert-roghair@uiowa.edu

Introduction

Cystic fibrosis (CF) is the most common life-limiting autosomal recessive disease [1]. It is caused by mutations of the gene encoding the cystic fibrosis transmembrane conductance regulator (CFTR), a cAMP-activated chloride channel. The predominant CFTR-F508del mutation, carried by 2–3% of individuals of European descent [2], disrupts the biosynthetic processing of CFTR such that the protein is retained in the endoplasmic reticulum and degraded [3], [4]. Individuals homozygous for the F508del mutation have classic CF-related morbidities, including pulmonary disease, gastrointestinal abnormalities, and pancreatic insufficiency. However, little is known about the direct effect of CFTR and the common CFTR mutations on cardiovascular physiology.

Patients with CF, as well as CFTR-F508del carriers, have decreased blood pressures [5–8]. As some have speculated [7], the F508del mutation's evolutionary persistence may be related in part to this antihypertensive effect. Alternatively, the cardiovascular effects of the CFTR-F508del mutation could contribute to morbidity and mortality if a hypotensive phenotype correlates with altered tissue perfusion or elicits a neurohumoral response that could exacerbate the secondary pulmonary hypertension seen in cystic fibrosis patients with chronic lung disease. Intriguingly, the lower blood pressure seen in heterozygous F508del women is most dramatic in those with the highest sweat chloride levels, suggesting a potential explanatory relationship between blood pressure and fluid or electrolyte status [8]. However, studies have consistently shown a lack of hypovolemia in CF patients [6], [9], and an increasing number of investigations have identified functional CFTR expression in non-epithelial cells, including human bronchial smooth muscle cells [10]. Interestingly, airway smooth muscle cells isolated from patients with the F508del mutation have reduced histamine-induced calcium release, a phenotype replicated by pharmacologic CFTR inhibition [10]. In a complementary neonatal piglet model, some of us have likewise shown the F508del mutation reduces aortic smooth muscle cell agonist-induced calcium release and aortic tone [11].

In order to further assess the cardiovascular effects of the F508del mutation, we have turned to a mouse model. Unlike CF piglets, CF mice do not develop co-morbid lung disease and arterial pressures can be measured while the mice are housed in their home environment, thereby clarifying the direct effect of CFTR on blood pressures [12], [13]. With human data suggesting a correlation between reduced chloride gating and decreased blood pressure [8] and cell culture data suggesting the F508del mutation interferes with agonist-induced calcium mobilization [10], [11], we hypothesized that the F508del mutation reduces arterial tone and lowers arterial pressures in the absence of hypovolemia.

Methods

Radiotelemetry

All procedures were performed within the guidelines of the Animal Welfare Act and the National Institutes of Health *Guide for the Care and Use of Laboratory Animals* and were approved by the University of Iowa Animal Care and Use Committee (Permit Number: 1306101). CFTR-F508del mice were generated at the University of Iowa Gene Therapy Center [14]. At 4 to 5 months, wild type (WT) and F508del mice were instrumented with carotid radiotelemeters (Data Sciences International, St Paul, MN) under isoflurane anesthesia with the transmitter housed in a subcutaneous pouch. Following 7 days of recovery, blood pressures and body temperature were sampled for 10 s every 5 min during an 84 h long uninterrupted series of dark and light cycles, as previously described [15]. The arterial waveforms were utilized to derive blood pressures and pulse rate with proprietary software (Dataquest A.R.T., Data Sciences International). During the subsequent light cycle, between 0900 and 1000, the mice were awoken and arterial pressures plus body temperature were recorded at a sampling rate of 1000 Hz. Normal saline (0.9% NaCl, 10 mL/kg) was administered by intraperitoneal injection 20 min into the continuous recording and the transmitters were turned-off after 2 h. At the same time the following day, the transmitters were turned on by passing a magnet under the home cage, and the same recordings were obtained, this time with intraperitoneal administration of the beta-adrenergic receptor agonist isoproterenol (2 mg/kg) plus epinephrine (2 mg/kg) 20 min into the 2 h recording [16], [17].

Blood Volume Determination

Jugular venous catheters were placed in an additional group of mice during isoflurane anesthesia. The following day, 500 μL of blood was obtained from a C57BL/6 donor mouse via cardiac puncture, and the harvested red blood cells (RBCs) were isolated by centrifugation. Utilizing methods analogous to those described for sheep [18], the RBCs were washed and re-suspended to a hematocrit of 25%, as measured by an automated hematology analyzer (Sysmex XE-2100, Sysmex Corp, Kobe, Japan). The washed RBCs were then biotinylated by adding 1 mg/mL Biotin-S-NHS (Thermo Scientific, Rockford, IL) and incubating at room temperature for 30 min. Donor RBCs were then washed, the RBC count determined, and 470 to 530 million biotinylated RBCs (50 μL) were transfused over 10 min via the jugular catheter. One hour after the transfusion, 40 μL of blood was sampled by cardiac puncture or from a free flowing tail vein incision. Hematocrit and mean corpuscular volume were measured with a Sysmex XE-2100. The ratio of biotinylated donor to non-biotinylated recipient RBCs was determined by flow cytometry (FACScan, Becton Dickinson, Franklin Lakes, NJ) after co-labeling all RBCs with FITC-Streptavidin. Blood volume was calculated using the following formula: (number of transfused RBC × mean corpuscular volume × 100) ÷ (ratio of biotinylated RBCs × hematocrit). To validate the technique, an additional 200 μL of blood was collected from the final four mice, and post-phlebotomy blood volumes were again measured after administering a second biotinylated RBC transfusion. Measured post-bleed blood volumes were compared to expected post-bleed blood volumes, as calculated using the following formula: (pre-bleed blood volume − phlebotomy losses) × pre-bleed hematocrit ÷ post-bleed hematocrit.

Wire Myography

Thoracic aortas were obtained from additional WT and CFTR-F508del adult mice and 2.5 mm segments were assessed by wire myography (Danish Myotechnology), as previously described [19]. Constriction to KCl and noradrenaline (NA) were examined in the presence of buffer alone, the inositol triphosphate receptor (IP_3R) antagonist 2-aminoethoxydiphenyl borate (2APB, 50 μM) [20], or the CFTR inhibitor 5-[(4-carboxyphenyl) methylene]-2-thioxo-3-[(3-trifluoromethyl) phenyl]-4-thiazolidinone (CFTRinh-172, 50 μM). Following a one hour equilibration at a resting tension of 5 mN, the aortic segments were constricted with cumulative concentrations of KCl (5 to 90 mM). After rinsing and re-equilibration, the vessels were constricted with cumulative concentrations of NA (10^{-9} to 10^{-6} M) to assess alpha-adrenergic receptor responsiveness (at low concentrations) and beta-adrenergic receptor responsiveness (at higher concentrations). All compounds were acquired from Sigma Chemical (St. Louis, MO).

Statistical Analysis

All data are expressed as means ± SE. Values were considered statistically significant when $p<0.05$ by Student's two-tailed *t*-test. Baseline hemodynamics, activity and temperature were analyzed by two way repeated measures ANOVA, factoring for genotype and time of day, followed by Bonferroni *post hoc* testing. Whenever a significant interaction was present between genotype and time of day, multiple comparison tests were utilized to evaluate for independent effects. The correlation between calculated and measured blood volumes was assessed by Pearson Product Moment Correlation. All analyses were performed by SigmaPlot 12.0 (Systat Software, Inc.).

Results

Perioperative Mortality

Despite maintenance on corn grit bedding and a high energy content diet (Teklad S-2335, 3.5 kcal/g), 7 out of 30 (23%) of the homozygous $CFTRF^{508del/F508del}$ mice died prior to 4 months of age, and necropsy confirmed the presence of distal intestinal obstruction. Other than a heterozygous $CFTRF^{508del/+}$ mouse that died on the same day as a $CFTRF^{508del/F508del}$ littermate, there was no further preoperative mortality. Radiotelemeters were readily implanted in three $CFTRF^{508del/F508del}$ mice, but all died by postoperative day 5. Given the high perioperative mortality of $CFTRF^{508del/F508del}$ mice and our overarching interest in the phenotype of F508del carriers, our subsequent studies focused exclusively on WT and F508del heterozygous mice. For these mice, intraoperative mortality was 9.5% (1 of 20 WT, 3 of 22 F508del), and postoperative mortality was 13.2% (2 of 19 WT, 3 of 19 F508del).

CFTR-induced Hypotension

Baseline blood pressures were influenced by a significant interaction between genotype and time of day ($P<0.001$). By post-hoc testing, F508del heterozygous mice had significantly lower systolic and diastolic pressures, and this was the most prominent at the 0600 transition from dark to light cycles (Figure 1A). Because human studies have shown the blood pressure lowering effect of F508del status may be specific to females [8], we performed *a priori* sex-specific subgroup analysis

(Table 1). Overall, female but not male blood pressures were reduced by the F508del mutation. Looking specifically at the key dark-to-light transition, dF508del mice had an overall reduction in mean arterial pressure of 9.3 mmHg (female mean difference: 9.7 mm Hg, $P<0.05$; male mean difference: 8.1 mm, $P = 0.23$). CFTR genotype did not significantly alter pulse rate, locomotor activity, or body temperature (Figure 1). Because CFTR is activated by cAMP, the key second messenger in β-adrenergic receptor activation, we speculated that the hemodynamic effects of the CFTR-F508del mutation may be further unmasked during pharmacologic β-adrenergic receptor activation.

Hemodynamic Responses to β-adrenergic Receptor Agonists

Other than a brief hypertensive response to the injection, normal saline had no demonstrable effect on blood pressures, pulse rate or body temperature (Figure 2A to 2C). Consistent with the baseline data, F508del mice had lower blood pressures immediately after the stress-inducing intraperitoneal injection (Figure 2A). While the initial stress responses to co-injection of isoproterenol and epinephrine were reminiscent of the responses elicited by the normal saline injection, the second hour of recording revealed a substantial hypotensive, tachycardic and hypothermic response in both WT and F508del mice (Figure 2D to 2F). Compared to WT mice, F508del mice had exaggerated hypotensive and tachycardic responses to the co-injected β-adrenergic receptor agonists (Figure 2D and 2E, respectively). These results suggest the presence of increased β-adrenergic receptor-mediated vasodilation in F508del mice that may underlie the lower baseline pressures. Because hypovolemia enhances the hemodynamic responses to vasodilators and the presence of CFTR mutations may enhance electrolyte and water losses, circulating blood volumes were determined.

Lack of Hypovolemia in F508del Mice

The ratio of biotinylated donor and non-biotinylated RBCs was accurately quantified (Figure 3A). CFTR genotype had no significant effect on mean corpuscular volume, hematocrit or circulating blood volume (Table 2). To validate the blood volume measurements, paired samples were obtained from 4 mice before and after removal of 15–17% of the circulating blood volume. Post-bleed sampling showed a 10–14% reduction in hematocrit and a 4–10% decrease in blood volume. This is consistent with partial fluid redistribution to maintain circulating volume (Table 2). Measured and calculated blood volumes were correlated ($R = 0.98$, $P = 0.02$) as indicated by the slope of the regression line approximating the line of identity (Figure 3B). This finding bolsters confidence that if a significant difference in blood volume had been present, it would have been identified.

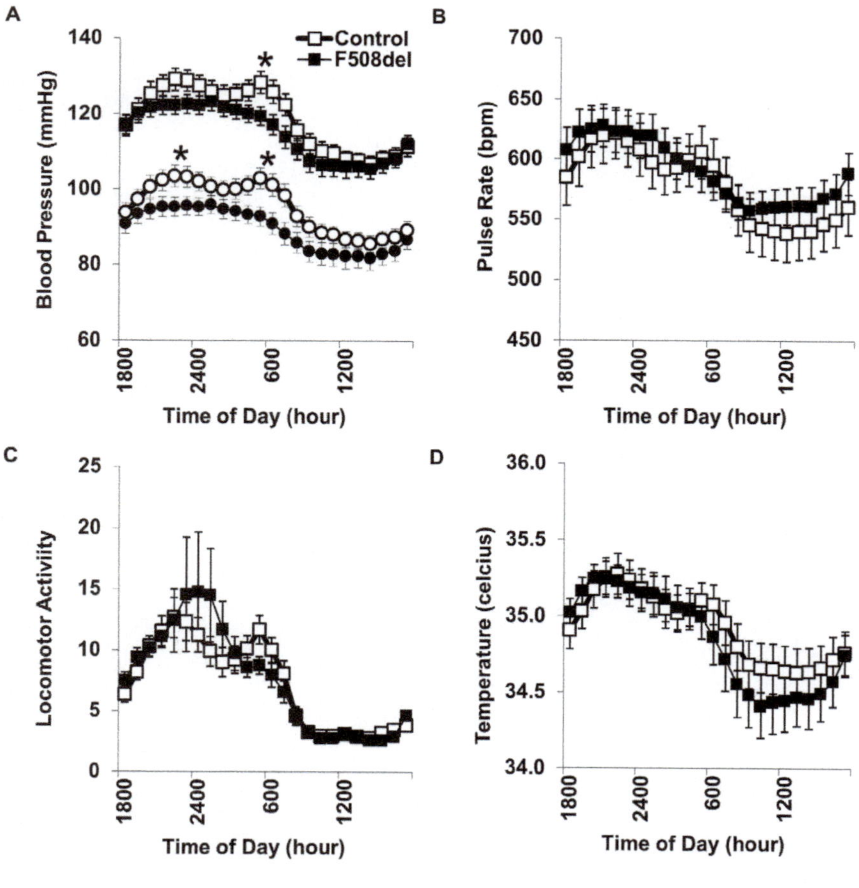

Figure 1. Carotid radiotelemetry. Systolic and diastolic blood pressures (squares and circles, respectively) were measured while mice were housed in their home cage during alternating cycles of darkness (1800 to 0600) and light (0600 to 1800) (A). Compared to wild-type mice (WT, open symbols), heterozygous F508del mice (solid symbols) had lower systolic and diastolic pressures at the dark-to-light transition. Pulse rate (B), locomotor activity (C), and body temperature (D) were not significantly influenced by F508del status. *$P<0.05$ versus WT; N = 17 WT and 16 F508del mice.

Table 1. Baseline radiotelemetry.

	Female		Male	
	WT	**F508del**	**WT**	**F508del**
N	10	8	7	8
Systolic blood pressure (mmHg)	119±2	112±1*	119±5	118±5
Diastolic blood pressure (mmHg)	98±3	90±3	92±5	89±4
Pulse rate (bpm)	560±35	582±25	605±11	599±22
Temperature (°C)	35.2±0.1	35.3±0.1	34.6±0.2	34.4±0.1

Arterial waveform-derived systolic blood pressure, diastolic blood pressure and pulse rate were recorded, along with subcutaneous body temperature, every 5 minutes over an 84 h interval while wild-type (WT) and heterozygous F508del mice freely explored their home cage. *P<0.05 versus WT.

CFTR-dependent Aortic Reactivity

Without evidence that the hypotensive phenotype of F508del mice is a consequence of hypovolemia, we went on to assess the effects of the F508del mutation on isolated vessel reactivity. Aortic constriction to KCl was not significantly altered by CFTR mutation status (Figure 4A). CFTRinh-172 significantly decreased the response of WT but not F508del aorta to 10–20 mM KCl (Figure 4B; 38+/−12% versus 14+/−18% decrease in constriction to 15 mM KCl, respectively), while the IP_3R antagonist 2APB significantly decreased the response of both WT and F508del aorta to >15 mM KCl (Figure 4C). Compared to WT aorta, aorta from F508del heterozygous mice had decreased constriction to the highest concentrations of NA (Figure 4D). Although preincubation with CFTRinh-172 did not significantly decrease NA-evoked constriction of aorta from WT or F508del mice (Figure 4E), IP_3R inhibition with 2APB decreased the NA responsiveness of WT more than F508del aorta (73+/−7% versus 3+/−59% decrease in constriction to 10^{-7} M NA, respectively), thereby replicating the vascular effects of the F508del mutation (Figure 4F).

Discussion

While the effects of CFTR expression on epithelial tissue are well described [21], [22], the effects of CFTR on muscle tissue are relatively undefined. Both human and murine studies have shown skeletal muscle dysfunction may be intimately linked with the respiratory insufficiency and exercise intolerance that contribute to the morbidity of patients with F508del mutations [23], [24]. Likewise, both human and murine studies suggest CFTR mutations directly interfere with cardiac myocyte function [25–27]. Utilizing a neonatal piglet CF model, we recently replicated

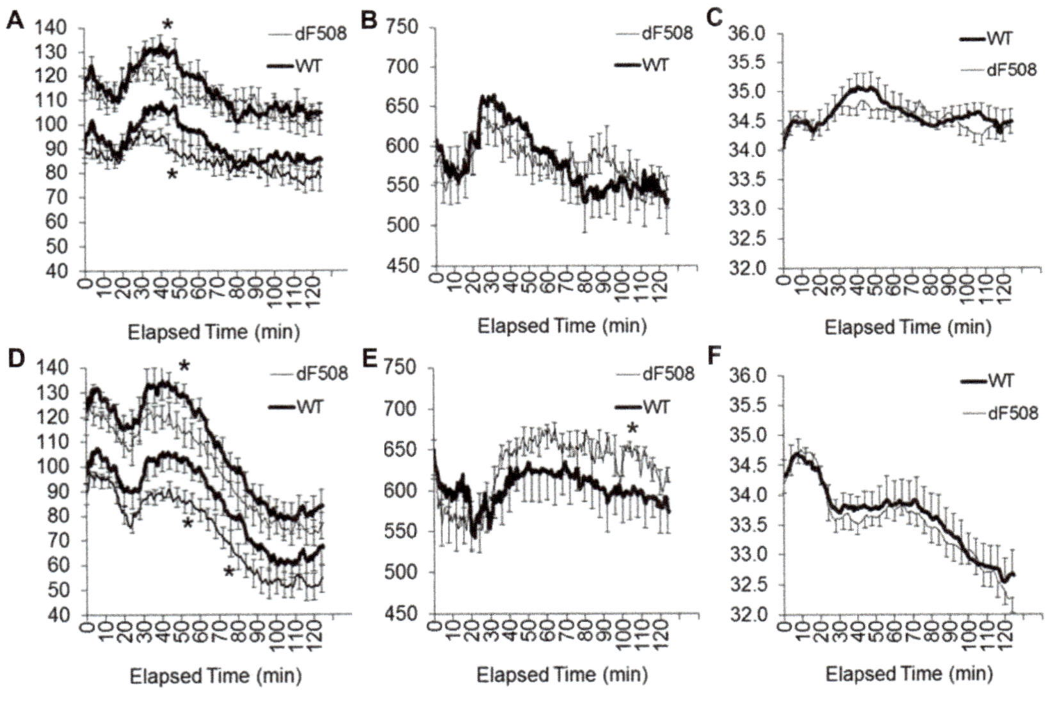

Figure 2. Physiological responses to β-adrenergic agonists. Twenty minutes after starting the continuous recording of arterial pressures (A), pulse rate (B) and body temperature (C), wild-type mice (WT, thick line) and heterozygous F508del mice (thin line) received normal saline (10 mL/kg i.p.). The following day, the same protocol was utilized with the injection of normal saline containing isoproterenol and epinephrine (2 mg/kg of each) (D to F). *P<0.05 versus WT; N = 14 WT and 16 F508del (injections were not given to the initial 3 WT female mice with baseline data reported in Figure 1).

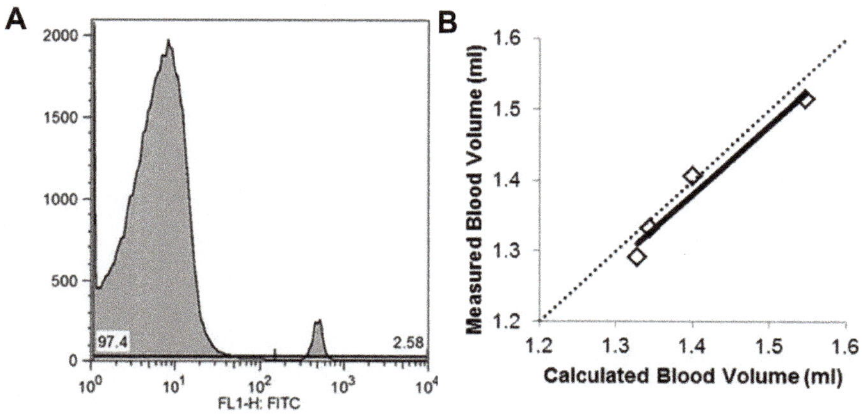

Figure 3. Circulating blood volume. One hour following the transfusion of biotinylated RBC, the ratio of biotinylated RBCs to native circulating RBCs was determined by flow cytometry (A, representative histogram showing 97.4% non-biotinylated RBC peak on the left and 2.6% biotinylated RBCs on the right). For 4 mice, 200 µL of blood was collected and repeat biotinylated RBC infusion was administered prior to the measurement of post-bleed blood volumes. The measured post-bleed blood volumes closely approximated the values expected based on the amount of blood removed (B, R = 0.98 and slope = 0.97 with dotted line indicating the line of identity).

human data showing decreased calcium transients in F508del expressing smooth muscle cells and further correlated this with impaired aortic constriction [11]. In that study, F508del heterozygous aortic smooth muscle cells had a phenotype intermediate between that of the WT and CF cells [11]. The present studies investigated whether a single copy of the F508del mutation is sufficient to reduce arterial pressure and arterial contractility.

As reported in human carriers, F508del heterozygous mice had significantly decreased baseline arterial pressures. In both cases, the phenotype is stronger in females than males. In the human studies, women with the lowest blood pressures tended to have the lowest level of CFTR activity, as measured by sweat chloride levels [8]. Similarly, the hypotensive effect of the mutation in mice was most pronounced during the transition between dark and light cycles, a time of heightened arousal associated with increased sympathetic tone and potentially increased CFTR activation [28]. In F508del male mice, a hypotensive phenotype was elicited during the administration of beta-adrenergic receptor agonists, compounds that increase cAMP levels and, at least theoretically, WT CFTR activity, thereby magnifying the phenotypic effect of endogenous CFTR expression. Among the intracellular processes that may contribute to the CFTR modulation of β-adrenergic signaling, there is experimental support for CFTR-mediated membrane depolarization leading to enhanced flux through voltage-dependent calcium channels [27].

To begin testing the hypothesis that cAMP-mediated WT CFTR co-activation facilitates myocyte contraction as a buffer against β-adrenergic receptor-mediated vasodilation, the reactivity of isolated aortic segments was assessed. There were no significant differences between WT and F508del aortic reactivity to depolarizing concentrations of KCl, possibly reflecting a low level of basal CFTR activation. Nevertheless, CFTR inhibition did significantly reduce the constriction of WT aorta to KCl. This contrasts with studies in epithelial cells where CFTR activation antagonizes IP_3-mediated smooth muscle cell constriction and promotes vasodilation, possibly by hyperpolarizing the endoplasmic reticulum membrane [21], [22]. This dichotomy may originate from the differing resting membrane potentials and intracellular chloride content of the 2 cells types. As reviewed by Matchkov and colleagues, vascular smooth muscle cells have a relatively depolarized resting potential and actively accumulate chloride, allowing for chloride efflux-induced membrane depolarization [29]. Because it is difficult to achieve consistent submaximal aortic preconstriction prior to the addition of β-adrenergic receptor-specific vasodilators, we instead chose to assess aortic responsiveness to NA, a catecholamine with mixed α- and β-adrenergic receptor activity.

Unlike the progressive vasoconstriction seen from WT aorta, the aorta from F508del mice had significantly diminished arterial tone at the highest NA concentrations. While pharmacologic CFTR inhibition of WT responsiveness largely recapitulated the F508del phenotype, it is possible the limiting effects of the F508del mutation on vasoconstriction may extend beyond the channels chloride gating properties. In particular, the expression of CFTR-

Table 2. Blood Volume.

	WT	F508del	Pre-bleed	Post-bleed
N	10	6	4	4
Mean corpuscular volume (fL)	48.6±0.2	46.9±0.5	47.8±0.7	47.6±0.8
Hematocrit (%)	44±2	39±4	49±1	43±1*
Blood Volume (ml/kg)	58±3	64±2	64±3	60±4*

One hour after infusion of biotinylated RBCs, mean corpuscular volume and hematocrit were measured along with flow cytometric determination of the percentage of donor and recipient RBCs. These values were utilized in calculating the circulating blood volume. In 4 mice (3 WT and 1 F508del), an additional 200 µl of blood was collected and a second biotinylated RBC transfusion administered prior to the measurement of post-bleed values. *$P<0.05$ versus pre-bleed values by paired t-test.

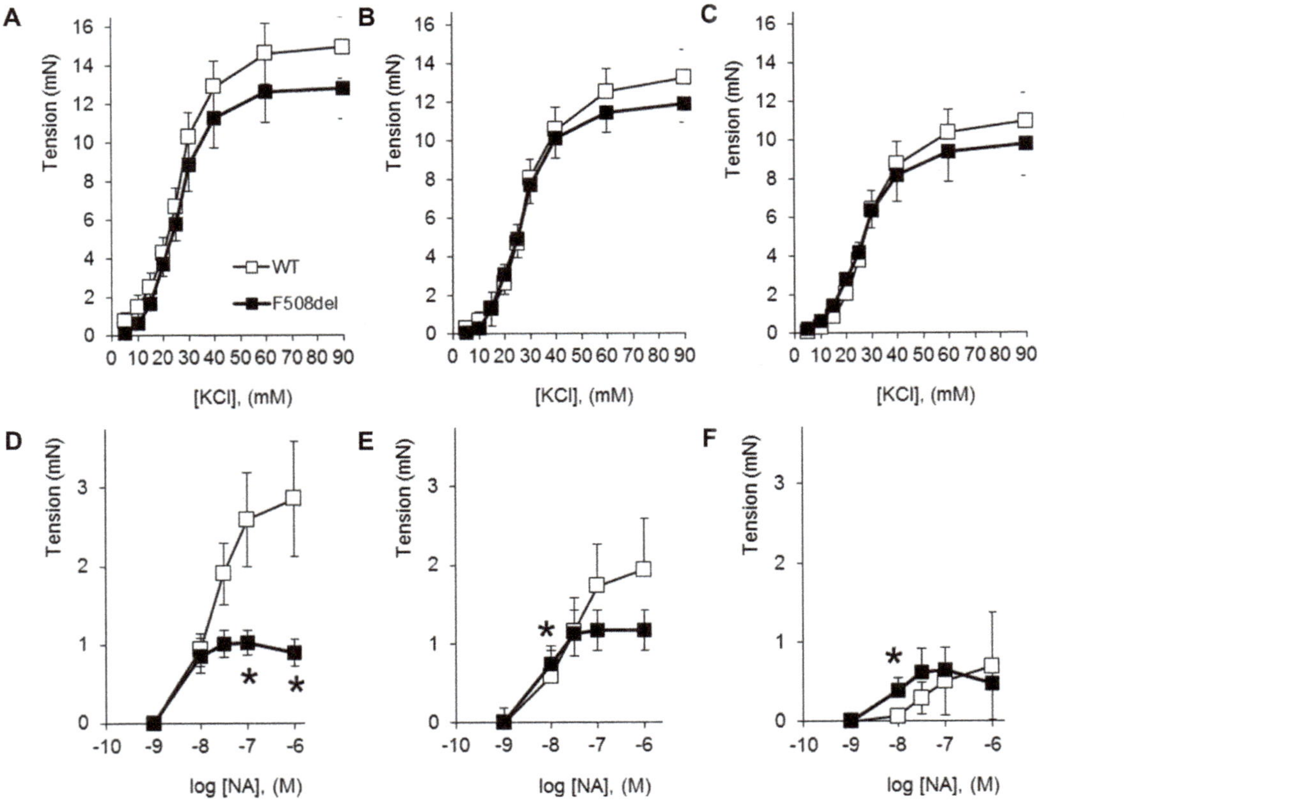

Figure 4. Aortic myography. Wild type (WT, open symbols, N = 9) and heterozygous F508del (closed symbols, N = 8) aortic constriction to KCl was assessed in the presence of buffer alone (A), CFTR inhibition (B, CFTRinh-172), or IP_3R antagonism (C, 2-APB). After rinsing the arterial segments, the responses were then assessed to cumulative concentrations of noradrenaline (NA). In buffer alone, F508del aorta had attenuated constriction to NA (D). This was blocked by preincubation of the aortic segments in either CFTRinh-172 (E), or 2-APB (F). *$P<0.05$ versus WT.

F508del may elicit an unfolded protein response that could alter endoplasmic reticulum structure and the activity of other proteins that are targets of the endoplasmic reticulum stress response, including the IP_3 receptor [30], [31]. The IP_3 receptor is intimately involved in the regulation of aortic reactivity, as demonstrated by the inhibitory effects of 2APB in the current study. Furthermore, the induction of an endoplasmic reticulum stress response to CFTR-F508del expression has been shown to transcriptionally repress WT CFTR [32]. A reduction in chloride gating, interference with IP_3 receptor expression and/or a decrease in expression of the WT CFTR allele could contribute to the cardiovascular phenotypes of mice expressing but a single copy of the F508del mutation.

The circulating blood volume data complemented the myography results. Our results are comparable to those reported for wild-type mice using an alternative radiolabelled RBC method [33]. While no significant differences in circulating blood volume were seen in F508del mice, it is notable that F508del mice tended to have an increase, rather than the theoretical decrease in blood volume. This is consistent with human data showing an increase in total body water among CF patients with congestive heart failure and even relatively healthy adolescents with F508del mutations [6], [9]. The etiology of this relative hypervolemia does not appear to correlate with dietary sodium intake, but could be influenced by renin-angiotensin system activation [6].

Our studies are limited by the lack of hemodynamic measurements on CFTR-F508del homozygous mice. As previously reported, CF mice have increased mortality, primarily attributed to a distal intestinal obstruction syndrome [14]. Further investigations are needed to reconcile the demonstrated reduction in vascular reactivity with clinical data showing increased aortic stiffness and impaired flow mediated vasodilation in F508del homozygous patients [34], [35]. In both studies, the increase in aortic stiffness or decrease in vasodilation correlated with inflammatory markers and the severity of lung disease, and it is thus difficult to extrapolate from homozygous to heterozygous individuals. As an endothelium-dependent process, the reduction in flow-mediated dilation suggests the need to further assess the effects of endothelial cell-restricted CFTR-F508del expression [36]. Likewise, because adult blood pressures are influenced by factors other than arterial tone, further investigations centered on vascular smooth muscle-specific F508del expression are needed to clarify the causal relationship between CFTR mutations and the observed reductions in arterial pressure. While CFTR null mice might serve well as a genetic background to introduce vascular-specific F508del expression, studies on murine aortic smooth muscle cells and cardiomyocytes show the loss of CFTR in these cells strongly upregulates alternative chloride channels, as well as voltage-dependent calcium channels [27], [37].

In an autosomal dominant inheritance pattern, mice with an F508del mutation have decreased aortic responsiveness and lower arterial blood pressures. The pathophysiological implications of these findings are unknown. While the hypotensive phenotype may be considered an advantage, if it is a manifestation of dysregulated vascular tone, the exaggerated hypotensive response to adrenergic stimulation may interfere with the regulation of blood flow at times of sympathetic activation. Reassuringly, young adults with relatively mild cystic fibrosis do not appear to have basal or exercise-induced sympathetic over-activation, as measured by circulating norepinephrine levels [5]. With studies showing increased urinary and adrenal catecholamines in patients with late-stage cystic fibrosis [38], further studies are needed to track the state of sympathetic activation, vascular tone, blood pressure and tissue perfusion during the evolution of cystic fibrosis-induced lung disease. There are active clinical trials of small molecules capable of stabilizing CFTR-F508del and enhancing plasma membrane CFTR expression [1], [39]. As these systemically administered medications are increasingly used to modify CFTR expression or activation, our understanding of the physiological effects of extra-pulmonary CFTR expression must keep pace.

Acknowledgments

Dr. John Widness provided invaluable support throughout the investigations.

Author Contributions

Conceived and designed the experiments: VAP PB KAV RDR. Performed the experiments: VAP PB UO KAV RDR. Analyzed the data: VAP PB UO KAV RDR. Contributed to the writing of the manuscript: VAP PB RDR.

References

1. Rogan MP, Stoltz DA, Hornick DB (2011) Cystic fibrosis transmembrane conductance regulator intracellular processing, trafficking, and opportunities for mutation-specific treatment. Chest 139: 1480–1490.
2. Bobadilla JL, Macek M, Fine JP, Farrell PM (2002) Cystic fibrosis: a worldwide analysis of CFTR mutations-correlation with incidence data and application to screening. Hum Mutat 19: 575–606.
3. Cheng SH, Gregory RJ, Marshall J, Paul S, Souza DW, et al. (1990) Defective intracellular transport and processing of CFTR is the molecular basis of most cystic fibrosis. Cell 63: 827–834.
4. Kartner N, Augustinas O, Jensen TJ, Naismith AL, Riordan JR (1992) Mislocalization of delta F508 CFTR in cystic fibrosis sweat gland. Nat Genet 1: 321–327.
5. Lake CR, Davis PB, Ziegler M, Kopin IJ (1979) Electrolytes and norepinephrine levels in blood of patients with cystic fibrosis. Clin Chim Acta 92: 141–146.
6. Legris GJ, Dearborn D, Stern RC, Geiss CL, Hopfer U, et al. (1998) Sodium space and intravascular volume: dietary sodium effects in cystic fibrosis and healthy adolescent subjects. Pediatrics 101: 48–56.
7. Lieberman J, Rodbard S (1975) Low blood pressure in young adults with cystic fibrosis: an effect of chronic salt loss in sweat? Ann Intern Med 82: 806–808.
8. Super M, Irtiza-Ali A, Roberts SA, Schwarz M, Young M, et al. (2004) Blood pressure and the cystic fibrosis gene: evidence for lower pressure rises with age in female carriers. Hypertension 44: 878–883.
9. Rosenthal A, Button LN, Khaw KT (1977) Blood volume changes in patients with cystic fibrosis. Pediatrics 59: 588–594.
10. Michoud MC, Robert R, Hassan M, Moynihan B, Haston C, et al. (2009) Role of the cystic fibrosis transmembrane conductance channel in human airway smooth muscle. Am J Respir Cell Mol Biol 40: 217–222.
11. Guo JJ, Stoltz DA, Zhu V, Volk KA, Segar JL, et al. (2013) Genotype-specific alterations in vascular smooth muscle cell function in cystic fibrosis piglets. J Cyst Fibros doi:10.1016/j.jcf.2013.10.009.
12. Grubb BR, Boucher RC Pathophysiology of gene-targeted mouse models for cystic fibrosis. (1999) Physiol Rev 79: S193–S214.
13. Ostedgaard LS, Meyerholz DK, Chen JH, Pezzulo AA, Karp PH, et al. (2011) The ΔF508 mutation causes CFTR misprocessing and cystic fibrosis-like disease in pigs. Sci Transl Med 3: 74ra24.
14. Zeiher BG, Eichwald E, Zabner J, Smith JJ, Puga AP, et al. (1995) A mouse model for the delta F508 allele of cystic fibrosis. J Clin Invest 96: 2051–2064.
15. Haskell SE, Hermann GM, Reinking BE, Volk KA, Peotta VA, et al. (2103) Sertraline exposure leads to small left heart syndrome in adult mice. Pediatr Res 2013; 73: 286–293.
16. Denegri M, Avelino-Cruz JE, Boncompagni S, De Simone SA, Auricchio A, et al. (2012) Viral gene transfer rescues arrhythmogenic phenotype and ultrastructural abnormalities in adult calsequestrin-null mice with inherited arrhythmias. Circ Res 110: 663–668.
17. Dirksen WP, Lacombe VA, Chi M, Kalyanasundaram A, Viatchenko-Karpinski S, et al. (2007) A mutation in calsequestrin, CASQ2D307H, impairs Sarcoplasmic Reticulum Ca2+ handling and causes complex ventricular arrhythmias in mice. Cardiovasc Res 75: 69–78.
18. Mock DM, Mock NI, Lankford GL, Burmeister LF, Strauss RG, et al. (2008) Red cell volume can be accurately determined in sheep using a nonradioactive biotin label. Pediatr Res 64: 528–532.
19. Roghair RD, Segar JL, Kilpatrick RA, Segar EM, Scholz TD, et al. (2007) Murine aortic reactivity is programmed equally by maternal low protein diet or late gestation dexamethasone. J Matern Fetal Neonatal Med 20: 833–841.
20. Maruyama T, Kanaji T, Nakade S, Kanno T, Mikoshiba K (1997) 2APB, 2-aminoethoxydiphenyl borate, a membrane-penetrable modulator of Ins(1,4,5) P3-induced Ca2+ release. J Biochem 122: 498–505.
21. Antigny F, Norez C, Becq F, Vandebrouck C (2011) CFTR and Ca Signaling in Cystic Fibrosis. Front Pharmacol 2: 67.
22. Martins JR, Kongsuphol P, Sammels E, Dahimène S, Aldehni F, et al. (2011) F508del-CFTR increases intracellular Ca(2+) signaling that causes enhanced calcium-dependent Cl(−) conductance in cystic fibrosis. Biochim Biophys Acta 1812: 1385–1392.
23. Dassios T, Katelari A, Doudounakis S, Mantagos S, Dimitriou G (2013) Respiratory muscle function in patients with cystic fibrosis. Pediatr Pulmonol 48: 865–873.
24. Divangahi M, Balghi H, Danialou G, Comtois AS, Demoule A, et al. (2009) Lack of CFTR in skeletal muscle predisposes to muscle wasting and diaphragm muscle pump failure in cystic fibrosis mice. PLoS Genet 5: e1000586.
25. Baño-Rodrigo A, Salcedo-Posadas A, Villa-Asensi JR, Tamariz-Martel A, Lopez-Neyra A, et al. (2012) Right ventricular dysfunction in adolescents with mild cystic fibrosis. J Cyst Fibros 11: 274–280.
26. Ozcelik N, Shell R, Holtzlander M, Cua C (2013) Decreased right ventricular function in healthy pediatric cystic fibrosis patients versus non-cystic fibrosis patients. Pediatr Cardiol 34: 159–164.
27. Sellers ZM, De Arcangelis V, Xiang Y, Best PM (2010) Cardiomyocytes with disrupted CFTR function require CaMKII and Ca(2+)-activated Cl(−) channel activity to maintain contraction rate. J Physiol 588: 2417–2429.
28. Makino M, Hayashi H, Takezawa H, Hirai M, Saito H, et al. (1997) Circadian rhythms of cardiovascular functions are modulated by the baroreflex and the autonomic nervous system in the rat. Circulation 96: 1667–1674.
29. Matchkov VV, Secher Dam V, Bødtkjer DM, Aalkjær C (2013) Transport and function of chloride in vascular smooth muscles. J Vasc Res 50: 69–87.
30. Bartoszewski R, Rab A, Jurkuvenaite A, Mazur M, Wakefield J, et al. (2008) Activation of the unfolded protein response by deltaF508 CFTR. Am J Respir Cell Mol Biol 39: 448–457.
31. Lu JP, Wang Y, Sliter DA, Pearce MM, Wojcikiewicz RJ (2011) RNF170 protein, an endoplasmic reticulum membrane ubiquitin ligase, mediates inositol 1,4,5-trisphosphate receptor ubiquitination and degradation. J Biol Chem 286: 24426–24433.
32. Rab A, Bartoszewski R, Jurkuvenaite A, Wakefield J, Collawn JF, et al. (2007) Endoplasmic reticulum stress and the unfolded protein response regulate genomic cystic fibrosis transmembrane conductance regulator expression. Am J Physiol Cell Physiol 292: C756–C766.
33. Sluiter W, Oomens LW, Brand A, Van Furth R (1984) Determination of blood volume in the mouse with 51chromium-labelled erythrocytes. J Immunol Methods 73: 221–225.
34. Hull JH, Garrod R, Ho TB, Knight RK, Cockcroft JR, et al. (2009) Increased augmentation index in patients with cystic fibrosis. Eur Respir J 34: 1322–1328.
35. Poore S, Berry B, Eidson D, McKie KT, Harris RA (2013) Evidence of vascular endothelial dysfunction in young patients with cystic fibrosis. Chest 143: 939–945.
36. Tousson A, Van Tine BA, Naren AP, Shaw GM, Schwiebert LM (1998) Characterization of CFTR expression and chloride channel activity in human endothelia. Am J Physiol 275: C1555–C1564.
37. Robert R, Norez C, Becq F (2005) Disruption of CFTR chloride channel alters mechanical properties and cAMP-dependent Cl- transport of mouse aortic smooth muscle cells. J Physiol 568: 483–495.
38. Barbero GJ, Braddock LI (1967) Catecholamines in cystic fibrosis. Lancet 290: 158.
39. Clancy JP, Rowe SM, Accurso FJ, Aitken ML, Amin RS, et al. (2012) Results of a phase IIa study of VX-809, an investigational CFTR corrector compound, in subjects with cystic fibrosis homozygous for the F508del-CFTR mutation. Thorax 67: 12–18.

14

Swimming Motility in a Longitudinal Collection of Clinical Isolates of *Burkholderia cepacia* Complex Bacteria from People with Cystic Fibrosis

James E. A. Zlosnik*, Paul Y. Mori, Derek To, James Leung, Trevor J. Hird, David P. Speert

Centre for Understanding and Preventing Infection in Children, Department of Pediatrics, Faculty of Medicine, University of British Columbia, Vancouver, British Columbia, Canada

Abstract

Chronic bacterial lung infections in cystic fibrosis (CF) are the leading cause of morbidity and mortality. While a range of bacteria are known to be capable of establishing residence in the CF lung, only a small number have a clearly established link to deteriorating clinical status. The two bacteria with the clearest roles in CF lung disease are *Pseudomonas aeruginosa* and bacteria belonging to the *Burkholderia cepacia* complex (BCC). A number of common adaptations by *P. aeruginosa* strains to chronic lung infection in CF have been well described. Typically, initial isolates of *P. aeruginosa* are nonmucoid and display a range of putative virulence determinants. Upon establishment of chronic infection, subsequent isolates ultimately show a reduction in putative virulence determinants, including swimming motility, along with an acquisition of the mucoid phenotype and increased levels of antimicrobial resistance. Infections by BCC are marked by an unpredictable, but typically worse, clinical outcome. However, in contrast to *P. aeruginosa* infections in CF, studies describing adaptive changes in BCC bacterial phenotype during chronic lung infections are far more limited. To further enhance our understanding of chronic lung infections by BCC bacteria in CF, we assessed the swimming motility phenotype in 551 isolates of BCC bacteria from cystic fibrosis (CF) lung infections between 1981 and 2007. These data suggest that swimming motility is not typically lost by BCC during chronic infection, unlike as seen in *P. aeruginosa* infections. Furthermore, while we observed a statistically significant link between mucoidy and motility, we did not detect any link between motility phenotype and clinical outcome. These studies highlight the need for further work to understand the adaptive changes of BCC bacteria during chronic infection in the CF lung.

Editor: Tom Coenye, Ghent University, Belgium

Funding: This work was supported by a Cystic Fibrosis Canada (www.cysticfibrosis.ca) operating grant to DPS (20R32976) and a fellowship to JZ. The funders had no role in study design, data collection and analysis, decision to publish, or preparation of the manuscript.

Competing Interests: The authors have declared that no competing interests exits.

* Email: jzlosnik@cfri.ubc.ca

Introduction

People with cystic fibrosis (CF) experience chronic lung infections, lasting years and sometimes decades. These lung infections are the main cause of morbidity and mortality in CF, leading to either lung transplantation or death through cumulative damage to the lungs. A number of bacterial species are associated with chronic infection in the CF endobronchial space [1,2]. Bacteria belonging to the *Burkholderia cepacia* complex (BCC) are particularly concerning to the CF community due to their well-documented capacity for inter-patient transmission and an association with an unpredictable but typically worse outcome [1,3,4]. The BCC comprises at least 18 distinct species of bacteria and all, except for *B. ubonensis*, have been isolated from the lungs of people with CF [5,6]. Historically, *B. cenocepacia* has been the most common and problematic species in many CF centres. However, the epidemiology of BCC bacteria in CF appears to be changing, with *B. multivorans* becoming the most common cause of new BCC infection in CF in number of studies [1,7]

The most common pathogen in CF is *Pseudomonas aeruginosa* [1]. Numerous studies have described a range of common adaptations to chronic infection by *P. aeruginosa*. The current paradigm for *P. aeruginosa* infections in CF involves infection with a virulent nonmucoid strain, which, upon establishment of chronic infection, ultimately converts to the mucoid phenotype through the production of exopolysaccharide alginate [8]. In addition, a range of other adaptations have been described, which presumably enhance the capacity for survival in the CF lung [9,10]. These often include the loss of a range of putative virulence determinants such as a quorum sensing and swimming motility as well as acquisition of other traits such as increased antibiotic resistance, serum sensitivity through loss of LPS O-polysaccharide and hypermutability [10–15].

Currently published data suggest that the pathogenic mechanisms employed by BCC bacteria in chronic CF lung infections may in fact be distinct from those observed in *P. aeruginosa*. For instance, a recent survey of sequential clinical isolates from a number of CF patients attending the Vancouver CF clinics who had been chronically infected with BCC indicated that, unlike *P.*

aeruginosa, BCC maintain quorum sensing systems during chronic infection in the CF lung [16]. Recent transcriptomic and proteomic studies on isolates of *B. cenocepacia* from a single chronic infection have also suggested that virulence may be increased in isolates taken from later in chronic infection [17,18]. In addition to these experimental data, the apparent aggressiveness of BCC bacteria in CF is also consistent with BCC bacteria deploying differential pathogenic mechanisms during chronic infections. Most notable is the well described capacity for BCC to cause a typically fatal invasive necrotizing pneumonia known as 'cepacia syndrome', which has commonly been associated with *B. cenocepacia* but is also known to occur in other species including *B. multivorans* and *B. dolosa* [19–21]. Invasive disease is rarely, if ever, seen in *P. aeruginosa* infections in CF.

In contrast to *P. aeruginosa*, studies on adaptation to chronic lung infections in CF by BCC are very limited. We have previously shown that, unlike *P. aeruginosa*, the nonmucoid phenotype is associated with a worse outcome in terms of lung function decline and survival, while mucoid to nonmucoid transitions are common in adaptation to chronic infection [22,23]. Other studies have also documented BCC phenotypic colonial morphology variation in the context of chronic CF lung infections [24]. Variation in some other phenotypic traits has been described in clinical isolates of BCC bacteria, most notably, in antimicrobial susceptibility profiles, in the context of chronic CF infections [25,26]. Recently, whole genome sequencing of sequential isolates from multiple patients in an outbreak of *B. dolosa* in the United States also revealed a number of candidate pathogenicity genes that appear to be commonly mutated during chronic infection and may confer elevated virulence on this species [27].

We have previously described an association between colonial morphology and motility, whereby increased flagellin protein production and swimming motility were detected in a shiny colony clonal variant that was obtained from an infection model where the infection had been established with an isolate that demonstrated a matte colony morphology [28,29]. The swimming motility phenotype is also of interest, due to the well described capacity for bacterial flagella to stimulate inflammation through the TLR5 pathogen recognition receptor as well as its involvement in epithelial invasion by BCC bacteria [30–34]. In this study we examine the clinical significance of motility in BCC bacteria. We report the largest assessment to date of swimming motility from a longitudinal collection of over 550 BCC isolates, collected at least annually from 100 CF patients attending the Vancouver clinics during the period June 1981–June 2007.

Materials and Methods

Bacterial isolates

Bacteria were collected from CF patients at least annually between June 1981 and June 2007 from the Vancouver CF clinics as described previously [23]. Briefly we examined 551 isolates from 100 patients. For patients culturing BCC this collection typically contains at least one isolate per year. Bacteria were routinely stored by freezing confluent growth, taken from a purity plate, at −80°C in Mueller Hinton broth (Oxoid) plus 8% dimethyl sulfoxide. For experiments, bacteria were revived on a Columbia Blood Agar plate, and a fresh culture was established the day prior to the experiment on a Luria Bertani (LB) agar plate (10 g l^{-1} tryptone, 5 g l^{-1} yeast extract, 10 g l^{-1} sodium chloride) containing 1.5% agar. All plates were incubated overnight at 35°C.

Swimming motility

Swimming motility for each isolate was individually assessed on LB supplemented with 0.3% agar plates as previously described [11]. Briefly, plates were poured on the bench with no drying time and then used the same day. Growth from the confluent area of a freshly cultured plate was inoculated into the center of the swimming motility agar plates using a sterilized wooden stick. Motility plates were then incubated for 48 hours at 35°C in stacks 4 plates high, the plates were kept upright and not inverted. At 48 hours the diameter of the colonial growth was measured. Isolates with less than or equal to 10 mm growth at 48 hours were classified as nonmotile, while those with >10 mm growth were classified as motile. Motile and nonmotile controls, *P. aeruginosa* PAK and *P. aeruginosa* PAK Δ*fliC* [35], were run in all experiments.

Western blotting

Whole protein extractions from BCC bacteria were prepared as described previously [11]. Briefly, bacterial growth was scraped from the confluent area of a freshly grown agar plate using a sterile wooden stick and resuspended in 1 ml of 1.5 mM Tris.Cl pH 7.5. The bacteria were then added to an equal volume of 0.1 mm diameter glass beads in a 2 ml screw cap centrifuge tube (Lysing Matrix B, MP Biomedicals). Bacterial cells were then broken with 3 rounds of beating in a FastPrep ribolyzer (ThermoSavant) set to speed 6.5 for 45 seconds. Cellular debris was pelleted by centrifugation at 18,400 x *g* in a Hettich Mikro 200 microcentrifuge. 250 µl of supernatant was then removed to harvest the extracted protein. Protein concentration was determined using the Micro BCA protein assay kit (Pierce). 15 or 25 µg of protein was separated on a 12% acrylamide gel, proteins were transferred to a PVDF membrane by electroblotting and then probed using a 1 in 10,000 dilution of an anti-*Burkholderia pseudomallei* flagellin antibody [36] as described previously [37]. Blots were visualized either using chemiluminensce (Amersham ECL detection kit, GE Healthcare) with a 1 in 10,000 dilution of an anti-rabbit HRP linked secondary antibody (Cell Signalling) or green fluorescence using a 1 in 10,000 dilution of a goat anti-rabbit IRDye 800CW secondary antibody (Licor) on an Odyssey (Licor) infrared imaging system. Blots were performed in at least triplicate for all isolates examined.

TLR5 stimulatory assays

TLR5 activation was assessed using a TLR5-NF-κB luciferase reporter system as described previously [32]. Briefly, bacterial cells were grown overnight in 3 mls of LB broth at 37°C on an orbital rotator. Bacterial cells were harvested by centrifugation (2,340 x *g* for 5 minutes) and washed twice in phosphate buffered saline and adjusted to 2.5×10^6 CFU ml^{-1}. Heat killed bacteria (30 mins at 65°C) were then added to 5×10^4 freshly cultured CHO-K1 cells containing the TLR5-NF-κB luciferase reporter, representing an MOI of 50:1, and incubated for 4 hrs in 96-well plates. CHO-K1 cells were routinely cultured both before and during experiments in F-12 K media (Gibco). Activation of the TLR5-NF-κB luciferase reporter was then assessed using a luciferase assay (Promega) and a Tecan Infinite M200 plate reader. Luminescence was measured by injecting 50 µl of substrate into each well, with an injection speed of 200 µl sec^{-1}, and luminescence was measured over an integration time of 5 seconds. All values are expressed relative to an unstimulated control containing only the reporter cell line and no bacteria. TLR5 activation assays were performed on five separate occasions for each isolate and in triplicate on each occasion.

Clinical data

Clinical data were previously collected for all patients included in the study [22]. We employed the same inclusion/exclusion criteria in this study. The clinical data included in this manuscript was obtained following approval the Providence Healthcare Research Ethics Board - part of the UBC Research Ethics Boards (H07-01396). Informed consent was not required as the data was analysed in aggregate and de-linked from any patient identifiers.

Statistical analysis

All motility data were collected and stored in a Microsoft Access 2010 database. For analysis, data were exported initially to Microsoft Excel 2010 and then transferred to GraphPad Prism V.4. Data were graphed using either Microsoft Excel 2010 directly or exported to GraphPad Prism V.4. All statistical analyses were performed with appropriate statistical tests using GraphPad Prism V.4.

Results

Prevalence of the motile phenotype in clinical isolates of BCC in the Vancouver CF population 1981–2007

Isolates from people with CF infected with BCC are routinely collected and stored in our laboratory at least annually. We have previously reported data from this collection, describing the prevalence of the mucoid phenotype in Vancouver isolates of BCC from CF infections between June 1981 and June 2007 [23]. Given the well-described loss of swimming motility in *P. aeruginosa* during chronic CF lung infections, we assessed our isolate collection for swimming motility in order to understand the significance of swimming motility during chronic BCC infections in CF. An examination of the full isolate collection revealed that both motile and nonmotile isolates of all species were present, with the exception of *B. cepacia* for which there were only four isolates that were all motile and *B. metallica* for which the sole isolate was motile (Table 1). In total we examined 551 isolates from 100 patients. *B. cenocepacia* is traditionally considered the most virulent of the BCC species, so it is notable that a larger percentage - 38% - of *B. cenocepacia* isolates examined were nonmotile as opposed to 14% of *B. multivorans* (Table 1). We also assessed the extent of motility displayed by these isolates, in terms of the diameter of the resultant colony when *B. cenocepacia* and *B. multivorans* were grown on swimming motility agar. These data show that, consistent with this trend, *B. cenocepacia* isolates on average exhibit considerably smaller diameter of colonial growth than *B. multivorans* on swim plates (Fig 1). In fact only 1% of *B. cenocepacia* isolates in our collection possessed the capacity to swim across the entire plate, whereas 16% of *B. multivorans* isolates possessed this capacity (Fig 1).

Motility and the mucoid phenotype

Previous studies of clonal variants in *B. cenocepacia* taken from a CF lung infection have found that nonmucoid variants demonstrated loss of swimming motility capacity [24,38]. Unlike *P. aeruginosa*, the mucoid phenotype is not visually detectable on LB-agar motility plates [23]. Therefore any differences observed in the diameter of growth on swimming motility plates used in this study is due to the swimming motility phenotype, rather than excess elaboration of exopolysaccharide in mucoid isolates. Even though the mucoid phenotype does not manifest itself visually on LB agar plates it is conceivable there still could be a link between EPS production capacity and swimming motility. As we have previously assessed the mucoid phenotype in these isolates [23], we examined the swimming motility phenotype in relation to the mucoid phenotype. These data support previous observations, showing a general, but not absolute, correlation between the extent of mucoidy, scored from – to +++ and capacity for swimming motility as measured by the diameter of bacterial growth after 48 hours at 35°C (Fig 2). This trend was statistically significant (Kruskal-Wallis $p<0.0001$). Breaking down these data into species, the same trend was observable for both *B. multivorans* and *B. cenocepacia* (Fig 2), which was statistically significant for both species (data not shown).

The motility phenotype in relation to clinical outcome in BCC lung infections in people with cystic fibrosis

Given that initial colonizing isolates of *P. aeruginosa* infection in CF are typically motile, while phenotype switches to nonmotility are commonly seen in later isolates, we were interested in assessing the clinical significance of the BCC swimming motility phenotype. In the context of the 89 clinical infections where there was infection by a single clone, 51/89 infections only ever had motile BCC isolated while 19/89 were only ever nonmotile, indicating that nonmotile isolates of BCC may be competent to initiate and maintain infection (Fig. 3A). We also examined the dataset to look at infections where there was clear evidence of chronic infection (defined as the presence in our collection of at least three different isolates of the same strain type over the period of at least a year, $n = 48$). Swimming motility phenotype switches were detected during chronic infection, but only in a minority of cases (11/48). Like *P. aeruginosa*, these switches were always motile to nonmotile, although they were often accompanied by subsequent isolation of motile variants (data not shown). Previous RAPD typing of these isolates [23] indicated that all cases of swimming motility phenotype switching took place in sequential clonal isolates and therefore were not replacement infections (data not shown). In total these data represent over 214 patient years of BCC infection data and an average of 8.5 isolates per patient for chronic infections.

We also sought to assess the clinical impact of the different phenotypes (Fig 3B). Patient data were previously collected and this study was approved by the UBC research ethics boards [22]. For cases for which we have suitable follow up clinical data ($n = 52$), as defined by our previous criteria [22], we assessed the post infection decline in lung function, using Forced Expiratory Volume in one second (FEV1), % predicted. The mean annual post-infection lung function decline was 4.0% FEV1 % predicted for those infected with motile BCC bacteria ($n = 32$), while those only infected with nonmotile BCC bacteria ($n = 5$) had a mean annual decline of 8.2% FEV1% predicted. Patients who were colonized with either mixed motile phenotypes ($n = 5$) or those where there was clear evidence of a motile to nonmotile phenotype switch ($n = 10$) had annual post-infection FEV1% predicted declines of 4.4% and 3.0% respectively. Among all groups, these data demonstrated no significant differences between patients infected with motile or nonmotile BCC, irrespective of whether we examined all cases (Kruskal-Wallis $p = 0.273$, Fig. 3B) or just those for whom chronic infection (defined as the presence in our collection of 3 or more isolates over a period of a year or more) was documented ($n = 34$, Kruskal-Wallis $p = 0.174$, data not shown).

The effects of loss of motility on the biological properties of BCC bacteria during chronic infection

To assess the biological consequence of the motile to nonmotile switches, we investigated the production of flagellum protein by Western blot using a polyclonal antibody [36] raised against *B.*

Table 1. Prevalence of swimming motility in isolates of *B. cepacia complex* from cystic fibrosis infections in Vancouver from 1981–2008.

	Total number of isolates tested, *n*	Nonmotile, *n* (%)	Motile, *n* (%)
B. cepacia	4	0 (0)	4 (100)
B. multivorans	207	29 (14)	178 (86)
B. cenocepacia	294	111 (38)	183 (62)
B. stabilis	10	3 (30)	7 (70)
B. vietnamiensis	35	23 (66)	12 (34)
B. metallica	1	0 (0)	1 (100)

pseudomallei flagellin, as described previously [37]. We examined isolates from 5 patients in whom there was a switch from motility to nonmotility in later isolates. These cases were selected to represent *B. multivorans* as well as most of the major epidemic lineages of *B. cenocepacia* (RAPD types 01, 04 and 06). In addition, we also examined a well-described isolate of the RAPD02/ET-12 lineage, K56-2. In most cases, lack of motility was associated with a loss of detectable flagellin protein, however flagellin protein was detected in 2 nonmotile isolates (C9343 and VC8402) from two patients in which there had been a phenotype switch from motile to nonmotile (Table 1). Given the role flagella play in activating inflammation through the pattern recognition receptor TLR5, we also assessed TLR5 activation in these isolates using a TLR5-NF-κB luciferase reporter assay system as described previously [32]. Motile isolates demonstrated significantly increased TLR5 activation compared to nonmotile isolates (2.88 vs 2.10 fold compared to unstimulated controls, unpaired one tailed *t*-test $p = 0.0092$).

Discussion

Chronic bacterial infections in CF are particularly difficult to model *ex-vivo*, in part due to the length of time that bacteria are resident in the CF lung, making it hard to mimic conditions of the CF lung using either *in vitro* or animal/plant model systems. The inability to effectively model CF lung infections in the laboratory makes it challenging to understand the contribution any given bacterial trait may have towards disease severity or to understand the adaptive mechanisms bacteria use to facilitate chronic residence in the CF lung. There are a large range of putative virulence determinants now described for BCC bacteria, for a recent review see [39], however, for the most part, the clinical significance of these determinants is unclear. In addition, there is a growing range of *ex-vivo* models for BCC infection, however there is little consistency among these models in terms of conserved virulence determinants and in any case none of the models truly mimics CF infection [40].

Swimming motility is well described as an adaptive trait in *P. aeruginosa* infections in CF whereby initial infection is typically by

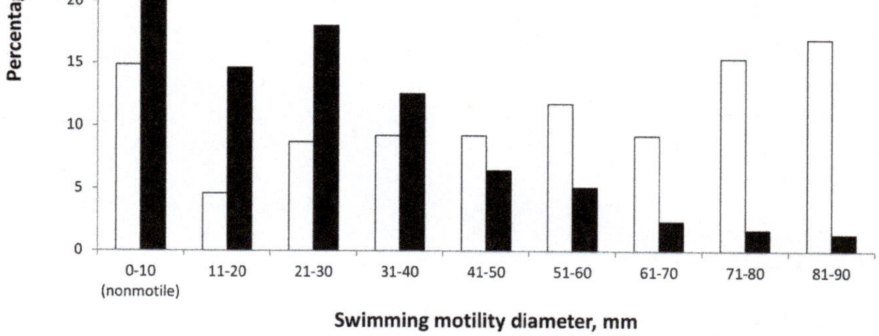

Figure 1. Analysis of swimming motility capacity of *B. multivorans* (white bars) and *B. cenocepacia* (black bars) isolates from cystic fibrosis lung infections in Vancouver between 1981 and 2008. Motility was assessed by inoculating bacteria into the center of a motility agar plate and incubating for 48 hrs, after which the diameter was measured. Isolates were classified as motile if colonial diameter was >10 mm and nonmotile if the diameter was less than or equal to 10 mm.

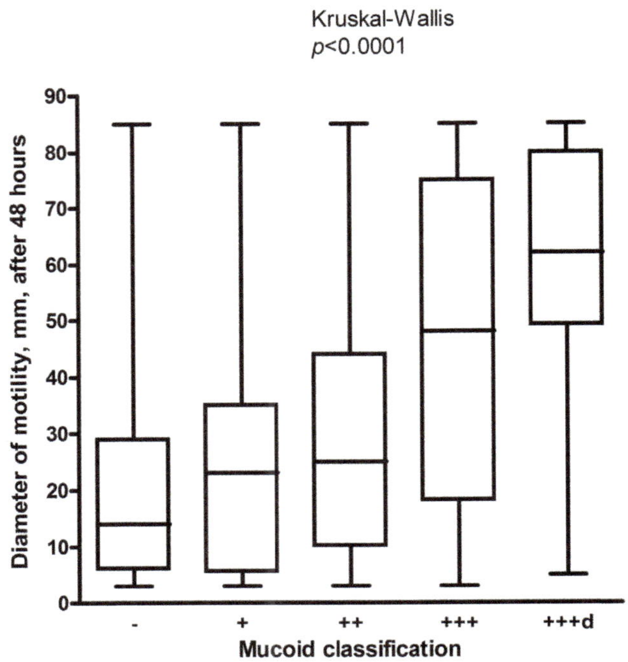

All BCC isolates, median (IQR)	14 (6-29)	23 (5.5-35)	25 (10-44)	48 (18-75)	62 (49-80)
B. cenocepacia, median (IQR)	14 (5-28.5)	25.5 (10.5-37)	25 (9-38)	24 (7.5-51)	49 (27.5-62.5)
B. multivorans, median (IQR)	29 (13-52)	38 (6-56)	38.5 (14.5-65.5)	64.5 (7.5-51)	70 (53.5-84)
BCC other species, median (IQR)	11.5 (6.5-19.5)	4 (3.5-10.5)	9 (5-13)	8 (-)	85 (-)

Figure 2. Motility and the mucoid phenotype in BCC. Box and Whisker plot of motility phenotype compared to the mucoid phenotype (as previously assessed: [23]) in all isolates of *B. cepacia* complex assessed for which we had corresponding mucoid scores ($n = 541$). Statistical significance was assessed by the non parametic Kruskal-Wallis one-way analysis of variance in GraphPad Prism v.4. Data were also analyzed separately for *B. cenocepacia* ($n = 288$) and *B. multivorans* ($n = 203$) as well as all the remaining species examined ($n = 50$) and the medians and inter-quartile range (IQR) are provided in the box below the figure. IQRs could not be calculated for BCC other species scored +++ and +++d because there were only 3 and 1 isolates in those categories respectively.

a motile isolate which can convert to a nonmotile phenotype later in chronic infection [11,14]. The swimming motility phenotype is also well described in BCC bacteria and is mediated by a single polar flagellum [41–43]. *In-vitro* experiments have shown that the BCC flagellum facilitates invasion into epithelial cells *in-vitro* and promotion of inflammatory markers [34,44]. The clinical significance of motility in chronic BCC lung infections in CF, however, is not clear.

In order to describe the significance of motility in clinical isolates of BCC we examined our collection of BCC taken on a regular basis from people with CF. Aside from the longitudinal nature of our BCC collection, a strength of this study is that our collection contains large numbers of the two most commonly isolated species from the BCC: *B. cenocepacia* and *B. multivorans*. Our data reveal that both motile and nonmotile isolates can be recovered from CF lung infections for all species examined, except for *B. cepacia* for which we only had 4 isolates from a single infection and *B. metallica* for which we had only one isolate (Table 1). Stratifying infections into 'motility phenotypes' revealed that isolates from the majority of chronic infections most commonly display the motile phenotype throughout the infection and do not normally switch to nonmotile (Fig 3A). We identified a limited number of infections where nonmotile isolates were the only phenotype ever isolated, suggesting that nonmotile BCC bacteria are also competent to initiate infection. However, these data must be understood in the context that although they were the first recovered isolates, the duration of colonization prior to the first positive culture cannot be determined. Additionally, although there was minimal passage of the bacteria between the lung and storage, it is still conceivable that phenotype switching may have already taken place as a consequence of adaptation to growth either in the lung or in the lab. Nonetheless, by examining archived bacterial isolates, the approach we have taken in this study is identical to that used by us to describe the evolution of *P. aeruginosa* motility in the CF lung [11].

A number of studies have examined adaptation of BCC bacteria to various *in-vitro* growth environments [45–49]. However, there are currently little data on adaptive strategies of BCC bacteria to chronic pulmonary infection in CF. This study adds to other evidence [16,22] which suggest that at least some of the mechanisms of pathogenesis in BCC bacterial lung disease are distinct from those described for *P. aeruginosa*. Our data indicate

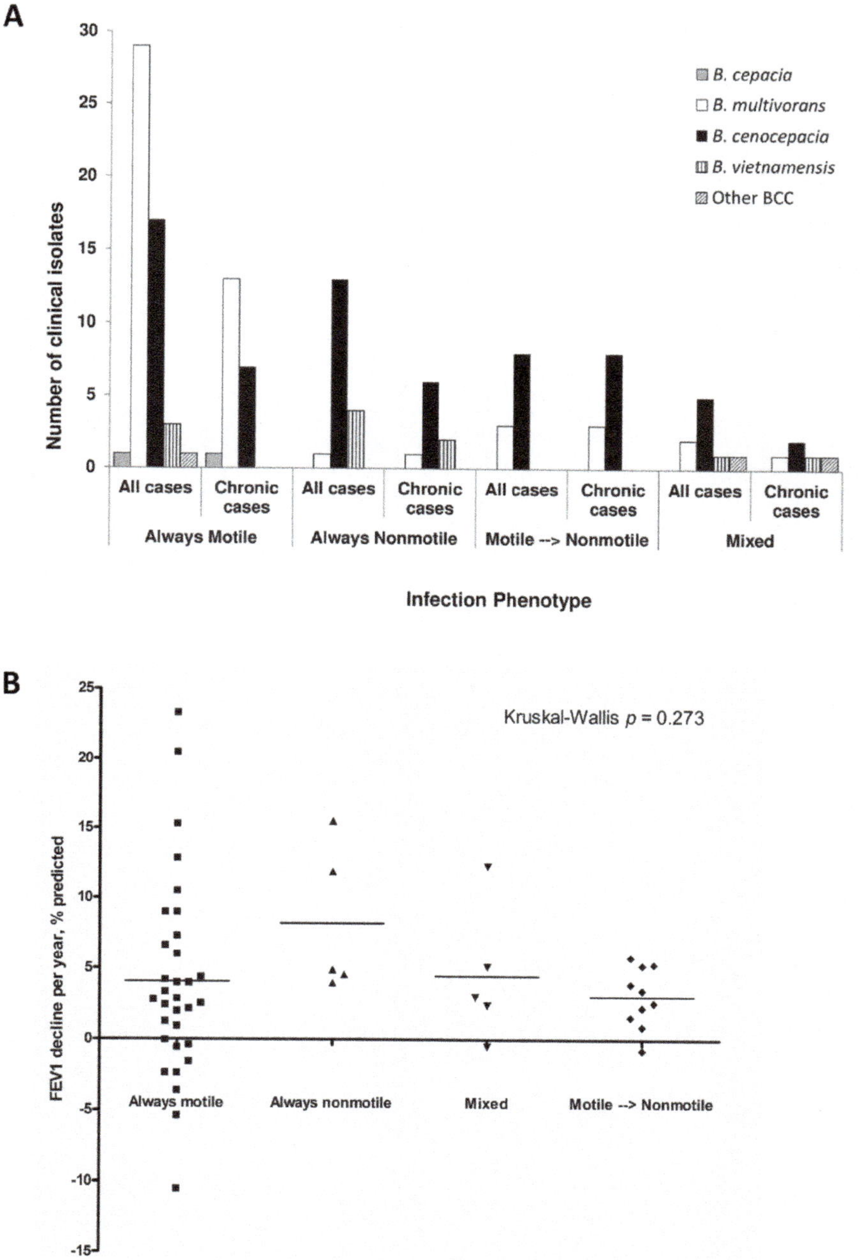

Figure 3. Assessment of clinical significance of swimming motility in BCC bacteria. A) CF lung infections categorized by species and motility phenotype. Data are displayed for all cases ($n = 89$) and for cases where chronic infection ($n = 48$) was clearly established (defined as the presence in our collection of at least 2 or more isolates of the same strain type that were collected at least a year apart). Grey bars = *B. cepacia*, white bars = *B. multivorans*, black bars = *B. cenocepacia*; vertical striped bars = *B. vietnamiensis* and diagonal striped bars = other BCC species. Infections were categorized as: isolates were always motile; always nonmotile; motile to nonmotile phenotype switches detected during infection (as defined by an initial isolation of at least 2 separate motile isolates on separate months followed by a nonmotile isolate at any point thereafter) or mixed (there was no clear established initial swimming motility phenotype as the first two isolates stored for patients on separate months demonstrated both motile and nonmotile phenotypes). One case was also classified as mixed (FEV1% predicted decline −0.5%) as most isolates were nonmotile, however several marginally motile (diameter 11 and 12 mm) isolates were detected during the course of the patients' infection. B) Assessment of the impact of motility phenotype on FEV1 decline following initial infection with BCC. FEV1 data were collected from the patient charts as described previously. Criteria for inclusion were established previously [22]. Data were analyzed in GraphPad Prism v.4 and the non-parametric Kruskal-Wallis test calculated to assess difference.

that loss of motility is not a common adaptive feature in BCC bacteria to chronic lung infection, as opposed to *P. aeruginosa* (Fig 3A). Examination of the biological properties of sequential clonal isolates from infections where there was switch from motile to nonmotile phenotypes (Table 2), revealed that loss of motility is often, but not always, associated with a loss of detectable flagellin protein by Western blot. Consistent with published data [33], we also show that conversion to the nonmotile phenotype was associated with a reduction in TLR-5 stimulator capacity (Table 2).

Table 2. Biological characteristics of motile and nonmotile CF clinical isolates of *Burkholderia cepacia* complex bacteria.

Patient	Isolate	Species	Date of isolation	Strain type (RAPD)	Motility	Flagella Western blot	TLR5 activity
A	C3921	BC	Oct 1990	001	+	+	1.95 (0.44)
	C8963	BC	Jan 2000	001	−	−	2.00 (0.27)
	C9343	BC	Oct 2000	001	−	+	2.99 (0.56)
B	VC3868	BC	Aug 1990	004	+	+	3.35 (0.69)
	VC9670	BC	Jun 1999	004	−	−	1.82 (0.26)
	VC13450	BC	Jul 2006	004	−	−	1.99 (0.29)
C	VC6432	BC	Jul 1994	006	+	+	3.38 (0.78)
	VC8402	BC	Sep 1997	006	−	+	2.47 (0.59)
D	VC2307	BC	Apr 1987	006	+	+	3.71 (1.00)
	VC6905	BC	Mar 1995	006	−	−	1.82 (1.00)
E	VC12201	BC	Jan 2004	009	+	+	3.10 (0.58)
	VC13307	BC	Mar 2006	009	−	−	1.87 (0.25)
F	VC12539	BM	Sep 2004	BM-044	+	+	1.86 (0.25)
	VC13732	BM	Mar 2007	BM-044	−	−	1.85 (0.32)
n/a	K56-2	BC	−	002	+	+	3.03 (0.41)

Date of isolation = month/year. Species: BC = *B. cenocepacia*, BM = *B. multivorans*. Strain types were determined previously for these isolates by RAPD [23,50]. Western blotting was performed on whole cell extracts using a polyclonal anti-*B. pseudomallei* flagella antibody [36] as we have described previously [37]. Results are representative of three independent experiments and are positive or negative for the presence of a band at either 45 kDa or 55 kDa – the variants of flagella known to be produced by BCC bacteria [41]. TLR5 activation values are the mean of assays performed in triplicate on five separate occasions, with standard error of the mean in brackets.

These data further support the contention that the adaptive strategies used by BCC in chronic CF lung infections are distinct from those described for *P. aeruginosa* and therefore BCC merits separate consideration. While phenotype conversion, from motile to nonmotile, did occur during chronic infection, it was not common and was often accompanied by the subsequent isolation of motile isolates from the same infection (Figure 3A). Other data from this isolate collection also supports this suggestion. One study has shown that BCC maintain functional quorum sensing signaling systems during chronic infection, whereas isolation of quorum sensing mutants during chronic *P. aeruginosa* infections in CF is common [16,22]. Meanwhile we have also shown that conversion to the nonmucoid phenotype in BCC infections is common, while the extent of mucoidy is inversely related to survival and outcome, also in contrast to *P. aeruginosa* [22,23].

Our data are supportive of a link between motility and the mucoid phenotype as has previously been described by others [24,38]. This correlation was seen both when all isolates were examined and in both *B. multivorans* and *B. cenocepacia* isolates when examined separately (Figure 2). Nonetheless, it is notable that there is considerable variation in all mucoid classes in their capacity for swimming motility and we identified both nonmotile and motile nonmucoid isolates (considered as mucoid scores – and +) as well as nonmotile and motile mucoid isolates (considered as mucoid scores ++/+++/+++d) (Fig 2). Therefore our data indicate that, while there is a significant trend, the connection between swimming motility and the mucoid colonial morphology phenotype is not absolute. Given our previously described link between mucoidy and outcome [22,23], the link described here between mucoidy and motility might suggest that there would be a link with patient outcome in terms of lung function decline. However, we did not observe a link between motility and clinical outcome (Fig 3B). Conclusions from these data are limited by the small numbers of cases in the nonmotile group in particular ($n = 5$) and therefore this question requires further investigation in another population containing larger numbers of nonmotile infections.

We believe this study is the most comprehensive analysis to date of the swimming motility phenotype in clinical isolates of BCC bacteria. Based on these data, it appears that differences in the motility phenotype do not contribute significantly to the severity of BCC lung disease in CF. We suggest, however, that these data and others indicate that the pathogenic mechanisms of BCC bacteria in CF lung disease need to be considered separately from those that have been observed for *P. aeruginosa*. The assertion is supported by the clinical picture, where BCC have a well-established elevated risk of mortality/lung transplantation and can result in an invasive necrotizing pneumonia known as 'cepacia syndrome' rarely if ever seen in *P. aeruginosa* infections [3,20]. As a consequence further studies on adaptation to the CF lung, using clinical isolates with matched clinical data from patients are merited.

Acknowledgments

We would like to thank Don Woods for the generous provision of the anti-*Burkholderia pseudomallei* flagellum antibody. We would also like to thank Stuart Turvey for the provision of reagents and the TLR-5 reporter cell line. This work was supported by a Cystic Fibrosis Canada operating grant to DPS (20R32976) and a Cystic Fibrosis Canada Postdoctoral Fellowship to JEAZ.

Author Contributions

Conceived and designed the experiments: JZ DS. Performed the experiments: JZ PM DT JL TH. Analyzed the data: JZ. Contributed to the writing of the manuscript: JZ DS.

References

1. Lipuma JJ (2010) The changing microbial epidemiology in cystic fibrosis. Clin Microbiol Rev 23: 299–323. doi:10.1128/CMR.00068-09.
2. Hauser AR, Jain M, Bar-Meir M, McColley SA (2011) Clinical Significance of Microbial Infection and Adaptation in Cystic Fibrosis. Clin Microbiol Rev 24: 29–70. doi:10.1128/CMR.00036-10.
3. Corey M, Farewell V (1996) Determinants of mortality from cystic fibrosis in Canada, 1970–1989. Am J Epidemiol 143: 1007–1017.
4. LiPuma JJ, Dasen SE, Nielson DW, Stern RC, Stull TL (1990) Person-to-person transmission of Pseudomonas cepacia between patients with cystic fibrosis. Lancet 336: 1094–1096.
5. Vandamme P, Dawyndt P (2011) Classification and identification of the Burkholderia cepacia complex: Past, present and future. Syst Appl Microbiol 34: 87–95. doi: 10.1016/j.syapm.2010.10.002.
6. Peeters C, Zlosnik JEA, Spilker T, Hird TJ, Lipuma JJ, et al. (2013) Burkholderia pseudomultivorans sp. nov., a novel Burkholderia cepacia complex species from human respiratory samples and the rhizosphere. Syst Appl Microbiol 36: 48–489. doi: 10.1016/j.syapm.2013.06.003.
7. Govan JR, Brown AR, Jones AM (2007) Evolving epidemiology of Pseudomonas aeruginosa and the Burkholderia cepacia complex in cystic fibrosis lung infection. Futur Microbiol 2: 153–164. doi: 10.2217/17460913.2.2.153.
8. Martin DW, Schurr MJ, Mudd MH, Govan JR, Holloway BW, et al. (1993) Mechanism of conversion to mucoidy in Pseudomonas aeruginosa infecting cystic fibrosis patients. Proc Natl Acad Sci U S A 90: 8377–8381.
9. Ciofu O, Mandsberg L, Hengzhuag W, Hoiby N (2012) Phenotypes selected during chronic lung infection in cystic fibrosis patients: implications for the treatment of Pseudomonas aeruginosa biofilm infections. FEMS Immunol 65: 215–225. doi:10.1111/j.1574-695X.2012.00983.x.
10. Folkesson A, Jelsbak L, Yang L, Johansen HK, Ciofu O, et al. (2012) Adaptation of Pseudomonas aeruginosa to the cystic fibrosis airway: an evolutionary perspective. Nat Rev Microbiol 10: 841–851. doi:10.1038/nrmicro2907.
11. Mahenthiralingam E, Campbell ME, Speert DP (1994) Nonmotility and phagocytic resistance of Pseudomonas aeruginosa isolates from chronically colonized patients with cystic fibrosis. Infect Immun 62: 596–605.
12. Huse HK, Kwon T, Zlosnik JEA, Speert DP, Marcotte E, et al. (2013) Pseudomonas aeruginosa Enhances Production of a Non-alginate Exopolysaccharide During Long-term Colonization of the Cystic Fibrosis Lung. PLoS One 8: e82621. doi:10.1371/journal.pone.0082621.
13. Rau MH, Hansen SK, Johansen HK, Thomsen LE, Workman CT, et al. (2010) Early adaptive developments of Pseudomonas aeruginosa after the transition from life in the environment to persistent colonization in the airways of human cystic fibrosis hosts. Environ Microbiol 12: 1643–1658. doi:10.1111/j.1462-2920.2010.02211.x.
14. Smith EE, Buckley DG, Wu Z, Saenphimmachak C, Hoffman LR, et al. (2006) Genetic adaptation by Pseudomonas aeruginosa to the airways of cystic fibrosis patients. Proc Natl Acad Sci U S A 103: 8487–8492. doi: 10.1073/pnas.0602138103.
15. Ciofu O, Riis B, Pressler T, Enghusen H, Høiby N, et al. (2005) Occurrence of Hypermutable Pseudomonas aeruginosa in Cystic Fibrosis Patients Is Associated with the Oxidative Stress Caused by Chronic Lung Inflammation Occurrence of Hypermutable Pseudomonas aeruginosa in Cystic Fibrosis Patients Is Associated with the. Antimicrob Agents Chemother 49: 2276–2282. doi:10.1128/AAC.49.6.2276.
16. McKeon SA, Nguyen DT, Viteri DF, Zlosnik JEA, Sokol PA (2011) Functional quorum sensing systems are maintained during chronic Burkholderia cepacia complex infections in patients with cystic fibrosis. J Infect Dis 203: 383–392. doi:10.1093/infdis/jiq054.
17. Mira NP, Madeira A, Moreira AS, Coutinho CP, Sá-Correia I (2011) Genomic Expression Analysis Reveals Strategies of Burkholderia cenocepacia to Adapt to Cystic Fibrosis Patients' Airways and Antimicrobial Therapy. PLoS One 6: e28831. doi:10.1371/journal.pone.0028831.
18. Madeira A, Dos Santos SC, Santos PM, Coutinho CP, Tyrrell J, et al. (2013) Proteomic Profiling of Burkholderia cenocepacia Clonal Isolates with Different Virulence Potential Retrieved from a Cystic Fibrosis Patient during Chronic Lung Infection. PLoS One 8: e83065. doi:10.1371/journal.pone.0083065.
19. Nash EF, Thomas A, Whitmill R, Rashid R, Barker B, et al. (2011) "Cepacia syndrome" associated with Burkholderia cepacia (genomovar I) infection in an adolescent with cystic fibrosis. Pediatr Pulmonol 46: 512–514. doi: 10.1002/ppul.21404.
20. Isles A, Maclusky I, Corey M, Gold R, Prober C, et al. (1984) Pseudomonas cepacia infection in cystic fibrosis: an emerging problem. J Pediatr 104: 206–210.
21. Kalish LA, Waltz DA, Dovey M, Potter-Bynoe G, McAdam AJ, et al. (2006) Impact of Burkholderia dolosa on lung function and survival in cystic fibrosis. Am J Respir Crit Care Med 173: 421–425. doi: 10.1164/rccm.200503-344OC.

22. Zlosnik JEA, Costa PS, Brant R, Mori PYB, Hird TJ, et al. (2011) Mucoid and Nonmucoid Burkholderia cepacia Complex Bacteria in Cystic Fibrosis Infections. Am J Respir Crit Care Med 183: 67–72. doi:10.1164/rccm.201002-0203OC.
23. Zlosnik JEA, Hird TJ, Fraenkel MC, Moreira LM, Henry DA, et al. (2008) Differential mucoid exopolysaccharide production by members of the Burkholderia cepacia complex. J Clin Microbiol 46: 1470–1473. doi:10.1128/JCM.02273-07.
24. Coutinho CP, de Carvalho CCCR, Madeira A, Pinto-de-Oliveira A, Sá-Correia I (2011) Burkholderia cenocepacia phenotypic clonal variation during a 3.5-year colonization in the lungs of a cystic fibrosis patient. Infect Immun 79: 2950–2960. doi:10.1128/IAI.01366-10.
25. Larsen GY, Stull TL, Burns JL (1993) Marked phenotypic variability in Pseudomonas cepacia isolated from a patient with cystic fibrosis. J Clin Microbiol 31: 788–792.
26. Leitão JH, Sousa S A, Cunha MV, Salgado MJ, Melo-Cristino J, et al. (2008) Variation of the antimicrobial susceptibility profiles of Burkholderia cepacia complex clonal isolates obtained from chronically infected cystic fibrosis patients: a five-year survey in the major Portuguese treatment center. Eur J Clin Microbiol Infect Dis 27: 1101–1111. doi:10.1007/s10096-008-0552-0.
27. Lieberman TD, Michel J-B, Aingaran M, Potter-Bynoe G, Roux D, et al. (2011) Parallel bacterial evolution within multiple patients identifies candidate pathogenicity genes. Nat Genet 43: 1275–1280. doi:10.1038/ng.997.
28. Chung JW, Altman E, Beveridge TJ, Speert DP (2003) Colonial morphology of Burkholderia cepacia complex genomovar III: implications in exopolysaccharide production, pilus expression, and persistence in the mouse. Infect Immun 71: 904–909.
29. Chung JW, Speert DP (2007) Proteomic identification and characterization of bacterial factors associated with Burkholderia cenocepacia survival in a murine host. Microbiology 153: 206–214. doi: 10.1099/mic.0.2006/000455-0.
30. Smith KD, Andersen-Nissen E, Hayashi F, Strobe K, Bergman MA, et al. (2003) Toll-like receptor 5 recognizes a conserved site on flagellin required for protofilament formation and bacterial motility. Nat Immunol 4: 1247–1253. doi:10.1038/ni1011.
31. de C Ventura GM, Le Goffic R, Balloy V, Plotkowski MC, Chignard M, et al. (2008) TLR 5, but neither TLR2 nor TLR4, is involved in lung epithelial cell response to Burkholderia cenocepacia. FEMS Immunol Med Microbiol 54: 37–44. doi: 10.1111/j.1574-695X.2008.00453.x.
32. Blohmke CJ, Victor RE, Aaron F, Elias IM, Hancock DG, et al. (2008) Innate immunity mediated by TLR5 as a novel antiinflammatory target for cystic fibrosis lung disease. J Immunol 180: 7764–7773.
33. Urban TATAA, Griffith A, Torok AMAM, Mark E, Burns JL, et al. (2004) Contribution of Burkholderia cenocepacia flagella to infectivity and inflammation. Infect Immun 72: 5126–5134. doi:10.1128/IAI.72.9.5126.
34. Tomich M, Herfst CA, Golden JW, Mohr CD (2002) Role of flagella in host cell invasion by Burkholderia cepacia. Infect Immun 70: 1799–1806. doi: 10.1128/IAI.70.4.1799-1806.2002.
35. Simpson DA, Ramphal R, Lory S (1992) Genetic analysis of Pseudomonas aeruginosa adherence: distinct genetic loci control attachment to epithelial cells and mucins. Infect Immun 60: 3771–3779.
36. Brett PJ, Mah DCW, Woods DE (1994) Isolation and Characterization of Pseudomonas pseudomallei Flagellin Proteins. Infect Immun 62: 1914–1919.
37. Zlosnik JEA, Speert DP (2010) The Role of Mucoidy in Virulence of Bacteria from the Burkholderia cepacia Complex: A Systematic Proteomic and Transcriptomic Analysis. J Infect Dis 202: 770–781. doi:10.1086/655663.
38. Silva IN, Ferreira AS, Becker JD, Zlosnik JEA, Speert DP, et al. (2011) Mucoid morphotype variation of Burkholderia multivorans during chronic cystic fibrosis lung infection is correlated with changes in metabolism, motility, biofilm formation and virulence. Microbiology: 3124–3137. doi:10.1099/mic.0.050989-0.
39. Loutet SA, Valvano MA (2010) A decade of Burkholderia cenocepacia virulence determinant research. Infect Immun 78: 4088–4100. doi:10.1128/IAI.00212-10.
40. Uehlinger S, Schwager S, Bernier SP, Riedel K, Nguyen DT, et al. (2009) Identification of specific and universal virulence factors in Burkholderia cenocepacia strains by using multiple infection hosts. Infect Immun 77: 4102–4110. doi:10.1128/IAI.00398-09.
41. Hales BA, Morgan JAW, Hart CA (1998) Variation in Flagellin Genes and Proteins of Burkholderia cepacia Variation in Flagellin Genes and Proteins of Burkholderia cepacia. J Bacteriol 180: 1110–1118.
42. Montie T, Stover G (1983) Isolation and characterization of flagellar preparations from Pseudomonas species. J Clin Microbiol 18: 452–456.
43. Mahenthiralingam E, Urban TA, Goldberg JB (2005) The multifarious, multireplicon Burkholderia cepacia complex. Nat Rev Microbiol 3: 144–156. doi: 10.1038/nrmicro1085.
44. Urban TA, Goldberg JB, Forstner JF, Sajjan US (2005) Cable pili and the 22-kilodalton adhesin are required for Burkholderia cenocepacia binding to and transmigration across the squamous epithelium. Infect Immun 73: 5426–5437. doi: 10.1128/IAI.73.9.5426-5437.2005.
45. Traverse CC, Mayo-smith LM, Poltak SR, Cooper VS (2012) Tangled bank of experimentally evolved Burkholderia biofilms reflects selection during chronic infections. 110. doi: 10.1073/pnas.1207025110.
46. Ellis CN, Cooper VS (2010) Experimental adaptation of Burkholderia cenocepacia to onion medium reduces host range. Appl Environ Microbiol 76: 2387–2396. doi:10.1128/AEM.01930-09.
47. O'Grady EP, Sokol PA (2011) Burkholderia cenocepacia differential gene expression during host-pathogen interactions and adaptation to the host environment. Front Cell Infect Microbiol 1: 15. doi:10.3389/fcimb.2011.00015.
48. Pessi G, Braunwalder R, Grunau A, Omasits U, Ahrens CH, et al. (2013) Response of Burkholderia cenocepacia H111 to Micro-Oxia. PLoS One 8: e72939. doi:10.1371/journal.pone.0072939.
49. Drevinek P, Holden MTG, Ge Z, Jones AM, Ketchell I, et al. (2008) Gene expression changes linked to antimicrobial resistance, oxidative stress, iron depletion and retained motility are observed when Burkholderia cenocepacia grows in cystic fibrosis sputum. BMC Infect Dis 8: 121. doi:10.1186/1471-2334-8-121.
50. Mahenthiralingam E, Campbell ME, Henry DA, Speert DP (1996) Epidemiology of Burkholderia cepacia infection in patients with cystic fibrosis: analysis by randomly amplified polymorphic DNA fingerprinting. J Clin Microbiol 34: 2914–2920.

T Helper Cell Subsets Specific for *Pseudomonas aeruginosa* in Healthy Individuals and Patients with Cystic Fibrosis

Hannah K. Bayes[1], Stephen Bicknell[2], Gordon MacGregor[2], Tom J. Evans[1]*

1 Institute of Infection, Immunology and Inflammation, College of Medical, Veterinary and Life Sciences, University of Glasgow, Glasgow, United Kingdom, **2** West of Scotland Cystic Fibrosis Centre, Gartnavel General Hospital, Glasgow, United Kingdom

Abstract

Background: We set out to determine the magnitude of antigen-specific memory T helper cell responses to *Pseudomonas aeruginosa* in healthy humans and patients with cystic fibrosis.

Methods: Peripheral blood human memory $CD4^+$ T cells were co-cultured with dendritic cells that had been infected with different strains of *Pseudomonas aeruginosa*. The T helper response was determined by measuring proliferation, immunoassay of cytokine output, and immunostaining of intracellular cytokines.

Results: Healthy individuals and patients with cystic fibrosis had robust antigen-specific memory $CD4^+$ T cell responses to *Pseudomonas aeruginosa* that not only contained a Th1 and Th17 component but also Th22 cells. In contrast to previous descriptions of human Th22 cells, these Pseudomonal-specific Th22 cells lacked the skin homing markers CCR4 or CCR10, although were $CCR6^+$. Healthy individuals and patients with cystic fibrosis had similar levels of Th22 cells, but the patient group had significantly fewer Th17 cells in peripheral blood.

Conclusions: Th22 cells specific to *Pseudomonas aeruginosa* are induced in both healthy individuals and patients with cystic fibrosis. Along with Th17 cells, they may play an important role in the pulmonary response to this microbe in patients with cystic fibrosis and other conditions.

Editor: Dominik Hartl, University of Tübingen, Germany

Funding: The work was funded by the Wellcome Trust through the award of a Clinical Research Fellowship to HB under the Scottish Translational Medicine and Therapeutics Initiative. The funders had no role in study design, data collection and analysis, decision to publish, or preparation of the manuscript

Competing Interests: The authors have declared that no competing interests exist.

* E-mail: tom.evans@glasgow.ac.uk

Introduction

Cystic fibrosis (CF) typically results in recurrent pulmonary infections and inflammation that produces progressive respiratory failure [1,2]. The most common pathogen in these patients is *Pseudomonas aeruginosa* (PA), which produces a neutrophil dominated host response that does not, however, clear the infection [3]. Indeed, this persistent inflammatory response contributes to progressive lung injury [4,5] and thus pulmonary immune responses to *P. aeruginosa* are a potential therapeutic target.

Colonization with this bacterium results in an antibody response, which is not, however, protective [6]. In contrast, cell-mediated immunity to *P. aeruginosa* is important in host defence [7]. Recently, attention has focused on the novel T helper 17 (Th17) subset of Th cells [8]. These produce the signature cytokine IL-17 that plays a critical role in the generation and recruitment of neutrophils to sites of infection. In experimental murine models of acute pulmonary *P. aeruginosa* infection, there is evidence that Th17 cells play a key role in vaccine-induced protection [9]. Human studies have shown IL-17 is produced in CF lung, and that Th17 cells are present in the submucosa of airways from CF patients, although IL-17 is also produced from innate immune cells [10,11]. Humans typically have a very strong Th17 memory response to *Candida albicans* as well as *Staphylococcus aureus* [12,13]. However, it is not known whether there are similar memory responses to PA or whether these are altered in patients with CF.

IL-17 is commonly co-expressed with IL-22 in classic Th17 cells. IL-22 is a cytokine of the IL-10 family that has important effects on non-immune cells, promoting repair of epithelial surfaces and inducing an anti-microbial state [14]. More recently, a distinct lineage of Th cells producing IL-22 in the absence of IL-17 has been discovered, termed Th22 cells [15–18]. These cells have been found to possess a skin homing phenotype and infiltrate the skin in inflammatory disorders such as psoriasis in which IL-22 has been proposed to play a pathogenic role. In contrast, IL-22 also induces a variety of antimicrobial peptides and is important in host defence against pulmonary pathogens such as *Klebsiella pneumonia* [19]. Additionally, in a murine model of gut inflammation following infection with *Citrobacter rodentium*, IL-22 plays an important role in host defence [20,21]. In this model, IL-22 is produced both by innate lymphoid cells as well as Th22 cells [18]. IL-22 is also required to prevent dissemination of the commensal enteric bacteria from the genus *Alcaligenes* [22]. As yet, no specific pathogen or antigen has been demonstrated to elicit a human memory Th22 response.

Given that IL-22 promotes epithelial repair and induces an antimicrobial state, we hypothesised that Th22 cells could play an important role in host defence against lung infection with *P. aeruginosa* in CF and other clinical settings. Additionally, given the proposed role of Th17 cells in protection against PA infection, we hypothesized that PA-specific Th17 cells would be found in patients with CF. In order to test these hypotheses, we set out to examine the Th22, Th17 and Th1 cell responses to *P. aeruginosa* in both control and healthy individuals as well as patients with cystic fibrosis. We found that both healthy individuals as well as those with cystic fibrosis had robust antigen-specific Th17, Th1 and Th22 responses to *P. aeruginosa.* The PA-specific Th22 cells were $CCR6^+$ but lacked the skin-homing receptors CCR4 and CCR10 that have previously been found on human Th22 cells. PA-specific Th17 cells were reduced in patients with CF. These PA-specific Th cell subsets represent novel effector cells that can modulate the host anti-bacterial and inflammatory response to this pathogen and hence could be targets for novel therapeutic interventions in PA infection in CF and other conditions.

Materials and Methods

Ethics

All subjects gave informed written consent. The study was approved by West of Scotland Research Ethics Committee Number 2, a committee of the West of Scotland Research Ethics Service (WoSRES) that oversees ethical review of studies carried out on patients of the National Health Service Greater Glasgow and Clyde Health Board.

Participants and Cell Isolation

Peripheral blood samples were collected from adult CF patients attending the West of Scotland Adult CF Unit, Glasgow. Healthy individuals (controls) had no history of respiratory disease or intercurrent illness. Participant characteristics are shown in Table 1. Patients with CF attending the West of Scotland Adult CF Unit are deemed to be chronically colonized with *Pseudomonas aeruginosa* if sputum cultures remain positive for the organism after two attempts to clear the organism with combination antibiotic eradication therapy. Intermittent infection is deemed to exist when PA has been isolated and eradicated via antibiotic therapy.

PBMCs were obtained by Ficoll-Paque gradient centrifugation (GE Healthcare). $CD14^+$ monocytes were then magnetically isolated by a positive selection kit (Miltenyi Biotech). Memory $CD4^+$ T cells (purity for $CD4^+CD45RO^+$ >98%) were magnetically isolated by a negative selection kit (Miltenyi Biotech). Memory $CD4^+$ T cells were further sorted into CCR6-enriched and CCR6-depleted populations using positive selection microbeads (Stemcell Technologies). Proliferation was measured with CFSE (carboxyfluorescein diacetate succinimidyl ester; Invitrogen) or proliferation dye eFluor®450 (eBioscience) incorporated prior to cell culture.

Bacteriology

Laboratory *P. aeruginosa* (PA) strains PA103ΔpcrV and PA103-ΔUΔT [23,24] were kind gifts of Dr. Dara Frank, University of Wisconsin. Both strains have modulation of the function of the type three secretion system (T3SS), a common finding amongst CF PA strains; PA103ΔpcrV lacks the pore-forming protein of the T3SS rendering it non-functional and PA103ΔUΔT lacks the major translocation proteins (exoU and exoT) of the T3SS. Clinical non-mucoid PA strains Yorkhill 1 and Yorkhill 2, and clinical mucoid PA strain Yorkhill 5 were from CF samples (provided by Dr Craig Williams, Royal Hospital for Sick Children, Yorkhill). PA strains were grown to mid-log growth phase prior to infection.

Cell Culture

Dendritic cells (DCs) were derived from $CD14^+$ monocytes with IL-4 (500 IU/mL; Peprotech) and GM-CSF (50 ng/mL; Peprotech) for 7-days. DCs were infected with live PA strains as indicated. Ninety-minutes following infection, DCs were treated with bactericidal antibiotics (100 U/mL penicillin-streptomycin and 10 mg/mL gentamicin; both Sigma) followed by overnight incubation. Additionally, in some experiments, DCs were treated with tetanus toxoid (5 ug/mL; Calbiochem) or heat-killed preparation of Candida albicans (InvivoGen).

Infected DCs (1×10^4 cells) were cultured with autologous memory $CD4^+$ T cells (1×10^5 cells) in 96-well U-bottom plates in IMDM+Glutamax medium (Gibco Life Technologies) supplemented with 5% fetal bovine serum (Invitrogen) and 100 U/mL penicillin-streptomycin for 6-days. For polyclonal stimulation conditions, $CD4^+$ T cells were cultured with plate-bound anti-CD3 (5 ug/mL) and soluble anti-CD28 (1 ug/mL) (both eBioscience).

Measurement of $CD4^+$ T cell response

Following 6-days of co-culture, supernatants were harvested and cytokine levels measured via ELISA for IL-17A, IL-22, and IFN-γ (eBioscience).

Cell Staining and Analysis

Cells were stimulated for 5-hours with phorbol 12-myristate 13-acetate (50 ng/ml; Sigma) and ionomycin (500 ng/ml; Sigma) in

Table 1. Characteristics of participants providing peripheral blood specimens for the analysis of T helper cell responses to *Pseudomonas aeruginosa.*

	Patients with cystic fibrosis	Healthy controls
Participants (n)	8	10
Age, median (IQR), years	23 (23.5–30)	26 (24–29)
Male sex, n (%)	5 (62.5)	4 (40)
Chronic *Pseudomonas aeruginosa* colonization, n	7	na
FEV_1 median (IQR), % predicted	38.2 (35.2–44.4)	na
No. of patients with respiratory exacerbation at time of sample collection, n (%)	6 (75)	na

n, number in group; na, non-applicable; IQR, inter-quartile range; FEV_1, forced expiratory volume in 1 second.

the presence of Golgiplug (1 µl/ml; BD Pharmingen) at 37°C. Cells were fixed using 4% paraformaldehyde (VWR International) and made permeable, following extracellular staining, using Perm/Wash (BD Biosciences).

Extracellular staining was with phycoerythrin-labelled anti-CD4 (RPA-T4; eBioscience), phycoerythrin-labelled anti-αβTCR (IP26; eBioscience), phycoerythrin-Cy7-labelled anti-CCR4 (IGI; BD Pharminogen), AlexFluor®647-labelled anti-CCR9 (BL/CCR9; BioLegend), phycoerythrin-labelled anti-CCR10 (FAB 3478P; R&D), CD86 and CD40. Intracellular staining was with eFluor®660-labelled anti-IL-22 (22URTI; eBioscience), phycoerythrin-labelled anti-IL-22 (BG/IL-22; Biolegend), PerCP-Cy5.5-labelled anti-IFN-γ (4S.B3; eBioscience), and AlexFluor®488 anti-IL-17A (eBioDEC17; eBioscience). Corresponding isotype controls were used. Dead cell exclusion was achieved either by Boolean-gating based on cell scatter properties or labelling with Fixable Viability Dye eFluor®506 (eBioscience). Stained cells were analysed on either a FACSCalibur or CyAn flow cytometer (BD Biosciences). Collected data were analysed using FlowJo software (Tree Star).

Statistical analysis

Non-parametric statistical tests were used (Mann-Whitney, Kruskal-Wallis (KW), and, where appropriate, Dunn's multiple comparison test), using Prism Version 6.0 (GraphPad Software).

Results

Antigen-specific memory $CD4^+$ T cell responses exist against *P. aeruginosa* in Healthy Individuals

In order to examine antigen-dependent T cell memory responses from healthy controls and patients with CF, we isolated monocyte-derived dendritic cells (DCs) and $CD4^+CD45RA^-$C-$D45RO^+$ memory T cells from peripheral blood. Memory $CD4^+$ T cells were co-cultured with either uninfected DCs, DCs infected with PA, or the supernatant of such DCs, and the production of IL-17A, IL-22 and IFN-γ measured in the culture supernatant by ELISA (Figure 1).

Firstly, we examined the memory T cell responses of healthy controls. Small amounts of IL-17A were produced by T cells cultured with unstimulated DCs; this was abolished in the absence of DCs (Figure 1A). In the absence of DC infection, there was no significant production of either IL-22 (Figure 1B) or IFN-γ (Figure 1C). In contrast, co-culture of memory T cells with DCs infected with PA103 gave robust production of IL-17A, IL-22 and IFN-γ (Figure 1). This was almost completely abolished when T cells were cultured with infected DC supernatants alone (Figure 1); thus direct contact between T cells and DCs is required for cytokine production. No cytokines were produced when T cells were infected directly in the absence of DCs or when infected DCs were cultured alone in the absence of T cells (data not shown). Thus, the observed memory Th cell responses in healthy individuals were entirely dependent on physical contact between the DCs and T cells, as expected of an antigen-driven response. Cytokine production did not vary significantly following co-culture of memory T cells with DCs infected at multiplicities of infection (MOIs) between 10–60 (Figure 1D–F), suggesting even at the lowest MOI used the stimulating effect on memory T cells was already maximal.

Next, we compared this cytokine production by memory $CD4^+$ T cells in healthy individuals against different strains of PA. Similar levels of these three cytokines were produced following infection of DCs with strains of PA103 that differed in the possession of a functional type III apparatus (Figure S1). Additionally, these cytokine levels did not vary significantly between these laboratory strains and the response to PA strains isolated from patients with CF (Figure S1).

We then examined the proliferation of memory $CD4^+$ T cells of healthy individuals following co-culture with DCs alone or DCs infected with PA, using a flow cytometric method. As expected, little proliferation was seen with T cells cultured with uninfected DCs (Figure 2A). However, marked proliferation of $CD4^+$ T cell was seen in response to DCs infected with either laboratory PA103ΔUΔT (average proliferation [+/−SEM] 18.8% [+/−9.0%] for three donors) and clinical Yorkhill 5 (average proliferation [+/−SEM] 35.1% [+/−5.2%] for three donors) PA strains (Figure 2A). We also stained these cells for the presence of intracellular cytokines to determine which cells were producing the measured cytokines. IL-17 and IL-22 production in the co-cultures was predominantly by cells proliferating in response to PA (Figure 2B and C). Proliferating cells producing intracellular IL-17 and/or IL-22 were also confirmed to be αβ T cell receptor positive cells (data not shown). No intracellular cytokines were produced in DCs. Small amounts of intracellular IFN-γ were expressed by the non-proliferating $CD4^+$ memory cells following polyclonal stimulation; however, IFN-γ was only secreted from memory $CD4^+$ T cells in response to PA infected DCs (Figure 1). Collectively, these data show the existence of a classical antigen-specific memory $CD4^+$ T cell response to *P. aeruginosa* in healthy individuals with no previous history of pulmonary infection with this organism.

DC Activation following Infection with *P. aeruginosa*

To explore potential differential effects of the different PA strains on DC activation, we stained DCs for the activation markers CD86 and CD40 following infection with the different PA strains (Figure 3). Figure 3A shows representative plots of flow cytometric analysis of CD86 and CD 40 on the surface of DCs following infection with PA103ΔUΔT and Yorkhill 1 strains of PA as well as exposure to heat killed *Candida albicans*. These examples all show a marked upregulation of these activation markers on the surface of DCs. This was quantified for both CD86 and CD40 for a range of strains as shown in Figure 3B and 3C respectively. All strains tested produced an increase in expression of these markers. There was a trend towards slightly higher levels of expression in DCs infected with the PA103 strains, but this did not reach statistical significance.

Cytokine secretion by *P. aeruginosa*-specific $CD4^+$ T cells in patients with CF and controls

We then examined the cytokine responses of peripheral memory T cells in response to PA infected DCs in patients with CF compared to healthy individuals. All CF patients had a history of chronic or intermittent PA infection (Table 1). As seen in the experiments with T cells from healthy control individuals, memory $CD4^+$ T cells from patients with CF produce significant amounts of IL-17A, IL-22 and IFN-γ in response to DC infection with either laboratory or clinical PA strains compared with uninfected DCs (Figure 4A, B and C). However, the magnitude of this response between patients with CF with a history of *P. aeruginosa* infection and healthy controls was not significantly different for all three of the cytokines measured ($p>0.05$ for all strains, Kruskal Wallis).

P. aeruginosa-specific Th22, Th17 and Th1 responses in patients with CF and controls

Further to assess the Th cell subsets constituting the memory $CD4^+$ T cell response to PA, we used polyclonal re-stimulation

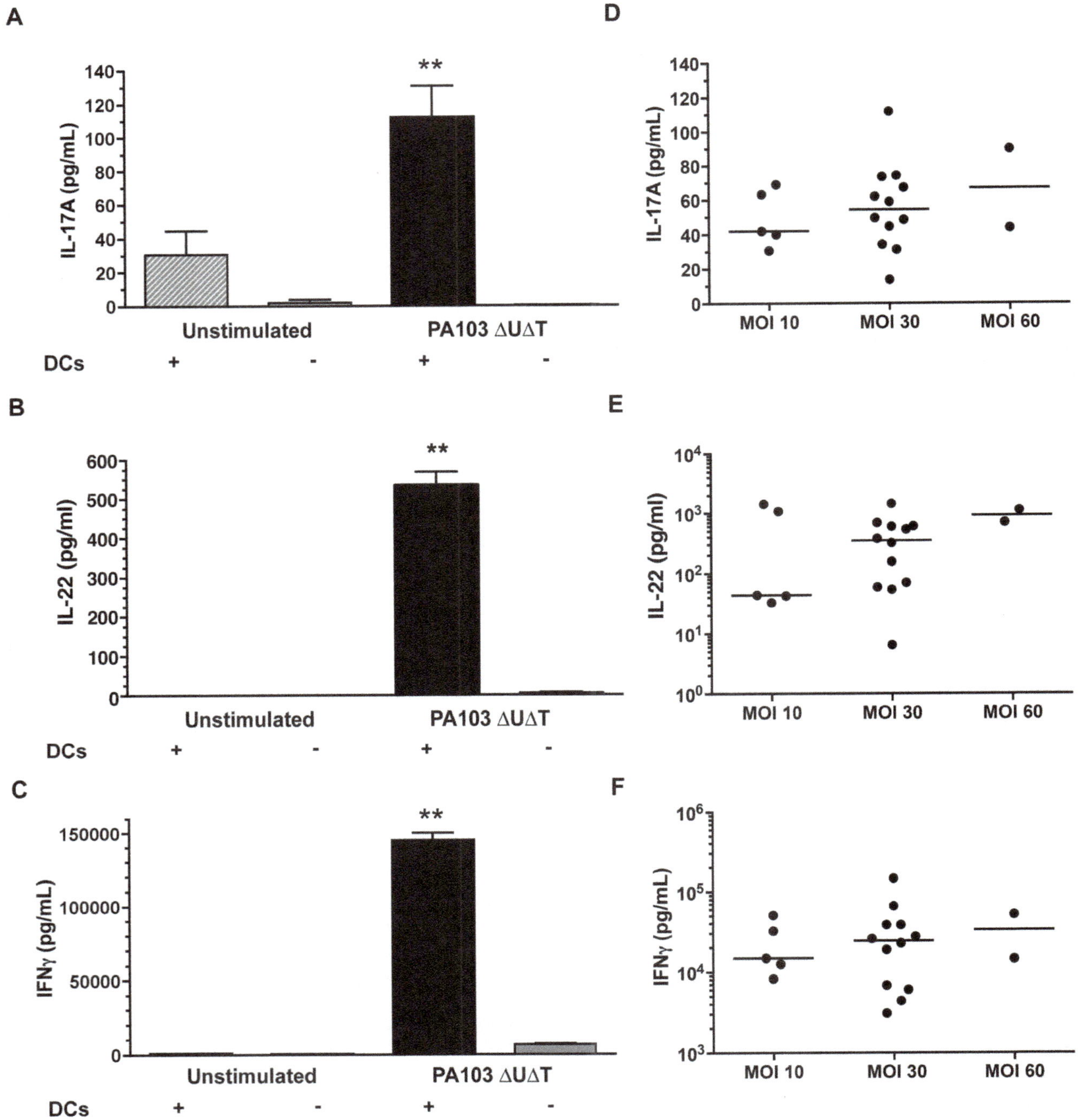

Figure 1. Cytokine production of human memory CD4$^+$ T cells in response to *P. aeruginosa*. A–C Sorted human memory CD4$^+$ T cells from healthy volunteers were co-cultured either with dendritic cells that had been infected with *P. aeruginosa* (DCs +) or with the supernatant from such infected DCs (DC −). Levels of IL-17A (**A**), IL-22 (**B**) and IFN-γ (**C**) were measured in supernatants after 6 days. DCs were infected at a MOI of 60 before culturing with T cells. Columns show the mean of triplicate determinations; error bars are ±1 standard error of mean. Results are representative of experiments in three separate individuals. **D–F**, secreted cytokine levels following DC infection at a variety of different MOIs. Each point represents a value from an individual healthy individual.

and intracellular staining of the resultant CD4$^+$ T cell populations present at the end of the co-cultures followed by flow cytometric analysis. Th1 cells are characterized by their production of IFN-γ on antigen stimulation. In humans, Th1 cells can co-produce IL-17 and IL-22, which was indeed initially classed as a Th1 cytokine [25]. To provide an unambiguous classification of the different cytokine producing cells, we adopted the following definitions. CD4$^+$ T cells expressing IFN-γ were designated as Th1 cells; Th17 cells were any IFN-γ negative cell producing IL-17A with/without IL-22; and Th22 cells were defined as those expressing IL-22 alone (Figure 5A). We used this gating strategy to quantify the proportions of memory CD4$^+$ T cells in each of these categories following stimulation with PA-infected DCs.

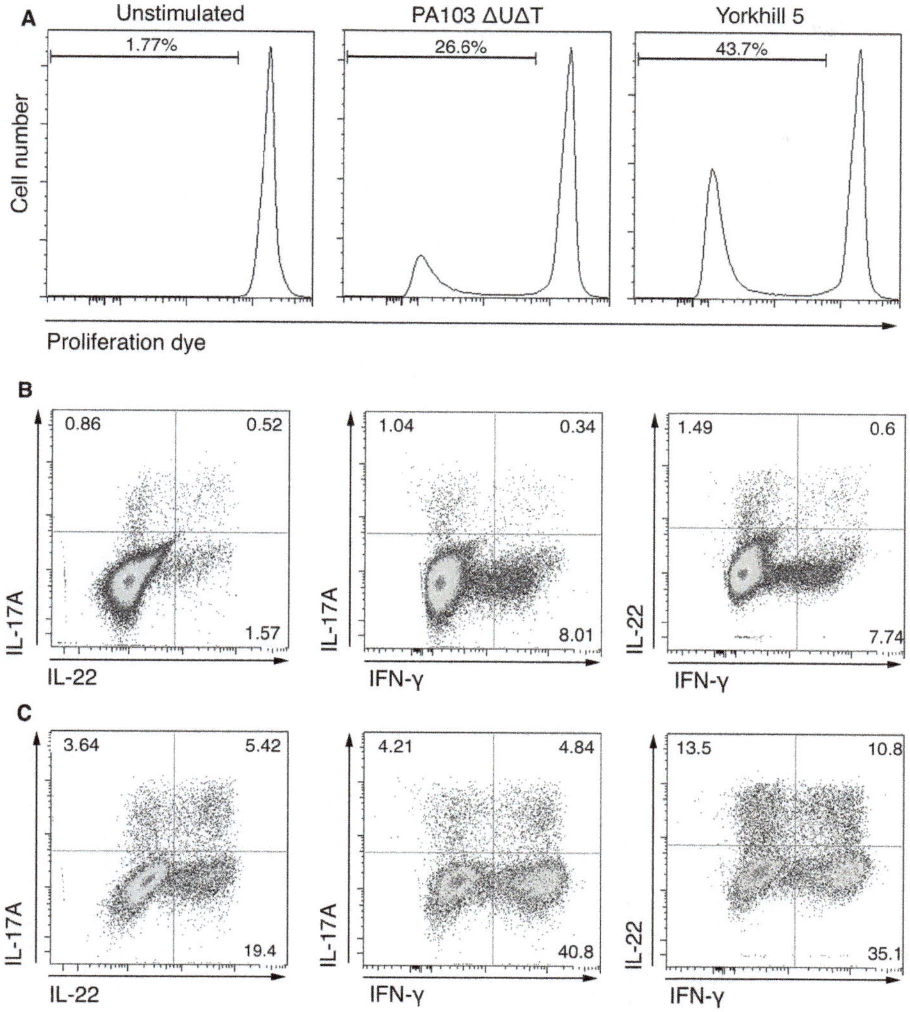

Figure 2. Cell proliferation of memory CD4⁺ T cells following co-culture with infected dendritic cells (DCs). (**A**) Memory $CD4^+$ T cells loaded with proliferation dye were co-cultured with unstimulated DCs, DCs infected with PA103ΔUΔT MOI 30 (PA103), or DCs infected with Yorkhill 5 MOI 30 (Yorkhill 5). Panels show the distribution of the proliferation dye fluorescence in the cell population after 6-days; inset figures show the percentage of the initial population that has undergone one or more cell divisions. (**B**) Patterns of cytokine expression by non-proliferating $CD4^+$ T cells following 6-days of culture with DCs infected with Yorkhill 5. (**C**) Patterns of cytokine expression by $CD4^+$ T cells proliferating in response to culture with DCs infected with Yorkhill 5. Numbers in plot represent per cent cells in each quadrant. The experiment was repeated in 3 independent individuals with the same result.

In healthy controls (Figure 5B) and patients with CF (Figure 5C) the predominant responding population was a memory Th1 response. Within the population of IFN-γ positive cells proliferating in response to PA infected DCs, there were cells that that co-produced IL-17 and/or IL-22 (Figure 2C). Significantly, however, there were clear populations of Th22 and Th17 cells, as defined above, i.e. $IFN\text{-}\gamma^-$ $IL\text{-}17^-$ $IL\text{-}22^+$ and $IFN\text{-}\gamma^-$ $IL\text{-}17^+$ respectively (Figure 5). The proportion of Th1 and Th22 cells detected following co-culture with PA infected DCs was similar in healthy controls and patients with CF (see Figure S2). However, although the observed IL-17A cytokine response was of a similar magnitude (Figure 4A), there was a significantly lower proportion of Th17 cells in CF patients compared with healthy controls (Figure 5D). This was particularly evident in response to the clinical PA strains, where median percentage of Th17 cells was 5.3% in healthy controls compared with 1.04% in CF patients ($p = 0.003$).

These cytokine profiles were in distinct contrast to those obtained from memory $CD4^+$ T helper cells that were stimulated with either tetanus-toxoid treated DCs (Figure S3A, B) or heat-killed *Candida albicans* (Figure S3C, D). Tetanus-toxoid induced, as predicted, an essentially pure Th1 response. *Candida albicans*, as has been previously described [26], induced a robust Th17 response, although Th1 and Th22 cells were also evident.

Tissue-homing characteristics of-specific memory Th22 and Th17 cells

Human memory Th17 and Th22 cells characteristically express the mucosal chemokine receptor CCR6 [13,16,17]. To further verify the existence of memory Th17 and Th22 populations against PA, we sorted memory $CD4^+$ T cells on the basis of their CCR6 expression prior to culture with PA-infected DCs. This confirmed that virtually all IFN-γ negative $CD4^+$ T cell producing IL-17A and/or IL-22 (i.e. Th17 and Th22 cells) in response to PA infection were in the CCR6-enriched population (Figure 6A, B and C).

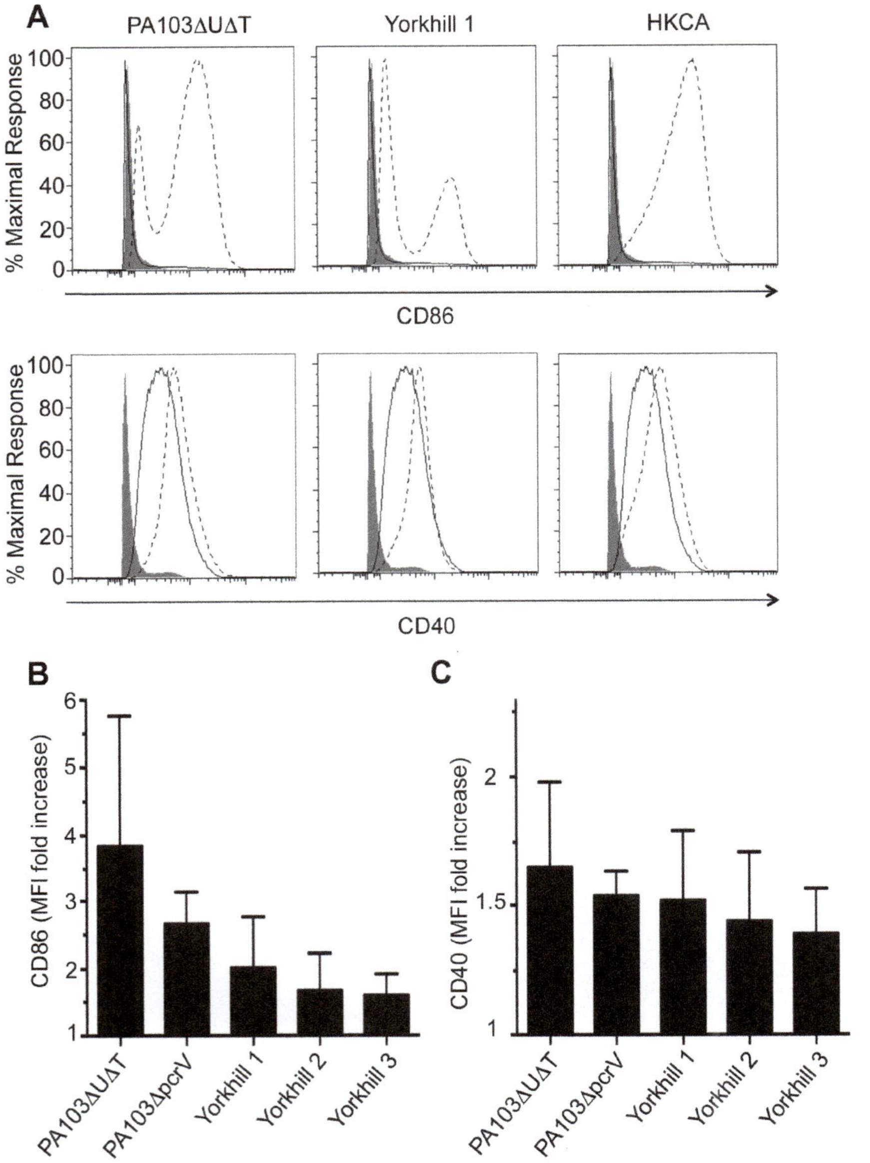

Figure 3. DC Activation following infection with different strains of *P. aeruginosa*. Levels of CD86 (**A**) and CD40 (**B**) following DC activation 24 hours following treatment with the indicated microbes. The panels show representative plots of isotype staining (solid shading), staining of unstimulated DCs (solid line) and staining following microbial treatment (dotted line). **B** and **C**, mean fold-increase in mean fluorescence intensity (MFI) of CD86 and CD40 respectively in 5 independent individuals. This was calculated as the fold-increase in MFI in infected DCs versus uninfected controls. Columns show mean and SEM.

We next addressed whether the PA-specific memory Th17 and Th22 populations demonstrated features of homing to specific tissues. Th22 cells have previously been found to demonstrate a skin-homing phenotype [13,16,17] and have been implicated in the pathogenesis of inflammatory skin conditions [15]. We thus analysed the PA-specific memory IL-22 secreting cell population for expression of the skin-homing receptors CCR4 and CCR10. In contrast to the reported properties of peripheral blood derived Th22 cells without a characterised antigen specificity [16,17], IL-22 production in response to PA infection was from memory $CD4^+$ T cells that did not express the skin-homing receptors CCR4 or CCR10 (Figure 6D). Additionally, we found that PA-specific IL-17A and IL-22 expressing memory T helper cells did not display the gut-homing receptor CCR9 (Figure 6D).

Discussion

The work described in this paper provides an important advance in our understanding of the human T helper response to *P. aeruginosa* and how this might influence the course of lung disease in individuals with CF who are chronically colonized with this microbe, as well as in other patients with PA infections. We found robust memory Th responses to *P. aeruginosa* in both normal individuals and in those with CF who have Pseudomonas colonization of the respiratory tract. These specific responses to *P. aeruginosa* contain Th1, Th17 and Th22 cells. This is the first time that an antigen-specific human Th22 response has been demonstrated. Moreover, these cells have a novel phenotype, lacking homing markers for skin and gut although retaining CCR6, which would allow them to respond to the ligands CCL20

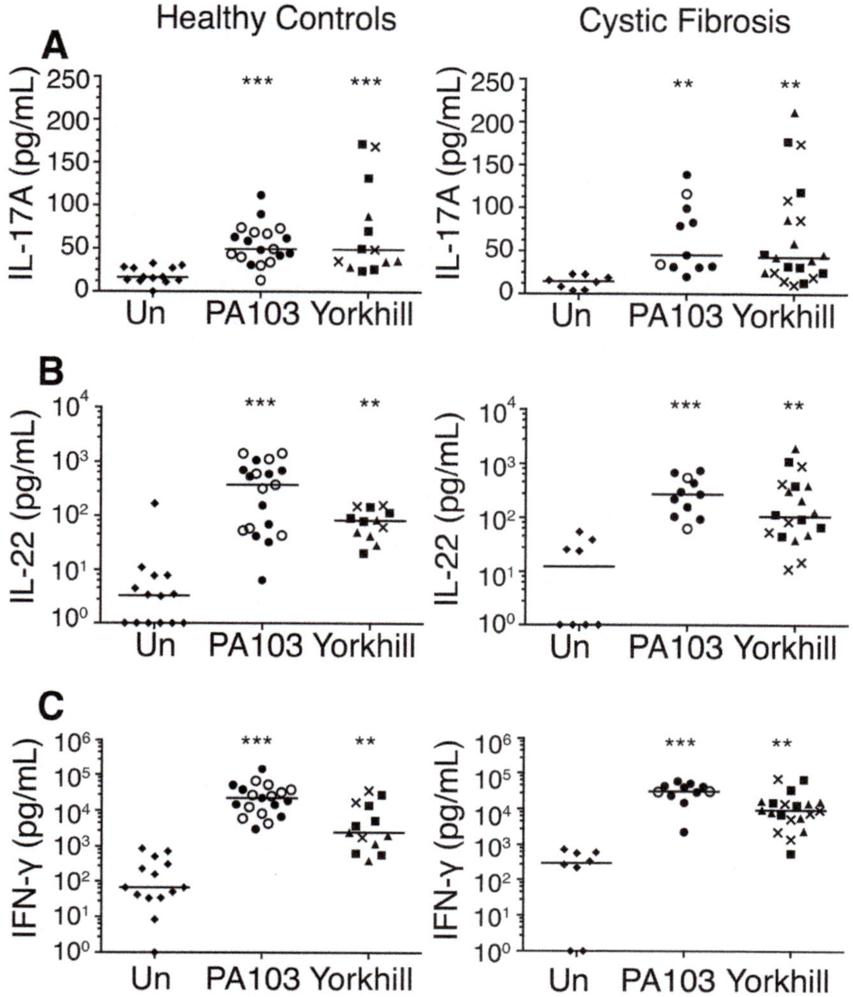

Figure 4. Cytokine production by human memory CD4$^+$ T cells in healthy controls and cystic fibrosis. Human memory CD4$^+$ T cells were exposed to unstimulated DCs or DCs infected with the laboratory strains (PA103) or clinical *Pseudomonas aeruginosa* strains (Yorkhill). After 6 days of co-culture levels of (**A**) IL-17, (**B**) IL-22 and (**C**) IFN-γ were measured. Each point represents the mean of triplicate wells and is the result from one individual. The different bacterial strains used are: ♦, unstimulated; ○, PA103 ΔpcrV; ●, PA103ΔUΔT; ▲, YH1; ■, YH2; ×, YH5. The line indicates the median value. Differences between infection conditions (**A–C**) were evaluated by a Kruskal-Wallis test all of which had p values <0.0009). Differences between unstimulated and infected conditions were then tested using Dunn's multiple comparison test. ** significant $p<0.01$ and *** significant $p<0.001$.

and β-defensins produced from damaged epithelia. We show that although Th22 and Th1 responses are similar in controls and patients with CF, the proportion of Th17 responding cells is significantly diminished in peripheral blood of patients with CF. Taken together, these data show that chronic airway colonization with *P. aeruginosa* could activate both Th17 and Th22 memory responses that would migrate to inflamed lung, and potentially alter the balance between inflammation, host defence and tissue repair.

The most striking finding of this study was the identification of Pseudomonal-specific Th22 cells in both healthy individuals and in those with CF. We were surprised that normal healthy controls had robust Th22 (and indeed Th1 and Th17) responses to *P. aeruginosa*, as it is generally only pathogenic in immunocompromised states. The microbe is found within the bowel flora of a minority of normal individuals, 4% in one report [27], so it would not seem likely that this is the source of bacteria to provoke a memory Th response. Indeed, the Pseudomonal-specific Th22 cells we identified did not have gut or skin homing receptors (Fig 6). Although *P. aeruginosa* is a common environmental organism, it remains unclear at what site this microbe triggers a memory T helper response. Others have also demonstrated cross-reactivity of Th17 cells against different bacterial serotypes and fungi [28,29]. We have not sought to define the antigenic component, of which there may be many, of *Pseudomonas aeruginosa* eliciting the observed Th17 and Th22 response, which might be shared with other infecting organisms and particularly with other Gram negative bacteria. The possibility of cross-reactivity of these Th cell responses remains, yet we have shown a lack of gut-homing and thus cross-reactivity with phylogenetically-related organisms in gut flora is unlikely.

In common with previous descriptions of Th22 cells in humans, the Pseudomonal-specific Th22 cells we identified were in the CCR6$^+$ population (Figure 6) [15–17]. Previous studies identified these cells as bearing skin-homing markers and a pathogenic role for these cells in psoriasis and other inflammatory skin disorders

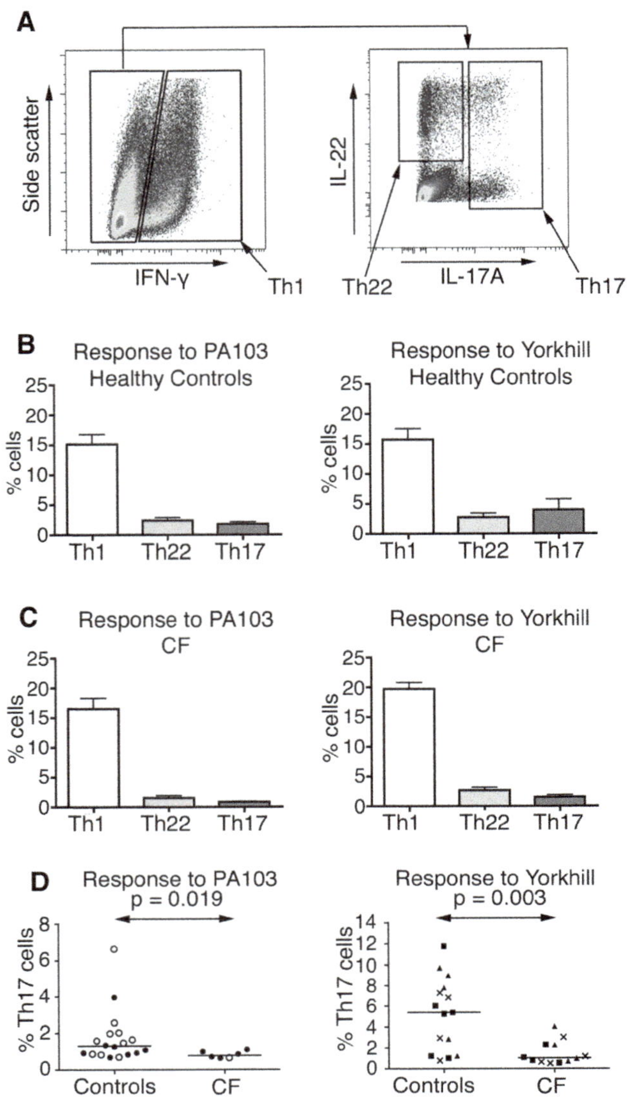

Figure 5. Memory CD4$^+$ T cells subset response to different Pseudomonas strains in CF and controls. Following co-culture with dendritic cells infected with laboratory Pseudomonas aeruginosa (PA) strains (PA103) or clinical PA strains (Yorkhill), CD4$^+$ T cells were classified into T helper cell subsets based on intracellular cytokine straining patterns, as shown for a representative patient in panel **A**. The Th1, Th17 and Th22 responses to both PA103 and Yorkhill PA strains is shown for healthy controls (**B**) and patients with CF (**C**), as a percentage of the total numbers of CD4$^+$ memory cells analysed. The columns show the mean values +/− SEM; n = 8 for CF patients and 10 for healthy controls. Panel **D** shows the proportions of PA-specific Th17 cells in CF patients compared with controls. Each point represents the result from one individual; different bacterial strains are indicated by the symbols as described in Figure 4. The line indicates the median value. Differences between controls and patients with CF (**D**) were evaluated by a Mann-Whitney test.

has been proposed. We propose that the pseudomonal-specific Th22 cells we have identified in healthy humans and patients with CF can migrate to inflamed lung, which will release the chemokines CCL20 and β-defensins, both ligands for CCR6. In relation to pulmonary recruitment, we have previously sought evidence of Th17 and Th22 recruitment within bronchoalveolar lavage (BAL) from CF patients, an approach that has significant technical limitations. We have, however, identified low level IL-22 production (IL-22 detectable in 5 of 14 CF patients, with median IL-22 levels of 12.39pg/mL) within the CF BAL and thus further implicating a potential Th22 response within the disease pathogenesis. Given its potent action in promoting epithelial repair, regulating fibrosis and mediating host defense [14,19,30], we believe that IL-22 is important in attenuating the effects of chronic pulmonary infection with *P. aeruginosa* and enhancing tissue repair. The action of IL-22 may well be modified by IL-17, as demonstrated in lung fibrosis [30]. Testing of this hypothesis will best be performed in an animal model of chronic *P. aeruginosa* lung infection. We found in general that IL-22 production in the T cell memory population was predominantly from Th22 cells more than Th17 cells (Figures 2 and 6). As outlined above, these cells would be able to migrate to inflamed tissue producing the CCR6 ligands CCL20 and β-defensins, both of which would be found in infected lung. The swift expansion of a PA-specific Th22 memory cell population would thus ensure a rapid production of an IL-22 producing cell that could migrate to the site of infection to mediate host defence and/or contribute to tissue repair.

A very recent study from Jay Kolls' group identified Pseudomonal-specific Th17 cells in the draining lymph nodes of patients with CF [31]. Intriguingly, we found a reduction in Pseudomonal-specific Th17 cells in peripheral blood of CF patients. These data suggest that this Th17 population translocates from blood to pulmonary system during the chronic pulmonary colonization with *P. aeruginosa*. Indeed, IL-17$^+$ T cells and IL-17 production has previously been observed within CF lung [10] and BAL [32], respectively. Alternatively, a recent study demonstrated that PA can induce myeloid-derived suppressor cells via flagellin stimulation [33]. These cells could act to down-regulate Th17 responses to PA, accounting for the observed reduction in PA-specific Th17 cells in CF patients.

Within the CF patient population exogenous and endogenous factors which may modulate immune function are common. For example, within our sampled CF population all patients were receiving long-term low-dose macrolide therapy and a quarter had CF-related diabetes mellitus. Nutritional status of CF patients will also be worse than age-matched controls. Controlling for such variables is problematic without a large sample size, which would be prohibitive for our described method of *ex vivo* T cell stimulation. We did however achieve adequate age matching of CF patients and controls, as well as ensuring that controls were healthy and free from conditions linked to pulmonary Th17 responses and pulmonary Pseudomonas infections, such as asthma and bronchiectasis. The data identifies and describes a previously uncharacterized Th cell response against *Pseudomonas aeruginosa* in both healthy controls and patients with CF, however generalizations to the whole heterogeneous CF population are preliminary at present.

Although this study has focussed on PA-specific Th cells in patients with cystic fibrosis, PA infections are significant in immunocompromised patients [34], in ventilator-associated pneumonia [35], following extensive burns and as a cause of infective exacerbations in patients with chronic obstructive airways disease [36]. Thus, the presence of Th22, Th17 and Th1 memory CD4$^+$ cells specific to PA may play a role in these situations as well. The balance of effects on host defence, tissue repair and systemic inflammation produced by Il-22 will likely differ between these different conditions, necessitating further experimental investigation to define the role of IL-22 and Th22 cells in each of these conditions.

In conclusion, our work has demonstrated the presence in peripheral blood of memory CD4$^+$ T cells of the Th22 lineage that are specific for *P. aeruginosa* antigens. They lack conventional skin

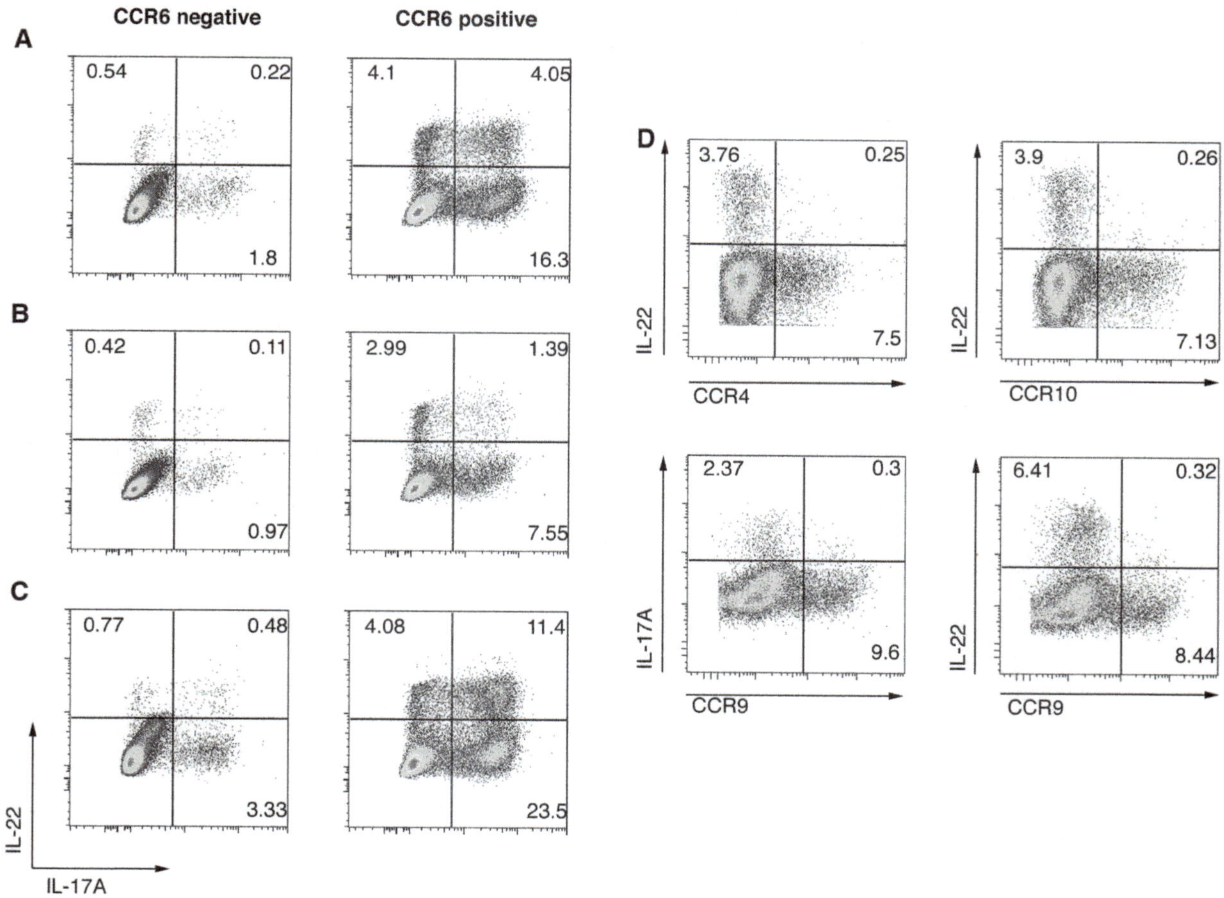

Figure 6. Tissue-homing characteristics of Pseudomonas aeruginosa-specific memory Th22 and Th17 cells. A–C Human memory CD4$^+$ T cells were sorted into CCR6-depleted (CCR6 negative) and CCR6-enriched (CCR6 positive) populations before being exposed to dendritic cells (DCs) infected with Yorkhill 5 MOI30 (**A**), DCs infected with PA103 ΔUΔT MOI30 (**B**), or stimulated with anti-CD3 and anti-CD28 which acted as a positive control by polyclonal T cell stimulation (**C**). Plots show CD4$^+$ IFN-γ negative T cells after 6-days of co-culture. **D** Memory CD4$^+$ T cells were cultured with DCs infected with PA103 ΔpcrV MOI30. Pseudomonas-specific memory CD4$^+$ T cells were analysed for expression of intracellular IL-22 or IL-17 as shown together with the skin-homing chemokine receptors CCR4, CCR10 and CCR9 as indicated. Numbers in each plot represent per cent cells in each quadrant. Results are representative of those seen in three independent individuals.

or gut homing markers but are CCR6$^+$. We propose that these cells will migrate to areas of inflamed lung under the influence of CCL20 or β-defensins. Local IL-22 within the lung could play a key role in host defence, epithelial repair and regeneration, and may be amenable to therapeutic intervention to promote healthy lung repair after damaging infection.

Supporting Information

Figure S1 Cytokine production by human memory CD4$^+$ T cells to different *Pseudomonas aeruginosa* strains. Human memory CD4$^+$ T cells from healthy volunteers (**A**, **B** and **C**) and patients with cystic fibrosis (CF) (**D**, **E** and **F**) were co-cultured with dendritic cells infected with different strains of (PA). Laboratory PA strains PA103 ΔpcrV and PA103 ΔUΔT, clinical non-mucoid strains Yorkhill 1 and 2, and the clinical mucoid strain Yorkhill 5 were used; clinical strains were derived from cystic fibrosis patients. Levels of cytokines were measured in the supernatant after 6-days of culture. Each point represents the result from one individual; an individual may be represented more than once by separate experiments. The line indicates the median value. Differences between strains were evaluated by a Kruskal-Wallis (KW) test with pairwise assessments of differences between groups made using Dunn's multiple comparison test. *, significance difference <0.05. Only minor differences were seen in the cytokine response to different strains of PA in both healthy controls and patients with CF.

Figure S2 Memory CD4$^+$ T cells subset response to different Pseudomonas strains in CF and controls. The proportion of PA specific CD4$^+$ T helper cell responses to PA103 (PA103 ΔpcrV and PA103 ΔUΔT) and Yorkhill strains (Yorkhill 1, 2 and 5) that are Th1 (**A**) or Th22 (**B**) was determined as outlined in Figure 5 in the main text. Each point represents the result from one individual; some individuals were tested against different bacterial strains as indicated by the symbols used in Figure 4. The line indicates the median value. Differences between controls and patients with CF were evaluated by a Mann-Whitney test with the p value as shown.

Figure S3 Cytokine production by human memory CD4$^+$ T cells to tetanus toxoid and heat-killed candida albicans. Human memory CD4$^+$ T cells from healthy were co-cultured with dendritic cells infected with tetanus toxoid or heat-killed candida albicans. (**A**) Patterns of cytokine expression by non-proliferating CD4$^+$ T cells following 6-days of culture with DCs infected with tetanus toxoid. (**B**) Patterns of cytokine expression by CD4$^+$ T cells proliferating in response to culture with DCs infected with tetanus toxoid. (**C**) Patterns of cytokine expression by non-proliferating CD4$^+$ T cells following 6-days of culture with DCs infected with heat-killed candida albicans (HKCA). (**D**) Patterns of cytokine expression by CD4$^+$ T cells proliferating in response to culture with DCs infected with HKCA. Numbers in plot represent percent cells in each quadrant.

Acknowledgments

We are grateful to Diane Vaughan, (Glasgow), for assistance in running the flow cytometry analyses.

Author Contributions

Conceived and designed the experiments: HKB SB GM TJE. Performed the experiments: HKB TJE. Analyzed the data: HKB TJE. Wrote the paper: HKB TJE.

References

1. Rowe SM, Miller S, Sorscher EJ (2005) Cystic fibrosis. N Engl J Med 352: 1992-2001.
2. Ratjen F, McColley SA (2012) Update in cystic fibrosis 2011. Am J Respir Crit Care Med 185: 933–936.
3. Sadikot RT, Blackwell TS, Christman JW, Prince AS (2005) Pathogen-host interactions in Pseudomonas aeruginosa pneumonia. Am J Respir Crit Care Med 171: 1209–1223.
4. Dubin PJ, Kolls JK (2007) Pseudomonas aeruginosa and the host pulmonary immune response. Expert Rev Respir Med 1: 121–137.
5. Downey DG, Bell SC, Elborn JS (2009) Neutrophils in cystic fibrosis. Thorax 64: 81–88.
6. Doring G (1989) Host response to Pseudomonas aeruginosa. Acta Paediatr Scand Suppl 363: 37–39; discussion 40.
7. Markham RB, Powderly WG (1988) Exposure of mice to live Pseudomonas aeruginosa generates protective cell-mediated immunity in the absence of an antibody response. J Immunol 140: 2039–2045.
8. Stockinger B, Veldhoen M, Martin B (2007) Th17 T cells: linking innate and adaptive immunity. Semin Immunol 19: 353–361.
9. Priebe GP, Walsh RL, Cederroth TA, Kamei A, Coutinho-Sledge YS, et al. (2008) IL-17 is a critical component of vaccine-induced protection against lung infection by lipopolysaccharide-heterologous strains of Pseudomonas aeruginosa. J Immunol 181: 4965–4975.
10. Tan HL, Regamey N, Brown S, Bush A, Lloyd CM, et al. (2011) The Th17 pathway in cystic fibrosis lung disease. Am J Respir Crit Care Med 184: 252–258.
11. Brodlie M, Corris PA, Lordan J, Ward C (2012) Interleukin-17 and cystic fibrosis lung disease. Am J Respir Crit Care Med 185: 108–109; author reply 109–110.
12. Zielinski CE, Mele F, Aschenbrenner D, Jarrossay D, Ronchi F, et al. (2012) Pathogen-induced human TH17 cells produce IFN-gamma or IL-10 and are regulated by IL-1beta. Nature 484: 514–518.
13. Acosta-Rodriguez EV, Rivino L, Geginat J, Jarrossay D, Gattorno M, et al. (2007) Surface phenotype and antigenic specificity of human interleukin 17-producing T helper memory cells. Nat Immunol 8: 639–646.
14. Wolk K, Witte E, Witte K, Warszawska K, Sabat R (2010) Biology of interleukin-22. Semin Immunopathol 32: 17–31.
15. Eyerich S, Eyerich K, Pennino D, Carbone T, Nasorri F, et al. (2009) Th22 cells represent a distinct human T cell subset involved in epidermal immunity and remodeling. J Clin Invest 119: 3573–3585.
16. Duhen T, Geiger R, Jarrossay D, Lanzavecchia A, Sallusto F (2009) Production of interleukin 22 but not interleukin 17 by a subset of human skin-homing memory T cells. Nat Immunol 10: 857–863.
17. Trifari S, Kaplan CD, Tran EH, Crellin NK, Spits H (2009) Identification of a human helper T cell population that has abundant production of interleukin 22 and is distinct from T(H)-17, T(H)1 and T(H)2 cells. Nat Immunol 10: 864–871.
18. Basu R, O'Quinn DB, Silberger DJ, Schoeb TR, Fouser L, et al. (2012) Th22 cells are an important source of IL-22 for host protection against enteropathogenic bacteria. Immunity 37: 1061–1075.
19. Aujla SJ, Chan YR, Zheng M, Fei M, Askew DJ, et al. (2008) IL-22 mediates mucosal host defense against Gram-negative bacterial pneumonia. Nat Med 14: 275–281.
20. Ota N, Wong K, Valdez PA, Zheng Y, Crellin NK, et al. (2011) IL-22 bridges the lymphotoxin pathway with the maintenance of colonic lymphoid structures during infection with Citrobacter rodentium. Nat Immunol 12: 941–948.
21. Zheng Y, Valdez PA, Danilenko DM, Hu Y, Sa SM, et al. (2008) Interleukin-22 mediates early host defense against attaching and effacing bacterial pathogens. Nat Med 14: 282–289.
22. Sonnenberg GF, Monticelli LA, Alenghat T, Fung TC, Hutnick NA, et al. (2012) Innate lymphoid cells promote anatomical containment of lymphoid-resident commensal bacteria. Science 336: 1321–1325.
23. Vallis AJ, Finck-Barbancon V, Yahr TL, Frank DW (1999) Biological effects of Pseudomonas aeruginosa type III-secreted proteins on CHO cells. Infect Immun 67: 2040–2044.
24. Sawa T, Yahr TL, Ohara M, Kurahashi K, Gropper MA, et al. (1999) Active and passive immunization with the Pseudomonas V antigen protects against type III intoxication and lung injury. Nat Med 5: 392–398.
25. Gurney AL (2004) IL-22, a Th1 cytokine that targets the pancreas and select other peripheral tissues. Int Immunopharmacol 4: 669–677.
26. Gaffen SL, Hernandez-Santos N, Peterson AC (2011) IL-17 signaling in host defense against Candida albicans. Immunol Res 50: 181–187.
27. Stoodley BJ, Thom BT (1970) Observations on the intestinal carriage of Pseudomonas aeruginosa. J Med Microbiol 3: 367–375.
28. Wuthrich M, Hung CY, Gern BH, Pick-Jacobs JC, Galles KJ, et al. (2011) A TCR transgenic mouse reactive with multiple systemic dimorphic fungi. J Immunol 187: 1421–1431.
29. Chen K, McAleer JP, Lin Y, Paterson DL, Zheng M, et al. (2011) Th17 cells mediate clade-specific, serotype-independent mucosal immunity. Immunity 35: 997–1009.
30. Sonnenberg GF, Nair MG, Kirn TJ, Zaph C, Fouser LA, et al. (2010) Pathological versus protective functions of IL-22 in airway inflammation are regulated by IL-17A. J Exp Med 207: 1293–1305.
31. Chan YR, Chen K, Duncan SR, Lathrop KL, Latoche JD, et al. (2012) Patients with cystic fibrosis have inducible IL-17(+)IL-22(+) memory cells in lung draining lymph nodes. J Allergy Clin Immunol.
32. Brodlie M, McKean MC, Johnson GE, Anderson AE, Hilkens CM, et al. (2011) Raised interleukin-17 is immunolocalised to neutrophils in cystic fibrosis lung disease. Eur Respir J 37: 1378–1385.
33. Rieber N, Brand A, Hector A, Graepler-Mainka U, Ost M, et al. (2013) Flagellin induces myeloid-derived suppressor cells: implications for Pseudomonas aeruginosa infection in cystic fibrosis lung disease. J Immunol 190: 1276–1284.
34. Pier GB, Ramphal R (2005) Pseudomonas aeruginosa. In: Mandell GL, Bennett JE, Dolin R, editors. Principles and Practice of Infectious Diseases. 6th ed. Philadelphia: Elsevier Churchill Livingstone. pp. 2587–2615.
35. Wunderink RG (2005) Nosocomial pneumonia, including ventilator-associated pneumonia. Proc Am Thorac Soc 2: 440–444.
36. Martinez-Solano L, Macia MD, Fajardo A, Oliver A, Martinez JL (2008) Chronic Pseudomonas aeruginosa infection in chronic obstructive pulmonary disease. Clin Infect Dis 47: 1526–1533.

16

Testing Two Different Doses of Tiotropium Respimat® in Cystic Fibrosis: Phase 2 Randomized Trial Results

Judy M. Bradley[1], Paul Koker[2], Qiqi Deng[2], Petra Moroni-Zentgraf[3], Felix Ratjen[4], David E. Geller[5], J. Stuart Elborn[6]* on behalf of the Tiotropium Cystic Fibrosis Study Group¶

1 Institute of Nursing and Health Research, University of Ulster, Ulster, Northern Ireland, **2** Boehringer Ingelheim Pharmaceuticals Inc, Ridgefield, Connecticut, United States of America, **3** Boehringer Ingelheim Pharma GmbH & Co KG, Ingelheim, Germany, **4** The Hospital for Sick Children, Toronto, Ontario, Canada, **5** Florida State University College of Medicine, Orlando, Florida, United States of America, **6** Centre for Infection and Immunity, Queen's University Belfast, Belfast, Northern Ireland

Abstract

Background: Tiotropium is a once-daily, long-acting anticholinergic bronchodilator with the potential to alleviate airway obstruction in cystic fibrosis. Our objective was to evaluate the efficacy and safety of 2.5 and 5 µg once-daily tiotropium delivered via the Respimat Soft Mist Inhaler vs. placebo in people with cystic fibrosis.

Methods: This phase 2, 12-week, randomized, double-blind, placebo-controlled parallel-group study of tiotropium Respimat as add-on to usual cystic fibrosis maintenance therapy included people with cystic fibrosis with pre-bronchodilator forced expiratory volume in 1 second (FEV_1) ≥25% predicted. Co-primary efficacy end points were change from baseline in percent-predicted FEV_1 area under the curve from 0 to 4 hours (FEV_1 AUC_{0-4h}), and trough FEV_1 at the end of week 12.

Findings: A total of 510 subjects with cystic fibrosis aged 5–69 years were randomized. Both doses of tiotropium resulted in significant improvement compared with placebo in the co-primary efficacy end points at the end of week 12 (change from baseline in percent-predicted FEV_1 AUC_{0-4h}: 2.5 µg: 2.94%, 95% confidence interval 1.19–4.70, $p = 0.001$; 5 µg: 3.39%, 95% confidence interval 1.67–5.12, $p = 0.0001$; in percent-predicted trough FEV_1:2.5 µg: 2.24%, $p = 0.2$; 5 µg: 2.22%, $p = 0.02$). There was a greater benefit with tiotropium 5 vs. 2.5 µg. No treatment-related adverse events or unexpected safety findings were observed in patients taking tiotropium.

Conclusions: Tiotropium significantly improved lung function in people with cystic fibrosis. The improvement was greater with the higher dose than the lower dose, with no difference in adverse events.

Trial Registration: ClinicalTrials.gov NCT00737100 EudraCT 2008-001156-43.

Editor: Leonardo M. Fabbri, University of Modena and Reggio Emilia, Italy

Funding: This study was funded by Boehringer Ingelheim. Boehringer Ingelheim was involved in the study design, data collection and analysis, decision to publish, and preparation of the manuscript.

Competing Interests: JSE acted as a consultant for Boehringer Ingelheim and was principal investigator for this study; JMB declares no conflicts; PK, QD, and PMZ are employees of Boehringer Ingelheim; FR acts as a consultant for Boehringer Ingelheim and is the principal investigator for the phase 3 study of tiotropium in CF; DEG declares no conflicts related to bronchodilators in CF.

* Email: s.elborn@qub.ac.uk

¶Membership of the Tiotropium Cystic Fibrosis Study Group is provided in the Acknowledgments.

Introduction

Respiratory disease is the major cause of death in people with cystic fibrosis (CF), and new therapies addressing important pathophysiologic aspects of CF are urgently needed [1]. Treatments targeting airflow obstruction may provide clinical benefit to people with CF. Current standard therapy includes antibiotics, airway clearance techniques, dornase alfa, hypertonic saline, and inhaled bronchodilators [2]. Approximately 80% of people with CF use short- and/or long-acting bronchodilators, although their place as long-term therapy is not clearly defined and there are no bronchodilators with an approved indication for CF [3,4].

Bronchodilator agents improve pulmonary function and lessen wheezing in many people with CF [4]. The similar effectiveness of β_2 agonists and anticholinergics suggests that a significant proportion of airflow obstruction in CF is parasympathetically mediated [5]. Anticholinergic treatment may therefore prove a valuable add-on to current CF treatments.

A single dose of ipratropium bromide, a short-acting anticholinergic compound, has demonstrated lung function improvements in people with CF [6]. However, the long-term effects of maintenance therapy with ipratropium bromide have not been studied in CF. Tiotropium bromide (hereafter referred to as tiotropium), a long-acting anticholinergic compound delivered as an aqueous solution using the Respimat Soft Mist Inhaler, has consistently shown superior efficacy to ipratropium [7], and is well tolerated in the treatment of chronic obstructive pulmonary disease (COPD); these findings are consistent with those observed with the tiotropium 18 μg HandiHaler [8]. Tiotropium Respimat therefore has the potential to alleviate airflow obstruction in people with CF. Tiotropium Respimat was selected because the inhaler and formulation are suitable for populations of all ages. The inhaler is an active device that releases drug substance as an aerosol; hence, no minimal inspiratory flow is required by the patient. Suitability of the Respimat Soft Mist Inhaler was demonstrated in children aged <5 years using Respimat with a valved holding chamber and facemask [9,10]. Results from a phase 1 study *(manuscript in press)* showed that safety and tolerability of tiotropium are acceptable when compared with placebo in people with CF. Based on available data, tiotropium delivered by Respimat was tested at doses of 2.5 and 5 μg in this phase 2 study.

The primary objective was to evaluate the efficacy and safety of 12 weeks' treatment with tiotropium Respimat 2.5 or 5 μg once daily compared with placebo in people with CF. We hypothesized that treatment with tiotropium for 12 weeks is more effective in improving lung function compared with placebo, and that the higher dose of tiotropium (5 μg) is more effective than the 2.5 μg dose.

Methods

The protocol for this trial and supporting CONSORT checklist are available as supporting information; see Checklist S1 and Protocol S1.

Study Design

This was a double-blind, placebo-controlled, multicenter, multinational, parallel-group study to evaluate treatment with two doses of tiotropium (2.5 and 5 μg once daily, two inhalations at the same time of day) compared with placebo over 12 weeks (ClinicalTrials.gov identifier: NCT00737100). The trial period was from 23 September 2008 to 2 April 2010. The study was conducted at 94 centers in Australia, Europe, Canada, and the United States.

Ethical review was undertaken for each site/country by the local institutional review board/independent ethics committee and approval granted by the Competent Authority in each state.

Participants

Participants with documented CF had to be able to perform spirometric maneuvers according to American Thoracic Society (ATS) standards [11]. Patients of all ages were included, except in Russia, where patients aged <6 years were excluded. Subjects had to have a screening pre-bronchodilator forced expiratory volume in 1 second (FEV_1) ≥25% of predicted values [12,13] and inhale medication competently using the Respimat Soft Mist Inhaler. Patients were trained using a placebo Respimat device. They were to be clinically stable as defined by no evidence of acute respiratory tract infection or pulmonary exacerbation requiring use of antibiotics or oral corticosteroids within 4 weeks of screening. Pre-bronchodilator FEV_1 at week 0 or start of treatment had to be within 15% of FEV_1 at screening. All patients continued to receive their standard-of-care treatment during the study; tiotropium and placebo were considered add-on to usual therapy. If patients were diagnosed with a pulmonary exacerbation during the study period then this was recorded as an adverse event (AE) or serious AE, but there was no requirement to discontinue medication, and this decision was determined by the patient and physician. If taking long-term medication, participants had to agree to continue it throughout the study. Patients were allowed to continue using short-acting β-agonists (SABAs) and long-acting β-agonists (LABAs) if they were stabilized at least 4 weeks prior to randomization and throughout the study. Furthermore, patients taking SABAs and LABAs were required to have a 6-hour or 12-hour washout period, respectively, prior to all spirometry measurements.

Daily inhaled antibiotic use was allowed if stabilized for at least 6 weeks prior to and throughout the study period. Cyclic therapies (e.g., 4-week on/off tobramycin inhalation solution [TIS]) can impact treatment outcomes in short-term early phase trials. Cycled inhaled antibiotic use (e.g., TIS every other month) was allowed; however, the start of treatment had to be scheduled 2 weeks after the most recent TIS cycle and the last TIS cycle was to happen 2 weeks before the last treatment visit. This trial's 12-week design minimized the impact of cyclic medications by ensuring that baseline and final assessments were scheduled at a similar time point in the TIS cycle (i.e., both 2 weeks following completion of a TIS cycle). In order to comply with a 4-week on/off TIS regimen, the end-of-treatment visit may have been scheduled within 10–14 weeks after start of treatment to ensure baseline and end of study assessments occurred at mid-point of an off month in participants cycling TIS on alternate months. Physicians were advised to follow similar timing for other cycled medication use as for TIS, although this was not an official protocol procedure. Written informed consent was obtained from each patient or the patient's legal representative. Exclusion criteria (see Protocol S1 and File S1) included previous intolerance to tiotropium.

End Points

The co-primary end points for this trial were: i) the change from baseline (30 min prior to administration of first tiotropium dose at randomization; week 0) in percent-predicted FEV_1 area under the curve from time 0–4 hours (AUC_{0-4h}) at the end of week 12; and ii) the change from baseline (30 min prior to administration of first tiotropium dose at randomization; week 0) in percent-predicted trough FEV_1 at the end of week 12. The secondary outcomes in this study were changes from baseline in forced vital capacity (FVC), residual volume/total lung capacity (RV/TLC), forced expiratory flow (FEF) from 25% to 75% of vital capacity (FEF_{25-75}), Respiratory and Systemic Symptoms Questionnaire (RSSQ), and health-related quality of life (Cystic Fibrosis Questionnaire-Revised [CFQ-R]) at the end of week 12 [14]. AEs were also recorded. To measure exposure to the study drug, all patients were asked to return all dispensed Respimat inhalers.

Assessments

Pulmonary function tests (PFTs). The use of spirometers, including daily calibration, met ATS/European Respiratory Society criteria [15]. The qualifying PFTs (FEV_1 and FVC) were conducted at the screening visit. At weeks 0 and 12, PFTs were performed pre-dose (−10 minutes prior to study drug inhalation), at 30 minutes, and at 1, 2, 3, and 4 hours after inhalation of study drug. FEV_1 AUC_{0-4h} was calculated using the trapezoidal rule [16], divided by the duration (4 hours) reported in liters. Trough FEV_1 was defined as the FEV_1 value performed at −30 minutes prior to study drug inhalation. At weeks 4 and 8, PFTs were performed 30 minutes prior to drug administration. During the follow-up visit, after 30 days post-treatment (or at the time of premature study discontinuation), a single PFT was performed. Percent-predicted FEV_1 was calculated using the reference equations by Wang and colleagues [12] for pediatric/adolescents (aged 6–18 years) and by Knudson and colleagues [13] for adults (aged >18 years). RV/TLC measurements were performed as described in File S1.

Patient-reported outcomes. The proportion of patients with at least one pulmonary exacerbation during the double-blind period was analyzed using the RSSQ [17,18]. Health-related quality of life was assessed as the change from baseline in CFQ-R score [14]. Both methods are described in detail in File S1. For patients aged 6–13 years and depending on the patient's age and reading ability, the CFQ-R was administered to the patient directly, indirectly, or administered to their parent or caregiver. No patient under the age of 6 years completed the CFQ-R.

Safety. Medical history was recorded at screening. All patients were reviewed at screening and baseline entry into the study and at 2, 4, 8, and 12 weeks of therapy, and then at 30 days' post-treatment. Health status of patients who withdrew prematurely from the treatment period was followed up until their predicted study completion date. At each visit, all AEs and serious AEs, regardless of causality, were recorded.

Statistical Analyses

The primary analyses were performed in all randomized patients who received at least one dose of study drug and had both baseline and at least one post-dose PFT measurement at or before 12 weeks for either co-primary efficacy variable. Mean change from baseline in the co-primary efficacy variables (FEV_1 AUC_{0-4h} and trough FEV_1) was analyzed using a restricted maximum likelihood–based mixed-effect model with repeated measures (MMRM). To model the within-patient errors, an unstructured covariance matrix was used. Analyses were implemented using Statistical Analysis System software version 8.2 (SAS Institute Inc., Cary, NC, USA). The primary comparisons were between treatments after 12 weeks. The first co-primary end point, FEV_1 AUC_{0-4h}, was also stratified by age group. The age variable was dichotomized into patients aged 12 years and older and patients aged 11 years and younger, and was included in the model as a fixed effect. Other terms in the model were "treatment," "visit," "treatment-by-visit interaction," "baseline" and "baseline-by-visit interaction," and "random effect of center." Prespecified subgroup analyses for both primary end points included age group and baseline LABA use. The subgroup analyses were performed by adding subgroup, treatment-by subgroup, visit-by-subgroup, and treatment-by-visit-by subgroup interaction into the primary model.

All secondary end points on additional PFT parameters were analyzed as in the primary analysis, using the same MMRM model. For exacerbation analyses, Mantel-Haenszel test was adjusted for age group; treatment and age group were covariates for logistic regression analysis. The duration of pulmonary exacerbation was calculated based on the AE listings. Safety end points were summarized descriptively.

Data considered to be missing at random were not imputed, but handled in the analysis via the use of the MMRM model; only data that could be considered not missing at random were imputed. Randomly missing data with no subsequent non-missing values for that visit were imputed using the last observation carried forward technique (FEV_1, FVC, and FEF_{25-75} measurements).

In order to detect a difference of five units in the percentage change from baseline in FEV_1 values between tiotropium and placebo with 80% power at a two-sided significance level of 5%, a minimum of 465 patients in the full analysis set were required (155 in each treatment group). Based on a previous study [19], an approximate estimate of the expected standard deviation for FEV_1 percent-predicted value at screening was used (15.66). In this study, the ratio of adult to pediatric patients was approximately 2:1.

A detailed description of blinding and randomization and handling of missing data can be found in File S1.

Results

The study flow for this trial is summarized in Figure 1 [20].

Demographics and Other Baseline Characteristics

Of 620 recruited patients, a total of 510 patients (54% male) were randomized and treated (placebo, n = 168; tiotropium 2.5 μg, n = 166; tiotropium 5 μg, n = 176). Mean (SD) age was 20.9 (11.6) years (range, 5–69 years) and 27.1% were aged ≤11 years (range, 5–11 years). There were no clinically relevant differences between treatment groups (overall or by age group) in any demographic or baseline characteristic (Table 1).

Co-primary Efficacy End Points

For percent-predicted FEV_1 AUC_{0-4h} at the end of week 12, adjusted changes (improvements) from baseline were greater for both doses of tiotropium compared with placebo (tiotropium 2.5 μg: 1.20%; tiotropium 5 μg: 1.65%; placebo: –1.74%. Tiotropium 2.5 μg difference from placebo [95% CI]: 2.94% [1.19, 4.70], $p = 0.001$; tiotropium 5 μg difference from placebo [95% CI]: 3.39% [1.67, 5.12], $p = 0.0001$) (Fig. 2). The adjusted mean change was larger in the tiotropium 5 μg group than in the tiotropium 2.5 μg group (Fig. 2). The additional bronchodilator efficacy observed in the tiotropium 5 μg group was driven by the results obtained in patients younger than 12 years (Table 2). Both tiotropium dose groups had estimated mean changes (improvements), measured in liters at the end of week 12 (Table 2), that were statistically significantly greater than that of placebo.

Adjusted changes (improvements) from baseline in percent-predicted trough FEV_1 (at end of week 12) were greater for both doses of tiotropium compared with placebo (tiotropium 2.5 μg: 0.81%; tiotropium 5 μg: 0.78%; placebo: –1.44%. Tiotropium 2.5 μg difference from placebo [95% CI]: 2.24% [0.38, 4.11], $p = 0.02$; tiotropium 5 μg difference from placebo [95% CI]: 2.22% [0.38, 4.06], $p = 0.02$; Table 3). The mean adjusted change was similar between the tiotropium 2.5 μg and 5 μg groups and was not affected by age.

Other Lung Function Measures

Both the 2.5 and 5 μg doses of tiotropium had adjusted mean improvements from baseline in percent-predicted FVC AUC_{0-4h} response that were greater than placebo (tiotropium 2.5 μg: 0.53%; tiotropium 5 μg: 1.81%; placebo: –1.30%. Tiotropium 2.5 μg difference from placebo [95% CI]: 1.83% [–0.19, 3.86], $p = 0.08$; tiotropium 5 μg difference from placebo [95% CI]: 3.12% [1.12, 5.12], $p = 0.002$). The mean adjusted change was greater for tiotropium 5 than 2.5 μg and was only statistically significant for the tiotropium 5 μg group. The observed improvement for FVC AUC_{0-4h} in the tiotropium 5 μg group was largely driven by results in patients aged ≤11 years (described in detail in File S1).

Both doses of tiotropium had estimated adjusted mean improvements in percent-predicted trough FVC response that were greater than placebo, but not statistically significant (tiotropium 2.5 μg: 0.47%; tiotropium 5 μg: 0.81%; placebo: –0.39%. Tiotropium 2.5 μg difference from placebo [95% CI]: 0.85% [–1.08, 2.79], $p = 0.4$; tiotropium 5 μg difference from placebo [95% CI]: 1.19% [–0.72, 3.11], $p = 0.2$). FEF_{25-75} results were consistent with these results; static lung hyperinflation as measured by RV/TLC showed no difference between dose groups (described in detail in File S1).

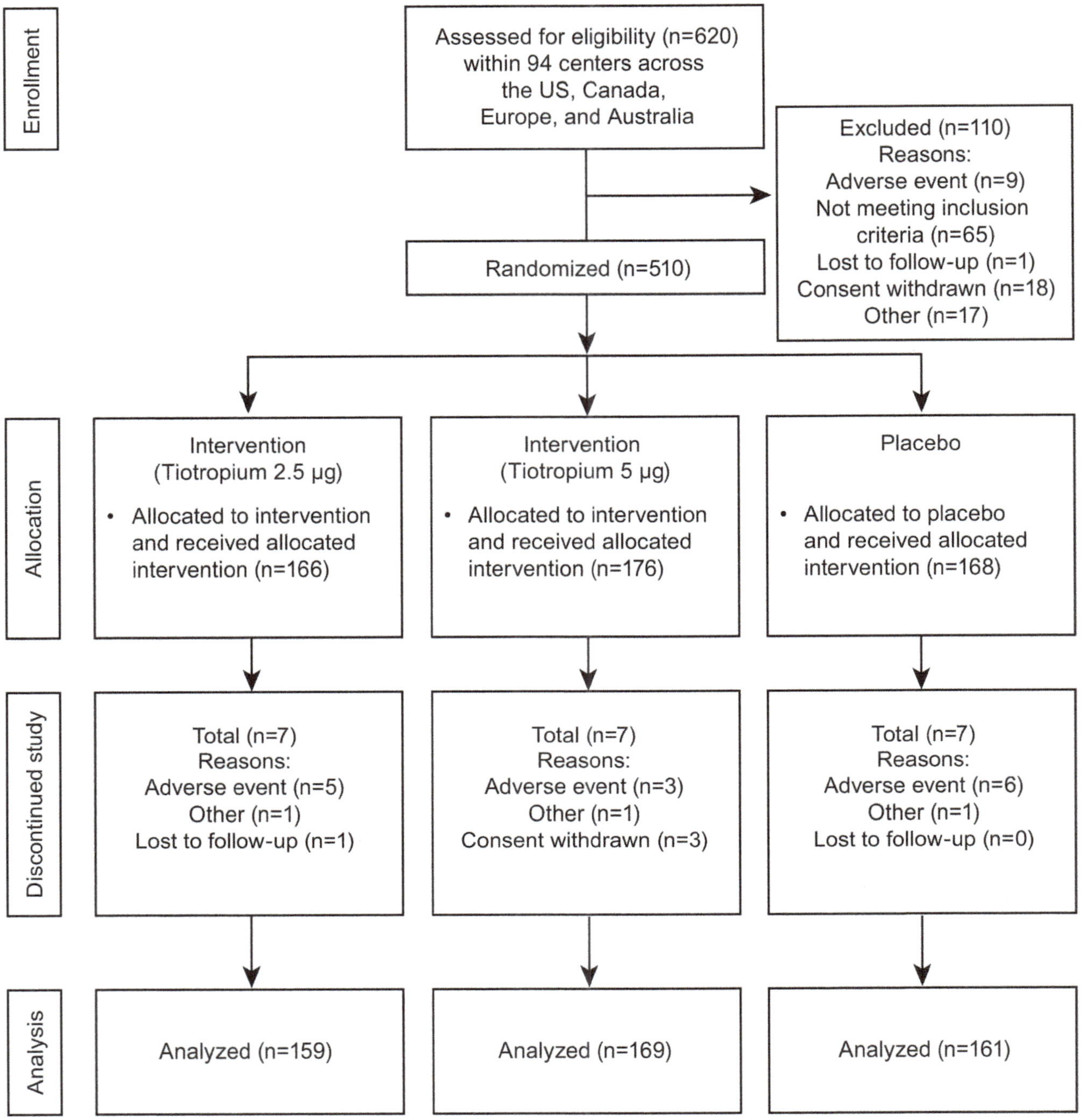

Figure 1. Flow diagram of participant recruitment and randomization [20].

Exposure

Overall exposure to study drug was acceptable, with a mean (SD) duration of treatment of 85.6 days (12.1); 87.5% of patients (446/510) took their study drug between >10 and ≤14 weeks. Approximately 9% of patients (47/510) took their study drug for ≥14 weeks.

Pulmonary Exacerbation as Assessed by RSSQ and Health-Related Quality of Life by CFQ-R

The proportions of patients who had at least one pulmonary exacerbation as determined by the RSSQ and intravenous antibiotic use were lower in the tiotropium 2.5 μg (7.8%) and 5 μg (6.9%) groups compared with the placebo group (9.6%; not statistically significant; $p = 0.9$ and $p = 0.6$ vs. placebo for tiotropium 2.5 μg and 5 μg respectively). Except for one pulmonary exacerbation in each treatment group, all events occurred in patients aged ≥12 years. The CFQ-R scores did not differ from baseline throughout the study period and no difference between the treatment groups was observed (additional results detailed in File S1).

Table 1. Patient demographics and characteristics of the study population at baseline.

	Placebo	Tiotropium 2.5 μg	Tiotropium 5 μg	Total
No. of patients	168	166	176	510
Male sex, n (%)	96 (57.1)	85 (51.2)	94 (53.4)	275 (53.9)
Age, years (mean, SD)	20.4 (11.6)	21.5 (12.0)	20.7 (11.3)	20.9 (11.6)
Age group, n (%)				
≤11 years	44 (26.2)	42 (25.3)	52 (29.5)	138 (27.1)
≥12 years	124 (73.8)	124 (74.7)	124 (70.5)	372 (72.9)
Percent-predicted FEV_1, (mean, SD)	76.6 (23.8)	75.4 (26.7)	75.9 (22.6)	76.0 (24.3)
≤11 years	94.9 (16.7)	98.8 (16.1)	90.3 (15.5)	94.3 (16.3)
≥12 years	70.1 (22.5)	67.5 (24.9)	69.9 (22.4)	69.2 (23.3)
BMI, kg/m^2 (mean, SD)	20.3 (4.4)	19.9 (4.0)	20.0 (4.1)	20.1 (4.2)
Baseline* concomitant pulmonary medications, n (%)	129 (76.8)	121 (72.9)	128 (72.7)	378 (74.1)
SABA	103 (61.3)	90 (54.2)	111 (63.1)	304 (59.6)
LABA	67 (39.9)	63 (38.0)	58 (33.0)	188 (36.9)

*Baseline includes all medications used on at least 1 day between informed consent and randomization (inclusive) and on at least 1 day between randomization and the first day of randomized drug intake (inclusive). BMI, body mass index; FEV_1, forced expiratory volume in 1 second; LABA, long-acting β-agonist; SABA, short-acting β-agonist; SD, standard deviation.

Subgroup Analysis

Differences in response to tiotropium by baseline LABA were explored by a prespecified subgroup analysis. In patients who used LABA at baseline, a larger difference compared with placebo (n = 64) was observed for the tiotropium 5 μg group (n = 56; 5.30% difference; 3.09% vs. –2.21%; 95% CI, 2.44–8.2; p = 0.0003) than for the tiotropium 2.5 μg (n = 60; 1.79% difference; –0.43% vs. –2.21%; 95% CI, –1.03 to –4.61; p = 0.2). In patients who did not use LABA at baseline, similar differences compared with placebo (n = 99) were observed for both tiotropium groups (tiotropium 2.5 μg: n = 98, 3.63% difference, 2.19% vs. –1.44%, 95% CI, 1.40–5.86, p = 0.002; tiotropium 5 μg: n = 113, 2.37% difference, 0.93% vs. –1.44%, 95% CI, 0.22–4.53, p = 0.03).

Adverse Events

The majority of patients (82.9%) reported one or more AE during the study. Most were mild to moderate in intensity and were primarily of respiratory nature; the most common AEs (defined as AE with an incidence >5% in any treatment group) were cough, exacerbation of CF, pyrexia, nasopharyngitis, and headache (Table 4). All deaths (two in the placebo group and one in the tiotropium 2.5 μg group) were due to exacerbation and/or complications of CF. An overall summary of AEs is provided in

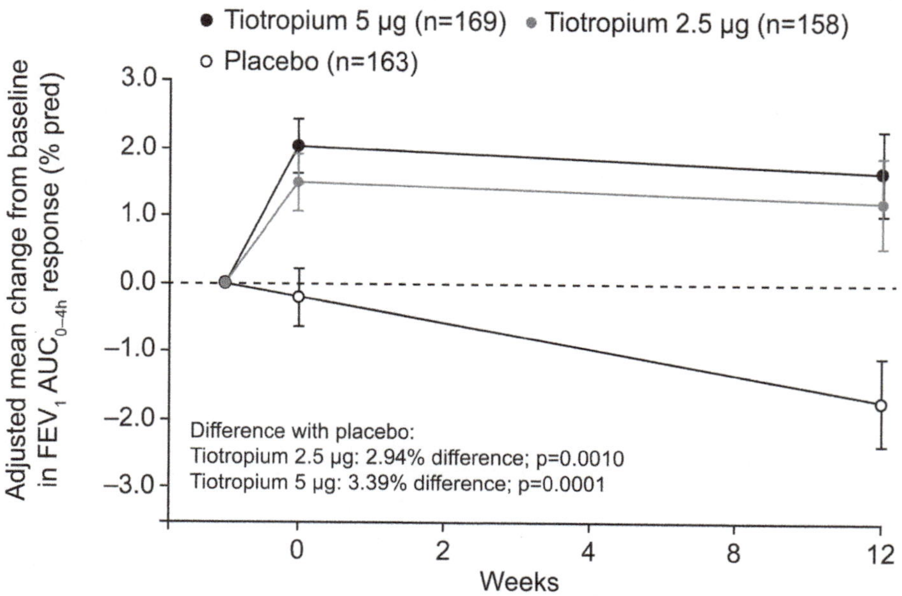

Figure 2. Adjusted mean FEV_1 AUC_{0-4h} (percent-predicted ± SE) change from baseline (full analysis set). AUC_{0-4h}, area under the curve from 0 to 4 hours; FEV_1, forced expiratory volume in 1 second.

Table 2. Adjusted mean (SE) changes from baseline in FEV_1 AUC_{0-4h} overall and in patients (aged ≤11 years and ≥12 years) treated with tiotropium (2.5 or 5 μg) or placebo after 12 weeks*.

Age group	Treatment	Difference from placebo		
Treatment	Mean (SE)	Mean (SE)	p value	95% CI
Overall, % predicted				
Placebo (n = 163)	−1.74 (0.65)			
Tiotropium 2.5 μg (n = 158)	1.20 (0.66)	2.94 (0.89)	0.0010	1.19–4.70
Tiotropium 5 μg (n = 169)	1.65 (0.63)	3.39 (0.88)	0.0001	1.67–5.12
Overall, L				
Placebo (n = 163)	−0.07 (0.02)			
Tiotropium 2.5 μg (n = 158)	0.02 (0.02)	0.09 (0.03)	0.0004	0.04–0.14
Tiotropium 5 μg (n = 169)	0.03 (0.02)	0.09 (0.02)	0.0002	0.05–0.14
≤11 years, % predicted				
Placebo (n = 43)	−0.32 (1.26)			
Tiotropium 2.5 μg (n = 42)	2.01 (1.29)	2.33 (1.74)	0.1801	−1.08 to 5.75
Tiotropium 5 μg (n = 50)	3.57 (1.16)	3.89 (1.67)	0.0199	0.62–7.17
≥12 years, % predicted				
Placebo (n = 120)	−2.55 (0.75)			
Tiotropium 2.5 μg (n = 116)	0.57 (0.76)	3.12 (1.04)	0.0028	1.08–5.17
Tiotropium 5 μg (n = 119)	0.55 (0.75)	3.11 (1.03)	0.0028	1.08–5.14

*Analysis of the full analysis set study group based on mixed-effect model with repeated measures model using unstructured covariance matrix.
AUC_{0-4h}, area under the curve from 0 to 4 hours; CI, confidence interval; FEV_1, forced expiratory volume in 1 second; SE, standard error.

Table 5 (and in File S1). Frequency of AEs was similar in all treatment arms and there was no evidence of a treatment relationship for any AE category; small differences between treatment groups were considered consequent to variability related to the overall small number of events.

Table 3. Adjusted mean (SE) changes from baseline in overall trough FEV_1 response and in patients (aged ≤11 years and ≥12 years) treated with tiotropium (2.5 or 5 μg) compared with placebo after 12 weeks*.

	Treatment	Difference from placebo		
Treatment	Mean change (SE)	Mean change (SE)	p value	95% CI
Overall, % predicted				
Placebo (n = 163)	−1.44 (0.71)			
Tiotropium 2.5 μg (n = 158)	0.81 (0.71)	2.24 (0.95)	0.0184	0.38–4.11
Tiotropium 5 μg (n = 169)	0.78 (0.69)	2.22 (0.93)	0.0179	0.38–4.06
Overall, L				
Placebo (n = 163)	−0.06 (0.02)			
Tiotropium 2.5 μg (n = 158)	−0.00 (0.02)	0.06 (0.03)	0.0330	0.00–0.11
Tiotropium 5 μg (n = 169)	−0.00 (0.02)	0.06 (0.03)	0.0281	0.01–0.11
≤11 years, % predicted				
Placebo (n = 43)	−0.83 (1.35)			
Tiotropium 2.5 μg (n = 42)	2.71 (1.38)	3.54 (1.86)	0.0577	−0.12 to 7.19
Tiotropium 5 μg (n = 50)	1.85 (1.24)	2.68 (1.78)	0.1322	−0.81 to 6.18
≥12 years, % predicted				
Placebo (n = 120)	−2.14 (0.80)			
Tiotropium 2.5 μg (n = 116)	−0.38 (0.81)	1.76 (1.11)	0.1128	−0.42 to 3.94
Tiotropium 5 μg (n = 119)	−0.11 (0.80)	2.03 (1.10)	0.0668	−0.14 to 4.20

*Analysis of the full analysis set study group based on mixed-effect model with repeated measures model using unstructured covariance matrix.
CI, confidence interval; FEV_1, forced expiratory volume in 1 second; SE, standard error.

Table 4. Summary of adverse events that occurred in >5% of patients in any treatment group (treated set).

	Placebo	Tiotropium 2.5 μg	Tiotropium 5 μg	Total
No. of patients, n	168	166	176	510
Cough, n (%)	34 (20.2)	35 (21.1)	46 (26.1)	115 (22.5)
Cystic fibrosis*, n (%)	17 (10.1)	23 (13.9)	25 (14.2)	65 (12.7)
Pyrexia, n (%)	17 (10.1)	9 (5.4)	18 (10.2)	44 (8.6)
Nasopharyngitis, n (%)	14 (8.3)	11 (6.6)	14 (8.0)	39 (7.6)
Headache, n (%)	18 (10.7)	7 (4.2)	14 (8.0)	39 (7.6)
Sputum increased	8 (4.8)	12 (7.2)	13 (7.4)	33 (6.5)
Abdominal pain	10 (6.0)	13 (7.8)	9 (5.1)	32 (6.3)
Hemoptysis	7 (4.2)	13 (7.8)	12 (6.8)	32 (6.3)
Oropharyngeal pain	13 (7.7)	5 (3.0)	11 (6.3)	29 (5.7)
Bronchitis	9 (5.4)	6 (3.6)	10 (5.7)	25 (4.9)
Upper respiratory tract infection	6 (3.6)	8 (4.8)	11 (6.3)	25 (4.9)
Rhinorrhea	9 (5.4)	6 (3.6)	9 (5.1)	24 (4.7)
Dyspnea	9 (5.4)	8 (4.8)	6 (3.4)	23 (4.5)
Nasal congestion	4 (2.4)	9 (5.4)	10 (5.7)	23 (4.5)
Sinusitis	6 (3.6)	3 (1.8)	9 (5.1)	18 (3.5)
Arthralgia	9 (5.4)	5 (3.0)	4 (2.3)	18 (3.5)

*The preferred adverse event term used for "CF exacerbation" was "cystic fibrosis."
A patient may have been counted in more than one preferred term. Percentages were calculated using the total number of patients per treatment as the denominator.
Medical Dictionary for Regulatory Activities (MedDRA) version used for reporting: 13.0.

Discussion

This is the first study to evaluate and provide evidence for the safety and efficacy of tiotropium in people with CF. Both doses of tiotropium resulted in statistically significant improvements compared with placebo in the co-primary efficacy end points of FEV_1 AUC_{0-4h} and trough FEV_1. Similarly, results for FEV_1 AUC_{0-4h} in liters and for FVC support the findings of the primary end points. Interestingly, a treatment benefit for respiratory symptoms (based on RSSQ) or health-related quality of life (based on CFQ-R) was not observed with either dose of tiotropium. Both doses of tiotropium were safe and well tolerated. The age subgroup analyses performed in our study demonstrate that tiotropium 5 μg is effective, with a favorable safety profile in children as well as in adults. The results from this study led to a phase 3 trial being performed using the 5 μg tiotropium dose [21].

Table 5. Overall summary of adverse events (treated set).

	Placebo	Tiotropium 2.5 μg	Tiotropium 5 μg	Total
No. of patients, n	168	166	176	510
Patients with any AE, n (%)	139 (82.7)	139 (83.7)	145 (82.4)	423 (82.9)
Patients with an SAE, n (%)	7 (4.2)	13 (7.8)	10 (5.7)	30 (5.9)
Patients with a study drug-related AE*, n (%)	14 (8.3)	15 (9.0)	18 (10.2)	47 (9.2)
Patients with other significant AE†, n (%)	3 (1.8)	2 (1.2)	3 (1.7)	8 (1.6)
Patients with AE leading to discontinuation of study drug, n (%)	6 (3.6)	6 (3.6)	3 (1.7)	15 (2.9)
Patients with SAEs, n (%)	21 (12.5)	28 (16.9)	21 (11·9)	70 (13.7)
Fatal, n	2	1	0	3
Immediately life-threatening, n	1	0	0	1
Disability/incapacity, n	0	0	1	1
Required hospitalization, n	21	28	21	70
Prolonged hospitalization, n	1	1	0	2
Congenital anomaly, n	0	0	0	0
Other, n	0	0	0	0

*As assessed by the study investigators. †As defined by International Conference on Harmonisation (ICH) E3 guidelines.
A patient may have been counted in more than one seriousness criterion. AE, adverse event; SAE, serious AE.

This study has a number of challenges in design, relating in particular to the use of cycled inhaled antibiotics. Study design was such that measurements were made on the off phase of inhaled antibiotic treatment for those on such treatment. The study was not sufficiently long to confidently determine the presence of any significant changes in symptoms or pulmonary exacerbations. The effects seen in the study should therefore be interpreted as demonstrating short- to medium-term effect of bronchodilator therapy by tiotropium. The study was, however, sufficiently powered to detect a meaningful change in FEV_1.

Despite widespread use, there is limited evidence supporting the use of bronchodilators in CF. A recent systematic review concluded that short-acting anticholinergics had no consistent effect on lung function tests in people with CF [22]. Efficacy of the LABA salmeterol in people with CF has only been investigated in several short-term (<1 week duration) clinical trials [23,24]. Results from one trial of longer-term use (24 weeks) showed improvement in FEV_1 in people with CF compared with treatment with salbutamol; however, no significant effect of salmeterol on other spirometric indices were detected in this trial, and therefore the clinical relevance of these results is debatable [25,22].

The highest tiotropium dose tested in this study, 5 µg daily, resulted in lung function improvement that was numerically above that observed for 2.5 µg. The study was not powered for differences between doses and no statistical comparison was performed; however, the effect of the 5 µg dose was about 15% greater than that of the 2.5 µg dose (percent-predicted FEV_1 AUC_{0-4h}) and the effect of the higher dose was more consistent across visits. Based on a numerically superior efficacy and a similar AE profile of both doses, 5 µg appeared to be the preferred dose for subsequent clinical development of tiotropium in people with CF. Longer term studies are required to evaluate the effect of tiotropium on symptoms.

Tiotropium Respimat 5 µg is also the approved dose for COPD patients, in whom evidence for improvements in lung function, exercise tolerance, and health-related quality of life, as well as reduction in the frequency of exacerbations, exists [26,27,28].

Effect sizes of lung function improvements for treatments used in CF patients vary widely [22] and it is difficult to compare the magnitude of improvement between different inhaled therapies such as mannitol [29,30], hypertonic saline [31], and TIS [32], as different variables are used (absolute change in FEV_1 from baseline vs. relative change). Currently, people with CF are recommended complex, time-intensive daily therapies that are often difficult to sustain over the long term, and the addition of new therapies usually increases that burden [33]. Drug delivery using the Respimat Soft Mist Inhaler is fast, easier than the more traditional metered-dose inhaler, and does not require a power source [34]. Furthermore, because it is effective over 24 hours, tiotropium only requires once-daily inhalation and therefore may ease the burden of the number of daily medications required in CF, contributing to improved compliance.

Conclusion

This study provides evidence of the efficacy and safety of inhaled tiotropium delivered by the Respimat Soft Mist Inhaler in people with CF and supports proceeding to further investigations in phase 3.

Supporting Information

File S1 Supporting information file.

Protocol S1 Trial Protocol.

Checklist S1 CONSORT checklist.

Acknowledgments

Writing and editorial assistance was provided by Sarah J Petit and Elena Garonna of PAREXEL. We also thank the Cystic Fibrosis Foundation Therapeutics - Therapeutic Development Network Coordinating Center and the European Cystic Fibrosis Society Clinical Trials Network for their support.

The principal investigators for the Tiotropium Cystic Fibrosis Study Group are (by country):

Australia: Barry Clements, Hugh Greville, Peter Middleton, David Serisier, Peter van Asperen;

Belgium: Lieven Dupont, Christiane Knoop, Anne Malfroot;

France: Chantal Belleguic, Raphael Chiron, Jocelyne Derelle, Stephane Dominique, Daniel Dusser, Jean-Louis Ginies, Marcel Guillot, Delphine Horeau-Langlard, Muriel Le Bourgeois, Sylvie Leroy, Christophe Marguet, Anne Munck, Jean-Claude Pautard, Philippe Reix, Marie-Laure Uffredi;

Germany: Manfred Ballmann, Joachim Bargon, Rainald Fischer, Felix Herth, Hans-Eberhard Heuer, Matthias Griese, Wolfgang Kamin, Martin Kohlhäufl, Lutz Nährlich, Joachim Riethmüller, Stephan Sorichter, Thomas Wagner;

United Kingdom: Lesley Bennett, Margaret Crawford, James Crossley, David Derry, Iolo Doull, J. Stuart Elborn, Mark Everard, Chris Groggins, Mary Johnson, Tim Lee, Rosemary Rayner, Alastair Reid, Alan Smyth, Kevin Southern, Douglas Thomas, Martin Walshaw, Joanna Whitehouse;

Italy: Cesare Braggion, Virginia De Rose, Rolando Gagliardini, Laura Minicucci;

Netherlands: M. Reijers, H.A.W.M. Tiddens;

New Zealand: Mark O'Carroll, Janice Wong;

Portugal: Celeste Barreto, Pilar Cardim, Mário Loureiro, Herculano Rocha, Maria Luisa Vaz;

Russia: Irina Asherova, Maria Chepurnaya, Alexander G. Chuchalin, Mikhail Ilkovich, Nikolay Kapranov, Alla Neretina; Alexander Orlov, Olga Simonova;

United States: Richard Ahrens, Ran Anbar, Julie Biller, Holly Carveth, Cori Daines, Stanley Fiel, Patrick Flume, Deborah Froh, James Harris III, Michelle Howenstine, Daniel Layish Susan Millard, Samya Nasr, H. Worth Parker, Mark Pian, James Royall, Carlos Sabogal, Matthias Salathe, Aruna Sannuti, David Schaeffer, Steven Strausbaugh, Debbie Toder, Santiago Reyes, Laurie Whittaker, Robert Zanni.

Author Contributions

Performed the experiments: JB PK QD PMZ FR DG JSE. Analyzed the data: JB PK QD PMZ FR DG JSE. Wrote the paper: JB PK QD PMZ FR DG JSE. Contributed to the planning and design of the trial: JB PK QD PMZ FR DG JSE.

References

1. Davis PB, Drumm M, Konstan MW (1996) Cystic fibrosis. Am J Respir Crit Care Med 154: 1229–1256.
2. Konstan MW, Butler SM, Schidlow DV, Morgan WJ, Julius JR, et al. (1999) Patterns of medical practice in cystic fibrosis: part II. Use of therapies. Investigators and Coordinators of the Epidemiologic Study of Cystic Fibrosis. Pediatr Pulmonol 28: 248–254.
3. Johnson C, Butler SM, Konstan MW, Morgan W, Wohl ME (2003) Factors influencing outcomes in cystic fibrosis: a center-based analysis. Chest 123: 20–27.

4. Colombo JL (2003) Long-acting bronchodilators in cystic fibrosis. Curr Opin Pulm Med 9: 504–508.
5. Cropp GJ (1996) Effectiveness of bronchodilators in cystic fibrosis. Am J Med 100: 19S–29S.
6. Avital A, Sanchez I, Chernick V (1992) Efficacy of salbutamol and ipratropium bromide in decreasing bronchial hyperreactivity in children with cystic fibrosis. Pediatr Pulmonol 13: 34–37.
7. Voshaar T, Lapidus R, Maleki-Yazdi R, Timmer W, Rubin E, et al. (2008) A randomized study of tiotropium Respimat Soft Mist inhaler vs. ipratropium pMDI in COPD. Respir Med 102: 32–41.
8. Bateman E, Singh D, Smith D, Disse B, Towse L, et al. (2010) Efficacy and safety of tiotropium Respimat SMI in COPD in two 1-year randomized studies. Int J Chron Obstruct Pulmon Dis 5: 197–208.
9. Kamin W, Bannemer-Schult K, Klemmer A, Schulze Schweinhorst P, Wachtel H, et al. (2010) Children below five years of age can handle Respimat Soft Mist inhaler [abstract]. Am J Respir Crit Care Med 181 A6254.
10. Kamin W, Bannemer-Schult K, Klemmer A, Schulze Schweinhorst P, Wachtel H, et al. (2011) Flow profile data indicate that Respimat with spacer is suitable for inhalation therapy of pre-school children. Presented at: International Society for Aerosols in Medicine Congress; 18–22 June 2011; Rotterdam, The Netherlands.
11. Farrell PM, Rosenstein BJ, White TB, Accurso FJ, Castellani C, et al. (2008) Guidelines for diagnosis of cystic fibrosis in newborns through older adults: Cystic Fibrosis Foundation consensus report. J Pediatr 153: S4–S14.
12. Wang X, Dockery DW, Wypij D, Gold DR, Speizer FE, et al. (1993) Pulmonary function growth velocity in children 6 to 18 years of age. Am Rev Respir Dis 148: 1502–1508.
13. Knudson RJ, Lebowitz MD, Holberg CJ, Burrows B (1983) Changes in the normal maximal expiratory flow-volume curve with growth and aging. Am Rev Respir Dis 127: 725–734.
14. Henry B, Aussage P, Grosskopf C, Goehrs JM (2003) Development of the Cystic Fibrosis Questionnaire (CFQ) for assessing quality of life in pediatric and adult patients. Qual Life Res 12: 63–76.
15. Miller MR, Hankinson J, Brusasco V, Burgos F, Casaburi R, et al. (2005) Standardisation of spirometry. Eur Respir J 26: 319–338.
16. Whittaker ET, Robinson G (1967) The trapezoidal and parabolic rules. The Calculus of Observations: an Introduction to Numerical Mathematics. 4th ed. Dover, New York, 156–158.
17. Goss CH, Burns JL (2007) Exacerbations in cystic fibrosis. 1: Epidemiology and pathogenesis. Thorax 62: 360–367.
18. Lymp J (2009) Pulmonary exacerbations in a phase 2 clinical trial of BIIL 284 BS in CF: development and implementation of a respiratory and systemic symptoms questionnaire (RSSQ) [abstract]. Pediatr Pulmonol S23 A221.
19. Koker P, Bhattacharya S, Staab A (2007) A randomized, double-blind, placebo controlled study to investigate the efficacy and safety of 24 weeks of oral treatment with BIIL 284 BS in adult (75 mg, 150 mg) and pediatric (75 mg) cystic fibrosis patients. Boeringher Ingelheim Report.
20. Moher D, Schulz KF, Altman DG (2001) The CONSORT statement: revised recommendations for improving the quality of reports of parallel group randomized trials. BMC Med Res Methodol 1: 2.
21. Ratjen F, Koker P, Geller D, Langellier-Cocteaux B, Maulf F Le, et al. (2013) Tiotropium Respimat in cystic fibrosis: efficacy and safety results of phase III randomized placebo-controlled trial [abstract]. J Cyst Fibros (Suppl 1): S64.
22. Halfhide C, Evans HJ, Couriel J (2005) Inhaled bronchodilators for cystic fibrosis. Cochrane Database Syst Rev: CD003428.
23. Hordvik NL, Sammut PH, Judy CG, Colombo JL (1999) Effects of standard and high doses of salmeterol on lung function of hospitalized patients with cystic fibrosis. Pediatr Pulmonol 27: 43–53.
24. Salvatore D, D'Andria M (2002) Effects of salmeterol on arterial oxyhemoglobin saturations in patients with cystic fibrosis. Pediatr Pulmonol 34: 11–15.
25. Hordvik NL, Sammut PH, Judy CG, Colombo JL (2002) Effectiveness and tolerability of high-dose salmeterol in cystic fibrosis. Pediatr Pulmonol 34: 287–296.
26. Ichinose M, Fujimoto T, Fukuchi Y (2010) Tiotropium 5 μg via Respimat and 18 μg via HandiHaler; efficacy and safety in Japanese COPD patients. Respir Med 104: 228–236.
27. van Noord JA, Cornelissen PJ, Aumann JL, Platz J, Mueller A, et al. (2009) The efficacy of tiotropium administered via Respimat Soft Mist Inhaler or HandiHaler in COPD patients. Respir Med 103: 22–29.
28. Spiriva RESPIMAT. Summary of Product Characteristics (2010) emc+ website. Available: http://www.medicines.org.uk/EMC/medicine/20134/SPC/Spiriva+Respimat+2.5+micrograms+solution+for+inhalation/. Accessed 9 June 2013.
29. Aitken ML, Bellon G, De BK, Flume PA, Fox HG, et al. (2012) Long-term inhaled dry powder mannitol in cystic fibrosis: an international randomized study. Am J Respir Crit Care Med 185: 645–652.
30. Bilton D, Bellon G, Charlton B, Cooper P, De BK, et al. (2013) Pooled analysis of two large randomised phase III inhaled mannitol studies in cystic fibrosis. J Cyst Fibros 12: 367–376.
31. Elkins MR, Robinson M, Rose BR, Harbour C, Moriarty CP, et al. (2006) A controlled trial of long-term inhaled hypertonic saline in patients with cystic fibrosis. N Engl J Med 354: 229–240.
32. Vandyke RD, McPhail GL, Huang B, Fenchel MC, Amin RS, et al. (2013) Inhaled tobramycin effectively reduces FEV1 decline in cystic fibrosis. An instrumental variables analysis. Ann Am Thorac Soc 10: 205–212.
33. Royce FH, Carl JC (2011) Health-related quality of life in cystic fibrosis. Curr Opin Pediatr 23: 535–540.
34. Kesser KC, Geller DE (2009) New aerosol delivery devices for cystic fibrosis. Respir Care 54: 754–767.

17

Nitrous Oxide Production in Sputum from Cystic Fibrosis Patients with Chronic *Pseudomonas aeruginosa* Lung Infection

Mette Kolpen[1,2], Michael Kühl[3,4,5], Thomas Bjarnsholt[1,2], Claus Moser[1], Christine Rønne Hansen[6], Lars Liengaard[3], Arsalan Kharazmi[1], Tanja Pressler[6], Niels Høiby[1,2], Peter Østrup Jensen[1]*

1 Department of Clinical Microbiology, Rigshospitalet, Copenhagen, Denmark, **2** Department of International Health, Immunology and Microbiology, Faculty of Health Sciences University of Copenhagen, Copenhagen, Denmark, **3** Marine Biological Section, Department of Biology, University of Copenhagen, Helsingør, Denmark, **4** Plant Functional Biology and Climate Change Cluster, University of Technology Sydney, Sydney, Australia, **5** Singapore Centre on Environmental Life Sciences Engineering, Nanyang Technological University, Singapore, Singapore, **6** Copenhagen CF Centre, Rigshospitalet, Copenhagen, Denmark

Abstract

Chronic lung infection by *Pseudomonas aeruginosa* is the major severe complication in cystic fibrosis (CF) patients, where *P. aeruginosa* persists and grows in biofilms in the endobronchial mucus under hypoxic conditions. Numerous polymorphonuclear leukocytes (PMNs) surround the biofilms and create local anoxia by consuming the majority of O_2 for production of reactive oxygen species (ROS). We hypothesized that *P. aeruginosa* acquires energy for growth in anaerobic endobronchial mucus by denitrification, which can be demonstrated by production of nitrous oxide (N_2O), an intermediate in the denitrification pathway. We measured N_2O and O_2 with electrochemical microsensors in 8 freshly expectorated sputum samples from 7 CF patients with chronic *P. aeruginosa* infection. The concentrations of NO_3^- and NO_2^- in sputum were estimated by the Griess reagent. We found a maximum median concentration of 41.8 µM N_2O (range 1.4–157.9 µM N_2O). The concentration of N_2O in the sputum was higher below the oxygenated layers. In 4 samples the N_2O concentration increased during the initial 6 h of measurements before decreasing for approximately 6 h. Concomitantly, the concentration of NO_3^- decreased in sputum during 24 hours of incubation. We demonstrate for the first time production of N_2O in clinical material from infected human airways indicating pathogenic metabolism based on denitrification. Therefore, *P. aeruginosa* may acquire energy for growth by denitrification in anoxic endobronchial mucus in CF patients. Such ability for anaerobic growth may be a hitherto ignored key aspect of chronic *P. aeruginosa* infections that can inform new strategies for treatment and prevention.

Editor: Erich Gulbins, University of Duisburg-Essen, Germany

Funding: This work was funded by Faculty of Health and Medical Sciences, University of Copenhagen. The funders had no role in study design, data collection and analysis, decision to publish, or preparation of the manuscript.

Competing Interests: The authors have declared that no competing interests exist.

* E-mail: Peter.Oestrup.Jensen@regionh.dk

Introduction

Cystic fibrosis (CF) is an autosomal recessive disease. It is caused by mutations in the cystic fibrosis trans-membrane conductance regulator gene [1] affecting apical ion transport. In the lungs, the defective ion transport results in endobronchial accumulation of thick, viscous mucus that prevents mucociliar cleaning of the lungs, and increases susceptibility to chronic respiratory infections [2,3]. *Pseudomonas aeruginosa* is a Gram-negative, gamma proteobacterium, which dominates chronic lung infections in CF patients and is considered the most serious complication of CF [4,5]. The chronic *P. aeruginosa* lung infection in CF patients is characterized by presence of endobronchial biofilm aggregates surrounded by numerous polymorphonuclear leukocytes (PMNs) [6,7]. Despite the bactericidal activity of the PMNs and intensive antibiotic therapy, these biofilms persist and grow in the endobronchial mucus of CF patients over many years [7,8]. *P. aeruginosa* can withstand the bactericidal activity of the PMNs by forming biofilms of the protective mucoid phenotype [9] and by quorum sensing (QS)-regulated production of leukolytic amounts of rhamnolipid [10–13]. The summoned PMNs produce reactive oxygen species (ROS) through a respiratory burst, which leads to intense depletion of molecular oxygen (O_2) [14], a common feature of infected endobronchial mucus in CF [6]. Biofilm formation may explain why *P. aeruginosa* survives the attacking PMNs, but it is not known how *P. aeruginosa* acquires the energy required for the observed growth in endobronchial secretions [8] when O_2 is absent. However, *P. aeruginosa* can grow anaerobically with alternative electron acceptors or by arginine fermentation [15], and it has been suggested that *P. aeruginosa* can respire by denitrification in anoxic CF mucus utilizing nitrate (NO_3^-) and nitrite (NO_2^-), which are both present in sufficient amounts [15,16]. Although the ability of *P. aeruginosa* to utilize reduction of NOx for anaerobic respiration is well known [17], denitrification in mucus and persistent biofilms present in the airways of CF patients remains to be demonstrated. Since N_2O is a natural intermediate belonging to the gases defining denitrification [17], we used electrochemical microsensors [18] to measure O_2 and

N_2O concentration gradients at high spatio-temporal resolution in freshly expectorated sputum from CF patients with chronic *P. aeruginosa* lung infection.

Further evidence for denitrification was obtained from nitrate (NO_3^-) and nitrite (NO_2^-) turnover measurements in the sputum samples. These measurements provided important new insights to the micro-environmental conditions and chemical dynamics associated with persistent *P. aeruginosa* lung infections in CF patients and indicate that nitrogen compounds can play an important role in the interaction between pathogenic bacteria and an active immune response.

Results

N_2O and O_2 in sputum from CF patients with chronic *P. aeruginosa* lung infection

Representative measurements of O_2 and N_2O in freshly expectorated sputum were acquired with O_2- and N_2O microsensors (Fig 1A). Measurements of O_2- and N_2O profiles in expectorated sputum from a CF patient with chronic *P. aeruginosa* lung infection showed the distribution of an upper oxygenated zone and a lower anoxic zone. The N_2O profile reached the maximal concentration of N_2O in the lower anoxic part of the sputum sample, suggesting that denitrification is mainly confined to the anoxic zone. A slow decline of O_2 was apparently detected above the sputum surface. This may be because the position of the sputum surface was estimated by visual inspection, which is associated with uncertainty due to small amounts of heterogeneous saliva (Fig 1B).

Sputum is composed of heterogeneously distributed bacterial aggregates surrounded by PMNs consuming O_2, and this respiratory burst creates local anoxic microenvironments in the sputum [14]. The metabolic mechanisms are thus compartmentalized according to the availability of O_2 with an oxygenated zone, wherein the majority of O_2 is reduced to superoxide by the summoned PMNs, and an anoxic zone, where *P. aeruginosa* can utilize nitrate as electron acceptor during oxidative phosphorylation (Fig. 1C).

NO_3^- and NO_2^- in sputum from CF patients with chronic *P. aeruginosa* lung infection

NO_3^- and NO_2^- concentrations in sputum samples were measured before N_2O profiling and 1 day later (Fig 2). The concentration of NO_3^- was significantly higher immediately before N_2O profiling as compared to 1 and 2 days after incubation indicating NO_3^- depletion due to ongoing denitrification (Fig 2A, B). The NO_2^- concentration was not changed significantly after one day (Fig 2C), but by including additional measurements of the NO_2^- concentration in 7 sputum samples a significantly decreased NO_2^- concentration was detected (Fig 2D).

Distribution of N_2O in sputum from CF patients with chronic *P. aeruginosa* lung infection

Vertical profiles of O_2 in sputum samples showed depletion of O_2, indicating the formation of anoxic zones below a mean depth of 3.1 mm (SD = 3.0 mm) from the sputum surface (Fig 3A) suggesting that the average depth of O_2 penetration of ~3 mm. A higher concentration of N_2O was observed in the anoxic zone as compared to the oxic zone ($p<0.026$, $n=8$) (Fig 3B). To verify that N_2O is related to *P. aeruginosa* we found significantly less N_2O in three control sputum samples from 1 CF patient and from 2

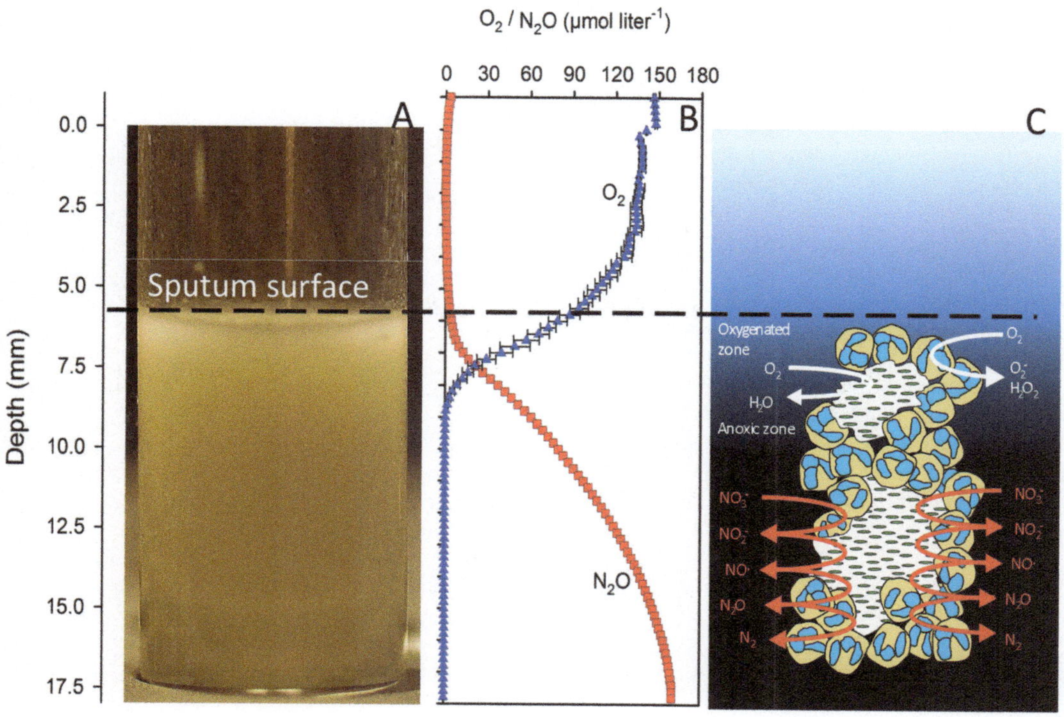

Figure 1. Microsensor measurements of chemical gradients in sputum. (A) Close up of a sputum sample from a cystic fibrosis patient with chronic *P. aeruginosa* lung infection with an inserted microsensor. (B) Representative microprofiles of N_2O and O_2 in a CF sputum sample. O_2 profiles are shown as the mean and SD of three microprofiles recorded in the beginning of the experiment and did not change significantly throughout the experimental period, while the N_2O profile represents the maximal N_2O levels measured about 6–7 h after beginning. (C) A schematic model of the involved PMN and biofilm processes in CF sputum explaining the microprofiles.

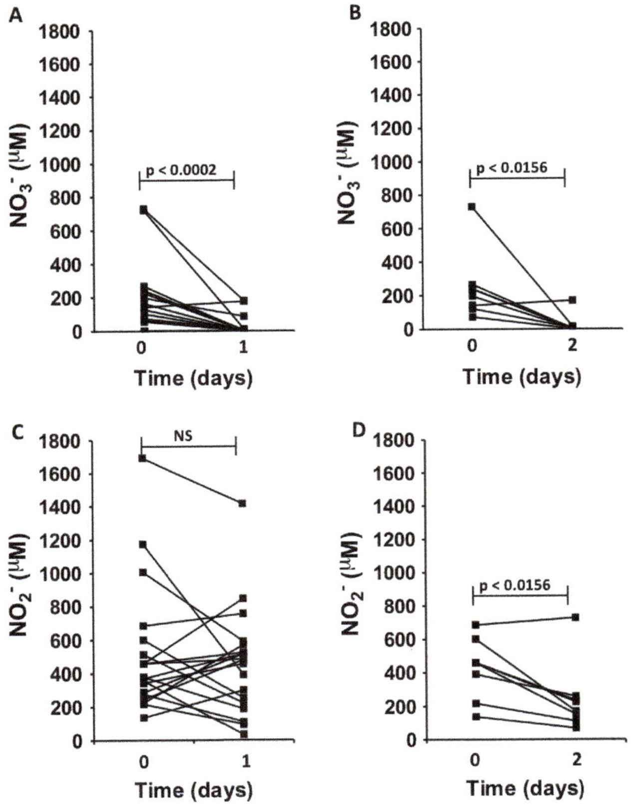

Figure 2. Consumption of NO3⁻ and NO2⁻ in sputum. (A, B) NO_3^- concentration in sputum samples from cystic fibrosis patients with chronic *P. aeruginosa* lung infection. (C, D) NO_2^- concentration in sputum samples from cystic fibrosis patients with chronic *P. aeruginosa* lung infection. Samples were collected immediately after expectoration and after 1 (n = 20) and 2 days (n = 7) of incubation. Data were analyzed by Wilcoxon signed rank test.

primary ciliary dyskinesia (PCD) patients without detectable *P. aeruginosa* ($p<0.030$).

Dynamics of N_2O in sputum from a CF patient with chronic *P. aeruginosa* lung infection

Figure 4 displays time series of representative N_2O profiles measured vertically through a sputum sample. The distribution of O_2 is displayed at 0 hr. During the initial measuring period, N_2O accumulated in the anoxic zone reaching a maximum concentration of 160 μM after 6.5 h incubation, which indicates ongoing production of N_2O. Within the subsequent 4 hours the accumulated N_2O decreased indicating consumption through reduction to N_2.

Rates of N_2O production and consumption in sputum samples

Measurements of the N_2O concentration dynamics over time in particular depths of a sputum sample showed an initial build-up of N_2O in layers below 7 mm (Fig. 5). In each layer, the slope of the net production curves was quasi-linear after ~180 min indicating a constant production of N_2O related to the particular layer and therefore that N_2O originates from immobile sources such as biofilm. The production ceased about 6–7 h after start of the sample incubation, and was then followed by a net consumption of N_2O over the following 4–5 h leading to N_2O depletion in the sputum sample after ~10–12 hours. In 4 sputum samples it was possible to estimate N_2O production and consumption rates (Table 1) and N_2O flux rates and cumulated emission (Figure 6) from measurements of such dynamic N_2O concentration microgradients. A substantial initial N_2O concentration was observed in the anaerobic zone of the remaining 4 assayed sputum samples. In these samples the N_2O concentration decreased steadily during incubation.

Discussion

The ability of microorganisms to exploit a wide range of electron acceptors for ATP generation by oxidative phosphorylation provides metabolic flexibility in transient environments as these organisms inhabit a variety of habitats ranging from soils, sediments to aquatic environments [19]. Even though several human pathogens, including *P. aeruginosa*, are equipped with the genetic setup for denitrification [20–22] including nitric oxide reductase (NOR) [22], we present the very first observations of N_2O production in clinical material from infected human airways demonstrating pathogenic metabolism based on denitrification. These data indicate that denitrification may serve as an alternative metabolic pathway allowing *P. aeruginosa* to thrive in O_2 depleted micro niches in the airways of CF patients. Besides our study, denitrification in humans has previously been demonstrated in human dental plaque [23] and has been related to infections of the gastrointestinal tract by the increased concentration of N_2O in exhaled breath from patients after oral intake of NO_3^- [24].

Seminal observations of O_2 depletion and the presence of OprF porin, which is involved in NO_3^- and NO_2^- diffusion, in habitats of *P. aeruginosa* during chronic lung infection of CF patients provided initial evidence for anaerobic respiration by denitrification [6,16]. To demonstrate denitrification we have included CF patients, who suffered from chronic *P. aeruginosa* infection in the endobronchial mucus as detected by routine culturing. We revealed a depletion of O_2 in CF sputum samples, which is in accordance with the steep O_2 gradients in endobronchial CF mucus [6] and due to O_2 consumption by activated PMNs for generation of ROS [14]. Our O_2 measurements in sputum confirmed the presence of O_2 concentration gradients reaching anoxia ~3 mm below the sputum surface.

The depletion of O_2 for microbial respiration in infected endobronchial CF mucus has motivated the present and several other studies of anaerobic metabolism by *P. aeruginosa* based on denitrification during chronic lung infection in CF. We demonstrated N_2O production and consumption in the sputum samples indicating the presence of active NOR and nitrous oxide reductase (N_2OR) for the reduction of nitric oxide (NO•) and N_2O [17]. Previously, NOR has been isolated from *P. aeruginosa* [25], the genes (*norCB*) have been sequenced [26] and functional NOR has been observed in clinical strains of *P. aeruginosa* by consumption of NO• [27].

In our study, the initial phase of N_2O production in the sputum samples was followed by a period of net N_2O consumption suggesting a depletion of NO• and a concomitant reduction of N_2O to N_2 by N_2OR. The N_2O consumption is in agreement with the demonstration of N_2OR activity and the identification of the *nos* genes in *P. aeruginosa* [28] as well as the induced genes for a N_2OR precursor in clinical isolates [29].

Our demonstration of significant N_2O production in sputum indicates ample presence of NO_3^- and NO_2^- that serve as electron acceptors for the denitrification pathway. We found high levels of NO_3^- and NO_2^- in the sputum, which are in agreement with previous findings [30–32]. It has been proposed that NO_3^-

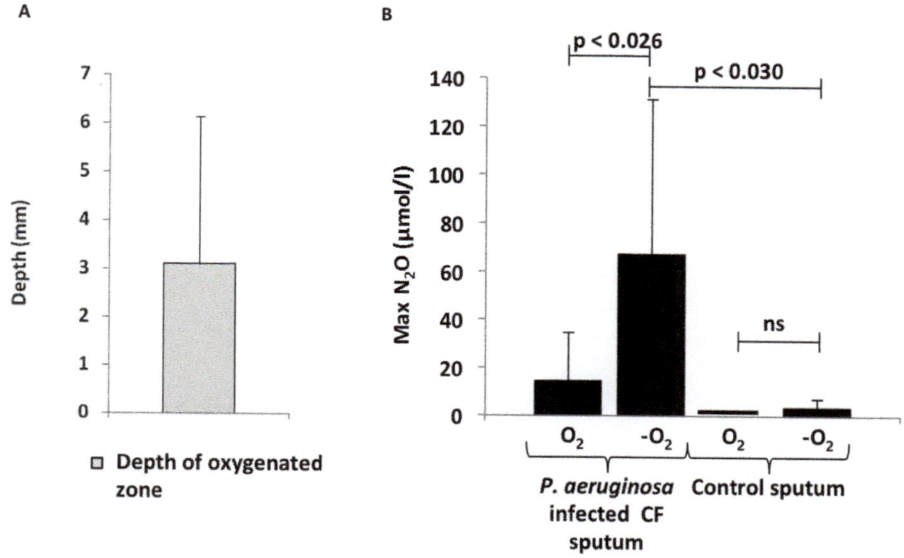

Figure 3. Distribution of O_2 and N_2O in sputum. (A) Depth of oxygenated zone in sputum samples from cystic fibrosis patients with chronic *P. eruginosa* lung infection (n = 8). (B) Maximal N_2O concentration in the oxic zone and anoxic zone in sputum samples from cystic fibrosis patients with chronic *P. aeruginosa* lung infection (n = 8). Control sputum without detectable *P. aeruginosa* was obtained from two PCD patients and one CF patient. Statistical analysis was performed by Student t-test.

and NO_2^- in CF sputum originates from the rapid reaction between superoxide (O_2^-) and NO• [15]. In this regard, we suggest the summoned activated PMNs [14] as a major source of O_2^-, while NO•, which is present in CF exhaled breath [33,34], may be produced by a variety of cells in the lungs. In fact, inhalation of NO• or incubation of sputum samples with NO• resulted in elevated levels of NO_3^- and NO_2^- in sputum from CF patients [35]. In addition, ongoing activity of the patients nitric oxide synthases was evidenced by the increased exhaled NO• from infected CF patients following supplementation with the substrate L-arginine [36,37].

As a consequence of our demonstration of N_2O production, we expected a consumption of the precursors NO_3^- and NO_2^-. Accordingly, NO_3^- was depleted in the sputum after incubation for 1 day, which likely is due to the membrane-bound nitrate reductase of *P. aeruginosa* [29]. NO_3^- consumption may also accompany assimilatory denitrification and ammonification resulting in the formation of ammonia (NH_4^+) [17], which has been detected in CF sputum [27]. However, assimilatory denitrification and ammonification does not involve production of N_2O [17,38,39] and NH_4^+ is also produced by several human cell types [40]. The concentration of NO_2^- was not changed during 1 day of incubation, but after 2 days of incubation the concentration of NO_2^- in the sputum was decreased significantly. This indicates that the production of NO• from NO_2^- is slower than the generation of NO_2^- resulting from reduction of NO_3^-. Indeed, during reduction of NO_3^- transient accumulation of NO_2^- is known from anaerobic cultures of *P. aeruginosa* growing by denitrification [16,41,42].

A further verification of ongoing dissimilatory denitrification in sputum is evident from the calculated rate of N_2O production (Fig. 6A), which easily can explain the depletion of NO_3^- during incubation (Fig. 2A). The depletion of NO_3^- in the sputum samples indicates that the NO_3^- in sputum samples is not replaced by the reaction between O_2^- and NO. This is possibly due to lack of contributions from immigrating PMNs and the epithelia as opposed to the conditions in the endobronchial mucus.

Since we calculated the rates of N_2O production by assuming linear changes between subsequent measurements in the beginning of incubation, the estimates are likely to reflect the situation in the endobronchial mucus, where reduced NO_3^- and NO_2^- is continuously being replaced as indicated by the high NO_3^- and NO_2^- content in fresh sputum. The estimated N_2O production, however, is calculated from the actual N_2O content and does not include the reduction of N_2O to N_2. Therefore, the actual rate of denitrification may be higher than our estimates.

We found the highest concentration of N_2O in the anoxic zone of the confined sputum samples indicating higher rate of denitrification without O_2 as previously demonstrated [43]. Accordingly, we suggest that the low concentration of N_2O found in the oxygenated zone is mainly due to diffusion from the active anoxic zone. Additionally, our estimate of the depth of the oxygenated zone implies that the bronchi, with diameters ranging from 0.8 to 13 mm [44,45], allow for numerous anoxic zones in the endobronchial mucus of the lungs and confirms the *in vivo* demonstration of O_2 depletion in the endobronchial mucus [6]. Consequently, our results propose the existence of several zones with N_2O production in the anoxic endobronchial mucus of the lungs of CF patients with chronic *P. aeruginosa* lung infection. However, such *in vivo* production of N_2O in CF patients still awaits direct experimental confirmation.

The involvement of denitrification enzymes as terminal oxidases that reduce nitrogen oxides in the highly branched respiratory chain of *P. aeruginosa* may enable anaerobic growth in the presence of nitrate or nitrite [19,46]. But the engagement of denitrification in *P. aeruginosa* may also contribute to virulence as evidenced by the finding of antibodies directed against components of denitrification in CF patients with *P. aeruginosa* lung infection [16,47] and the dependence on nitrite reductase for type III secretion [48]. In anaerobic cultures, denitrification promotes growth of *P. aeruginosa* [49], increases antibiotic tolerance of *P. aeruginosa* [50] and favors maintenance of the virulent mucoid phenotype [30].

A particular contribution to the pathogenesis of chronic lung infection in CF by NOR activity, is suggested by the induced *in vivo*

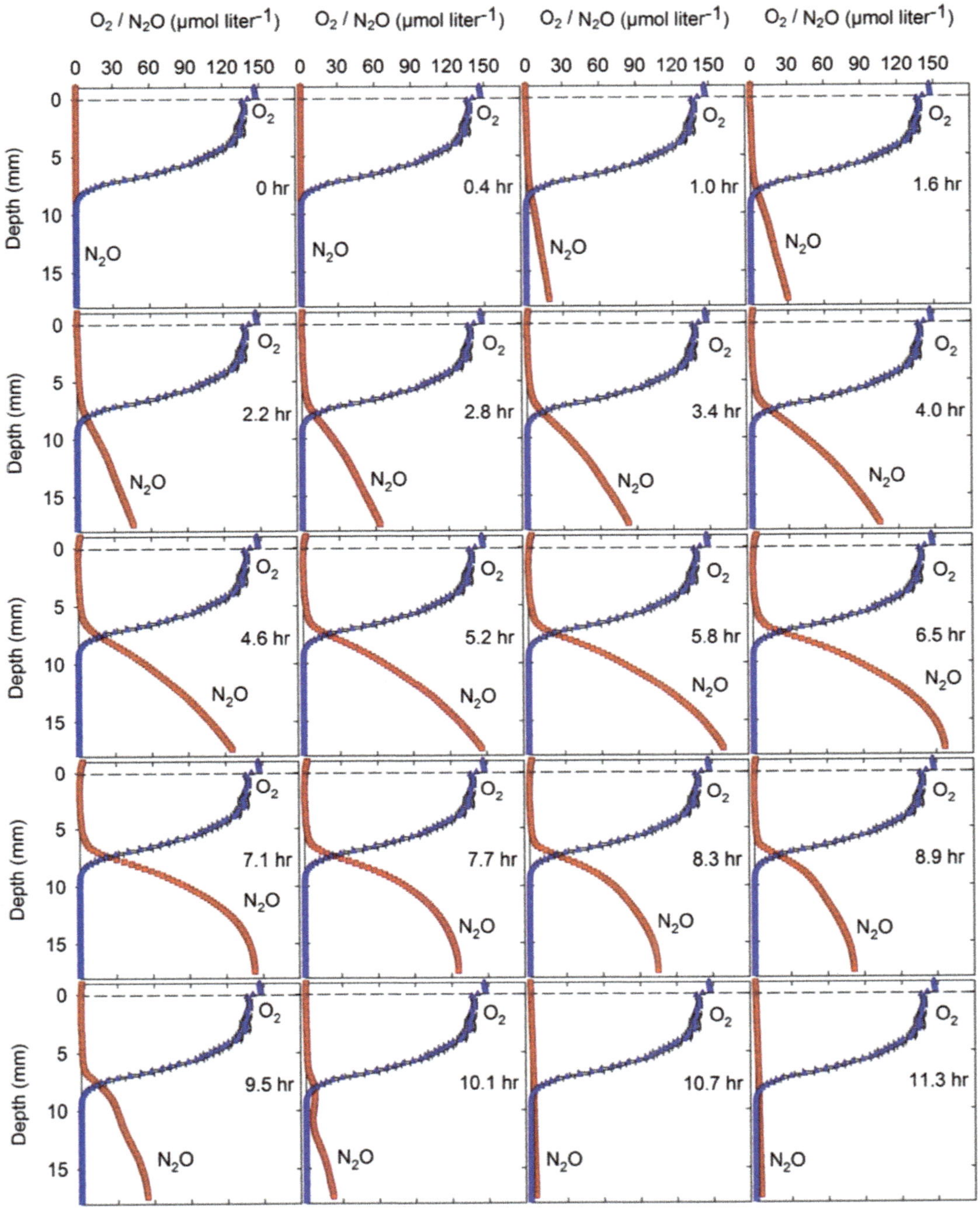

Figure 4. Generation and depletion of N_2O in sputum. Spatio-temporal dynamics of N_2O concentration profiles in a representative sputum sample from a cystic fibrosis patient with chronic *P. aeruginosa* lung infection showing initial accumulation of N_2O in the anoxic zone followed by total depletion. The O_2 concentration profile is shown as the mean and SD of three microprofiles recorded at the beginning of the experiment.

gene expression in clinical isolates [29] including the highly virulent mucoid isolates [51]. In this respect, the reduction of NO• to N_2O by active NOR may actually protect *P. aeruginosa* from the bactericidal action of NO• generated by the immune system. In fact, NOR-deficient *P. aeruginosa* is more susceptible to NO• generated by macrophages [52] and less virulent during infection of silkworm [53]. In addition, NOR activity increases the virulence of several pathogens [54–56].

In conclusion, this study points to the presence of anoxic microenvironments with strong spatio-temporal heterogeneity as well as a possible stratification of metabolic processes in the biofilm aggregates characteristic of chronic *P. aeruginosa* infections in the airways of CF patients. Such structural and metabolic heterogeneity may be a characteristic trait ensuring persistent infection. Indeed, spatio-temporal resolved measurements enabled the demonstrated of N_2O production in the anaerobic zones of freshly expectorated sputum samples from CF patients with chronic *P. aeruginosa* lung infection for the first time. Analysis of the N_2O production rates suggests ongoing generation of N_2O in the lungs of CF patients with chronic *P. aeruginosa* infection. N_2O production

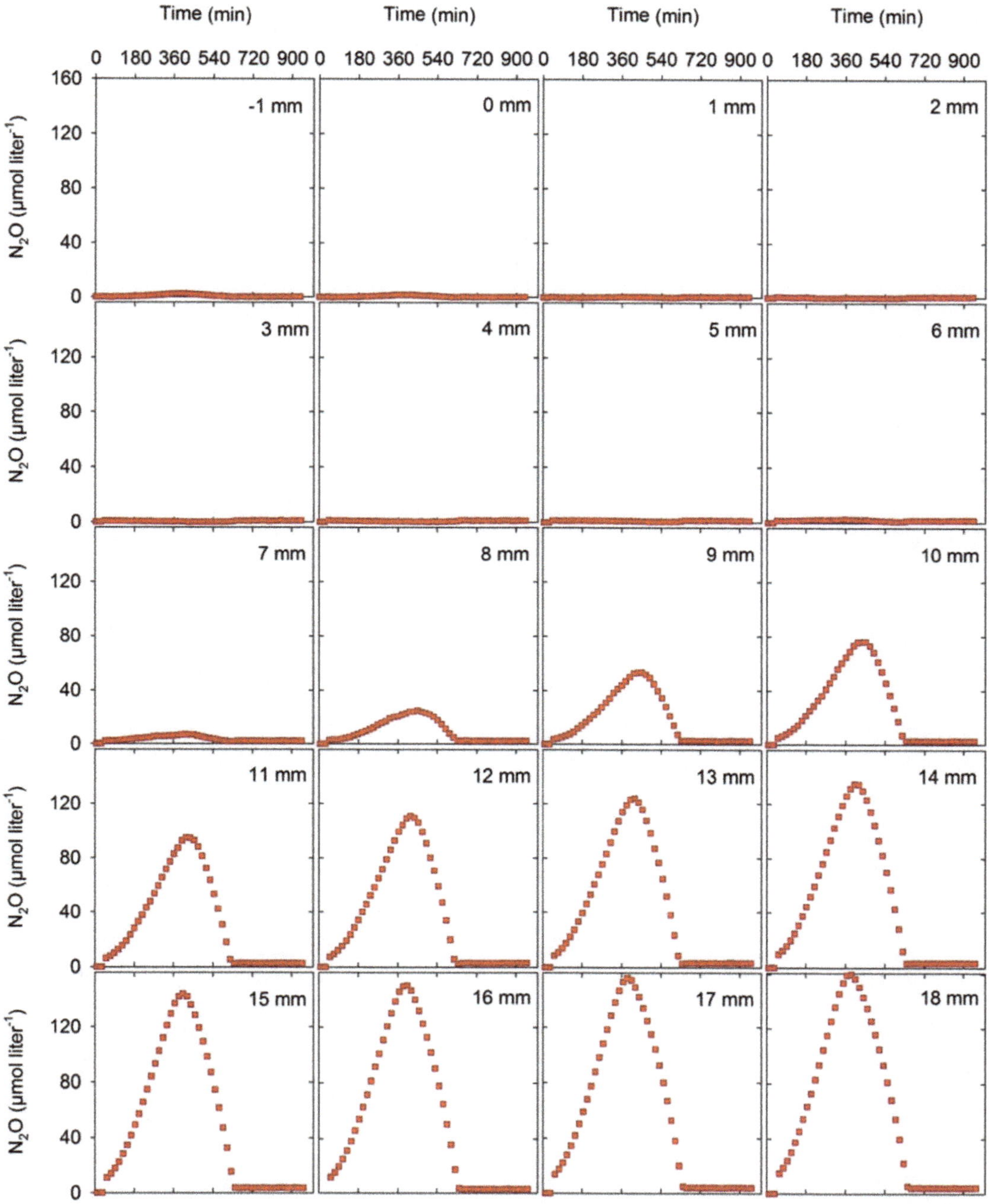

Figure 5. Rates of N2O production and consumption in sputum. Depth specific plots of N_2O concentration vs. time at particular measuring depths in the same sputum sample as displayed in Fig 4. Accumulation and thus net production of N_2O in all depths was observed until approximately 6 h, followed by net consumption of N_2O presumably due to depletion of nitrate around 6 h.

Table 1. N_2O production, consumption, max emission, and cumulated emission in 4 CF sputum samples.

	Net production rate (nmol cm^{-3}min^{-1})	Net consumption rate (nmol cm^{-3}min^{-1})	Max emission (nmol cm^{-2} min^{-1})	Cumulated emission (nmol cm^{-2})
Median	0.47	−0.39	5.06×10^{-5}	1.05×10^{-2}
Range	0.40–0.70	−0.77–−0.10	1.8×10^{-5}–6.78×10^{-5}	3.94×10^{-3}–1.46×10^{-2}

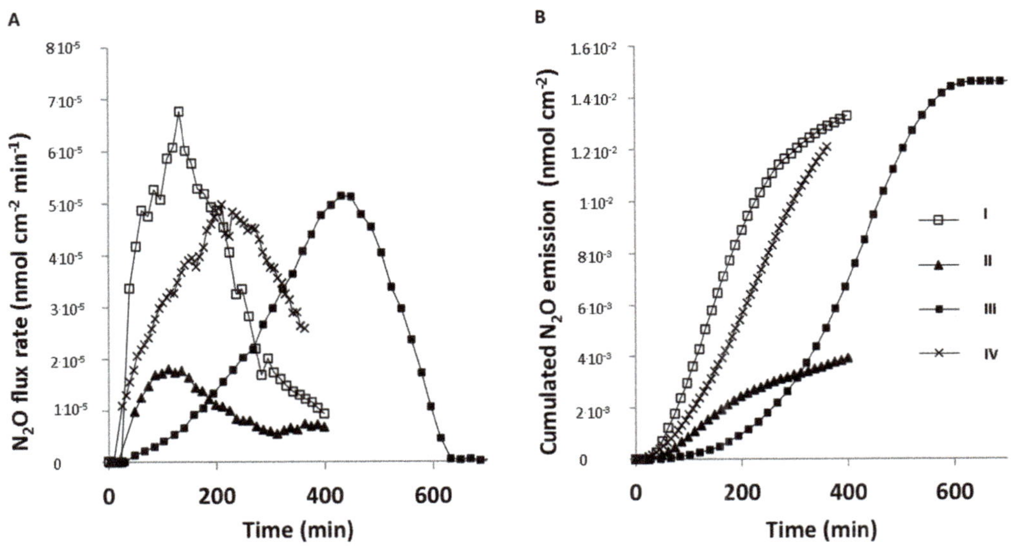

Figure 6. Efflux and cumulated emission of N_2O from sputum samples. (A) Estimated N_2O efflux rates in sputum samples from cystic fibrosis patients with chronic *P. aeruginosa* lung infection as calculated from N_2O microprofiles (n = 4). (B) Cumulated N_2O emission as calculated from N_2O microprofiles (n = 4). I, II, III and IV represents 4 different sputum samples.

by *P. aeruginosa* in this environment is associated with anaerobic growth, which can promote increased virulence and tolerance to antibiotic, as well as contribute to evasion of the host response. The chronic infected CF lung is in many ways a black box. By using the presented approach to elucidate the essential metabolites we may now open the black box and start mapping the micro-environment of infection which may inspire new strategies for prevention and treatment of chronic lung infections in CF.

Materials and Methods

Sputum Samples

As defined by the "Danish Act on Research Ethics Review of Health Research Projects" Section 2 the project does not constitute a health research project and was thus initiated without approval from The Committees on Health Research Ethics in the Capital Region of Denmark. Therefore, verbal informed consent was obtained using waiver of documentation of consent. The study was carried out on 21 anonymized samples of surplus expectorated sputum from 21 CF patients and 2 PCD patients (Table 2). Chronic *P. aeruginosa* infection was defined as the presence of *P. aeruginosa* in the lower respiratory tract at each monthly culture for >6 months, or for a shorter time in the presence of increased antibody response to *P. aeruginosa* (>2 precipitating antibodies, normal: 0–1) [57].

Microsensor Measurements of O_2 and N_2O. Each of 8 different sputum samples (1–2 ml) was added to a glass vial (35×12 mm) (Schuett Biotec, Germany) and allowed to settle for about 10 min. The glass vials were positioned in a heated metal rack, kept at 37°C. Vertical O_2-concentration profiles were recorded in the sputum with an amperometric O_2 microsensor (OX25, Unisense A/S, Århus, Denmark) mounted in a motorized PC-controlled profiling setup (MM33 and MC-232, Unisense A/S). Subsequently, vertical N_2O concentration profiles were recorded at defined time intervals for up to 12 hours with an amperometric N_2O microsensor [18] (N_2O-25, Unisense A/S) mounted in the micromanipulator.

The microsensors (tip diameter 25 μm) were connected to a picoammeter (PA2000, Unisense A/S) and positioned manually onto the upper surface of the sputum sample. Profile measurements were taken by movement of the sensor in vertical steps of 100 or 200 μm through the sputum sample. Positioning and data acquisition were controlled by dedicated software (Sensortrace Pro 2.0, Unisense A/S). The software was set to wait 3 seconds for the O_2-microprofile and 5 seconds for the N_2O-microprofile, before actual measurement and subsequent movement of the sensors to the next measuring depth. The interval between each cycle of profile measurements was 10 seconds.

The O_2-microsensor was linearly calibrated by measuring the sensor signal in an alkaline sodium ascorbate solution (zero O_2) and in air saturated free phosphate buffered saline (PBS) at experimental temperature and salinity. The O_2 concentration in air saturated water was determined from the known temperature and salinity according to [58]. The N_2O -microsensor was linearly calibrated according to [18] by measuring sensor signals in N_2O free PBS at experimental temperature and salinity and in PBS with sequential addition of a known volume of N_2O saturated PBS up

Table 2. Demographic data of the patients.

	CF patients		PCD patients
	Infectious status		
	P. aeruginosa	*S. aureus*	*H. influenzae*
Number (male)	20 (10)	1 (1)	2 (0)
Age (years)*	39 (24–50)	17	32 (27–36)
Duration of chronic infection (years)*, **	19 (4–38)		
FEV_1 (%)*	56 (23–96)	75	89 (70–109)
FVC (%)*	88 (46–139)	82	110 (95–125)

*Values are medians (range).
*Duration of chronic infection is only recorded for *P. aeruginosa* infections.
FEV_1, forced expiratory volume in 1 s.
FVC, forced vital capacity.

to a final concentration of 100 μM N_2O. The N_2O concentration in saturated PBS was determined according to [59].

NO_3^- and NO_2^- quantification. The concentration of NO_3^- and NO_2^- in sputum was measured in 20 samples. From each sputum sample, 0.1 ml was aspired with a syringe and was immediately diluted 10x in PBS and stored at -20°C for later analysis. The remaining sample was incubated in a glass vial at 37°C for 24 h before dilution 10x in PBS and storage at −20°C. The NO_3^- and NO_2^- levels in the sputum were measured using the Griess colorimetric reaction (no. 780001, Cayman Chemicals, USA) according to the manufacturer's recommendations. For this, sputum samples were transferred to a 96 well microtiter plate. NO_2^- concentration was estimated by addition of the Griess Reagent for 10 minutes, whereby NO_2^- was converted into a purple azo-compound, which was quantitated by the optical density at 540–550 nm measured with an ELISA plate reader (Thermo Scientific Multiskan EX, Thermo Fisher Scientific Inc, BioImage, Denmark). Total NO_3^- and NO_2^- levels were estimated by a two-step analysis process: The first step converted NO_3^- to NO_2^- utilizing NO_3^- reductase. After incubation for 2 hours, the next step involved the addition of the Griess Reagent, whereby NO_2^- was converted into a purple azo-compound. After incubation with Griess Reagent for 10 minutes, the optical density at 540–550 nm was measured with an ELISA plate reader (Thermo Scientific Multiskan EX, Thermo Fisher Scientific Inc, BioImage, Denmark). A NO_3^- standard curve was used for determination of total NO_3^- and NO_2^- concentration, while a NO_2^- standard curve was used for determination of NO_2^- alone. The concentration of NO_3^- was calculated as the difference between the NO_3^- concentration and the total NO_3^- and NO_2^- concentration.

Calculations of N_2O production rates. The local N_2O fluxes in sputum samples were calculated from the measured N_2O concentration gradient in the uppermost oxic sputum layer. It was assumed that no production or consumption of N_2O occurred in the presence of O_2. The flux was calculated using a modified version of Fick's 1st law of diffusion [60], where the slope of the profile in the sputum surface layer was calculated from the three uppermost measured concentrations (measurement a, b and c):

$$J = 0.5\left[-D\frac{C_a - C_b}{x_a - x_b}\right] + 0.5\left[-D\frac{C_b - C_c}{x_b - x_c}\right]$$

where J is the flux of N_2O (nmol N_2O cm^{-2} min^{-1}), D is the molecular diffusion coefficient of N_2O in water at 37°C (2.76×10^{-5} cm^2 s^{-1}) [61] and C is the concentration of N_2O (μmol liter^{-1}) at depth x_n, where n = a, b or c denote 3 subsequent depths of measurement. The cumulated N_2O emission was calculated by assuming linear changes between subsequent measurements. Net production and net consumption rates of N_2O in particular sputum layers were calculated from the slopes of linear increase and decrease of N_2O concentration at particular measuring depths in the sputum samples [62,63].

Statistical Analyses. Statistical significance was evaluated by Wilcoxon Signed Rank Test and by Students T-test. A p value <0.05 was considered statistically significant. The tests were performed with Prism 4.0c (GraphPad Software, La Jolla, California, USA).

Author Contributions

Conceived and designed the experiments: PØJ M. Kolpen M. Kühl. Performed the experiments: PØJ M. Kolpen M. Kühl CRH. Analyzed the data: PØJ M. Kolpen M. Kühl LL. Contributed reagents/materials/analysis tools: PØJ M. Kolpen M. Kühl CRH TP NH. Wrote the paper: PØJ M. Kolpen M. Kühl TB CM AK NH.

References

1. Riordan JR, Rommens JM, Kerem B, Alon N, Rozmahel R, et al. (1989) Identification of the cystic fibrosis gene: cloning and characterization of complementary DNA. Science 245: 1066–1073.
2. Knowles MR, Boucher RC (2002) Mucus clearance as a primary innate defense mechanism for mammalian airways. J Clin Invest 109: 571–577.
3. Boucher RC (2007) Evidence for airway surface dehydration as the initiating event in CF airway disease. J Intern Med 261: 5–16.
4. Koch C, Høiby N (1993) Pathogenesis of cystic fibrosis. Lancet 341: 1065–1069.
5. Koch C, Høiby N (2000) Diagnosis and treatment of cystic fibrosis. Respiration 67: 239–247.
6. Worlitzsch D, Tarran R, Ulrich M, Schwab U, Cekici A, et al. (2002) Effects of reduced mucus oxygen concentration in airway *Pseudomonas* infections of cystic fibrosis patients. J Clin Invest 109: 317–325.
7. Bjarnsholt T, Jensen PØ, Fiandaca MJ, Pedersen J, Hansen CR, et al. (2009) *Pseudomonas aeruginosa* biofilms in the respiratory tract of cystic fibrosis patients. Pediatr Pulmonol 44: 547–558.
8. Yang L, Haagensen JA, Jelsbak L, Johansen HK, Sternberg C, et al. (2008) In situ growth rates and biofilm development of *Pseudomonas aeruginosa* populations in chronic lung infections. J Bacteriol 190: 2767–2776.
9. Pedersen SS, Moller H, Espersen F, Sorensen CH, Jensen T, et al. (1992). Mucosal immunity to *Pseudomonas aeruginosa* alginate in cystic fibrosis. APMIS 100: 326–334.
10. Bjarnsholt T, Jensen PØ, Burmolle M, Hentzer M, Haagensen JA, et al. (2005) *Pseudomonas aeruginosa* tolerance to tobramycin, hydrogen peroxide and polymorphonuclear leukocytes is quorum-sensing dependent. Microbiology 151: 373–383.
11. Jensen PØ, Bjarnsholt T, Phipps R, Rasmussen TB, Calum H, et al. (2007) Rapid necrotic killing of polymorphonuclear leukocytes is caused by quorum-sensing-controlled production of rhamnolipid by *Pseudomonas aeruginosa*. Microbiology 153: 1329–1338.
12. van GM, Christensen LD, Alhede M, Phipps R, Jensen PØ, et al. (2009) Inactivation of the rhlA gene in *Pseudomonas aeruginosa* prevents rhamnolipid production, disabling the protection against polymorphonuclear leukocytes. APMIS 117: 537–546.
13. Alhede M, Bjarnsholt T, Jensen PØ, Phipps RK, Moser C, et al. (2009) *Pseudomonas aeruginosa* recognizes and responds aggressively to the presence of polymorphonuclear leukocytes. Microbiology 155: 3500–3508.
14. Kolpen M, Hansen CR, Bjarnsholt T, Moser C, Christensen LD, et al. (2010) Polymorphonuclear leucocytes consume oxygen in sputum from chronic *Pseudomonas aeruginosa* pneumonia in cystic fibrosis. Thorax 65: 57–62.
15. Hassett DJ, Cuppoletti J, Trapnell B, Lymar SV, Rowe JJ, et al. (2002) Anaerobic metabolism and quorum sensing by *Pseudomonas aeruginosa* biofilms in chronically infected cystic fibrosis airways: rethinking antibiotic treatment strategies and drug targets. Adv Drug Deliv Rev 54: 1425–1443.
16. Yoon SS, Hennigan RF, Hilliard GM, Ochsner UA, Parvatiyar K, et al. (2002) *Pseudomonas aeruginosa* anaerobic respiration in biofilms: relationships to cystic fibrosis pathogenesis. Dev Cell 3: 593–603. S1534580702002952 [pii].
17. Zumft WG (1997) Cell biology and molecular basis of denitrification. Microbiol Mol Biol Rev 61: 533–616.
18. Andersen K, Kjær T, Revsbech NP (2001) An oxygen insentitive microsensor for nitrous oxide. Sensors & Actuators B: Chemical 81: 42–48.
19. Richardson DJ (2000) Bacterial respiration: a flexible process for a changing environment. Microbiology 146 (Pt 3): 551–571.
20. Philippot L (2002) Denitrifying genes in bacterial and *Archaeal* genomes. Biochim Biophys Acta 1577: 355–376.
21. Philippot L (2005) Denitrification in pathogenic bacteria: for better or worst? Trends Microbiol 13: 191–192.
22. Zumft WG (2005) Nitric oxide reductases of prokaryotes with emphasis on the respiratory, heme-copper oxidase type. J Inorg Biochem 99: 194–215.
23. Schreiber F, Stief P, Gieseke A, Heisterkamp IM, Verstraete W, et al. (2010) Denitrification in human dental plaque. BMC Biol 8: 24.
24. Mitsui T, Kondo T (2004) Increased breath nitrous oxide after ingesting nitrate in patients with atrophic gastritis and partial gastrectomy. Clin Chim Acta 345: 129–133.
25. Hino T, Matsumoto Y, Nagano S, Sugimoto H, Fukumori Y, et al. (2010) Structural basis of biological N_2O generation by bacterial nitric oxide reductase. Science 330: 1666–1670.
26. Arai H, Igarashi Y, Kodama T (1995) The structural genes for nitric oxide reductase from *Pseudomonas aeruginosa*. Biochim Biophys Acta 1261: 279–284.
27. Gaston B, Ratjen F, Vaughan JW, Malhotra NR, Canady RG, et al. (2002) Nitrogen redox balance in the cystic fibrosis airway: effects of antipseudomonal therapy. Am J Respir Crit Care Med 165: 387–390.

28. SooHoo CK, Hollocher TC (1991) Purification and characterization of nitrous oxide reductase from *Pseudomonas aeruginosa* strain P2. J Biol Chem 266: 2203–2209.
29. Son MS, Matthews WJ Jr, Kang Y, Nguyen DT, Hoang TT (2007) In vivo evidence of *Pseudomonas aeruginosa* nutrient acquisition and pathogenesis in the lungs of cystic fibrosis patients. Infect Immun 75: 5313–5324.
30. Hassett DJ (1996) Anaerobic production of alginate by *Pseudomonas aeruginosa*: alginate restricts diffusion of oxygen. J Bacteriol 178: 7322–7325.
31. Jones KL, Hegab AH, Hillman BC, Simpson KL, Jinkins PA, et al. (2000) Elevation of nitrotyrosine and nitrate concentrations in cystic fibrosis sputum. Pediatr Pulmonol 30: 79–85.
32. Palmer KL, Brown SA, Whiteley M (2007) Membrane-bound nitrate reductase is required for anaerobic growth in cystic fibrosis sputum. J Bacteriol 189: 4449–4455.
33. Grasemann H, Michler E, Wallot M, Ratjen F (1997) Decreased concentration of exhaled nitric oxide (NO) in patients with cystic fibrosis. Pediatr Pulmonol 24: 173–177.
34. Linnane SJ, Keatings VM, Costello CM, Moynihan JB, O'Connor CM, et al. (1998) Total sputum nitrate plus nitrite is raised during acute pulmonary infection in cystic fibrosis. Am J Respir Crit Care Med 158: 207–212.
35. Ratjen F, Gartig S, Wiesemann HG, Grasemann H (1999) Effect of inhaled nitric oxide on pulmonary function in cystic fibrosis. Respir Med 93: 579–583.
36. Grasemann H, Grasemann C, Kurtz F, Tietze-Schillings G, Vester U, et al. (2005) Oral L-arginine supplementation in cystic fibrosis patients: a placebo-controlled study. Eur Respir J 25: 62–68.
37. Grasemann H, Tullis E, Ratjen F (2013) A randomized controlled trial of inhaled l-Arginine in patients with cystic fibrosis. J Cyst Fibros. Available: http://dx.doi.org/10.1016/j.jcf.2012.12.008.
38. Einsle O, Messerschmidt A, Stach P, Bourenkov GP, Bartunik HD, et al. (1999) Structure of cytochrome c nitrite reductase. Nature 400: 476–480.
39. Einsle O, Messerschmidt A, Huber R, Kroneck PMH, Neese F (2002) Mechanism of the six-electron reduction of nitrite to ammonia by cytochrome c nitrite reductase. J Am Chem Soc 124; 11737–11745.
40. Planelles G (2007) Ammonium homeostasis and human Rhesus glycoproteins. Nephron Physiol 105; 11–17.
41. Williams DR, Rowe JJ, Romero P, Eagon RG (1978) Denitrifying *Pseudomonas aeruginosa*: some parameters of growth and active transport. Appl Environ Microbiol 36: 257–263.
42. Hoffman LR, Richardson AR, Houston LS, Kulasekara HD, Martens-Habbena W, et al. (2010) Nutrient availability as a mechanism for selection of antibiotic tolerant *Pseudomonas aeruginosa* within the CF airway. PLoS Pathog 6: e1000712.
43. Thomas KL, Lloyd D, Boddy L (1994) Effects of oxygen, pH and nitrate concentration on denitrification by *Pseudomonas* species. FEMS Microbiol Lett 118: 181–186.
44. Seneterre E, Paganin F, Bruel JM, Michel FB, Bousquet J (1994) Measurement of the internal size of bronchi using high resolution computed tomography (HRCT). Eur Respir J 7: 596–600.
45. Hampton T, Armstrong S, Russell WJ (2000) Estimating the diameter of the left main bronchus. Anaesth Intensive Care 28: 540–542.
46. Arai H (2011) Regulation and Function of Versatile Aerobic and Anaerobic Respiratory Metabolism in *Pseudomonas aeruginosa*. Front Microbiol 2: 103.
47. Beckmann C, Brittnacher M, Ernst R, Mayer-Hamblett N, Miller SI, et al. (2005) Use of phage display to identify potential *Pseudomonas aeruginosa* gene products relevant to early cystic fibrosis airway infections. Infect Immun 73: 444–452.
48. Van Alst NE, Wellington M, Clark VL, Haidaris CG, Iglewski BH (2009) Nitrite reductase NirS is required for type III secretion system expression and virulence in the human monocyte cell line THP-1 by *Pseudomonas aeruginosa*. Infect Immun 77: 4446–4454.
49. Williams DR, Rowe JJ, Romero P, Eagon RG (1978) Denitrifying *Pseudomonas aeruginosa*: some parameters of growth and active transport. Appl Environ Microbiol 36: 257–263.
50. Borriello G, Werner E, Roe F, Kim AM, Ehrlich GD, et al (2004) Oxygen limitation contributes to antibiotic tolerance of *Pseudomonas aeruginosa* in biofilms. Antimicrob Agents Chemother 48: 2659–2664.
51. Lee B, Schjerling CK, Kirkby N, Hoffmann N, Borup R, et al (2011) Mucoid *Pseudomonas aeruginosa* isolates maintain the biofilm formation capacity and the gene expression profiles during the chronic lung infection of CF patients. APMIS 119: 263–274.
52. Kakishima K, Shiratsuchi A, Taoka A, Nakanishi Y, Fukumori Y (2007) Participation of nitric oxide reductase in survival of *Pseudomonas aeruginosa* in LPS-activated macrophages. Biochem Biophys Res Commun 355: 587–591.
53. Arai H, Iiyama K (2013) Role of nitric oxide-detoxifying enzymes in the virulence of *Pseudomonas aeruginosa* against the silkworm, *Bombyx mori*. Biosci Biotechnol Biochem 77: 198–200. DN/JST.JSTAGE/bbb/120656 [pii].
54. Shimizu T, Tsutsuki H, Matsumoto A, Nakaya H, Noda M (2012) The nitric oxide reductase of enterohaemorrhagic *Escherichia coli* plays an important role for the survival within macrophages. Mol Microbiol 85: 492–512.
55. Stevanin TM, Moir JW, Read RC (2005) Nitric oxide detoxification systems enhance survival of *Neisseria meningitidis* in human macrophages and in nasopharyngeal mucosa. Infect Immun 73: 3322–3329.
56. Loisel-Meyer S, Jimenez de Bagues MP, Basseres E, Dornand J, Kohler S, et al. (2006) Requirement of norD for *Brucella suis* virulence in a murine model of in vitro and in vivo infection. Infect Immun 74: 1973–1976.
57. Høiby N (2000) Microbiology of cystic fibrosis. In: Hodson ME GD, editors. Cystic fibrosis. London, UK: Arnold. pp. 83–107.
58. Gundersen JK, Glud RN, Ramsing NB (1998) Predicting the signal of O_2 microsensors from physical dimensions, temperature, salinity, and O_2 concentration. Limnol Oceanogr 43: 1932–1937.
59. Weiss RF, Price BA (1980) Nitrous oxide solubility in water and seawater. Marine Chemistry 8: 347–359.
60. de Beer D, Stoodley P (2006) Microbial biofilms. In: Dworkin M, Falkow S, Rosenberg E, Schleifer KH, Stackebrandt E, editors. The Prokaryotes. New York: Springer Science. pp. 904–937.
61. Broecker WS, Peng TH (1974) Gas-exchange rates between air and sea. Tellus 26: 21–35.
62. Markfoged R, Nielsen LP, Nyord T, Ottosen LDM, Revsbech NP (2013) Transient N_2O accumulation and emission caused by O_2 depletion in soil after liquid manure injection. European journal of soil science 62: 541–550.
63. Liengaard L, Nielsen LP, Revsbech NP, Priemé A, Elberling B, et al. (2013) Extreme emission of N_2O from tropical wetland soil (Pantanal, South America). Frontiers in Microbiology 3: 433. doi: 10.3389/fmicb.2012.00433.

18

Correcting the Cystic Fibrosis Disease Mutant, A455E CFTR

Liudmila Cebotaru[1,2], Daniele Rapino[1,2], Valeriu Cebotaru[3], William B. Guggino[2]*

1 Department of Ophthalmology, School of Medicine, The Johns Hopkins University, Baltimore, Maryland, United States of America, 2 Department of Physiology, School of Medicine, The Johns Hopkins University, Baltimore, Maryland, United States of America, 3 Department of Medicine, School of Medicine, The Johns Hopkins University, Baltimore, Maryland, United States of America

Abstract

Cystic fibrosis is caused by more than 1000 mutations, the most common being the ΔF508 mutation. These mutations have been divided into five classes [1], with ΔF508 CFTR in class II. Here we have studied the class V mutation A455E. We report that the mature and immature bands of A455E are rapidly degraded primarily by proteasomes; the short protein half-life of this mutant therefore resembles that of ΔF508 CFTR. A455E could be rescued by treatment of the cells with proteasome inhibitors. Furthermore, co-transfection of A455E with the truncation mutant Δ264 CFTR also rescued the mature C band, indicating that A455E can be rescued by transcomplementation. We found that Δ264 CFTR bound to A455E, forming a bimolecular complex. Treatment with the compound correctors C3 and C4 also rescued A455E. These results are significant because they show that although ΔF508 belongs to a different class than A455E, it can be rescued by the same strategies, offering therapeutic promise to patients with Class V mutations.

Editor: Effie C. Tsilibary, National Center for Scientific Research Demokritos, Greece

Funding: This work was supported in part by a CFTR Folding Consortium Grant from the Cystic Fibrosis Foundation. The funders had no role in study design, data collection and analysis, decision to publish, or preparation of the manuscript.

Competing Interests: The authors have declared that no competing interests exist.

* E-mail: wguggino@jhmi.edu

Introduction

Cystic fibrosis (CF) is caused by mutations in the cystic fibrosis transmembrane conductance regulator (CFTR) [2]. Symptoms of CF include higher-than-normal sweat chloride, thick airway mucus, persistent lung infections, pancreatic enzyme insufficiency, intestinal blockage, and infertility in males [3]. These classic symptoms of CF can range in severity from mild to severe. Extensive effort has been made to understand the genotype of CF patients, with over 1000 gene mutations identified thus far [4]. These mutations in the CF gene have been divided into five different classes: Class I mutations result in defective protein production. Class II mutations result in a protein whose processing is blocked in the ER. The most common CFTR mutation, ΔF508 CFTR [2], is a class II mutation. Like other class II mutations, ΔF508 CFTR is retained in the ER, incompletely glycosylated, and rapidly degraded in proteasomes [5]. Class III mutations produce a protein that has defective regulation; the most common is the G551D mutation, which reaches the cell surface but does not conduct chloride [6,7]. Class IV mutations cause defects in channel conductance. Finally, class V mutations affect protein synthesis or splicing, causing less protein to be made. One of these class V mutations is A455E.

The A455E mutation is located in NBD1. It was originally found in French Canadian patients and is associated with a mild phenotype, with borderline high sweat, moderate lung disease, and sufficient pancreatic function [8,9]. Unlike other mild missense mutations such as R117H that have altered channel conductance [10] and are considered class IV mutations, the single-channel characteristics of A445E resemble those of wild-type CFTR [11,12] . Thus, because the mild disease resulting from A455E is thought to arise from reduced protein expression, it is considered a class V mutation. Thus, an effective pharmacological approach to treating this mutation should involve increasing the protein levels of A455E.

Our group has been interested in transcomplementation [13,14] using Δ264 CFTR, which is a truncated version of CFTR missing the first four transmembrane domains. When monkey lungs are infected with an adeno-associated viral vector rAAV-Δ264 CFTR, the Δ264 CFTR produced can increase the levels of endogenous wild-type CFTR protein [15]. We have also shown in cotransfection studies that Δ264 CFTR increases wild-type CFTR protein levels and increases the degree of maturation of the immature band B to the mature C band of ΔF508 CFTR. The purpose of the current study was to determine whether analogous transcomplementation can be used to enhance the protein processing of A455E.

Experimental Procedures

Cell culture

African green monkey kidney cells (Cos7) were maintained in Dulbecco's modified Eagle's medium-high glucose 1x (DMEM), penicillin (100 U/ml), streptomycin (100 μg/ml), and 10% fetal bovine serum as described previously [14]).

Plasmids and constructs

The construct pEGFP A455E was a gift from Dr. Gary Cutting at Johns Hopkins U. The plasmids were transfected into Cos 7 cells using Lipofectamine 2000 (Invitrogen) as we have previously described. After 48 h of transfection, the cells were harvested and used for immunoprecipitation and immunoblotting.

Immunoblotting and immunoprecipitation

Cells were harvested and processed as described previously [16] using the (C-terminus) antibody (1:1500; R&D Systems, Inc.). Glyceraldehyde 3-phosphate dehydrogenase (GAPDH), used as a loading control, was detected with monoclonal anti-GAPDH antibody (1:10,000; US Biological).

For immunoprecipitation, cells were harvested and processed as described previously. For pull-down experiments, 10 µl of anti-GFP antibody (Roche) were added to the lysate and allowed to incubate for 30 min. with 50 µl of A/G-agarose beads (Santa Cruz Biotechnology, Inc.). CFTR was detected as described above.

Statistics

Western blots were evaluated by one-way ANOVA followed by LSD post hoc tests. Statistical significance was set at $P<0.05$, and data are presented as mean±2SEM. All experiments were normalized for the control. SPSS (version 17.0 SPSS, Inc, Chicago, Ill) was used for data analysis

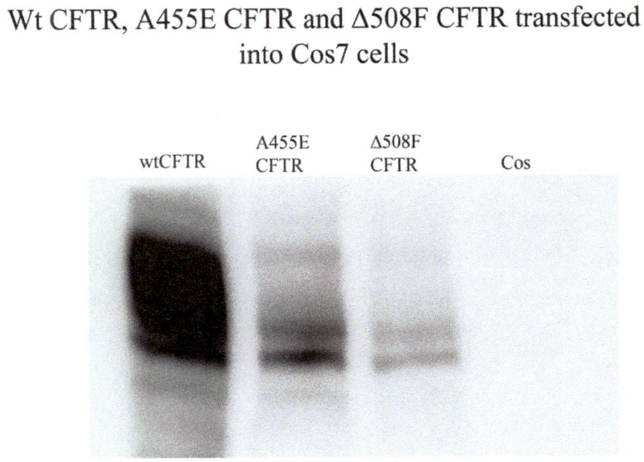

Figure 1. A455E has reduced expression of mature CFTR. Cos7 cells were transfected with 2 µg of wild-type, A455E, or ΔF508 CFTR constructs. After 48 h, the cells were lysed, and the total lysate was analyzed by western blotting with anti-human CFTR antibodies. Note that there is much less mature C band in the A455E sample than in the wild-type sample. In this and subsequent blots, some mature C band was detected with A455E (n = 8).

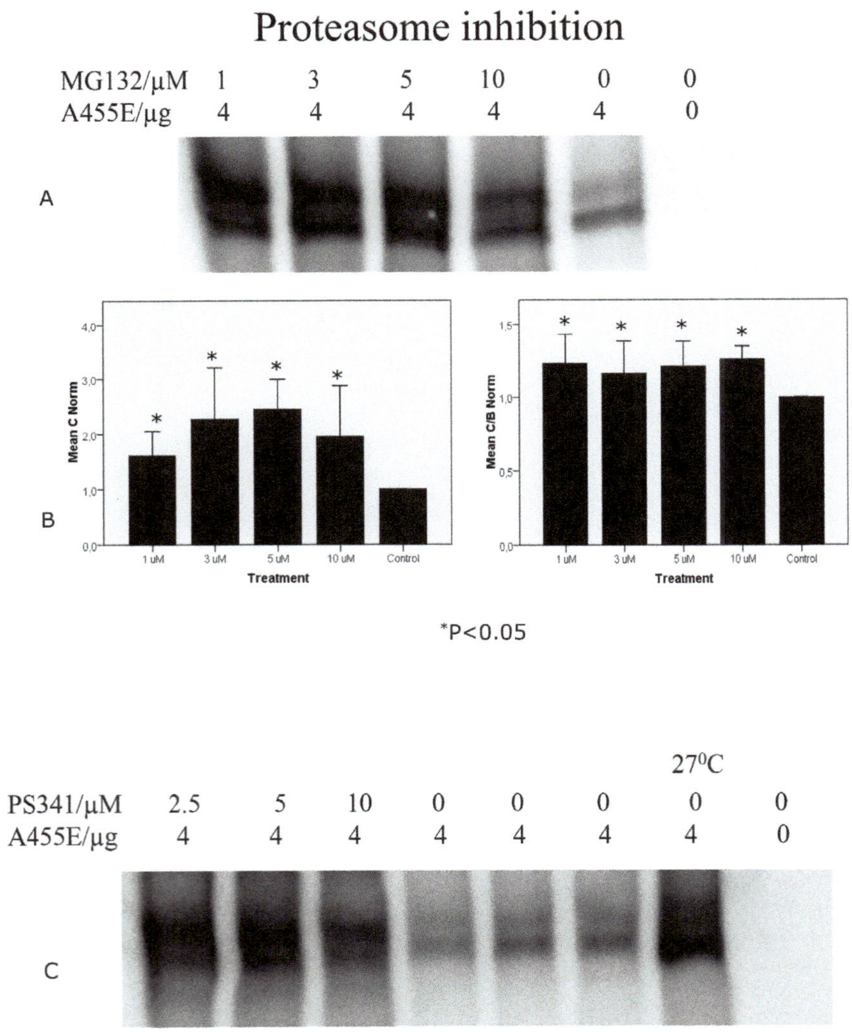

Figure 2. Proteasome inhibition. Cells transfected with A455E cDNA were treated either with MG132, a more general inhibitor (n = 6) (**A, B**), or the more specific inhibitor of proteasomes, PS341 (n = 2) (**C**). Note that in both cases, proteasome inhibition caused an increase in both the immature B and mature C bands of A455E.

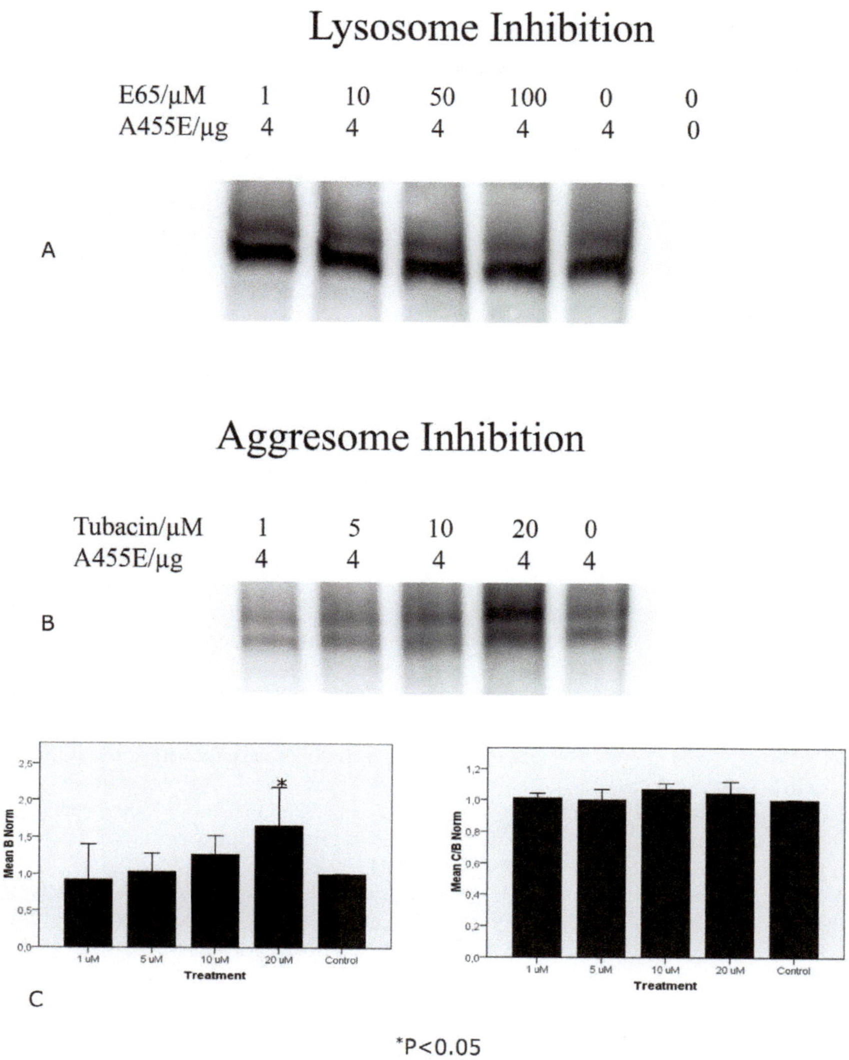

Figure 3. Lysosome/aggresome inhibition. Cos7 cells were transfected with A455E CFTR cDNA and treated for 16 h with the lysosome inhibitor E64 (n = 4) (**A**) There was very little change in band density in any of the treated groups or in the presence of the inhibitors when compared to the control or the HDAC6 inhibitor tubacin to inhibit aggresomes (n = 3) (**B, C**). Note that there is a significant increase with the highest concentration used.

Results

Expression of A455E

When we compared the expression of the A455E mutant to that of both wild-type and ΔF508 CFTR (Fig. 1) by western blotting, we found that the amount of CFTR protein was greatly reduced in the Cos7 cells transfected with the A455E mutant. To evaluate the degradation of A455E CFTR, we treated the cells with MG132, a non-specific inhibitor of proteasomal degradation. Fig. 2 shows that in the presence of MG132, the protein expression of both the B and C bands of A455E CFTR increased dramatically. A similar effect was seen when we used the more specific proteasome inhibitor, PS341. PS341 also caused an increase in both the B and C bands of A455E. Furthermore, we noted that A455E could be rescued by growing the cells at a reduced temperature, as had previously been observed for ΔF508 [13]. In sharp contrast, there was no increase in the protein expression of A455E CFTR when the cells were treated with the aggresome inhibitor tubacin or the lysosomal inhibitor E64 (Fig. 3). These data suggest that A455E is degraded primarily in proteasomes.

To evaluate how rapidly the A455E CFTR protein is degraded, we treated the transfected cells with cycloheximide for between 1 and 7 hours (Fig 4). Surprisingly, both the B and C bands of A455E CFTR rapidly disappeared in the cells treated with cycloheximide (Fig. 4), suggesting that it is rapidly degraded, as is ΔF508 CFTR (see [13]).

Δ264 CFTR increases the processing of band B to band C of A455E CFTR

We then tested whether the truncation mutant, Δ264 CFTR, was capable of transcomplementation with A455E (Fig. 5). In order to determine whether Δ264 CFTR affects the maturation of A455E CFTR, we cotransfected Δ264 CFTR and A455E CFTR into Cos7 cells and found that the mature C band from A455E CFTR was increased in cells cotransfected with Δ264 CFTR, as compared to cells transfected with A455E cDNA alone (Fig. 5).

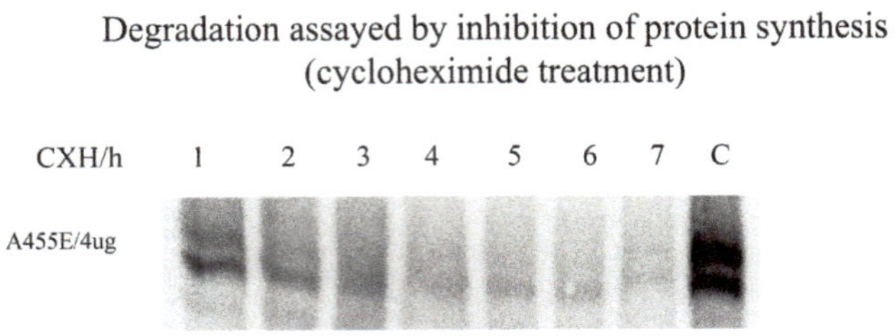

Figure 4. Effect of protein synthesis inhibition on the degradation of A455E. Cos7 cells were transfected with A455E cDNA and treated with cycloheximide (25 µg/ml) for the indicated times. Note the rapid decay of both the mature C and immature B bands of A455E. (n = 4).

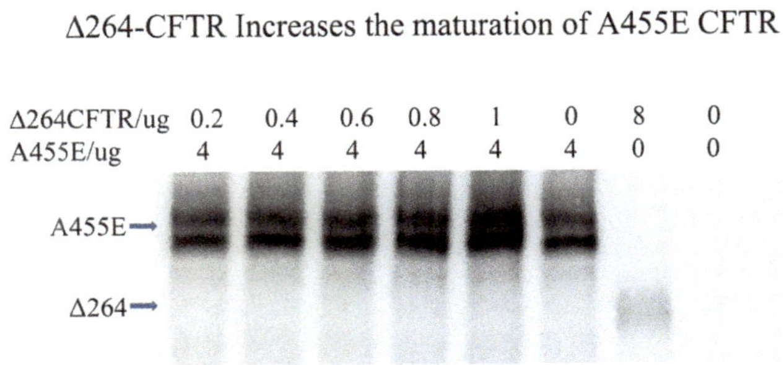

Figure. 5. Transcomplementation of A455E by Δ27-264 CFTR. Both the C and B bands of A455E CFTR were increased when cells were cotransfected with Δ27-264 CFTR, showing that A455E could be rescued by transcomplementation. (n = 11).

Δ264 CFTR binds to A455E CFTR, forming a biomolecular complex

We and others have shown that transcomplementation can occur via direct binding of truncated forms of CFTR to ΔF508-CFTR and via chaperone displacement [17]. In order to assess these possibilities in A455E CFTR, we conducted co-immunprecipitation experiments. Fig. 6 shows that Δ264-CFTR did indeed bind to A455E, in both the absence and presence of the proteasome inhibitor MG123.

Correctors 4A (C4) and VX325 (C3) increase the processing of band B to band C of A455E CFTR

We next asked whether small-molecule correctors might be effective in rescuing A455E CFTR (Fig. 7). We chose two well-known correctors, 4A (C4) [18] and VX325 (C3) [19]. We found that corrector C4 does have a robust effect on A455E CFTR; in contrast, C3 had only a minimal effect on A455E (Fig. 7).

Discussion

Transcomplementation of ΔF508-CFTR by fragments of CFTR has been observed [13,14,17,20,20]. These fragments are themselves extremely efficiently degraded; they bind to ΔF508 CFTR and improve the maturation from the immature band B to mature band C. Although transcomplementation has been observed by at least three different groups, it has never been demonstrated with other mutations. Here we show that A455E can also be rescued by transcomplementation. This finding is significant because it provides a new way to treat mutations other than ΔF508 CFTR and also provides insight into the mechanism of transcomplementation.

ΔF508 CFTR is associated with a least two major problems, an unstable NBD1 and defective interactions with intracellular loops (ICL), especially ICL4 [21–23]. These two defects disrupt both trafficking and channel activity. The A455E mutation, on the other hand, is located within the F1-type ATP-binding core subdomain near to the ABC protein signature, the Walker A domain [24]. Given the proximity to the Walker A domain, one might expect that A455E would have alterations in gating. However, electrophysiological studies have shown that its single-channel properties are similar to those of wild-type CFTR [11]. A455E also functions well as a regulator of other channels [25]. Thus, its ability to act as a conductance regulator is intact. What appears to be causing the disease, then, is a drastic reduction in the processing of the mature protein. At least two studies have failed to detect mature band C from A455E [11,26], although the results of their electrophysiological studies suggested that some mature band C must have been present at the plasma membrane in order to generate chloride currents [11]. In our study, we do detect some mature band C at the plasma membrane, but when the cells are treated with cycloheximide to evaluate protein degradation, it is clear that the mature band C of A455E is rapidly degraded along with the immature B band. This situation is similar to that in ΔF508 CFTR, in which both the immature mature bands of temperature-rescued ΔF508 CFTR are rapidly degraded. Van Oene et al. 2000.] have shown that A455E has a pattern of degradation that is clearly different from that of ΔF508 CFTR. A455E appears to be proteolytically cleaved within the NBD1-R domain to form C-terminal aggregates. This cleavage does not appear to occur via the 26S proteasome, but perhaps within the cytosol [26]. Clearly, these results show that the A455E mutant is distinctly different from ΔF508 CFTR.

Nevertheless, A455E shows some similarity to ΔF508 CFTR. Although A455E is uniquely cleaved in the cytoplasm, our results show that it is still degraded in the proteasome, because treatment with two types of proteasome inhibitors led to significant increases in steady-state protein levels. In fact, we saw a rather large increase in the mature band of A455E after proteasome inhibition. This result is in contrast to the response of A455E to lysosomal inhibitors, which were without effect. Inhibiting the aggresome

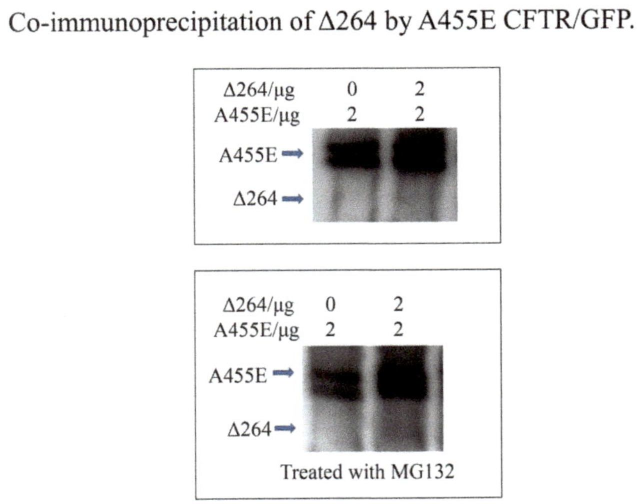

Figure 6. A455E binds to Δ27-264 CFTR. Cos7 cells were transfected with both Δ27-264 CFTR and an A455E CFTR construct bearing a GFP tag. Anti-GFP antibodies were used to pull down A455E, and the gels were blotted with anti-CFTR antibody. (n = 3).

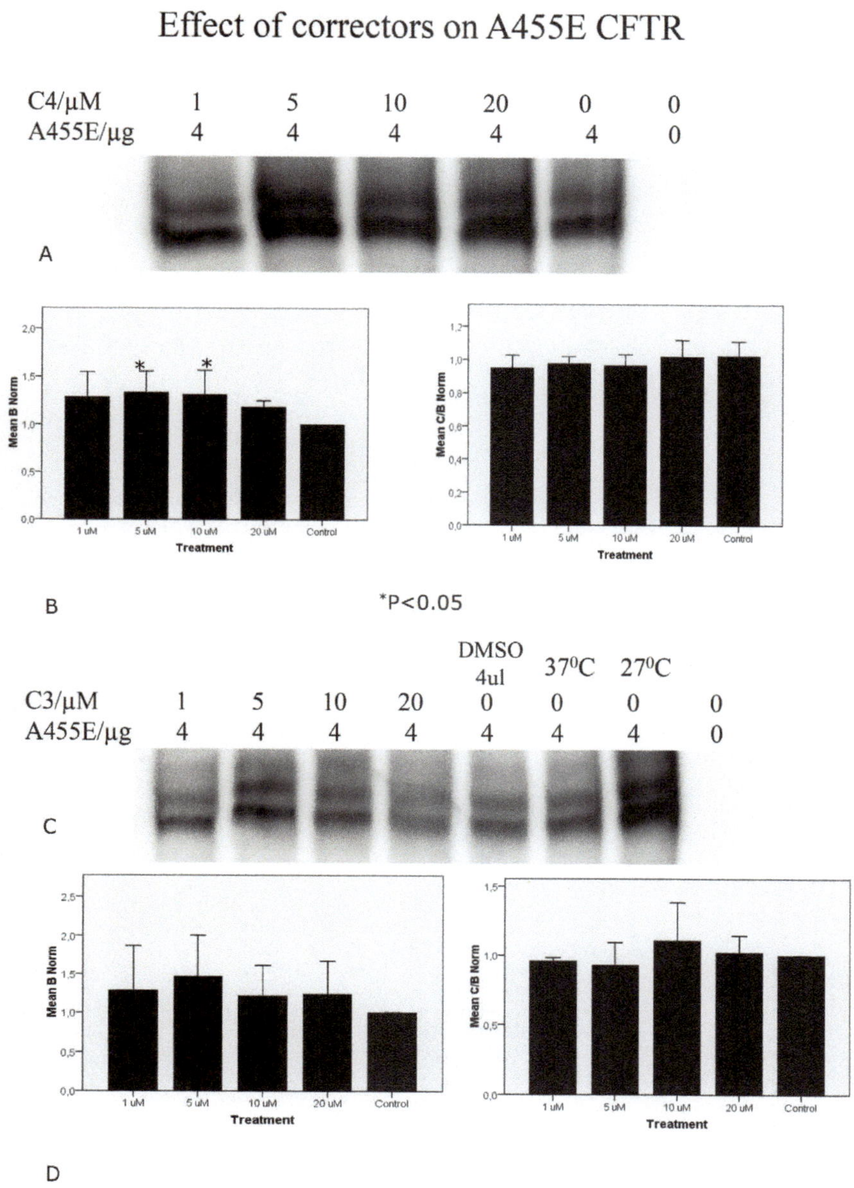

Figure 7. Correctors can rescue A455E. Cos7 cells were transfected with A455E and treated with the correctors C3 or C4 for 16 h at the specified concentrations. Note that C4 had a profound effect on the immature B band of A455E as well as causing an increase in the mature C band (**A, B**). C3 did not have a significant effect (**C, D**). (n = 3).

was also without effect. Taken together, our data suggest that A455E, like ΔF508 CFTR, is processed by proteasomes.

Δ264 CFTR rescues A455E and forms a molecular complex between the two molecules. It has been shown that CFTR forms an intramolecular dimer through an interaction between the Walker sites in the two NBDs that involves ATP. Indeed, Lewis et al. [27] have shown that the crystal structure indicates that two isolated NBD1s of CFTR readily form a head-to-tail dimer when both the regulatory insert and extension are removed. It is possible that a similar interaction occurs between Δ264 and A455E. Two other groups have shown that small fragments of CFTR can rescue ΔF508 CFTR, through either a bimolecular interaction [20] or chaperone displacement [17]. One group used a truncation that included TMD1 and NBD1 [20], and the other NBD1 plus the R domain [17]. What these truncations have in common with ours is that each contains NBD1. Thus, it is plausible to suggest that the transcomplementation most likely occurs by an interaction between the NBD1 moieties of the truncated and the mutant proteins. The observation that A455E is readily rescued by Δ264 CFTR suggests that transcomplementation may be influencing NBD1 in the region of the Walker sites. One then may ask why the interaction with the normal NBD2 of A455E does not rescue its own NBD1. One reason may be that NBD2 is translated much later than NBD1 [28]. By the time NBD2 is translated, the mutant NBD1 may already doom the molecule to be degraded by endoplasmic reticulum-associated degradation (ERAD). One might envision that the truncated and mutant CFTRs immediately form a complex during cotranslation of the NBD1s from the two molecules. Thus, the truncated NBD1 could act as a molecular chaperone to rescue the other molecule.

Therapeutic transcomplementation to rescue A455E would require gene transfer via a virus or non-viral particle. Several gene therapy approaches are currently being developed for both purposes [29].

Another way to rescue mutant CFTR is with corrector compounds that either bind to mutant CFTR or alter some component of the ERAD pathway. Several groups utilizing high-throughput methods to screen large compound libraries have identified correctors that rescue ΔF508 CFTR. For example, the C4 corrector utilized here was identified in an academic laboratory [30], whereas C3 was developed commercially [19]. Although many compounds have been identified, only VX 809 has reached clinical trials [31]. Although it has shown promise in laboratory experiments in clinical trials involving patients bearing the ΔF508 mutation, VX-809 [31] had a small effect on sweat chloride and no effect on pulmonary function or rescue of ΔF508 CFTR in rectal biopsies. Our demonstration that both C3 and C4 can rescue A455E suggests that A455E CFTR may be a better candidate for correction with either compound correctors or transcomplementation than is ΔF508 CFTR.

Acknowledgments

The authors thank Dr. Deborah McClellan for editorial assistance and Rahul Grover and Miqueias Lopes-Pacheco for help with experimental setups.

Author Contributions

Conceived and designed the experiments: LC WBG. Performed the experiments: VC. Analyzed the data: LC WBG DR. Contributed reagents/materials/analysis tools: VC. Wrote the paper: WBG.

References

1. Welsh MJ, Smith AE (1993) Molecular mechanisms of CFTR chloride channel dysfunction in cystic fibrosis. Cell 73: 1251–1254.
2. Rommens JM, Iannuzzi MC, Kerem B-S, Drumm ML, Melmer G, et al. (1989) Identification of the cystic fibrosis gene: Chromosome walking and jumping. Science 245: 1059–1065.
3. Rosenstein BJ, Cutting GR (1998) The diagnosis of cystic fibrosis: a consensus statement. Cystic Fibrosis Foundation Consensus Panel. J Pediatr 132: 589–595.
4. Cutting GR (1993) Spectrum of mutations in cystic fibrosis. J Bioenerg Biomembr 25: 7–10.
5. Cheng SH, Gregory RJ, Marshall J, Paul S, Souza DW, et al. (1990) Defective intracellular transport and processing of CFTR is the molecular basis of most of cystic fibrosis. Cell 63: 827–834.
6. Mickle JE, Cutting GR (2000) Genotype-phenotype relationships in cystic fibrosis. Med Clin North Am 84: 597–607.
7. Van GF, Hadida S, Grootenhuis PD, Burton B, Cao D, et al. (2009) Rescue of CF airway epithelial cell function in vitro by a CFTR potentiator, VX-770. Proc Natl Acad Sci U S A 106: 18825–18830. 0904709106 [pii];10.1073/pnas.0904709106 [doi].
8. Stansberg PM, Noreau D, McGlynn-Steele L, Koultchitski G, Ray PN (1997) PCR-based test for two cystic fibrosis mutations (A455E, 711+1G-->T) common among French Canadians. Clin Chem 43: 1083–1084.
9. De BM, Allard C, Leblanc JP, Simard F, Aubin G (1997) Genotype-phenotype correlation in cystic fibrosis patients compound heterozygous for the A455E mutation. Hum Genet 101: 208–211.
10. Sheppard DN, Rich DP, Ostedgaard LS, Gregory RJ, Smith AE, et al. (1993) Mutations in CFTR associated with mild-disease-form Cl- channels with altered pore properties. Nature 362: 160–164. 10.1038/362160a0 [doi].
11. Sheppard DN, Ostedgaard LS, Winter MC, Welsh MJ (1995) Mechanism of dysfunction of two nucleotide binding domain mutations in cystic fibrosis transmembrane conductance regulator that are associated with pancreatic sufficiency. EMBO J 14: 876–883.
12. Fulmer SB, Schwiebert EM, Morales MM, Guggino WB, Cutting GR (1995) Two cystic fibrosis transmembrane conductance regulator mutations have different effects on both pulmonary phenotype and regulation of outwardly rectified chloride currents. Proc Natl Acad Sci U S A 92: 6832–6836.
13. Cebotaru L, Woodward O, Cebotaru V, Guggino WB (2013) Transcomplementation by a truncation mutant of CFTR enhances {triangleup}F508 processing through a biomolecualr interaction. J Biol Chem . M112.420489 [pii];10.1074/jbc.M112.420489 [doi].
14. Cebotaru L, Vij N, Ciobanu I, Wright J, Flotte T, Guggino WB (2008) Cystic fibrosis transmembrane regulator missing the first four transmembrane segments increases wild type and DeltaF508 processing. J Biol Chem 283: 21926–21933.
15. Fischer AC, Smith CI, Cebotaru L, Zhang X, Askin FB, et al. (2007) Expression of a truncated cystic fibrosis transmembrane conductance regulator with an AAV5-pseudotyped vector in primates. Mol Ther 15: 756–763.
16. Cheng J, Moyer BD, Milewski M, Loffing J, Ikeda M, et al. (2002) A Golgi-associated PDZ domain protein modulates cystic fibrosis transmembrane regulator plasma membrane expression. J Biol Chem 277: 3520–3529.
17. Sun F, Mi Z, Condliffe SB, Bertrand CA, Gong X, Lu X, et al. (2008) Chaperone displacement from mutant cystic fibrosis transmembrane conductance regulator restores its function in human airway epithelia. FASEB J .
18. Pedemonte N, Lukacs GL, Du K, Caci E, Zegarra-Moran O, et al. (2005) Small-molecule correctors of defective DeltaF508-CFTR cellular processing identified by high-throughput screening. J Clin Invest 115: 2564–2571.
19. Van GF, Straley KS, Cao D, Gonzalez J, Hadida S, et al. (2006) Rescue of DeltaF508-CFTR trafficking and gating in human cystic fibrosis airway primary cultures by small molecules. Am J Physiol Lung Cell Mol Physiol 290: L1117–L1130. 00169.2005 [pii];10.1152/ajplung.00169.2005 [doi].
20. Cormet-Boyaka E, Jablonsky M, Naren AP, Jackson PL, Muccio DD, et al. (2004) Rescuing cystic fibrosis transmembrane conductance regulator (CFTR)-processing mutants by transcomplementation. Proc Natl Acad Sci U S A 101: 8221–8226.
21. Mendoza JL, Schmidt A, Li Q, Nuvaga E, Barrett T, et al. (2012) Requirements for efficient correction of DeltaF508 CFTR revealed by analyses of evolved sequences. Cell 148: 164–174. S0092-8674(11)01367-5 [pii];10.1016/j.cell.2011.11.023 [doi].
22. Du K, Sharma M, Lukacs GL (2005) The DeltaF508 cystic fibrosis mutation impairs domain-domain interactions and arrests post-translational folding of CFTR. Nat Struct Mol Biol 12: 17–25.
23. He L, Aleksandrov LA, Cui L, Jensen TJ, Nesbitt KL, et al. (2010) Restoration of domain folding and interdomain assembly by second-site suppressors of the DeltaF508 mutation in CFTR. FASEB J 24: 3103–3112. fj.09-141788 [pii];10.1096/fj.09-141788 [doi].
24. Lewis HA, Buchanan SG, Burley SK, Conners K, Dickey et al. (2004) Structure of nucleotide-binding domain 1 of the cystic fibrosis transmembrane conductance regulator. EMBO J 23: 282–293.
25. Schwiebert EM, Benos DJ, Egan ME, Stutts MJ, Guggino WB (1999) CFTR is a conductance regulator as well as a chloride channel. Physiol Rev 79: S145–S166.
26. Van Oene M, Lukacs GL, Rommens JM (2000) Cystic fibrosis mutations lead to carboxyl-terminal fragments that highlight an early biogenesis step of the cystic fibrosis transmembrane conductance regulator. Journal of Biological Chemistry 275: 19577–19584.
27. Atwell S, Brouillette CG, Conners K, Emtage S, Gheyi T, et al. (2010) Structures of a minimal human CFTR first nucleotide-binding domain as a monomer, head-to-tail homodimer, and pathogenic mutant. Protein Eng Des Sel 23: 375–384. gzq004 [pii];10.1093/protein/gzq004 [doi].
28. Kim SJ, Skach WR (2012) Mechanisms of CFTR Folding at the Endoplasmic Reticulum. Front Pharmacol 3: 201. 10.3389/fphar.2012.00201 [doi].
29. Boucher RC (1996) Current status of CF gene therapy. Trends Genet 12: 81–84.
30. Pedemonte N, Sonawane ND, Taddei A, Hu J, Zegarra-Moran O, et al. (2005) Phenylglycine and sulfonamide correctors of defective delta F508 and G551D cystic fibrosis transmembrane conductance regulator chloride-channel gating. Mol Pharmacol 67: 1797–1807.
31. Clancy JP, Rowe SM, Accurso FJ, Aitken ML, Amin RS, et al. (2012) Results of a phase IIa study of VX-809, an investigational CFTR corrector compound, in subjects with cystic fibrosis homozygous for the F508del-CFTR mutation. Thorax 67: 12–18. thoraxjnl-2011-200393 [pii];10.1136/thoraxjnl-2011-200393 [doi].

Gene Mutation in MicroRNA Target Sites of CFTR Gene: A Novel Pathogenetic Mechanism in Cystic Fibrosis?

Felice Amato[1,2], Manuela Seia[3], Sonia Giordano[1,2], Ausilia Elce[1,2], Federica Zarrilli[1,2,4], Giuseppe Castaldo[1,2]*, Rossella Tomaiuolo[1,2]

1 CEINGE-Biotecnologie avanzate, Naples, Italy, **2** Dipartimento di Medicina Molecolare e Biotecnologie Mediche, Università di Napoli Federico II, Naples, Italy, **3** Laboratorio di Genetica Medica, Fondazione IRCCS Cà Granda - Ospedale Maggiore Policlnico, Mangiagalli e Regina Elena, Milan, Italy, **4** Dipartimento di Bioscienze e Territorio, Università del Molise, Isernia, Italy

Abstract

Cystic fibrosis (CF) is the most frequent lethal genetic disorder among Caucasians. It depends on alterations of a chloride channel expressed by most epithelial cells and encoded by *CFTR* gene. Also using scanning techniques to analyze the whole coding regions of *CFTR* gene, mutations are not identified in up to 10% of CF alleles, and such figure increases in *CFTR*-related disorders (*CFTR*-RD). Other gene regions may be the site of causing-disease mutations. We searched for genetic variants in the 1500 bp of *CFTR* 3′ untranslated region, typical target of microRNA (miRNA) posttranscriptional gene regulation, in either CF patients with the F508del homozygous genotype and different clinical expression (n = 20), CF (n = 32) and *CFTR*-RD (n = 43) patients with one or none mutation after *CFTR* scanning and in controls (n = 50). We identified three SNPs, one of which, the c.*1043A>C, was located in a region predicted to bind miR-433 and miR-509-3p. Such mutation was peculiar of a *CFTR*-RD patient that had Congenital Bilateral Absence of Vas Deferens (CBAVD), diffuse bronchiectasis, a borderline sweat chloride test and the heterozygous severe F508del mutation on the other allele. The expression analysis demonstrated that the c.*1043A>C increases the affinity for miR-509-3p and slightly decreases that for the miR-433. Both miRNAs cause *in vitro* a reduced expression of CFTR protein. Thus, the c.*1043A>C may act as a mild *CFTR* mutation enhancing the affinity for inhibitory miRNAs as a novel pathogenetic mechanism in CF.

Editor: Neeraj Vij, Johns Hopkins School of Medicine, United States of America

Funding: Grants from Ministero della Salute (Legge 548/93, 2007, 2008 and 2012) and from F.A.R.O.2010 project supported this work. The funders had no role in study design, data collection and analysis, decision to publish, or preparation of the manuscript.

Competing Interests: The authors have declared that no competing interests exist.

* E-mail: giuseppe.castaldo@unina.it

Introduction

Cystic fibrosis (CF) is the most frequent lethal genetic disorder among Caucasians with one child in every 3000 newborns affected by disease. It depends on alterations of a chloride channel expressed by most epithelial cells and encoded by cystic fibrosis transmembrane regulator (CFTR) gene [1]. The diagnosis of CF is based on symptoms, sweat chloride and on the identification of *CFTR* mutations [2]. However, also using scanning techniques to analyze the whole coding regions of *CFTR* [3] and large gene rearrangements [4] in up to 10% of CF alleles any mutations are not identified. Such figure increases in *CFTR*-related disorders (*CFTR*-RD, [5]. It is possible that such alleles bear mutations in regulatory sequences, like those at the 3′ untranslated regions (UTR) that encode RNA sequences that bind specific microRNA (miRNA)s. These mutations may modify the affinity and thus the binding of a miRNA to the CFTR transcript, or may cause the appearance of novel target sites for miRNAs thus impairing the levels of *CFTR* expression, acting as causative mutations, or contributing to modulate the heterogeneous phenotypic expression of the disease. MicroRNAs are evolutionarily conserved, endogenous, single-stranded non-coding RNAs, 18–25 nucleotides in length [6]. These molecules regulate the expression of specific genes at post-transscriptional level [7]. The most common outcome following the formation of the miRNA/mRNA complex is the reduced expression of the gene [6,7]. According to the miRBase, release 18 (www.mirbase.org), about 2000 miRNAs have been identified so far in humans. Recently, some miRNAs that specifically regulate *CFTR* expression have been described [8].

We searched for mutations, both in CF patients and controls, within the 3′UTR region of *CFTR* gene that could affect the interaction and therefore the regulatory activity of miRNAs, by acting as disease-causative mutations or as modifier factors of CF phenotype.

Materials and Methods

Ethics Approval

The study was approved by the Ethics Committee of Fondazione IRCCS Ca' Granda Ospedale Maggiore Policlinico, Milan, Italy. Written informed consent was obtained from each individual (legal guardians for minors) to use an anonymous DNA sample and clinical data for scientific studies.

Patients and controls

We studied 95 Italian patients (Table 1) affected by CF (52 cases) or by CFTR-RD (43 cases). In detail: i) 20 CF patients homozygous for the F508del mutation, aged >18 years and classified as: severe pulmonary and liver (n = 10) or mild pulmonary and no liver (n = 10) expression as previously described [4,9]; ii) 32 CF patients with one (28 cases) or both (4 cases) unidentified CFTR mutations after the scanning of CFTR coding regions; iii) 43 subjects with CFTR-RD (mainly CBAVD) of which 32 with one and 11 with both unidentified CFTR mutations after the whole sequencing of CFTR gene coding regions [5]. As controls, we studied 50 healthy subjects. All patients and control subjects were unrelated up to the third generation. This study was performed according to the ethical requirements of the institution, and written informed consent was obtained from each individual (legal guardians for minors) to use an anonymous DNA sample and clinical data for scientific studies.

CFTR molecular analysis

A DNA sample was obtained from each subject (in most cases at the time of molecular analysis for diagnostic purposes). DNA was extracted from peripheral blood by standard procedures. The analysis of all CFTR coding regions (27 exons and intron-exon boundaries) was performed by gene sequencing (protocols available on request). We studied by automated gene sequencing the 3′ UTR of CFTR (starting from the 4575 last translated nucleotide up to 4575+1553). Primers and PCR conditions are available on request.

miRNA selection

We used different computational algorithms (i.e., TargetScan, miRBase, miRanda, PITA and PicTar) to identify miRNA putative binding sites within the CFTR 3′untranslated region (3′UTR). These alghorithms are available online at: www.mirbase.org, www.targetscan.org, www.microrna.org, and www.pictar.mdc-berlin.de.

Luciferase constructs for the 3′UTR of human *CFTR*

We cloned the 3′UTR of *CFTR* into pGL3-Control vector. To this aim, it was designed a pair of primers, both containing the site for the restriction enzyme XbaI at 5′, to amplify the entire region of the 3′UTR of *CFTR* directly from genomic DNA. Then, the PCR product was digested by XbaI and cloned into plasmid pGL3-control (Promega, USA) downstream of the luciferase cDNA (construct pLuc-*CFTR*-3′UTR). After sequencing, the construct was transfected into eukaryotic cells (HEK 293, HeLa, A549). After checking the functioning of the construct, it was co-transfected with synthetic miRNA or anti-miRNA (Qiagen, USA). Both the c.*1043A>C mutation and the overlapping miR-433 and miR-509-3p seed region mutation were performed by Site-Directed Mutagenesis using the QuikChange® II XL Site-Directed Mutagenesis Kit (Agilent Technologies) obtaining respectively the pLuc-*CFTR*-c*1043A>C and pLuc-*CFTR*-mut433-509-3p constructs.

Table 1. Main features of patients under study.

Diagnosis	CFTR genotype	Sweat test	Clinical expression	N of cases
CF	F508del/F508del	positive	PI, severe L, severe P	10
CF	F508del/F508del	positive	PI, no L, mild P	10
CF	Mutation/U	positive	variable	28
CF	U/U	positive	variable	4
CBAVD	Mutation/U	negative	CBAVD alone	12
CBAVD	U/U	negative	CBAVD alone	11

(PI: pancreatic insufficiency; PS: pancreatic sufficiency; L: liver; P: pulmonary)

Western Blot analysis

Cells were lysed in 50 mM Tris, 1% Triton X-100, 150 mM NaCl and protease inhibitors (Complete tablets, Roche). Concentration of total protein extracts was determined by the BioRad method using BSA as standard. All samples, after 30 min at 37°C in Laemmli buffer, were separated by SDS-PAGE 8% gel and transferred on to Protran Nitrocellulose membrane (Whatman). The polyclonal CFTR antibody (Cell Signaling Technologies #2269) was used for CFTR protein detection and monoclonal anti-α-Tubulin (Sigma-Aldrich, T9026) for western normalization. Western blot quantification was performed using both PhotoShop and ImageJ softwares.

MicroRNA precursor constructs and lentivirus production

In order to overexpress miR-433 and miR-509-3p in cell lines, we cloned approximately 650 bp genomic region of miR-433 gene, HGNC: 32026, and miR-509-3p gene, HGCN: 33675, in the lentiviral construct pMIRNA1, Figure S2-A (SBI System Biosciences, CA - USA). For *in vivo* expression of interfering RNA we used the pmiRZip vector (Figure S2-B), where we cloned a double-stranded oligo under the control of the constitutive RNA polymerase III H1 promoter. Once checked by sequencing, the various microRNA precursor constructs were packaged into VSV-G pseudotyped viral particles using SBI's pPACKH1 packaging plasmid Mix. Both packaging and transduction of PANC-1 cells were performed according to the manufacturer's instruction.

Cell culture

Cell lines were purchased from ATCC (Manassas, USA). Human hepatocellular carcinoma cells (HepG2, ATCC number HB-8065), human cervix carcinoma cells (HeLa, ATCC number HB-8065), human lung carcinoma cells (A549, ATCC number CCL-185) and epithelioid carcinoma pancreatic ducts cells (PANC-1, ATCC number CRL-1469), embryonic kidney cells (HEK 293, ATCC number CRL-1573), were maintained in Dulbecco's modified Eagle's medium (Gibco Invitrogen, USA) with 10% heat-inactivated fetal bovine serum (HyClone, USA) without the addition of antibiotics; colorectal adenocarcinoma cells (Caco2, ATCC number HTB-37), were maintained in Eagle's Minimum Essential Medium with 20% heat-inactivated fetal bovine serum, normal human bronchial epithelial (NHBE) cells were purchased by Lonza (Basel, SW). cells were cultured in BEGM medium (Clonetics, Walkersville, MD), renal proximal tubular epithelial cells (RPTEC) were purchased by Lonza (Basel, SW). cells were cultured in REGM medium (Clonetics, Walkersville, MD).

Transfection and Luciferase Assay

Transfection of HEK 293 cells with miRNA-mimics or anti-miRNA-mimics (Qiagen, Germany, EU) was performed with Attractene Transfection Reagent (Qiagen). Cells were seeded in 24-well plates and were cotransfected 24 hr after seeding with the Firefly reporter constructs described above (100 ng), the Renilla reporter plasmid pCMV-RL (50 ng), and the appropriate miRNA mimic at different concentrations (10 nM, and 30 nM). Twenty-four hours after transfection, cells were lysed and Firefly and Renilla luciferase activities were determined using the Dual-Glo Luciferase Assay System (Promega Corporation). The relative

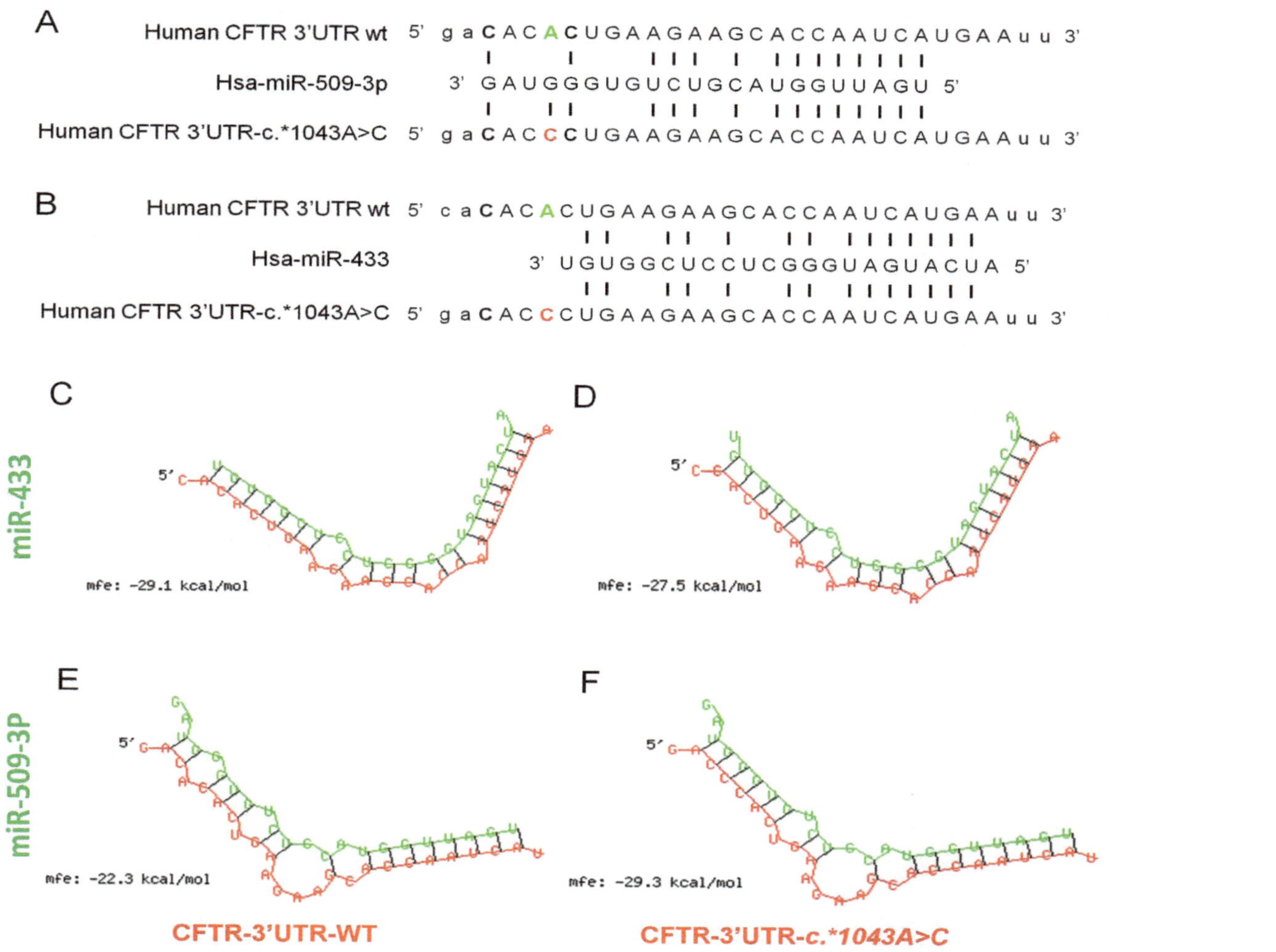

Figure 1. Bioinformatics prediction of c*1043A>C mutation position and effect on miRNA affinity. A–B) schematic diagram of the two *in silico* predicted miRNAs aligned with either wild-type (in green) or c.*1043A>C (in red) mutation of CFTR 3′UTR. C–D) predicted wild-type or CFTR 3′UTR-c.*1043A>C mutation Hybrid structure with miR-433. E–F) predicted wild-type or CFTR 3′UTR-c.*1043A>C mutaion Hybrid structure with miR-509-3p, for each hybrid structure is shown the mean free energy (mfe) calculated using the RNAHybrid server.

reporter activity was obtained by normalization to the Renilla luciferase activity. Each experiment was done in triplicate and at least three independent experiments were performed for each miRNA tested. Data are reported as mean (of all experiments performed)± St.Dev. Statistical significance was calculated using Student's t-test.

MiRNA expression analysis in cells and cell lines

Total RNA was extracted from the different cells the mirVana miRNA Isolation kit (Invitrogen) according to manufacturer's protocol. The total RNA was then reverse transcribed to cDNA using the miScript Reverse Transcription kit (Qiagen). The real-time PCR quantification of mature miRNA was performed using target-specific miScript primer assay (forward primer) and the miScript SYBR Green PCR Kit, which contains the miScript Universal Primer (reverse primer) and QuantiTect SYBR Green PCR Master Mix (Qiagen). The amount of target miRNA input was normalized by human U6 snRNA.

Results

Sequencing analysis of the 3′UTR of CFTR and screening for functional genetic variants

The 3′UTR (1553 bp) of the CFTR gene was sequenced from genomic DNA of 95 patients of which 52 with CF and 43 with CFTR-RD, and 50 control subjects (Table 1). We found three variants. The rs1042180 (c.*1251C>T) was found either in patients and in controls with no significant differences in the allelic frequency; the rs55831234 (c.*1283G>A) was found only in a control subject and the rs10234329 (c.*1043A>C) was identified only in a patient that had a CFTR-RD. We have focused our attention on this latter mutation present in one CFTR-RD patient, i.e., c.*1043A>C variant. First of all, because Gillen et al, have recently identified several miRNAs within the CFTR 3′UTR, we checked if any of these miRNAs fell at the site of the c*1043A>C mutation, but none of them fell on the site of our interest, so we used a variety of software available on the web to check for other miRNAs likely binding the CFTR 3′UTR close to the variant under study. The *in silico* analysis, using TargetScan5.2, predicted two putative binding sites for the miR-509-3p and miR-433. Specifically, the variant c.*1043A>C falls within the 3′ end of

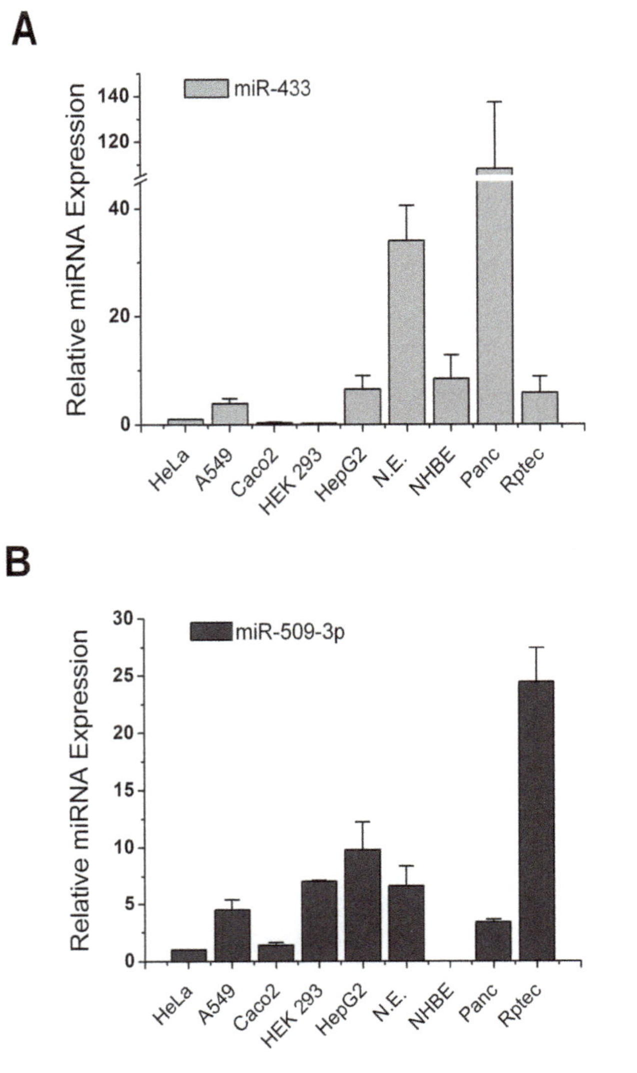

Figure 2. MiRNAs expression analysis. Relative expression of miR-433 A) and miR-509-3p B) in different cell line and brushed nasal epithelial cell (N.E.) compared to Hela cell line.

miR-509-3p region very close to the 3′end of miR-433 region (Figure 1, A–B). So, as the PITA algorithm [10] takes into account not only the strength of binding between miRNAs and the target-sites, but also the accessibility of the target-site, we used the PITA algorithm to analyze whether the genetic variant may change the affinity of the putative miRNAs to the target-site. The PITA algorithm predicted that the variant c.*1043A>C alters the binding of the miR-509-3p and miR-433. The same result was obtained using the RNAhybrid software (Figure 1, C–F). The two algorithms predicted about the same change in free energy between the miRNAs and the wild-type or variant form of CFTR 3′UTR. In particular, concerning the miR-433, the presence of the c.*1043A>C mutations causes a free energy lost of about 1.6 kcal/mol, while concerning the miR-509-3p, the presence of the c.*1043A>C mutation results in a free energy gain of about 7 kcal/mol (Figure 1, C–F).

Expression of miRNA-433 and miR-509-3p in different cell lines and primary human cells

Before starting experiments to validate in silico predictions, we verified the expression of miR-433 and miR-509-3p in different cell lines and primary nasal epithelial cells. As shown in Figure 2, the two miRNAs are differentially expressed in various cell lines and primary cells, the RPTEC cells are those showing a high expression level of miRNA 509-3p compared to other cells, even the HepG2, HEK 293, A549 and nasal epithelial cells showed expression levels of 5–10 times higher than HeLa cells. Concerning the miRNA-433, Panc-1 cells and nasal epithelial cells showed expression levels of 40–120 times higher compared to HeLa cells. The other cell types showed levels similar to each other and approximately 5-fold compared to HeLa cells.

Validation of miRNA Target Sites in the CFTR 3′UTR

Functional validation of the 2 predicted miRNA target sites containing the identified genetic variants was performed using a dual-luciferase assay in HEK 293 and in Panc1 cell lines. A luciferase-reporter construct containing the wild-type 3′UTR of CFTR was co-transfected with the miRNAs mimics of interest. As shown in Figure 3A, a statistically significant reduction of the luciferase activity was observed for both the miRNAs used (miR-509-3p, miR-433) when compared with control mimics. The down regulation observed ranged from a reduction of the luciferase expression of about 50% in the case of miR-433, up to 60% for the miR-509-3p. A western blot analysis was performed to check the levels of CFTR protein in Panc1 cells transient transfected with the two miRNAs. Both miRNAs were able, although to a different extent, to significantly reduce the endogenous levels of CFTR protein (Figure 3B). To further validate and to mimic a more physiological context, where different miRNAs may be expressed at high levels from their genomic loci, we cloned the genes of miR-433 and miR-509-3p in lentiviral vectors. We also constructed a lentiviral vector expressing a short hairpin RNA (shRNA) against the target region of both miR-433 and miR-509-3p (Figure 4A). Then, we produced lentiviral particles with which we transduced Panc 1 cells. So we obtained Panc 1 cells stably expressing each of the two miRNAs of interest or the shRNA (Panc-miR-433, Panc-miR-509-3p, Panc-sh-3′UTR). Thus, we transient transfected each of these cell lines with the wild-type construct of CFTR 3′UTR. The levels of luciferase in cells expressing high levels of miR-433 or miR-509 compared to not transduced cells were comparable to those obtained using the miRNA mimics (Figure 4B, white rectangles), the residual luciferase activity in Panc-sh-3′UTR was close to 10% compared to the control. The same results were obtained in HEK293 cell line.

Effect of the c.*1043A>C mutation on miRNA Target Sites in the CFTR 3′UTR

To verify the RNAhybrid and PITA *in silico* predictions on the effect of c.*1043A>C mutation on the miRNAs-target duplex, we introduced by site-directed mutagenesis the (C) variant within the 3′UTR region of the construct pLuc-CFTR-3′UTR. Thus, we transient transfected the pLuc-CFTR-c.*1043A>C, bearing the (C) variant, in different Panc 1 cells stably expressing the various miRNAs or shRNA. As shown in Figure 4B the (C) variant differentially affects the miRNAs-target duplex. In particular, the luciferase activity of pLuc-CFTR-c.*1043A>C was significant reduced up to 22% ($P<0.01$), in Panc-509-3p compared to the construct pLuc-CFTR-3′UTR. Instead, no significant change was observed between the two constructs transfected into Panc-433 cells. Similarly, either the construct pLuc-CFTR-3′UTR and the

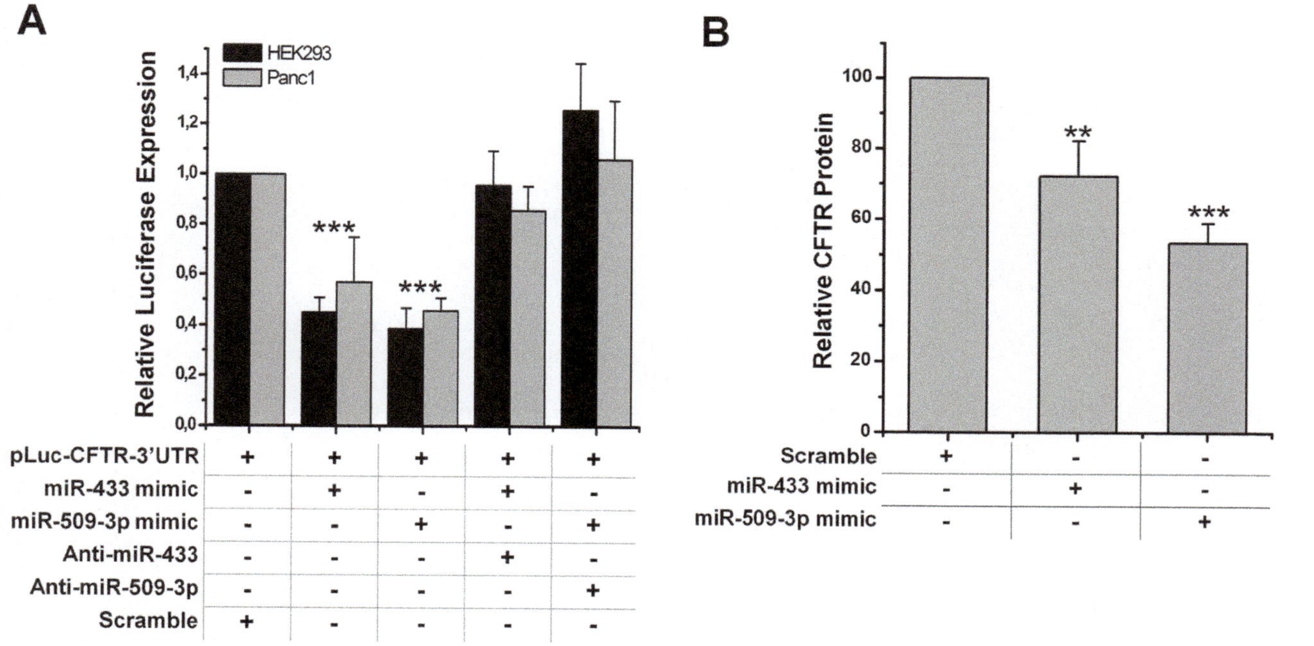

Figure 3. Effect of miR-433 and miR-509-3p on *CFTR*-3′UTR and CFTR protein expression.A: luciferase expression from pLuc-CFTR-3′UTR co-transfected with relative miRNA mimics and miRNA mimics plus anti-miRNA both in HEK293 and Panc1 cell lines, ***p<0.001 **B**: expression of CFTR protein is decreased to about 25% in Panc1 cells transfected with miR-433 mimic (** p<0.01) and about 45% in miR-509-3p (*** p<0.001) transfected cells.

construct pLuc-CFTR-c.*1043A>C have a residual luciferase activity of about 10% when transfected in Panc-sh-3′UTR. To further verify the specificity of action of the two miRNAs we have destroyed the two overlapping target seed regions through site-directed mutagenesis Figure 4A, (construct pLuc-CFTR-3′UTR-mut433-509-3p). The luciferase levels resulting from this construct were not affected by either miRNA or sh-3′UTR activity and was perfectly comparable to that resulting from transfected Panc 1 cells.

Discussion

We identified a SNP in a CFTR-RD patient, already known as rs10234329 that causes an A>C change at the 4575+1043 nucleotide within the 3′ UTR of the *CFTR* gene. The *in silico* prediction indicated that such mutation, the c.*1043A>C, variant is located in the target site of two miRNAs, i.e., the miR-433 and the miR-509-3p, even if two previous studies did not consider such miRNAs as CFTR transcript modulators [8,11]. The *in vitro* analysis demonstrated that the variant significantly enhances the affinity of the CFTR transcript for the miR-509-3p (that we demonstrated to inhibit CFTR expression). The patient had Congenital Bilateral Absence of Vas Deferens (CBAVD), diffuse bronchiectasis, pancreatic sufficiency and a borderline sweat chloride test (i.e., 41 mEq/L). He was heterozygous for the severe F508del mutation and the analysis of one parent revealed that the F508del was *in trans* with the c.*1043A>C mutation. Finally, the variant was not identified in alleles from 100 control subjects. All these data strongly suggest that the c.*1043A>C mutation may have a role in the pathogenesis of CF, impairing the regulation of gene expression, and thus acting as a mild causing disease mutation, since *CFTR-RD* patients typically are compound heterozygous for a severe and a mild CFTR mutation [5]. As regards the miR-433, the presence of the mutation c.*1043A>C, does not significantly influence its action, as expected from the *in silico* prediction. Even if this is the first report of such mechanism in cystic fibrosis (and more extensively in classic mendelian inherited diseases) similar mechanisms are becoming increasingly prevalent; in an attempt to find gene variants responsible for renal cell carcinoma (RCC), Wirsing et al. found that the rs11574744 SNP in the 3′UTR region of the HNF4A gene leads higher levels of HNF4A protein by destroying a target site for miR-34a [12]. Similarly, a SNP in a let-7 miRNA binding site in the KRAS 3′UTR increases Non-Small Cell Lung Cancer risk [13].

On the contrary, we did not identify mutations within the region at the 3′UTR of *CFTR* gene in none of 20 CF patients, homozygous for the F508del mutation, bearing a discordant pulmonary or liver expression. Of course, these data are preliminar because of the low number of patients (although carefully classified on the basis of the phenotype). Going to patients with one or both unidentified mutations, we did not identify peculiar variants within the 3′UTR CFTR region with the exception of the rs1042180, causing an C>T change at the 4575+1251 nucleotide in the 3′ UTR region, that was found in a large percentage of alleles from either CF and CFTR-RD patients and control subjects. Finally, we found the rs55831234 (c.*1283G>A) only in a control subject and in none chromosome from patients. Of course, both mutations c.*1251C>T and c.*1283G>A, even if present in control subjects, may nevertheless play a role in the expression of *CFTR* gene. This may be due not only to the action of miRNAs, but also to an effect on the accessibility to various factors involved in the conformation, translation and stability of CFTR mRNA. Of course, also for these mutations, it would be useful to understand whether they may have a pathological role.

Cystic fibrosis is characterized by a strong clinical heterogeneity. A number of factors affect this clinical variability; i.e: genotype, environmental factors, modifier genes. Our data suggest a new

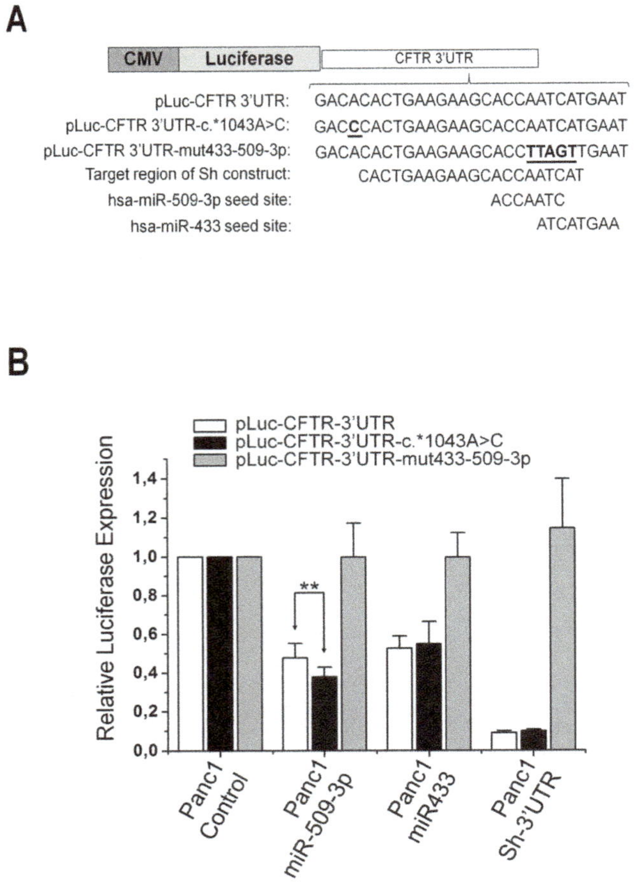

Figure 4. Experimental evaluation of c*1043A>C mutation effect on miRNAs affinity.A: luciferase reporter constructs derived from pGL3-Control vector. Underlined and in bold is shown the location of the variant c.*1043A>C or altered nucleotide bases to destroy the seed overlapping region of miR-433 and miR-509-3p in the CFTR 3'UTR. **B**: luciferase expression from pLuc-CFTR-3'UTR or mutated form constructs transient transfected in different Panc-1 cells stably espressing the miR-433, miR-509-3p or the sh-3'UTR. Data reported here are the means ± St.Dev., **P<0.01

possible molecular mechanism in its pathogenesis. The presence of SNPs in the 3′UTR may cause a variable phenotype, not only in terms of severity but also in terms of organ specificity. In particular, at least two different mechanisms lead to this variability. First, the aberrant expression of miRNAs, whose target sequence is present in the 3′UTR of the *CFTR* gene, may decrease the expression of CFTR protein in specific organs. Secondly, as supported by our data, a decrease of CFTR protein expression can be caused by the presence of SNPs that increase the affinity for a specific miRNA in the 3′UTR of the *CFTR* gene. In addition, our data suggest that the molecular analysis of the 3′UTR region should be performed in all cases in which clinical symptoms are present but no mutation has been identified.

Supporting Information

Figure S1 Repression of CFTR protein expression in Panc1 cells. Western blot analysis of CFTR protein expression in Panc1 cells using a Cell Signaling CFTR antibody after transient transfection of the indicated miRNA mimics. The molecular mass in kDa is indicated on the left-hand side.

Figure S2 Plasmids used for pre-miR and Sh expression. In panel A is shown the pMIRNA1 vector for the miR-433 and miR-509-3p expression, while in the panel B is shown the pmiRZip vector for the interfering RNA expression. Both plasmids were purchased from System Biosciences, SBI, CA–USA. In panel C are shown the oligos used for the amplification of the genomic region of both miR-433 and miR-509-3p, containing the XbaI restriction site at the 5′ end and the XhoI restriction site at the 3′ end. Further, the oligos pair for the interfering RNA is shown, with the sense region in red-bold and the antisense region in bold characters.

Author Contributions

Coordinator: GC. Collection of DNA samples: MS AE RT. Conceived and designed the experiments: FA. Performed the experiments: FA SG. Analyzed the data: FA FZ. Contributed reagents/materials/analysis tools: RT MS. Wrote the paper: FA GC.

References

1. McIntosh I, Cutting GR (1992) Cystic fibrosis transmembrane conductance regulator and the etiology and pathogenesis of cystic fibrosis. FASEB J 6: 2775–2782.
2. Castellani C, Cuppens H, Macek M Jr, Cassiman JJ, Kerem E, et al. (2008) Consensus on the use and interpretation of cystic fibrosis mutation analysis in clinical practice. J Cyst Fibros 7: 179–196.
3. Castaldo G, Polizzi A, Tomaiuolo R, Cazeneuve C, Girodon E, et al. (2005) Comprehensive cystic fibrosis mutation epidemiology and haplotype characterization in a southern Italian population. Ann Hum Genet 69: 15–24.
4. Tomaiuolo R, Sangiuolo F, Bombieri C, Bonizzato A, Cardillo G, et al. (2008) Epidemiology and a novel procedure for large scale analysis of CFTR rearrangements in classic and atypical CF patients: a multicentric Italian study. J Cyst Fibros 7: 347–351.
5. Amato F, Bellia C, Cardillo G, Castaldo G, Ciaccio M, et al. (2011) Extensive molecular analysis of patients bearing CFTR-related disorders. J Mol Diagn 14: 81–89.
6. Castaldo G, Lembo F, Tomaiuolo R (2010) Molecular diagnostics: between chips and customized medicine. Clin Chem Lab Med 48: 973–982.
7. Singh SK, Pal Bhadra M, Girschick HJ, Bhadra U (2008) MicroRNAs--micro in size but macro in function. FEBS J 275: 4929–4944.
8. Gillen AE, Gosalia N, Leir SH, Harris A (2011) MicroRNA regulation of expression of the cystic fibrosis transmembrane conductance regulator gene. Biochem J 438: 25–32.
9. Salvatore F, Scudiero O, Castaldo G (2002) Genotype-phenotype correlation in cystic fibrosis: the role of modifier genes. Am J Med Genet 111: 88–95.
10. Kertesz M, Iovino N, Unnerstall U, Gaul U, Segal E (2007) The role of site accessibility in microRNA target recognition. Nat Genet 39: 1278–1284.
11. Megiorni F, Cialfi S, Dominici C, Quattrucci S, Pizzuti A (2011) Synergistic post-transcriptional regulation of the Cystic Fibrosis Transmembrane conductance Regulator (CFTR) by miR-101 and miR-494 specific binding. PLoS One 6: e26601.
12. Wirsing A, Senkel S, Klein-Hitpass L, Ryffel GU (2011) A systematic analysis of the 3′UTR of HNF4A mRNA reveals an interplay of regulatory elements including miRNA target sites. PLoS One 6: e27438.
13. Chin LJ, Ratner E, Leng S, Zhai R, Nallur S, et al. (2008) A SNP in a let-7 microRNA complementary site in the KRAS 3′ untranslated region increases non-small cell lung cancer risk. Cancer Res 68: 8535–8540.

20

Phenotypic Heterogeneity of *Pseudomonas aeruginosa* Populations in a Cystic Fibrosis Patient

Matthew L. Workentine[1,2], Christopher D. Sibley[4], Bryan Glezerson[4], Swathi Purighalla[4], Jens C. Norgaard-Gron[4], Michael D. Parkins[4,5,6], Harvey R. Rabin[4,5,6], Michael G. Surette[1,2,3,4]*

1 Farncombe Family Digestive Health Research Institute, McMaster University, Hamilton, Ontario, Canada, **2** Department of Medicine, McMaster University, Hamilton, Ontario, Canada, **3** Department of Biochemistry and Biomedical Sciences, McMaster University, Hamilton, Ontario, Canada, **4** Department of Microbiology, Immunology and Infectious Diseases, University of Calgary, Calgary, Alberta, Canada, **5** Department of Medicine, University of Calgary, Calgary, Alberta, Canada, **6** Adult Cystic Fibrosis Clinic, University of Calgary, Calgary, Alberta, Canada

Abstract

The opportunistic pathogen *Pseudomonas aeruginosa* chronically infects the lower airways of patients with cystic fibrosis. Throughout the course of infection this organism undergoes adaptations that contribute to its long-term persistence in the airways. While *P. aeruginosa* diversity has been documented, it is less clear to what extent within-patient diversity contributes to the overall population structure as most studies have been limited to the analysis of only a few isolates per patient per time point. To examine *P. aeruginosa* population structure in more detail we collected multiple isolates from individual sputum samples of a patient chronically colonized with *P. aeruginosa*. This strain collection, comprised of 169 clonal isolates and representing three pulmonary exacerbations as well as clinically stable periods, was assayed for a wide selection of phenotypes. These phenotypes included colony morphology, motility, quorum sensing, protease activity, auxotrophy, siderophore levels, antibiotic resistance, and growth profiles. Each phenotype displayed significant variation even within isolates of the same colony morphotype from the same sample. Isolates demonstrated a large degree of individuality across phenotypes, despite being part of a single clonal lineage, suggesting that the *P. aeruginosa* population in the cystic fibrosis airways is being significantly under-sampled.

Editor: John R. Battista, Louisiana State University and A & M College, United States of America

Funding: This work was supported by grants from Cystic Fibrosis Canada to M.G.S and to M.D.P. and a postdoctoral fellowship to M.L.W. M.G.S. is also supported as a Canada Research Chair in Interdisciplinary Microbiome Research. C.D.S. was supported by a Canada Graduate Scholarship from the Canadian Institutes of Health Research. The funders had no role in study design, data collection and analysis, decision to publish, or preparation of the manuscript.

Competing Interests: The authors have declared that no competing interests exist.

* E-mail: surette@mcmaster.ca

Introduction

Cystic fibrosis (CF) is an autosomal recessive disorder where mutations in the CF transmembrane conductance regulator lead to altered ion flux and the reduction of fluid covering the surface of airway epithelial cells [1–3]. Compromised innate immunity including reduced mucociliary clearance in patients with CF, gives a variety of species the opportunity to colonize the lower airways, ultimately generating long-term complex bacterial infections [2,4–6]. The microbial community in the CF lung is known to be complex[7–15] and its changing dynamics can influence severity of disease [10,16]. However, *Pseudomonas aeruginosa* infection is traditionally considered to be the most common agent contributing to lung function decline and ultimate mortality in CF patients [17–19]. *P. aeruginosa* infections in the lower airways can be maintained for decades. Throughout this time *P. aeruginosa* exhibits genetic and phenotypic diversity thought to occur as the organism adapts to the lower airway environment [20,21]. Some factors considered to be the hallmarks of *P. aeruginosa* adaption to the CF airways include a switch to the mucoid phenotype [22] and loss of motility [23]. Diverse colony morphologies from clonal populations of *P. aeruginosa* are also routinely observed in clinical laboratories and some have been linked to increased antibiotic resistance and enhanced cytotoxicity [24–26]. It has been suggested that these colony variants have adaptations specific for persistence in the lower airways [27].

Although such genetic and phenotypic changes have been documented, cross-sectional studies are often limited to a small number time points from a large number of patients [28] and longitudinal studies by a large number of time points from a small number of patients [20] thus the full extent of micro-evolutionary dynamics that might be present throughout the course of infection is not yet well defined. Furthermore, most studies have analyzed a limited number of isolates per sample. Recent evidence suggests that this leads to an underestimation of the true diversity present in a sample. For example, Wilder and colleagues examined quorum-sensing phenotypes in clinical *P. aeruginosa* isolates and found very high within-patient diversity [29]. In addition, large variation in antibiotic resistance profiles was found for *P. aeruginosa* isolates with the same morphotype [30,31]. By way of screening multiple phenotypes Mowat *et al.* have demonstrated high intraspecific diversity in the *P. aeruginosa* Liverpool Epidemic Strain (LES) that is responsible for a significant burden of infection in both Europe and North America [32]. One implication of high intraspecific diversity in the CF airways is that analysis of only a few isolates may lead to a misrepresentation of the *P. aeruginosa* phenotype, such as oversimplified antibiotic resistance profiles. Therefore a clear understanding of *P. aeruginosa* evolutionary dynamics in the CF airways that includes intraspecific diversity is necessary.

In the present study we examined the population dynamics of a newly described transmissible strain of *P. aeruginosa* [33] in a single patient over the course of one year. A number of phenotypes linked to survival and persistence in the CF airways were measured including colony morphology, motility, quorum sensing, proteases, auxotrophy, siderophores, growth profiles and antibiotic resistance. This represents more phenotypes than have been previously examined in single studies of *P. aeruginosa* intraspecific diversity. We observed very high diversity across all phenotypes even within isolates of a single colony morphotype recovered from a single sputum sample, which has been noted previously in LES epidemic *P. aeruginosa* strain [32]. However, we find that each phenotype is highly variable between isolates and not accurately characterized as simply the presence or absence of a phenotype. No obvious patterns in phenotype prevalence or activity was strongly correlated with early exacerbation samples or periods of clinical stability. This suggests that *P. aeruginosa* contribution to acute exacerbation may arise in part through complex population interactions rather than fluctuations in specific virulent strains within the population.

Results

The source patient was a 31 year old male (genotype F508del/F508del) with advanced CF airways disease, whom had been chronically infected with *P. aeruginosa* for 20 years. Thirty-four expectorated sputum samples were collected from the patient over one year, and comprised 16 samples collected during periods of clinical stability and 18 samples collected through three acute pulmonary exacerbations during which the patient was hospitalized and treated with parenteral anti-pseudomonal therapies (Table S1). Multiple *P. aeruginosa* isolates were collected from each sample as well as multiple isolates with identical colony morphologies (representative plate image shown in Figure S1). To ensure that slow growing colonies were not overlooked the plates were allowed to incubate for 72 h, which is longer than usual for a clinical lab. Fourteen unique colony morphologies were identified in a total of 169 isolates and were comprised of equal numbers of mucoid and non-mucoid isolates (Figure 1A). The cell counts for each colony type varied greatly throughout the exacerbation periods and no associations between exacerbation and a particular colony type were observed (Figure 1B). We also noted for all three exacerbations that the total levels of *P. aeruginosa* did not show any decrease, despite antibiotic therapy and resolution of symptoms.

The genetic variability of this population was monitored using pulse field gel electrophoresis (PFGE). The pulse-field patterns reveal that all isolates belong to a single clonal group with only 2–3 band differences between them (Figure 2 and Figure S2), which is indicated by a Dice coefficient of greater than 80% for all the pairwise combinations of isolates. The PFGE patterns of the isolates matched the pattern of a recently identified epidemic strain (highlighted in yellow in Figure 2 and indicated in Figure S2), the Prairie Epidemic Strain (PES), which is known to be present in ~30% of the patients in the clinic that the source patient was attending [33].

To assemble phenotype profiles we measured 21 different phenotypes related to virulence, including swimming, swarming and twitching motility, activity of several proteases, quorum sensing signal molecule production, siderophore levels, antibiotic resistance to five antibiotics, and growth profiles in different media types, including nutrient rich medium, minimal medium, synthetic CF medium and medium lacking amino acids to measure the prevalence of auxotrophy. The most prominent feature that emerged from this analysis (summarized in Figure 3) is the large amount of variance within each phenotype. Each isolate demonstrated a high degree of individuality from the other isolates (i.e. no two isolates were the same) and we observed a large range in values for every phenotype measured beyond the normal variation inherent to the assays (Figure S3). We also noted that although some phenotypes, such as gelatinase and protease activity were highly correlated, for the most part, phenotypes behaved independently (Figure S4). Moreover, there were no significant changes in mean phenotype values over time (Figure S5). It is also interesting to note that there were approximately equal numbers of motile and non-motile organisms. In the swimming assay 51% of all the isolates were motile and in the swarming assay 56% were motile. There was also an approximately equal number of mucoid and non-mucoid colony types in both the motile and non-motile isolates (data not shown). That is to say, loss of motility was not correlated to mucoidy.

Disk diffusion assays were used to assess antibiotic susceptibility, which also showed a high level of variation (Figure 4). Many of the morphotypes had both sensitive and resistant isolates but even among the sensitive isolates there was large variability in the zone of clearing (colistin is a good example of this). Although all isolates were susceptible to colistin there was a range of zone sizes observed, with some approaching resistant. Importantly, this patient was exposed to colistin for only a few weeks during a clinically stable period and had no colistin exposure during exacerbation periods that samples were collected from (Table S1). In this set of isolates there was no association with acute antibiotic exposure during exacerbation and the abundance of resistant isolates in the population (Figure S6). We also noted that neither morphotype nor mucoidy were associated with any particular antibiotic resistance profile (Figure 4).

A clustering analysis of all the phenotypes measured (Figure 5) reveals a high level of individuality present in these isolates. What is noteworthy from the clustering is that the isolates do not cluster by morphotype or mucoidy or any of the other metadata variables, including date of isolation (not shown). Rather, the isolates clustered into 3 main phenotypic groups, which can also be seen in the principle components analysis (PCA) (Figure S7). To determine if there was any correlation between the genetic (PFGE profile) and phenotypic measures each isolate in the UPGMA tree was coloured according to the phenotypic groups it fell into (Figure 2). In general there was not good agreement between the genetic and phenotypic clustering with the exception of one group of isolates. The group is highlighted in purple in both the genetic (Figure 2) and phenotypic (Figure 5) data. The functional importance of any groups remains to be explored, however, these findings do highlight the depth of diversity even within a single morphotype.

The diversity present within a single sample was analyzed more in depth by selecting 44 individual isolates from each of two different morphotypes (4 and 5) from one sputum sample that was collected at later date. For these additional 88 isolates we measured a subset of phenotypes; antibiotic sensitivity, protease production and swimming motility. As shown in Figure 6 there was a large degree of phenotypic variation even within isolates from a single sample and of a single colony morphotype. Both morphotypes had motile and non-motile isolates and morphotype 5 had both protease positive and negative isolates. Both morphotypes also had a large distribution of antibiotic sensitive isolates and with the exception of colistin, a good number of resistant isolates. The large phenotypic variation observed in

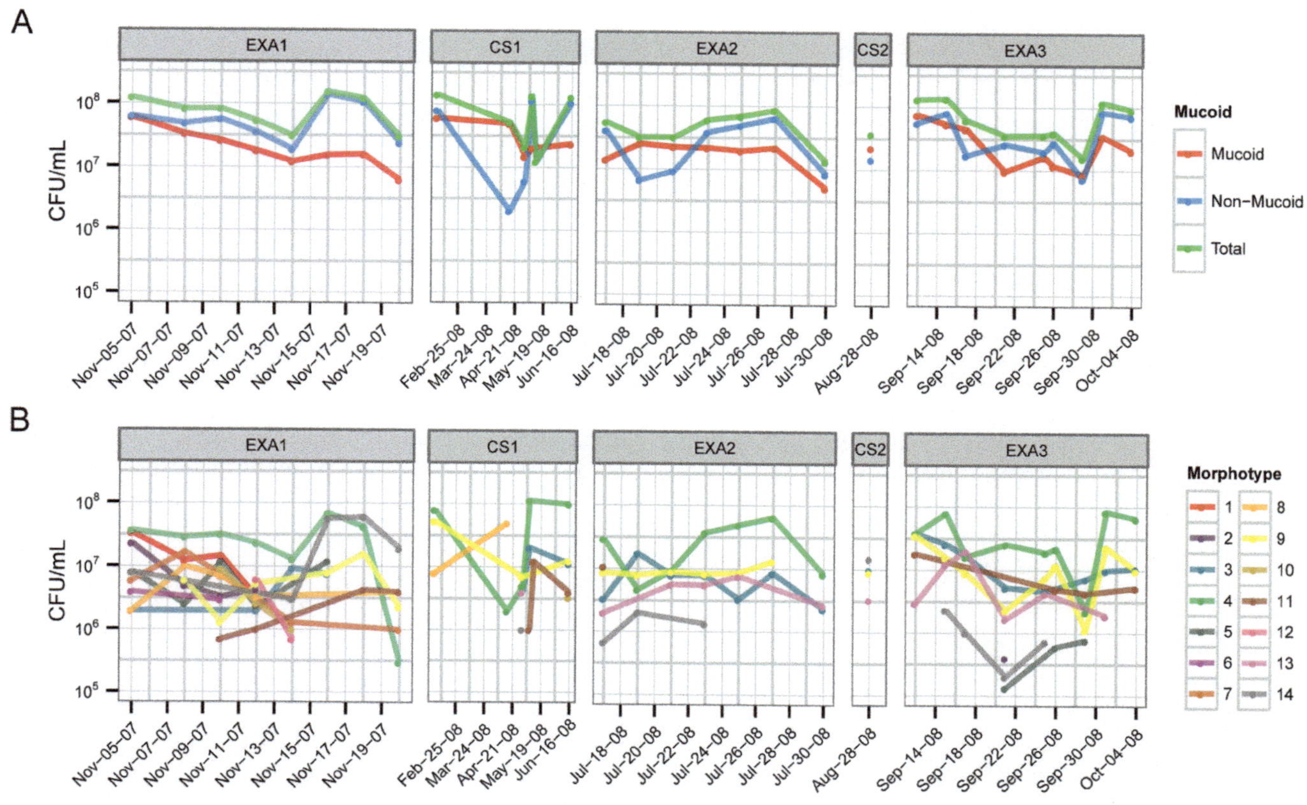

Figure 1. Levels of *P. aeruginosa* during three pulmonary exacerbation periods over the course of one year. A, Total levels, expressed as colony forming units (CFU) per mL of sputum are shown in green and the numbers of mucoid and non-mucoid isolates are indicated in red and blue, respectively. B, The CFU per ml for each of the 14 colony types are shown.

similar morphotypes was still present at a higher sampling depth, indicating that even with this number of isolates under-sampling is still occurring.

To verify that such high diversity is not limited to a single patient, samples were collected from an additional 3 patients during a single pulmonary exacerbation. We found high phenotypic diversity among the *P. aeruginosa* isolates from all patients

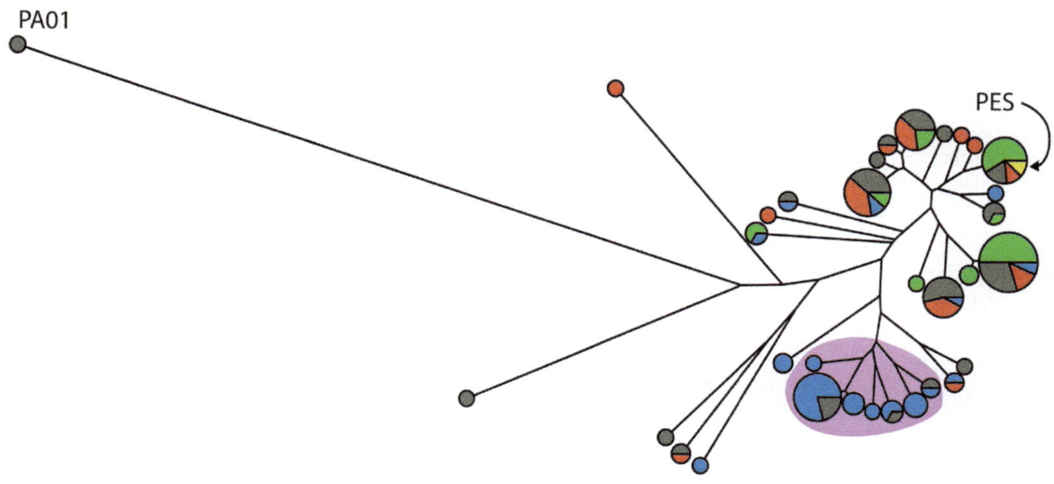

Figure 2. Genetic diversity present in collected *P. aeruginosa* isolates from a single patient. The Dice coefficient from pulse field gel electrophoresis patterns of each isolate was used to construct a UPGMA tree (unrooted). Isolates from this study were no more than 20% different from each other but were more than 40% different from PA01. Isolates with identical PFGE patterns are grouped into a single node where the size of that node represents the number of isolates. Colouring represents the phenotypic group that the isolate falls into and the colours match the colouring in Figure 5. Two PES strains were included in the analysis and are coloured in yellow. The cluster highlighted by purple is a cluster where the phenotypic and genetic groups are similar.

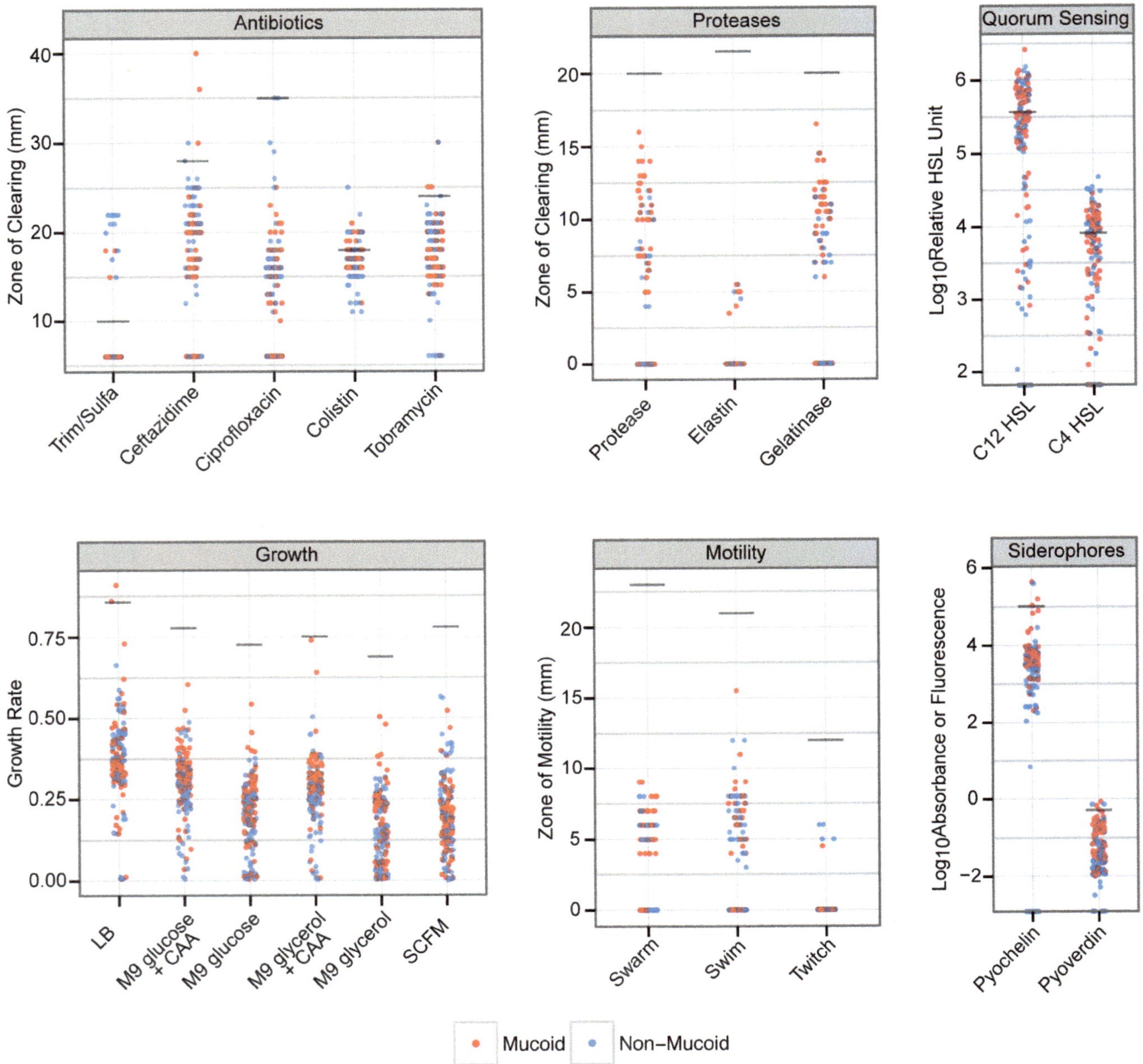

Figure 3. Phenotypic diversity present in collected *P. aeruginosa* isolates from a single patient. The data points are coloured according to whether the isolate was classified as mucoid or not. Grey lines indicate the phenotype value measured for the common lab strain, PA01.

examined, which were comprised of both PES and non-PES strains (Figure S8). Levels of *P. aeruginosa* were monitored throughout the course of the exacerbation and we found that in one of the three patients *P. aeruginosa* levels did not decrease (Figure S9C), as we observed for the main patient (Figure 1A and Figure S9D). However, in two of the patients there was a noticeable drop in *P. aeruginosa* levels near the end of the exacerbation period (Figure S9 A and B). For all patients examined we found that levels of mucoid and non-mucoid isolates were approximately the same and this did not change during exacerbation periods (Figure S9). Furthermore in the patients where the levels of *P. aeruginosa* dropped during the exacerbation we did not observe any corresponding decrease in measured antibiotic resistance (data not shown), however, deeper sampling will be required to fully resolve this.

Discussion

The phenotypic variability in *P. aeruginosa* isolates from chronic CF patients is documented in the literature. *P. aeruginosa* isolates, even clonal isolates from the same sample, have been shown to have large variations in motility [34,35], quorum sensing [29,34], virulence factor production [34–36], antibiotic susceptibility [30,31,36] and biofilm formation [34]. A recent study examined phenotypic and genetic variability in the *P. aeruginosa* Liverpool Epidemic Strain (LES) from 10 adult CF patients and found large diversity in virulence factors, auxotrophy, hypermutability, antibiotic resistance, presence of prophage, and colony morphotype [32]. Here we expand the range of phenotypes examined and identify high phenotypic diversity within a novel epidemic strain, PES. There are several key similarities between the LES and PES

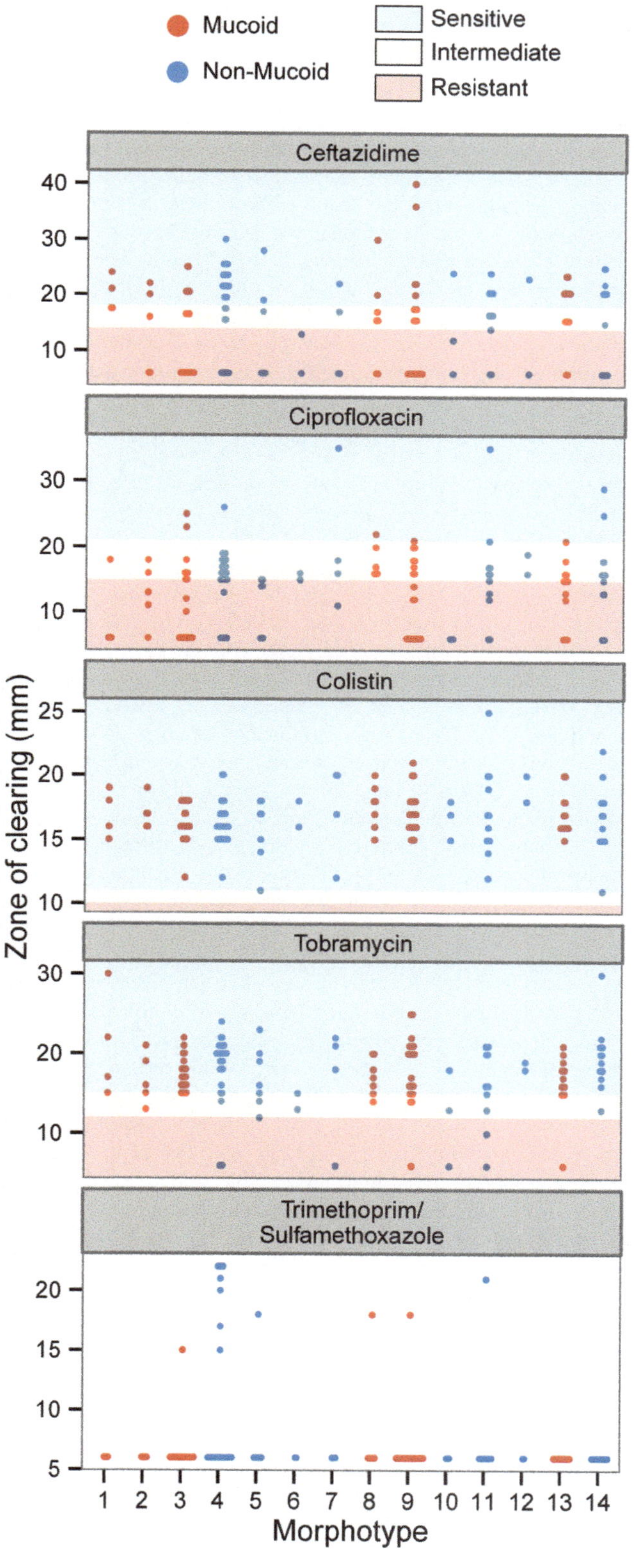

Figure 4. Distribution of antibiotic resistance among the analyzed isolates. Shown are zones of clearing from disc diffusion assays for five commonly used antibiotics in CF clinics and the resistance cutoffs for each antibiotic are given by the dashed lines. Resistance profiles for each colony morphotype are shown individually and coloured according to whether that colony type was initially identified as mucoid or not. Cutoff values for resistant, intermediate and sensitive are indicated by the colour of the background; red, yellow and blue, respectively. Cutoff values for trimethoprim/sulfamethoxazole are not published for *P. aeruginosa* by the CLSI.

isolate collections. First, both demonstrate a high degree of variability within isolates from a single sample, indicating the need for deeper sampling. In addition, the heterogeneity in antibiotic resistant profiles of both sets of isolates remained consistent during and after antibiotic treatment, indicating a lack of positive selection for resistance or negative selection for sensitivity. An important observation from our analysis of the PES isolates is that

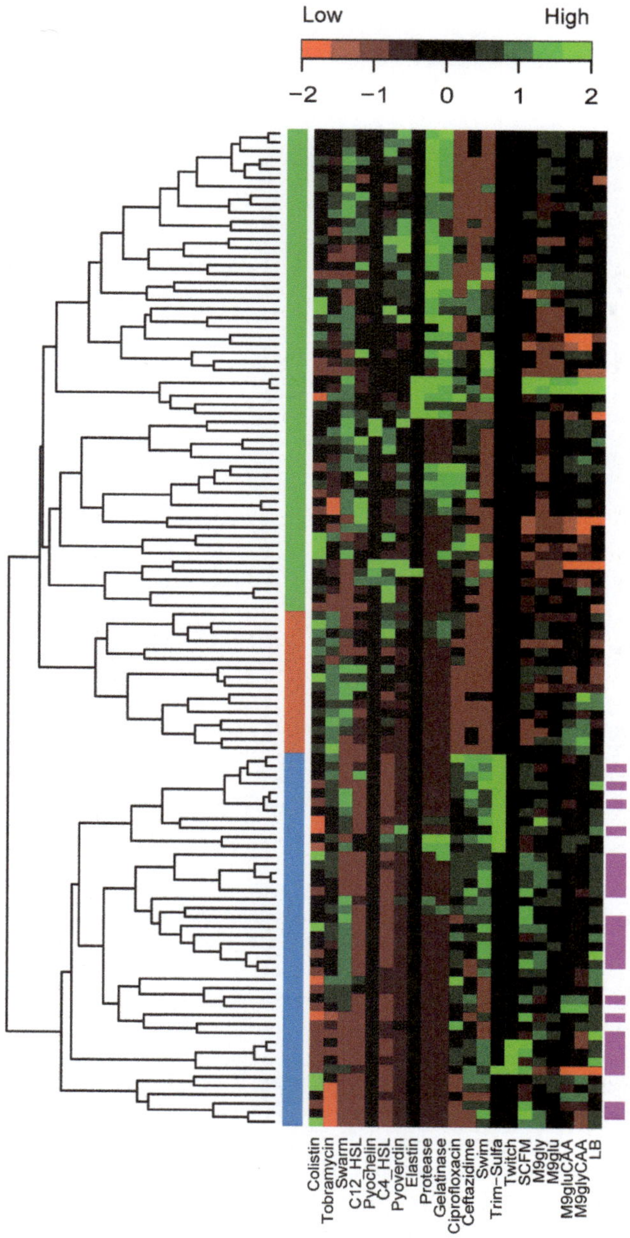

Figure 5. Hierarchical cluster analysis of the phenotype profiles. Green indicates a value above the mean and red indicates a value below the mean. The three colours on the left side indicate the three main cluster groups. Purple bars on the right side indicate the isolates that group closely in both the phenotypic and genetic analysis. Missing values were removed prior to analysis.

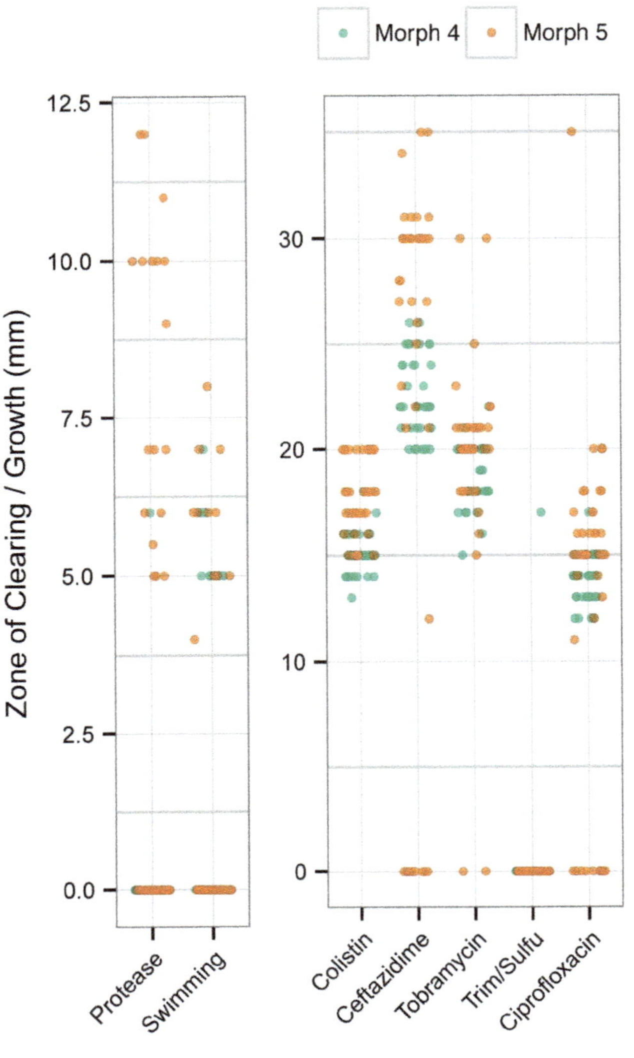

Figure 6. Phenotypic diversity of *P. aeruginosa* isolates from a single sample. Phenotype profiles were obtained from a total of 88 isolates and were comprised of two different colony morphologies, which are shown as orange and green on the plot.

binning a phenotype into categories such as 'high' or 'low' will lead to the underestimation of the true diversity in a sample. For example even though many of our isolates would be classified as sensitive to a number of antibiotics there was still variability within the measured zones of clearing. As such, if isolates are to be clustered for further analysis, as done by Mowat *et al.*, [32], binning the phenotypes will underestimate the diversity and may not represent an accurate population structure. What is clear however, from the current study and others [29,30,32,36] is that the *P. aeruginosa* population is being under-sampled based on morphotype assessment alone. How many isolates per sample are required to accurately describe the population structure and how best to measure diversity are significant challenges.

Many studies have also documented the genetic variability inherent to *P. aeruginosa* during chronic lower airway infections. Mutational targets often identified are *mexZ*, *lasR*, and *mucA*, a regulator of alginate biosynthesis [20,28,37–39]. For some time many *P. aeruginosa* adaptations have been associated with adaptation to and chronic persistence of the bacterium in the lower airways. Examples of this include loss of motility, thought to be associated with decreased immunogenicity [23,40], and conversion to the mucoid phenotype, a key indicator of poor prognosis [22,41,42]. Evidence presented in the current study suggests that non-mucoid isolates are just as prevalent as mucoid isolates. Similarly, we found both motile and non-motile isolates in relatively equal abundance, which has been observed previously [32,35,36]. The implication of this is that rather than a single phenotype dominating the lung environment, a number of phenotypes can evolve, including but not restricted to, mucoid phenotypes. Given that environmental heterogeneity is very good explanation for the maintenance of diversity [43], the rapid emergence of large diversity in the *Pseudomonas* population is suggestive of many diverse niches within the lower airways leading to a number of sub-populations [29]. It is also important to note that expectorated sputum by its very nature is not necessarily representative of the entire lung and we do not know whether it represents a sample from one lobe or a mixture (and will vary between samples). However, most of our samples were collected during physiotherapy and therefore may be more representative than single spontaneous sputum samples.

Adaptive radiation, the evolution of multiple lineages to fill available niches [44,45], is perhaps the most attractive theory to account for the emergence of such diversity in lower airway *Pseudomonas* populations. Lee *et al.*, observed large diversification of *E. coli* populations in monoassociated mice over a period of 1000 days, which corresponded to approximately 20,000 *E. coli* generations [46]. In a very reproducible manner, *P. fluorescens* rapidly diversifies into multiple niche specialists within a matter of days [47]. In *Salmonella*, laboratory passage leads to rapid loss of a spatial phenotype and accumulation of *rpoS* mutations [48]. The evolved populations exhibited a complex distribution of *rpoS* activity indicating that many different types of mutations were being generated even in the absence of spatial heterogeneity [48]. These examples highlight how spatial heterogeneity and niche partitioning can drive diversification, both of which are relevant in the complex and dynamic CF airways. It is important to note as well, that it is not clear if underlying cause of the phenotypic diversity is exclusively genetic in origin or partly a result of phenotypic plasticity. Although there were certainly genetic differences between the isolates, PFGE was not able to distinguish all the individual isolates due to inherent lack of resolution.

In conclusion, the high intraspecific diversity of *P. aeruginosa* populations demonstrated here and in other studies, indicates that caution is in order when making conclusions based on the analysis of a small number of samples. Assuming that one (or a few) isolates is representative of the entire population can lead to under-estimations of the true diversity present. This may also lead to inaccurate descriptions of *P. aeruginosa* phenotypes such as antibiotic resistance, which would have significant implications for antibiotic therapy [31]. There are also implications for detailed genetic and physiological studies that usually focus on a single isolate [27]. Such studies can provide useful information, however, to extend these conclusions to the whole population may not be accurate. Furthermore, from an ecological standpoint, under-estimating the diversity can also hinder attempts to fully understand the population structure and persistence of this organism in the lower airways. Given the polymicrobial nature of the CF lower airway infection it will be paramount to understand how *P. aeruginosa* diversity can influence the population structure of the whole polymicrobial community and vice versa. *P. aeruginosa* contribution to disease progression in CF may require an understanding of the interaction of a complex population of *P. aeruginosa* as a whole with the host and other microbes. Variants within the *P. aeruginosa* population may contribute to different aspects of disease progression such as the transition to a pulmonary exacerbation. Furthermore we know that other organisms in the lower airway community can modulate *P. aeruginosa* virulence [49,50] and it may be that the key to understanding these infections lies in the interplay between the various community members, including diverse *P. aeruginosa* sub-populations.

Materials and Methods

Ethics Statement

The research performed in this study including sample collection and subject consent procedures has been approved by the Conjoint Health Research Ethics Board of the Faculties of Medicine, Nursing and Kinesiology, University of Calgary (CHREB), approval number E-23087: Collection, Storage and Banking of Tissue Samples (Blood and Sputum) and Sputum Microbial Isolates of Patients Attending the Adult Cystic Fibrosis Clinic, University of Calgary Medical Clinic of the Foothills Medical Center for the purposes of CF research. Subject consent was provided in written format through an informed consent form approved by the CHREB.

Sample collection and bacterial isolation

Starting in the fall of 2007 serial sputum samples were collected from an adult CF patient from the Southern Alberta Adult CF clinic. After physical therapy targeting the four quadrants of the lungs, sputum was ptyalized four times and pooled into sterile containers. Within a period of two hours after collection, sputum samples were sheared by passage through a 1-cc needleless syringe to help emulsify the sample and then serially diluted in nutrient rich brain heart infusion (BHI) broth (BD). The 10^{-3}, 10^{-4} and 10^{-5} dilutions were first rigorously vortexed and 300 µL was plated on large (150 mm diameter, VWR) MacConkey (BD) (MAC) agar plates. After incubation for a minimum of 72 h and up to 96 h at 37°C, plates were visually inspected for growth of *P. aeruginosa* and morphotypes were identified based on colony size, pigment production, texture and mucoidy. A representative colony of each morphotype was purified three times on MAC plates and on Pseudomonas Isolation Agar (BD) (PIA) to confirm that the isolated colony was *P. aeruginosa.* Upon purification, colony morphology was compared to the morphology found on the initial sample plate. Morphotype stability of each isolate was checked by plating isolates on MAC plates and inspecting for changes in colony morphology after 48 hours of incubation at 37°C. Isolates were frozen at −80°C in 10% (w/v) skim milk powder (BD). One hundred sixty-nine *P. aeruginosa* isolates were collected through three exacerbations and 7 separate samples collected from routine visits to the CF clinic. An additional 88 isolates, comprised from two colony types, were collected at a later date from a single sputum sample.

For storage and routine assays the isolates were arrayed in multi-well plates containing TSB broth with 20% (w/v) glycerol and frozen at −80°C. For phenotyping, multi-well plates containing TSB or BHI were inoculated from the frozen storage plates using a pin replicator. Plates were then sealed with sealing tape and incubated for 24 or 48 hours with shaking at 37°C. After incubation, cultures were diluted (1/10) into 100 µl of fresh media and incubated for a further 4 hours at 37°C before being used as inoculants for phenotype assays. All isolates exhibited reproducible phenotypes when assayed as described. Many of the assays (e.g. motility) show day-to-day variability due to subtle differences in conditions but the relative phenotype measurements compared to control strains were consistent.

Phenotype Assays

Phenotype assays were performed according standard protocols previously described in the literature and summarized below. Full method details can be found in the supplementary information. Protease production was measured using dialyzed brain heart infusion (D-BHI) milk media [51]. Gelatinase and elastin activity were assayed using previously described assays [52,53]. Swimming motility of *P. aeruginosa* was investigated by using 0.3% (w/v) agar LB plates and swarming was assayed using nutrient glucose media solidified with 0.5% (w/v) agar [54]. Twitching was measured using thin LB media without salt (LBNS) [55]. *P. aeruginosa* was tested for resistance to commonly used anti-pseudomonal drugs using a modified Kirby Bauer disk diffusion method. Five common anti-pseudomonal antibiotics at clinically relevant concentrations were tested, ceftazidime 30 µg (CAZ, Sigma, Aldrich); ciprofloxacin 5 µg (CIP, Sigma, Aldrich), tobramycin 10 µg (NN, Sigma, Aldrich), trimethoprim/sulfamethoxazole 1.25 µg/23.75 µg (SXT, Sigma, Aldrich), colistin 10 µg (CL, Sigma, Aldrich). Zone diameters of clearing were measured and isolates were classified as described by the Clinical Laboratory Standards Institute, (formerly National Committee on Clinical Laboratory Standards) guidelines as resistant, intermediate or susceptible to the antibiotic [56]. Both 3-oxo-C12 HSL and C4 HSL autoinducer production of *P. aeruginosa* isolates were measured using previously described assays [57]. Growth in auxotrophic conditions was tested with M9 minimal media supplemented with either 0.5% (w/v) dextrose or glycerol, with and without 0.2% (w/v) casamino acids (CAA). Growth in high nutrient media was measured using LB media and growth was also measured in synthetic CF medium [58]. Siderophores were directly measured from spent media of cultures that were grown in M9 minimal media supplemented with glucose and CAA as described [59]. The presence of pyoverdin was assayed by measuring absorbance at 405 nm and pyochelin was assayed by measuring fluorescence with an excitation of 355 nm and emission at 460 nm. Raw data for the phenotype measurements is available upon request.

Data analysis

For comparison across different phenotypes mean measurements were normalized by unit variance scaling (dividing each value by the standard deviation of that phenotype) and then by mean centering. Principal component analysis and clustering using the Pearson correlation and un-weighted pair group average (UPGMA) was done in R [60]. Growth curves were fit using a spline method and growth parameters estimated from the fits [61]. Maximum growth rates were used for further analysis.

Pulse-field gel electrophoresis

Strains were inoculated from frozen stocks onto BHI agar and cultured at 37°C for 48 hours. A cell suspension equivalent to a 1.5 MacFarland standard was prepared in suspension buffer (1 M NaCl, 10 mM Tris-HCL, pH 7.6) and mixed with an equal volume of molton 1% (w/v) SeaKem Gold Agarose in TE_1 buffer (10 mM Tris-HCL, 1 mM EDTA, pH 7.6). This mixture was added immediately to a prepared PFGE plug mold (BioRad). Once the plugs were solidified the embedded cells were lysed for 4 h at 37°C in lysis solution (1 M NaCl, 100 mM EDTA, 0.5% Brij-58, 0.5% sarcosyl, 0.2% deoxycholate, 6 mM Tris-HCl [pH 7.6], 1 mg/mL lysozyme, 20 µg/mL RNase). This was followed by an overnight incubation at 50°C in ESP solution (0.5 M EDTA [pH 9], 1% sarcosyl, 70 µg/mL proteinase K) to digest proteins. Lysed plugs were washed 5 times in $TE_{0.1}$ (T10 mM Tris-HCL, 0.1 mM EDTA, pH 7.6) to remove all traces of lysis and ESP solutions. Plugs were stored temporarily at 4°C in

$TE_{0.1}$. Prior to restriction digest the plugs were incubated with 1X reaction buffer (NEBuffer 4) for 15 min at room temperature to allow the buffer to fully penetrate the plug. Each plug was digested with 20U *SpeI* (New England Biolabs) for 4 h at 37°C in 1X reaction buffer with agitation every hour to ensure complete restriction.

Electrophoresis was performed using the BioRad CHEF Mapper PFGE system according to manufacturers instructions. 1% agarorse gels were prepared with SeaKem Gold agarose in 0.5X TBE. Plugs were loaded along with the lambda ladder (New England Biolabs) and overlayed with more agarose. Running conditions were as follows: running buffer: 0.5X TBE, temperature: 10°C, initial switch time: 5 sec, final switch time: 45 sec, included angle: 120°, cell voltage: 6 V/cm, run time: 20 hours. Gels were stained for 60 min with 0.5X GelRed fluorescent nucleic acid stain (Biotium), rinsed 3X in distilled water and imaged on a UV transilluminator.

Gel images were inverted and the contrast and brightness optimized in Adobe Photoshop using the 'Curves' tool. Optimized images were analyzed with BioNumerics (Applied Maths). After gel normalization bands were assigned manually. Sample lanes were compared using the Dice coefficient, allowing for a 1% tolerance in band matching. Hierarchical clustering was performed using the un-weighted pair group average (UPGMA) linkage and selecting the highest scoring tree from 200 permutations.

Supporting Information

Figure S1 Representative plate showing the diversity of colony morphologies of *P. aeruginosa* isolates from a single sputum sample.

Figure S2 Pulse-field gel electrophoresis. A UPGMA tree based on PFGE patterns across all the isolates compared using the Dice coefficient. The tree is identical to the one shown in Figure 2, but has been rooted to allow for display of the gel images.

Figure S3 Variation in growth measures. Growth rates for each isolate under different media types are shown with error bars (standard deviation). Isolates were sorted according to their growth in M9 minimal media with glucose and case amino acids.

Figure S4 Correlation matrix of the measured phenotypes. The Pearson correlation coefficient was calculated for each phenotype pair where the yellow represents a high correlation (close to 1) and blue represents no correlation (close to 0).

Figure S5 Changes in mean phenotype values over time. The mean of each phenotype was calculated for each sputum sample. The point are coloured according to the clinical status. A local smoothing function, shown with a blue line (shaded area represents 95% confidence intervals) was added to identify any trends present in the data.

Figure S6 Antibiotic susceptibility profiles of the collected isolates during the three pulmonary exacerbations. Isolates were classified based on zone sizes from disk diffusion assays. For each sputum sample the relative proportion of resistant (red), intermediate (blue), and sensitive (green) isolates is shown for the four antibiotics where standardized cutoff values for *P. aeruginosa* are available.

Figure S7 PCA analysis of the measured phenotype profiles. The first two components are shown and the data points are coloured according to the cluster pattern observed in the hierarchical cluster analysis. The amount of variation (in percent) explained by each principle component is shown on the axis.

Figure S8 Phenotypic diversity of *P. aeruginosa* isolates from multiple CF patients. Isolates were collected from an additional 3 CF patients to determine the extent of phenotypic diversity. Samples were collected during a single exacerbation period and processed as before. Multiple isolates were collected from each sample, which often contained both mucoid (red) and non-mucoid (blue) isolates. Patient 1 was colonized with a non-PES strain while both patients 2 and 3 were colonized with PES.

Figure S9 Responders versus non-responders. Cell counts for mucoid (red), non-mucoid (blue), and total (green) *P. aeruginosa* in 4 CF patients throughout the course of a pulmonary exacerbation. Patient 4 is the patient from which the isolates in the current study were collected. Patients 2, 3 and 4 were colonized with the PES strain while the Patient 1 had a non-PES strain. Patients 1 and 2 showed a decline in total *P. aeruginosa* levels and are defined as 'responders', i.e. the drop in cell count corresponded with administration of antibiotic therapy. Patients 3 and 4 did not show any drop in *P. aeruginosa* levels despite resolution of exacerbation symptoms and can defined as 'non-responders'.

Table S1 Sample Details.

Acknowledgments

We acknowledge the Southern Alberta CF Clinic for their contribution, in particular Julie Wilson, for efforts to coordinate specimen processing. We would also like to thank the patient for his participation in this study.

Author Contributions

Conceived and designed the experiments: MLW CDS HRR MGS. Performed the experiments: MLW CDS BG SP JCN. Analyzed the data: MLW CDS MDP MGS. Wrote the paper: MLW MDP MGS.

References

1. Matsui H, Grubb BR, Tarran R, Randell SH, Gatzy JT, et al. (1998) Evidence for periciliary liquid layer depletion, not abnormal ion composition, in the pathogenesis of cystic fibrosis airways disease. Cell 95: 1005–1015.
2. Lipuma JJ (2010) The changing microbial epidemiology in cystic fibrosis. Clinical Microbiology Reviews 23: 299–323. doi:10.1128/CMR.00068-09.
3. Davis PB, Drumm M, Konstan MW (1996) Cystic fibrosis. Am J Respir Crit Care Med 154: 1229–1256.
4. Lyczak JB, Cannon CL, Pier GB (2002) Lung infections associated with cystic fibrosis. Clinical Microbiology Reviews 15: 194–222.
5. Hauser AR, Jain M, Bar-Meir M, McColley SA (2011) Clinical significance of microbial infection and adaptation in cystic fibrosis. Clinical Microbiology Reviews 24: 29–70. doi:10.1128/CMR.00036-10.
6. Sibley CD, Surette MG (2011) The polymicrobial nature of airway infections in cystic fibrosis: Cangene Gold Medal Lecture. Can J Microbiol 57: 69–77. doi:10.1139/w10-105.
7. Stressmann FA, Rogers GB, van der Gast CJ, Marsh P, Vermeer LS, et al. (2012) Long-term cultivation-independent microbial diversity analysis demonstrates that bacterial communities infecting the adult cystic fibrosis lung show stability and resilience. Thorax. doi:10.1136/thoraxjnl-2011-200932.

8. Zhao J, Schloss PD, Kalikin LM, Carmody LA, Foster BK, et al. (2012) Decade-long bacterial community dynamics in cystic fibrosis airways. P Natl Acad Sci Usa 109: 5809–5814. doi:10.1073/pnas.1120577109.
9. Tunney MM, Klem ER, Fodor AA, Gilpin DF, Moriarty TF, et al. (2011) Use of culture and molecular analysis to determine the effect of antibiotic treatment on microbial community diversity and abundance during exacerbation in patients with cystic fibrosis. Thorax. doi:10.1136/thx.2010.137281.
10. Sibley CD, Parkins MD, Rabin HR, Duan K, Norgaard JC, et al. (2008) A polymicrobial perspective of pulmonary infections exposes an enigmatic pathogen in cystic fibrosis patients. P Natl Acad Sci Usa 105: 15070–15075. doi:10.1073/pnas.0804326105.
11. Sibley CD, Grinwis ME, Field TR, Eshaghurshan CS, Faria MM, et al. (2011) Culture enriched molecular profiling of the cystic fibrosis airway microbiome. PLoS ONE 6: e22702. doi:10.1371/journal.pone.0022702.
12. Parkins MD, Sibley CD, Surette MG, Rabin HR (2008) The Streptococcus milleri group–an unrecognized cause of disease in cystic fibrosis: a case series and literature review. Pediatr Pulmonol 43: 490–497. doi:10.1002/ppul.20809.
13. Rogers GB, Carroll MP, Serisier DJ, Hockey PM, Jones G, et al. (2004) Characterization of bacterial community diversity in cystic fibrosis lung infections by use of 16 s ribosomal DNA terminal restriction fragment length polymorphism profiling. Journal of Clinical Microbiology 42: 5176–5183. doi:10.1128/JCM.42.11.5176–5183.2004.
14. Stressmann FA, Rogers GB, Klem ER, Lilley AK, Donaldson SH, et al. (2011) Analysis of the bacterial communities present in lungs of patients with cystic fibrosis from American and British centers. Journal of Clinical Microbiology 49: 281–291. doi:10.1128/JCM.01650–10.
15. van der Gast CJ, Walker AW, Stressmann FA, Rogers GB, Scott P, et al. (2010) Partitioning core and satellite taxa from within cystic fibrosis lung bacterial communities. ISME J. doi:10.1038/ismej.2010.175.
16. Sibley CD, Parkins MD, Rabin HR, Surette MG (2009) The relevance of the polymicrobial nature of airway infection in the acute and chronic management of patients with cystic fibrosis. Curr Opin Investig Drugs 10: 787–794.
17. Emerson J, Rosenfeld M, McNamara S, Ramsey B, Gibson RL (2002) Pseudomonas aeruginosa and other predictors of mortality and morbidity in young children with cystic fibrosis. Pediatr Pulmonol 34: 91–100. doi:10.1002/ppul.10127.
18. Kerem E, Corey M, Gold R, Levison H (1990) Pulmonary function and clinical course in patients with cystic fibrosis after pulmonary colonization with Pseudomonas aeruginosa. J Pediatr 116: 714–719. doi:10.1016/S0022-3476(05)82653–8.
19. Kosorok MR, Zeng L, West SE, Rock MJ, Splaingard ML, et al. (2001) Acceleration of lung disease in children with cystic fibrosis after Pseudomonas aeruginosa acquisition. Pediatr Pulmonol 32: 277–287.
20. Smith EE, Buckley DG, Wu Z, Saenphimmachak C, Hoffman LR, et al. (2006) Genetic adaptation by Pseudomonas aeruginosa to the airways of cystic fibrosis patients. P Natl Acad Sci Usa 103: 8487–8492. doi:10.1073/pnas.0602138103.
21. Hogardt M, Heesemann J (2010) Adaptation of Pseudomonas aeruginosa during persistence in the cystic fibrosis lung. Int J Med Microbiol. doi:10.1016/j.ijmm.2010.08.008.
22. Govan JR, Deretic V (1996) Microbial pathogenesis in cystic fibrosis: mucoid Pseudomonas aeruginosa and Burkholderia cepacia. Microbiol Rev 60: 539–574.
23. Mahenthiralingam E, Campbell ME, Speert DP (1994) Nonmotility and phagocytic resistance of Pseudomonas aeruginosa isolates from chronically colonized patients with cystic fibrosis. Infection and Immunity 62: 596–605.
24. Drenkard E, Ausubel FM (2002) Pseudomonas biofilm formation and antibiotic resistance are linked to phenotypic variation. Nature 416: 740–743. doi:10.1038/416740a.
25. Götz von F, Häussler S, Jordan D, Saravanamuthu SS, Wehmhöner D, et al. (2004) Expression analysis of a highly adherent and cytotoxic small colony variant of Pseudomonas aeruginosa isolated from a lung of a patient with cystic fibrosis. J Bacteriol 186: 3837–3847. doi:10.1128/JB.186.12.3837–3847.2004.
26. Häussler S, Ziegler I, Löttel A, Götz von F, Rohde M, et al. (2003) Highly adherent small-colony variants of Pseudomonas aeruginosa in cystic fibrosis lung infection. J Med Microbiol 52: 295–301.
27. Starkey M, Hickman JH, Ma L, Zhang N, de Long S, et al. (2009) Pseudomonas aeruginosa rugose small-colony variants have adaptations that likely promote persistence in the cystic fibrosis lung. J Bacteriol 191: 3492–3503. doi:10.1128/JB.00119–09.
28. Feliziani S, Luján AM, Moyano AJ, Sola C, Bocco JL, et al. (2010) Mucoidy, Quorum Sensing, Mismatch Repair and Antibiotic Resistance in Pseudomonas aeruginosa from Cystic Fibrosis Chronic Airways Infections. PLoS ONE 5. doi:10.1371/journal.pone.0012669.
29. Wilder CN, Allada G, Schuster M (2009) Instantaneous within-patient diversity of Pseudomonas aeruginosa quorum-sensing populations from cystic fibrosis lung infections. Infection and Immunity 77: 5631–5639. doi:10.1128/IAI.00755–09.
30. Foweraker JE, Laughton CR, Brown DFJ, Bilton D (2005) Phenotypic variability of Pseudomonas aeruginosa in sputa from patients with acute infective exacerbation of cystic fibrosis and its impact on the validity of antimicrobial susceptibility testing. J Antimicrob Chemother 55: 921–927. doi:10.1093/jac/dki146.
31. Foweraker JE, Laughton CR, Brown DF, Bilton D (2009) Comparison of methods to test antibiotic combinations against heterogeneous populations of multiresistant Pseudomonas aeruginosa from patients with acute infective exacerbations in cystic fibrosis. Antimicrob Agents Chemother 53: 4809–4815. doi:10.1128/AAC.00269–09.
32. Mowat E, Paterson S, Fothergill JL, Wright EA, Ledson MJ, et al. (2011) Pseudomonas Aeruginosa Population Diversity and Turnover in Cystic Fibrosis Chronic Infections. Am J Respir Crit Care Med: 201009–1430OCv1. doi:10.1164/rccm.201009–1430OC.
33. Glezerson BA, Sibley CD, Sibley KE, Surette MG, Rabin HR, et al. (2012) A twenty-five year outbreak of Pseudomonas aeruginosa: identification of the Prairie Epidemic Strain (PES). Journal of Cystic Fibrosis 11(S1) :S41.
34. Lee B, Haagensen JAJ, Ciofu O, Andersen JB, Høiby N, et al. (2005) Heterogeneity of biofilms formed by nonmucoid Pseudomonas aeruginosa isolates from patients with cystic fibrosis. Journal of Clinical Microbiology 43: 5247–5255. doi:10.1128/JCM.43.10.5247–5255.2005.
35. Leone I, Chirillo MG, Raso T, Zucca M, Savoia D (2008) Phenotypic and genotypic characterization of Pseudomonas aeruginosa from cystic fibrosis patients. Eur J Clin Microbiol Infect Dis 27: 1093–1099. doi:10.1007/s10096–008–0551–1.
36. Fothergill JL, Mowat E, Ledson MJ, Walshaw MJ, Winstanley C (2010) Fluctuations in phenotypes and genotypes within populations of Pseudomonas aeruginosa in the cystic fibrosis lung during pulmonary exacerbations. J Med Microbiol 59: 472–481. doi:10.1099/jmm.0.015875–0.
37. D'Argenio DA, Wu M, Hoffman LR, Kulasekara HD, Déziel E, et al. (2007) Growth phenotypes of Pseudomonas aeruginosa lasR mutants adapted to the airways of cystic fibrosis patients. Mol Microbiol 64: 512–533. doi:10.1111/j.1365–2958.2007.05678.x
38. Mena A, Smith EE, Burns JL, Speert DP, Moskowitz SM, et al. (2008) Genetic adaptation of Pseudomonas aeruginosa to the airways of cystic fibrosis patients is catalyzed by hypermutation. J Bacteriol 190: 7910–7917. doi:10.1128/JB.01147–08.
39. Ciofu O, Mandsberg LF, Bjarnsholt T, Wassermann T, Høiby N (2010) Genetic adaptation of Pseudomonas aeruginosa during chronic lung infection of patients with cystic fibrosis: strong and weak mutators with heterogeneous genetic backgrounds emerge in mucA and/or lasR mutants. Microbiology (Reading, Engl) 156: 1108–1119. doi:10.1099/mic.0.033993–0.
40. Amiel E, Lovewell RR, O'Toole GA, Hogan DA, Berwin B (2010) Pseudomonas aeruginosa evasion of phagocytosis is mediated by loss of swimming motility and is independent of flagellum expression. Infection and Immunity 78: 2937–2945. doi:10.1128/IAI.00144–10.
41. Henry RL, Mellis CM, Petrovic L (1992) Mucoid Pseudomonas aeruginosa is a marker of poor survival in cystic fibrosis. Pediatr Pulmonol 12: 158–161.
42. Li Z, Kosorok MR, Farrell PM, Laxova A, West SEH, et al. (2005) Longitudinal development of mucoid Pseudomonas aeruginosa infection and lung disease progression in children with cystic fibrosis. JAMA 293: 581–588. doi:10.1001/jama.293.5.581.
43. Kassen R (2002) The experimental evolution of specialists, generalists, and the maintenance of diversity. J Evolution Biol 15: 173–190.
44. Schluter D (2000) The Ecology of Adaptive Radiation. Oxford Univ Press.
45. Kassen R (2009) Toward a general theory of adaptive radiation: insights from microbial experimental evolution. Annals of the New York Academy of Sciences 1168: 3–22. doi:10.1111/j.1749–6632.2009.04574.x.
46. Lee SM, Wyse A, Lesher A, Everett ML, Lou L, et al. (2010) Adaptation in a mouse colony monoassociated with Escherichia coli K-12 for more than 1,000 days. Appl Environ Microbiol 76: 4655–4663. doi:10.1128/AEM.00358–10.
47. Rainey PB, Travisano M (1998) Adaptive radiation in a heterogeneous environment. Nature 394: 69–72.
48. Davidson CJ, White AP, Surette MG (2008) Evolutionary loss of the rdar morphotype in Salmonella as a result of high mutation rates during laboratory passage. ISME J 2: 293–307. doi:10.1038/ismej.2008.4.
49. Duan K, Dammel C, Stein J, Rabin H, Surette MG (2003) Modulation of Pseudomonas aeruginosa gene expression by host microflora through interspecies communication. Mol Microbiol 50: 1477–1491.
50. Sibley CD, Duan K, Fischer C, Parkins MD, Storey DG, et al. (2008) Discerning the Complexity of Community Interactions Using a Drosophila Model of Polymicrobial Infections. PLoS Pathog 4: e1000184. doi:10.1371/journal.-ppat.1000184.
51. Sokol PA, Ohman DE, Iglewski BH (1979) A more sensitive plate assay for detection of protease production by Pseudomanas aeruginosa. Journal of Clinical Microbiology 9: 538–540.
52. Smith HL, Goodner K (1958) Detection of bacterial gelatinases by gelatin-agar plate methods. J Bacteriol 76: 662–665.
53. Sokol PA, Cox CD, Iglewski BH (1982) Pseudomonas aeruginosa mutants altered in their sensitivity to the effect of iron on toxin A or elastase yields. J Bacteriol 151: 783–787.
54. Rashid MH, Kornberg A (2000) Inorganic polyphosphate is needed for swimming, swarming, and twitching motilities of Pseudomonas aeruginosa. P Natl Acad Sci Usa 97: 4885–4890. doi:10.1073/pnas.060030097.
55. Baynham PJ, Ramsey DM, Gvozdyev BV, Cordonnier EM, Wozniak DJ (2006) The Pseudomonas aeruginosa ribbon-helix-helix DNA-binding protein AlgZ (AmrZ) controls twitching motility and biogenesis of type IV pili. J Bacteriol 188: 132–140. doi:10.1128/JB.188.1.132–140.2006
56. CLSI (2009) Performance Standards for Antimicrobial Susceptibility Testing; Nineteenth Informational Supplement. Wayne, PA: Clinical and Laboratory Standards Institute.

57. Duan K, Surette MG (2007) Environmental regulation of Pseudomonas aeruginosa PAO1 Las and Rhl quorum-sensing systems. J Bacteriol 189: 4827–4836. doi:10.1128/JB.00043-07
58. Palmer KL, Aye LM, Whiteley M (2007) Nutritional cues control Pseudomonas aeruginosa multicellular behavior in cystic fibrosis sputum. J Bacteriol 189: 8079–8087. doi:10.1128/JB.01138-07
59. Wagner T, Soong G, Sokol S, Saiman L, Prince A (2005) Effects of azithromycin on clinical isolates of Pseudomonas aeruginosa from cystic fibrosis patients. Chest 128: 912–919. doi:10.1378/chest.128.2.912
60. Core R Team (2012) R: A Language and Environment for Statistical Computing. R Foundation for Statistical Computing. Available: http://www.R-project.org/
61. Kahm M, Hasenbrink G, Lichtenberg-Fraté H, Ludwig J, Kschischo M (2010) grofit: fitting biological growth curves with R. Journal of Statistical Software 33: 1–21.

21

Stochastic Tracking of Infection in a CF Lung

Sara Zarei[1*], Ali Mirtar[2], Forest Rohwer[3], Peter Salamon[4]

1 Computational Science Research Center, San Diego State University, San Diego, California, United States of America, **2** Electrical and Computer Eng. Dep/University of California San Diego, San Diego, California, United States of America, **3** Department of Biology, San Diego State University, San Diego, California, United States of America, **4** Department of Mathematics and Statistics, San Diego State University, San Diego, California, United States of America

Abstract

Magnetic Resonance Imaging (MRI) and Computed Tomography (CT) scan are the two ubiquitous imaging sources that physicians use to diagnose patients with Cystic Fibrosis (CF) or any other Chronic Obstructive Pulmonary Disease (COPD). Unfortunately the cost constraints limit the frequent usage of these medical imaging procedures. In addition, even though both CT scan and MRI provide mesoscopic details of a lung, in order to obtain microscopic information a very high resolution is required. Neither MRI nor CT scans provide micro level information about the location of infection in a binary tree structure the binary tree structure of the human lung. In this paper we present an algorithm that enhances the current imaging results by providing estimated micro level information concerning the location of the infection. The estimate is based on a calculation of the distribution of possible mucus blockages consistent with available information using an offline Metropolis-Hastings algorithm in combination with a real-time interpolation scheme. When supplemented with growth rates for the pockets of mucus, the algorithm can also be used to estimate how lung functionality as manifested in spirometric tests will change in patients with CF or COPD.

Editor: Wayne Iwan Lee Davies, University of Western Australia, Australia

Funding: This material is based upon work supported by the National Institutes of Health under Grant no. 56586B. The funders had no role in study design, data collection and analysis, decision to publish, or preparation of the manuscript.

Competing Interests: The authors have declared that no competing interests exist.

* Email: sara.zarei@alumni.ucsd.edu

Introduction

Patients with chronic obstructive pulmonary disease (COPD) or cystic fibrosis (CF) have chronic lung inflammation which causes airflow limitation and the scarring of lung tissues. Their airways are generally inflamed and produce excess amounts of mucus that impair the flow of air into and out of their lungs.

Our hypothesis is that the scarring, and ultimate remodeling of a CF lung is mostly due to the contact between the lung lining and the mucus. Inflammatory cytokines induce scars in lung tissue [1]. This contact between mucous biofilm and lung tissue facilitates virulent microbes that also play a role in remodeling a CF lung. In comparison with a normal lung, the airway fluids of CF patients contain large amounts of neutrophils as a result of the inflammatory response [2]. Thus our hypothesis is that mucus accumulation is primarily responsible for damage to the lung and therefore tracking its propagation is a crucial task for better diagnosis and treatment.

Spirometry, the measurement of a patient's breathing, is the standard clinical tool for monitoring lung disease. The two most common spirometric indicators are the forced expiratory volume in one second, FEV_1, and the forced vital capacity, FVC. FEV_1 measures the volume of air that can forcibly be blown out in one second while FVC measures the volume of air that can forcibly be blown out after a full inspiration maneuver. Although these tests provide a global measure of airflow obstruction and restriction, they do not give detailed information about the location of mucus blockage. Additional information is available from the repeated imaging of CF patients' lungs. This is usually in the form of chest x-ray, computed tomography (CT) or magnetic resonance imaging (MRI). Despite the fact that CT is an optimal morphological assessment of CF lung changes, the associated exposure to ionizing radiation is a serious obstacle. Therefore, MRI might be the appropriate method for imaging CF patient's lungs [3,4].

MRI was first introduced as an alternative imaging tool for patients with CF in 1987 [5]. There are numerous methods for the analysis of chest MRI. Theilmann et al. proposed a new MRI imaging method that can spatially locate the pockets of infection and measure the amount of mucus located within each pocket. This information is obtained with a resolution of approximately 1.0 cm^3 [6]. This resolution is equivalent to the last 10 generations of airways combined. Despite the accuracy level of MRI images, they do not contain any micro-level information on smaller airways. Hence the precise location of infection cannot be obtained from the MRI data.

There have been research studies on mesoscopic modeling of Cystic Fibrosis [7]. Such studies however did not address the micro level information about mucus propagation through the airways. The goal of this research is to provide the clinician with an algorithm that can track the location and propagation of mucus in a CF patient's lungs. Tracking the growth, or shrinkage of these pockets can be correlated to the efficacy of different treatment regimens on each pocket. Assuming further progress in metagenomic and transcriptomic analyses of sputum samples, tracking may allow also correlating the growth or shrinkage of these pockets and the composition of the local microbial community structure within the pocket.

The central tool introduced in the present article for tracking pockets of inflammation is based on using our airflow model [8] in reverse, i.e., as the main ingredient in an inverse problem. Our airflow model can calculate the flow and the total resistance corresponding to a given distribution of mucus obstructions in respiratory airways. The solution of the inverse problem is achieved by randomly sampling the many possible mucus configurations consistent with the current information regarding a patient. Many micro-scale distributions match any observed MRI and spirometric data. The fortuitous finding in the calculations described below is that a large majority of the possible distributions fall within narrow ranges of certain parameters such as which generations of airways contain how much mucus. Can we be certain of these most likely locations being the actual mucus distribution? The fact that most of the distributions consistent with the spirometric and MRI data have these features makes them a good bet while not giving us certainty that any *one* configuration is of this form. In fact, however, repeated MRI measurements separated by small challenges such as coughing or even just taking a few deep breaths reveal that mucus inside the lungs of CF patients show small but discernible movements in response to such challenges. Given this dynamic picture, the possibility that all of the configurations of mucus would avoid the configurations that can be realized the largest number of ways is extremely unlikely. We describe below how to construct such distributions that best represent the state of airways corresponding to the patients lung functionality test values (FEV_1 and FVC) and any available MRI or CT data. We use a maximum entropy approach to construct such estimates by sampling all consistent distributions and choosing the one that can be realized the largest number of ways. We find that the predicted microscopic distribution of mucus is generally sharply peaked, allowing us to estimate the distribution of mucus as the one that appears the most frequently in our simulation. The entire computation process can take a long time and would require enormous computational space to run the simulation for the entire 2^{23} airways in a lung. However after running the simulation once for a patient, we can store most of the data so the next simulations only take a few minutes to complete.

Given the micro-scale distribution obtained from our inverse problem, we can use our physiological model [9] to predict the growth and propagation of this distribution, thereby predicting the progression of the disease. This second model requires a rate for the growth of the mucus volume at each location. Currently only one overall average growth rate is available, a growth rate that was estimated based on a forty year CF population average [9]. Predictions of this model with the average growth rate can nonetheless be compared to actual observed disease progression between exacerbations. For predictions during exacerbations, a database of treatment and community specific growth rates are needed and in-principle available from multiple MRI and metagenomic/transcriptomic analyses. Two such datasets allow the extraction of pocket specific growth rates and corresponding linear extrapolation for the mucus volume in each pocket. This can at least lengthen the times between imaging sessions.

Methods

Inverse Problem Using Metropolis-Hastings Algorithm

Our algorithm uses CF patients' spirometry test values of FVC, FEV_1 and any available mucus distribution data from CT scans or MRI as its input. It then identifies the distribution of mucus obstructed bronchioles throughout different airway generations. The model assumes the lung airways to be binary branching trees [10] extending over 23 generations from the bronchus down to the alveoli. It further assumes a fractal structure [11–13] for the parameters of the binary airway tree.

Considering the fact that there are 2^{23} bronchioles in a human lung, there are astronomically many possible configurations for a certain amount of mucus distributed in an airway tree, even given the mucus in each voxel. In fact many of these configurations will result in the same FEV_1 and FVC values. Since exhaustive sampling of these configurations is impossible, we use the Metropolis-Hastings Markov chain Monte Carlo algorithm to sample a few hundred million and base our estimates on such a sample. The goal of this section is to introduce this method.

Our algorithm proceeds from an assumed amount of mucus to be distributed into the 2^{23} airways. It starts from a random distribution and obtains an unbiased sample of configurations satisfying certain requirements. These requirements are implemented as soft constraints via an energy function

$$E=(\alpha)(\text{Calculated } FEV_1-\text{Patient } FEV_1)^2+ (1-\alpha)(\text{Calculated FVC}-\text{Patient FVC})^2 \quad (1)$$

where (α) and $(1-\alpha)$ are weight factors. In our algorithm we set $\alpha=0.5$. The energy function is used as a way to force the sampling to stay near values with low energy, i.e. configurations with approximately correct spirometric readings.

We then examine successive samples by performing a random walk on the space of mucus configurations. Each move in our random walk reallocates the location of some of the mucus. The resulting distribution of mucus configurations turns out to be sharply peaked in certain natural parameters, a fact exploited by our algorithm.

The Metropolis algorithm is a widely used procedure for sampling a sequence from a specified distribution on a large finite set. It describes equilibrium for systems whose configurations have probability proportional to the Boltzmann factor ($e^{-E/T}$). This is a weighting factor which determines the relative probability that the system will be found in a particular configuration at energy E when the temperature of the environment is T [14]. We used a constant temperature, $T=1$, making the probability of a configuration with energy E proportional to $\exp(-E)$.

The following steps describe the Metropolis algorithm [15].

- Initiate the sampling from an arbitrary configuration A, with known energy E_A.
- Define a new neighbor configuration B from configuration A.
- Calculate the new configuration energy, E_B. This trial move is then either accepted or rejected according to the following simple probabilistic rule.
- If $E_B<E_A$ we accept the new configuration.
- if $E_B>E_A$, we may accept configuration B with the following probability.

$$p=e^{-(E_B-E_A)/T} \quad (2)$$

- Repeat until sufficient number of configurations have been collected.

To apply the Metropolis algorithm to our model, we need to define neighboring configurations. Our definition moves a certain amount of mucus between a few chosen bronchioles. This keeps the energy re-evaluation step computationally cheap and, provided we allow such rearrangement between all types of airways, we avoid the problems created by local minima. This assures that the system settles into and stays near the lowest energy configurations as the simulation proceeds [16].

Two-Dimensional Probability Density Function Estimation (PDFE-2D) of Mucus Obstructions

Imaging provides us with the data that corresponds to the spatial location of infection pockets and the amount of mucus within each pocket. Both MRI and CT images can have various resolutions and our approach is scalable to any resolution. For concreteness below we work with a resolution of 1 cm^3 and refer to this smallest volume as a voxel - a volume element.

Since on average the total lung capacity of an adult human is about 6 liters [17], an image will have about 6000 voxels. Using the binary tree structure of the lung airway, we set these voxels at the end of the 13th generation to approximately match the number of these elements to the number of subtrees that remain. Since $2^{13} = 8192 \approx 6000$, we can identify the mucus in the voxel with the mucus in the subtree of $2^{23-13} = 2^{10}$ bronchioles terminating in the alveoli. Thus each voxel in our lung model represents a binary tree structure that has a total of 10 bifurcations, from generation 13 to 23, with a known total amount of mucus obtained from imaging data.

Using a three-dimensional model of the human airway tree that was developed by [18], we are able to map each MRI or CT scan voxel into our lung model's voxels with their corresponding mucus content. The main task of our algorithm is to locate the infection in the airway tree structure of a CF lung. To achieve this goal, we use two summary features for each voxel: (1) the percent of alveoli that are accessible, i.e., not totally blocked and (2) the total resistance to flow from the alveoli to the 13th generation brochiole bronchiole assigned to the voxel. These two microscopic features correspond loosely to the spirometric indicators FVC and FEV_1, respectively.

In order for us to calculate each voxel's resistance and the percent of accessible alveoli (for simplicity, we refer to this as the AA%), we first have to define how mucus is distributed in a voxel's binary tree structure. There is an astronomical number of configurations for filling a binary tree of 10 generations with a given amount of mucus. Approximately, it is given by $(2^{10})^{M/m}$ where M is the total mucus volume and m is the volume of the smallest bronchiole. Thus even at this level, we used Metropolis-Hastings to sample many mucus configurations, recording the values of AA% and resistance for each configuration. We set the amount of mucus within each voxel and calculate the distribution of AA% and resistance: our PDFE-2D distribution.

Hence if a voxel contains 5% mucus, the first step is randomly filling up the voxel's airway tree with the specified mucus amount. Then using the Metropolis algorithm, at each state we move only a fraction of the mucus within a bronchiole that is equivalent to the smallest bronchiole's volume in a lung airway tree. We refer to this as the "unit volume". Once a unit volume is moved to a different location, the corresponding voxel's parameters (AA% and resistance) are recalculated.

In order to expedite the computational process; Dulcinea computing clusters from the Computational Science Research Center at San Diego State University were used for collecting almost 54 million samples. The Dulcinea computing clusters contains 12 workstations each with Dual-Quad Xeon central processing unit (CPU) (E5520 2.27GHz) and Dual Tesla graphic processing unit (GPU) (M1060) which provides the total of 96 CPU cores. The cluster system utilizes 3GB of memory per CPU core for nodes 1 to 10 and utilizes 6GB of memory per CPU core for nodes 11 and 12. After obtaining these samples the probability distributions for different amount of mucus are calculated. Figure 1A to Figure 1D illustrate the probability density function for (5%, 30%, 65%, and 75%) mucus respectively. As shown in Figure 1A, when there is only 5% mucus in a voxel, the most likely configuration has 86% of its alveoli accessible and the voxel's resistance increases by a factor of almost 1.1. When the mucus level reaches almost 30% there are only 27% accessible alveoli and the voxel resistance is almost 2.2 times a healthy voxel with no mucus. On the other hand in Figure 1C and 1D the number of accessible alveoli value approaches zero while the resistance value reaches infinity. This refers to a case that a voxel is almost completely filled with mucus to an extent that no more air can pass through and therefore blocks all the corresponding alveoli at the end of the branching tree.

Figure 2 displays the maximum likelihood combinations of AA% and resistance ratio for different amount of mucus in a voxel. As the mucus reaches almost 60% of the available airway volume in the voxel, there is no remaining access to the alveoli and as a result there is no gas exchange taking place in that particular part of the airway tree. After collecting these distributions, the model can initiate the prediction steps as well as providing the microlevel information about the location of obstructed bronchioles. We will discuss each outcome in the next two sections. Please note that all data underlying the findings of this section have been discussed in the manuscript. Other than the massive computing power needed to produce the findings in Figure 1 and Figure 2, all the relevant data have been shared.

Results

Micro-Level Information on Obstructed Bronchioles

In order to spatially locate each bronchiole in a human airway tree we used Kitaoka et al.'s three-dimensional model [18]. Once we receive the imaging data for each voxel, we need to map the values to our model's voxel using spatial location coordinates. Next we use the probability density function that we found in the previous section to determine the corresponding voxel parameters, AA% and resistance ratio, sampled according to the PDFE-2D distributions. The model randomly select a combination of percent accessible alveoli and resistance for each voxel in a way that the total resistance and number of accessible alveoli from these voxels provide the same value as the patient's FEV_1 and FVC. There is a complex calculation taking place in parallel to obtain the rate of flow (FEV_1) from the total resistance of all the voxels. To find the distribution of voxel parameters we use the Metropolis algorithm to focus the Markov chain to sample many configurations meeting our constraints. This is achieved by choosing the configuration energy provided in Eq(1).

At this stage we have mapped the voxels from imaging data into our model in a way that the total rate of airflow and the accessible alveoli of the lung model resemble the corresponding patient's FEV_1 and FVC values respectively. Once the current state of a CF lung is implemented we can obtain clinically useful information, such as mucus distribution within each voxel or predicted future states of each voxel and associated FEV_1 and FVC values as described in the next section.

Figure 3 displays the flowchart of this process. As shown in this flowchart, once we have all the voxels' parameters, we can select certain voxels for further analysis. We again apply the Metropolis algorithm on the selected voxel in order to visualize the distribution of mucus in its airway tree structure. For the chosen voxel, we have its mucus volume, its resistance and its AA%. We randomly fill out the voxels' airway tree to reach their

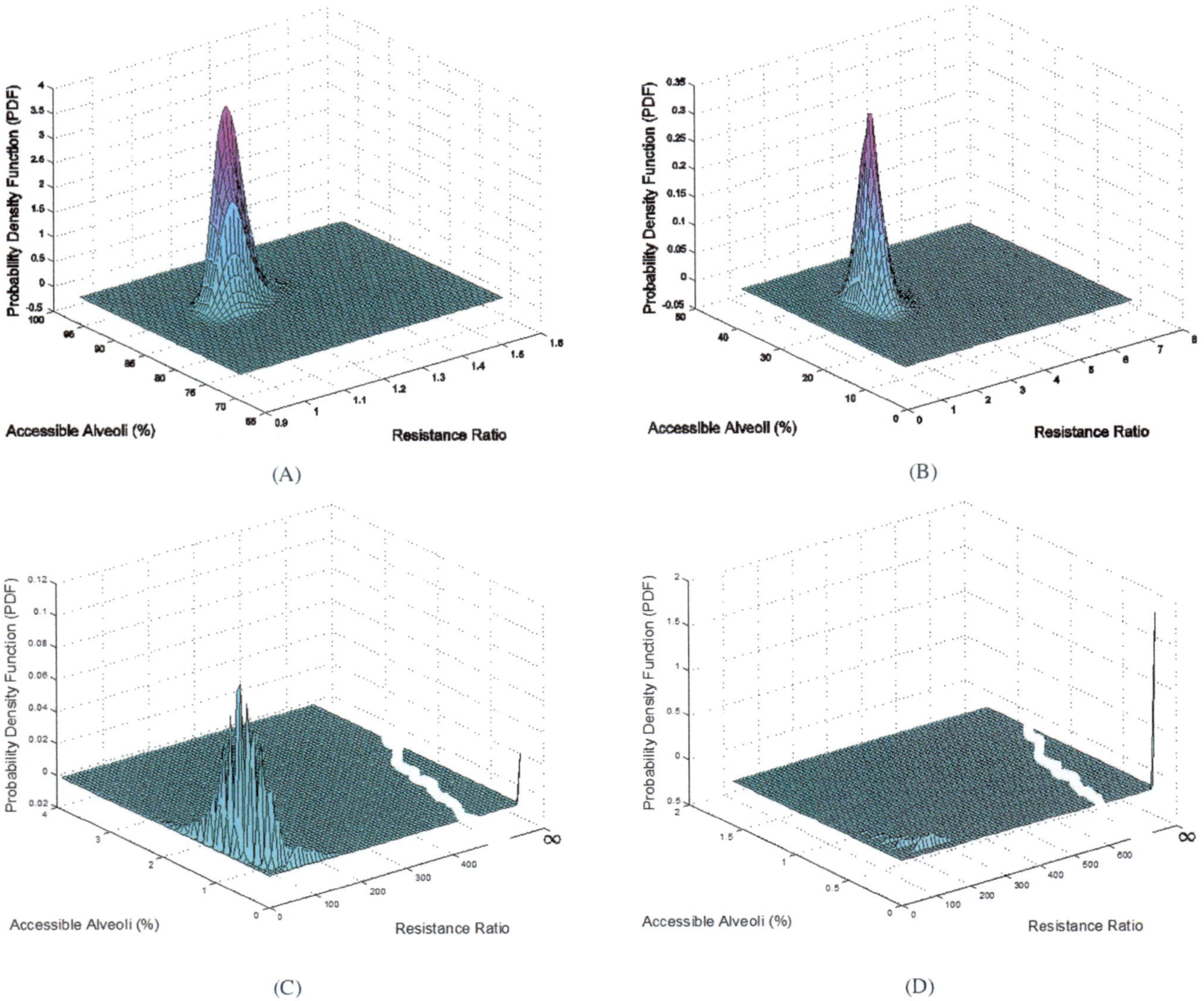

Figure 1. Probability density function for different percent volume of mucus in a small voxel of the lung. (A) 5%, **(B)** 30%, **(C)** 65% **and (D)** 75% Each voxel represents a subtree from generation 13 to 23 of the binary tree structure of lung. The x-axis is the corresponding airflow resistance and the y-axis shows the percent accessible alveoli.

corresponding mucus volume. At each iteration the new resistance and AA% are collected. To move to the neighbor configuration we move a unit volume of mucus in a bronchiole to keep the total mucus volume of the voxel fixed. The state energy we use for this step is as follows:

$$E = (\alpha)(\text{Resistance of the current state} - \text{Target voxel's resistance})^2 + (1-\alpha)(\text{AA\% of the current state} - \text{Target voxel's AA\%})^2 \quad (3)$$

where $\alpha = 0.5$. After we obtained enough samples we constructed the corresponding mucus distribution for the selected voxels. Figures 4 displays two examples of the mucus distribution for voxels that contained (5%) and (30%) mucus. As shown in these figures, as the percent mucus increases, the dominantly filled generation moves to bigger bronchioles. The y axis repressnts represents % normalized mucus where:

$$\text{Normalized mucus in generation n} = \frac{\left(\frac{\text{Mucus Volume in generation } n}{\text{Total mucus volume in voxel}}\right)}{\left(\frac{\text{Airway volume in generation } n}{\text{Total airway volume in voxel}}\right)} \quad (4)$$

Predicting future values of FEV_1 and FVC

In this section we use the mucus distribution and growth model presented in [9] to make predictions about the lung functionality of a CF patient. As can be seen in Figure 5 we use the imaging voxels' data and the constant mucus growth rate from [9], or, if available, infection and treatment specific growth rates specific to each voxel to predict the mucus growth in each pocket of infection. The model again resorts to the Monte Carlo method to randomly select the AA% and resistance from our model described in the

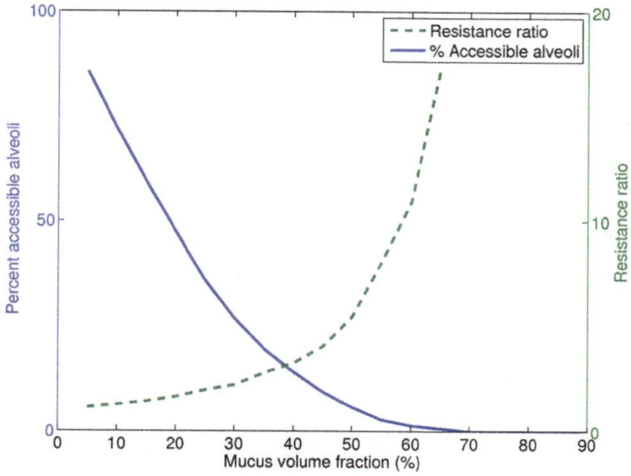

Figure 2. Maximum likelihood of percent of accessible alveoli AA% and airflow resistance for a given mucus volume fraction inside a voxel. The x-axis is mucus volume% and the two y-axes show the most probable combination of the airflow resistance ratio and percent of accessible alveoli. The resistance value increases as the mucus amount rises. Number of accessible alveoli decreases as the mucus volume grows, which leads to a lower lung functionality test value or FVC value.

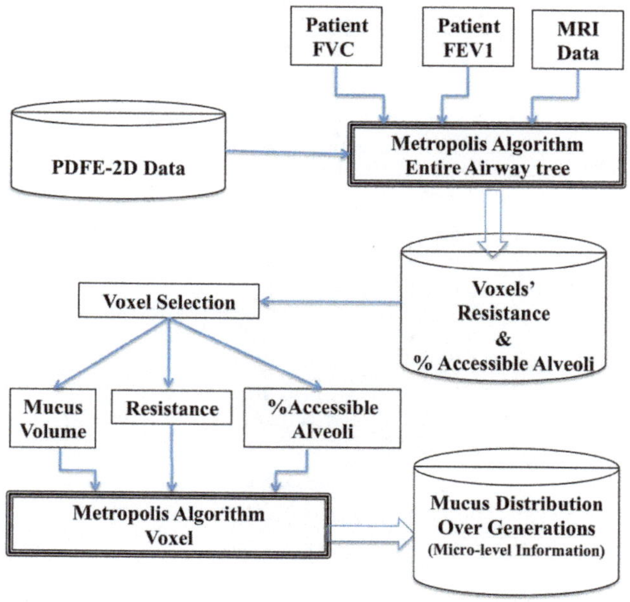

Figure 3. Generating the Micro-level information on obstructed bronchioles. This flowchart shows how the algorithm produces the mucus distribution of a selected voxel. Using the lung functionality test values: FEV1 and FVC and the data obtained from MRI lung imaging we can obtain the corresponding mucus distributions among the different generations of lung.

PDFE-2D section and calculates the new FEV_1 and FVC at each iteration and stores their values. After collecting enough samples we can predict the FEV_1 and FVC distributions for a patient after the indicated time period. For example, Figure 6 displays the probability density function of the predicted FEV_1 and FVC. As shown in the figure it is predicted that FEV_1 and FVC of our CF patient are approximately 61% and 78% respectively.

This method can even be applied to follow a patient's progress with out fewer imaging tests. Since most CF patients take spirometry test more often than any imaging tests, we can use our model without recourse to imaging data. This time the model takes only the FEV_1 and the FVC values of a patient as input. After applying the Metropolis algorithm (using additional rearrangements of mucus between voxels) the model can still provide an estimate of the distribution of mucus throughout the airway tree. This can be propagated using the constant any hypothetical growth rates to predict the next spirometric test. We have created a Matlab GUI version of the algorithm; its sample output is shown in Figures 7, 8 and 9.

Since the mean mucus growth rate was estimated based on years of data from many CF patients, such predictions should work reasonably well for a patient between exacerbations. Our model can also be used to predict the progression during exacerbations, albeit with voxel specific growth rates informed by much more data than we currently possess. Using one mean mucus growth rate is a shortcoming not of our algorithm but rather of the paucity of data to which our predictions have been applied. There is every indication that soon we will have reasonable metagenomic [19–22] and metabolomic [23] tools to assess the microbial composition present in a CF lung and will be able to infer growth rates that are specific to the community composition as well as the antibiotic administered. Entering voxel specific growth rates based on more information than we at present possess and using our program to test predictions can move our understanding of the patient's state to a new and quantitative level.

We can improve the accuracy level of the model by extending the resolution of our PDFE-2D distributions. The current PDFEs were constructed with 5% bins as described in PDFE-2D model section.

Discussion

With current research studies about cystic fibrosis, CF treatment is poised for great strides. Non-genetic treatments such as Ivacaftor (trade name Kalydeco, developed as VX-770) only works on patients with a certain mutation of cystic fibrosis which accounts for 4–5% of cystic fibrosis cases [24].

While an eventual cure for the disease by replacement of the defective gene is likely, we expect such treatment not to be available anytime soon. Rather we anticipate that new observational tools such as metagenomics, transcriptomics, metabolomics and MRI imaging coupled with our modeling approach will give the clinician unprecedented ability to follow and treat the disease. The models will provide quantitative predictions of responses to various drug regimens and prescribe adaptively implemented optimal controls for treatment. Predicting the impact of mucus growth on lung functionality will correlate the current stage of the disease with how infection has been propagating throughout different generations of lung. This will enable the physician with a tool to track this propagation of infection.

The various sub-models required here will soon be informed by data characterizing the microbial communities present. Such data comes from metagenomic and transcriptomics analyses of sputum samples and metabolomic analyses of exhaled air. In our current model we predict the dynamic distribution of mucus in a CF lung in the absence of treatment as a stepping stone for eventually eventual treatment and microbial community specific modeling of the treatment response.

According to a research study done by Willner et al. [25] microbial diversity in a CF lung is much higher than suggested by culturing alone. They were able to characterize the diversity of

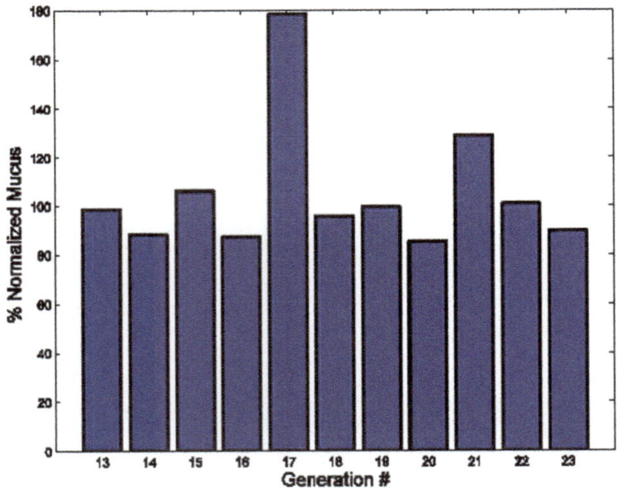

(A)

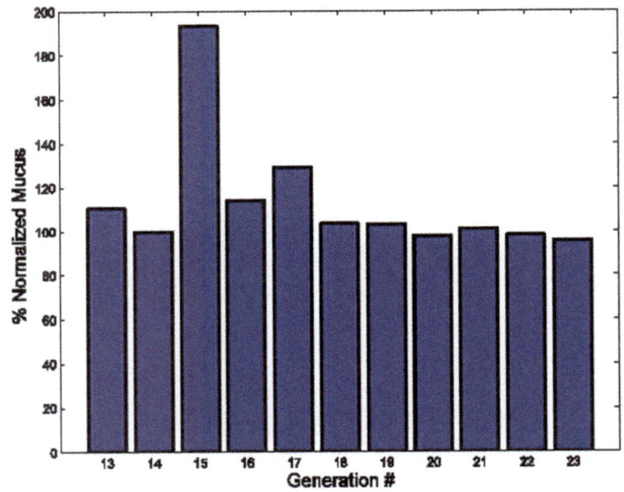

(B)

Figure 4. Mucus distribution among different generations of lung for two selected voxels. Figure (A) represents a voxel with 5% mucus volume that has 78% accessible alveoli: AA and resistance ratio of 1.22. Figure (B) repsresents represents a voxel with 30% mucus that has 19.45% AA and resistance ratio of 4.2. The x-axis is the generation number of the corresponding bronchioles in the selected voxel. The y-axis shows the normalized mucus present, which is equal to the ratio of the mucus amount in a generation to the total mucus volume in a voxel, divided by the ratio of the air volume in that generation to the total voxel volume.

microbial communities in tissue sections from anatomically distinct regions of the CF lung. Their result indicated that microbial communities in the Cystic Fibrosis lung are spatially heterogeneous.This Spatial heterogeneity will cause regional differences in microbial biomass and antibiotic resistance. The next version of the model, can use their results to adjust the parameters according to the microbial communities found and the treatment administered (e.g., timing of antibiotic administration, types of antibiotics, steroids, etc). The present model should be taken as a proof-of-concept step toward that goal. This will provide an opportunity for the researcher, and eventually the clinician, to access a framework for accurate quantitative predictions.

Our methods are completely scalable – the 1.0 cm^3 for the size of one voxel was for illustration. Any resolution scale however forces estimation of the distribution on spatial scales below this resolution. Since estimation of the distribution on finer spatial scales would perforce need the solution of an inverse problem with many possible solutions and since the movement of mucus hinted that the "right answer" would in any case not be a unique distribution, we were led naturally to using Monte Carlo

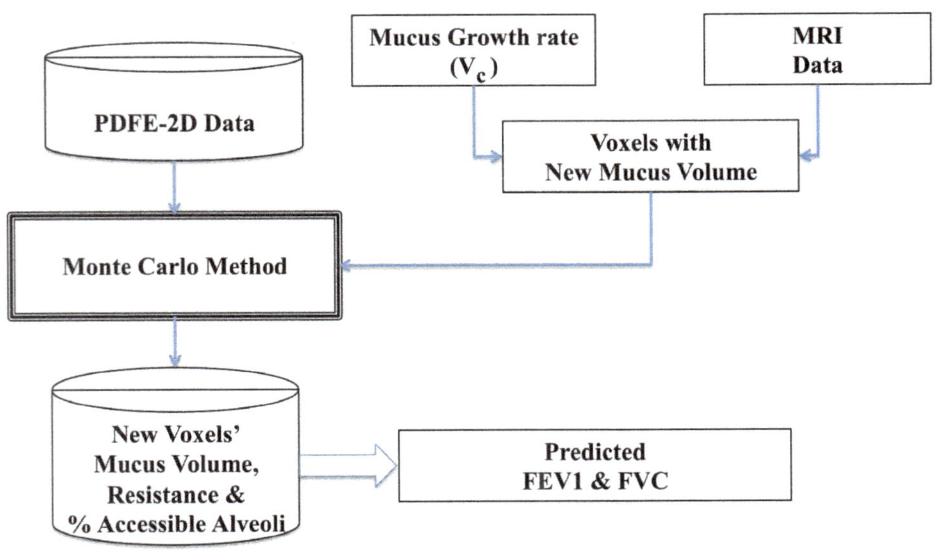

Figure 5. FEV_1 and FVC values predictions predicted from the lung model. This flowchart illustrates the process of how our lung model predicts the FVC and FEV_1 of a CF patient given the previous mucus content of each voxel along with a mucus growth rate.

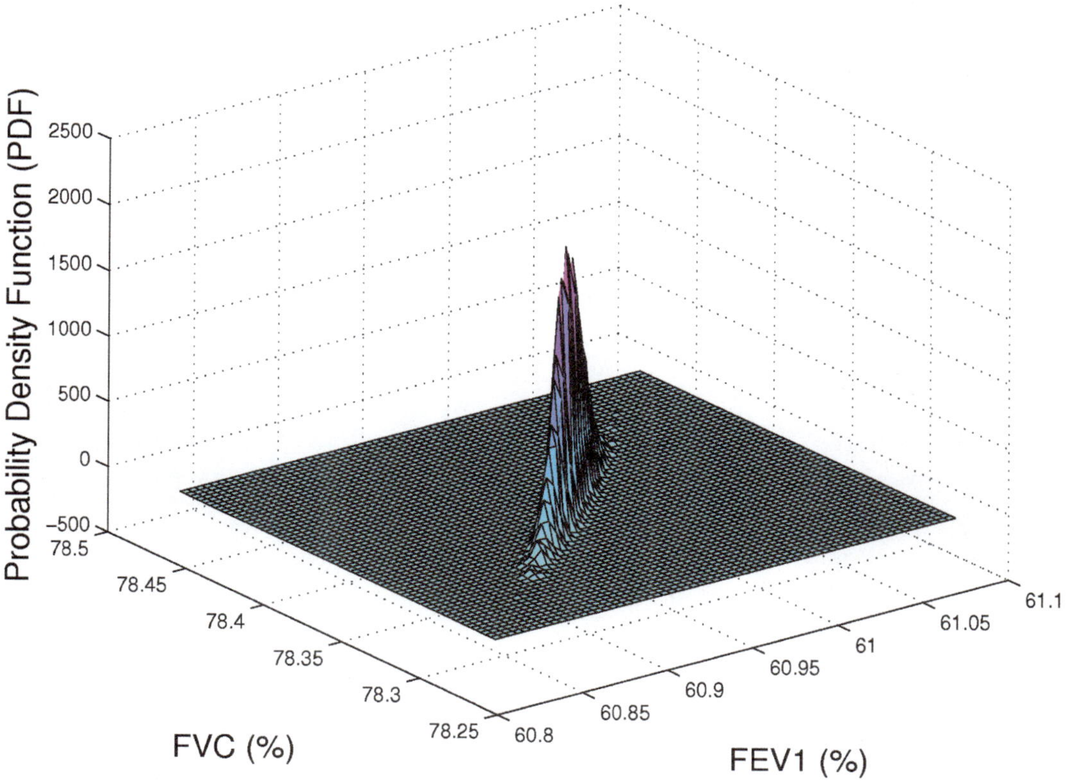

Figure 6. FEV_1 and FVC probability density function estimation. The x-axis shows the predicted FEV_1 values and the y-axis is the predicted FVC values for a hypothetical the synthetic lung example described in the text.

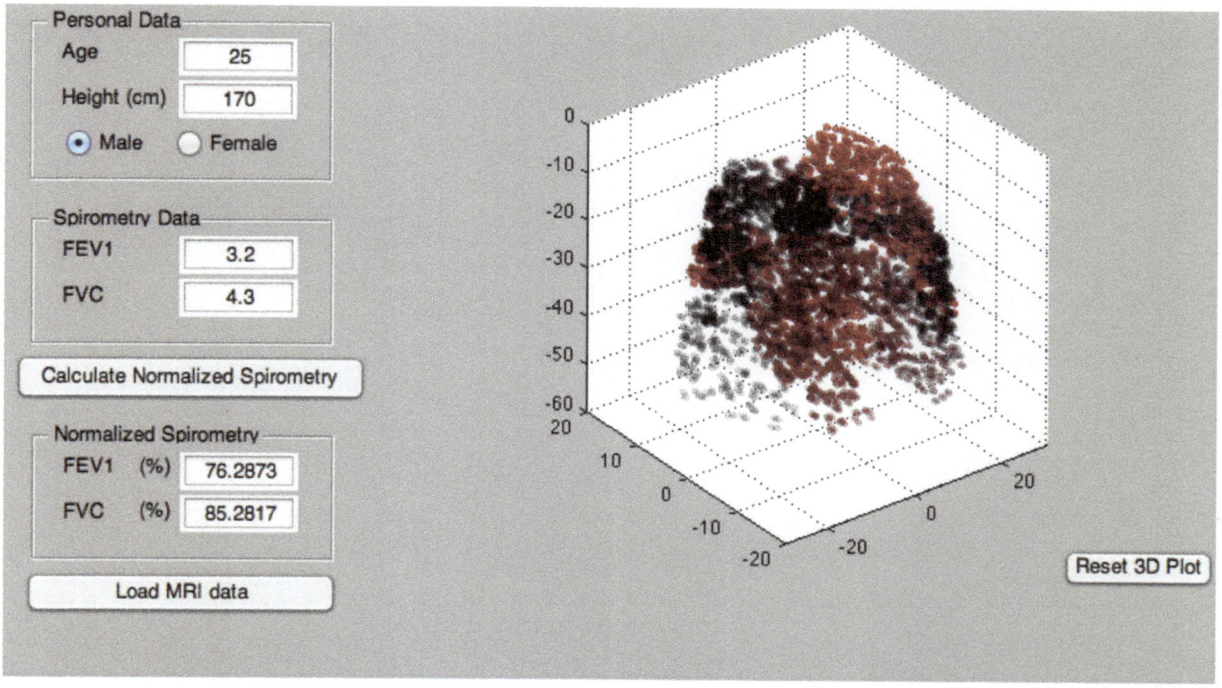

Figure 7. In this window user can enter the input parameters: patient's age, height, sex and Imaging data. The Model displays a 3D-lung that contains all the MRI/CT scan voxels.

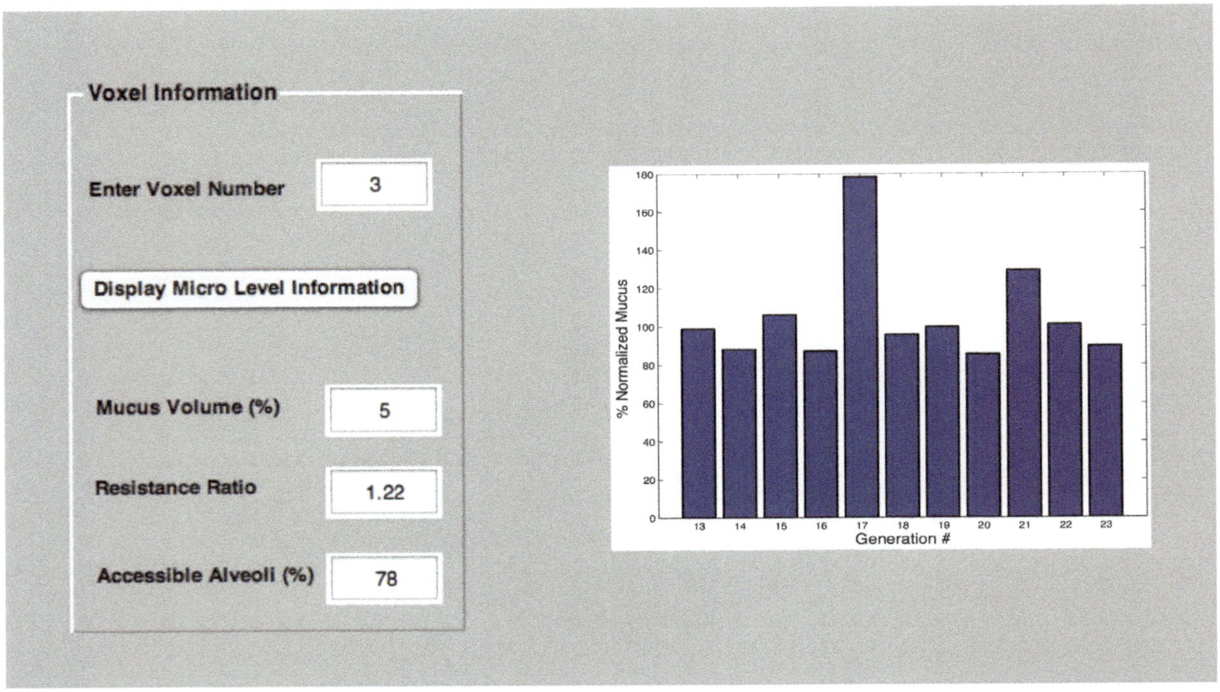

Figure 8. This window shows the mucus distribution among generations. The user selects a voxel and the model displays its corresponding parameters along with the micro-level information.

estimation methods for the most likely distribution and the corresponding spirometric observables. The resulting models and algorithms form a clinically useful tool with which to reassess the various simplest possible sub-models and assumptions used in our work so far. These models can play a crucial role in future treatments of the disease.

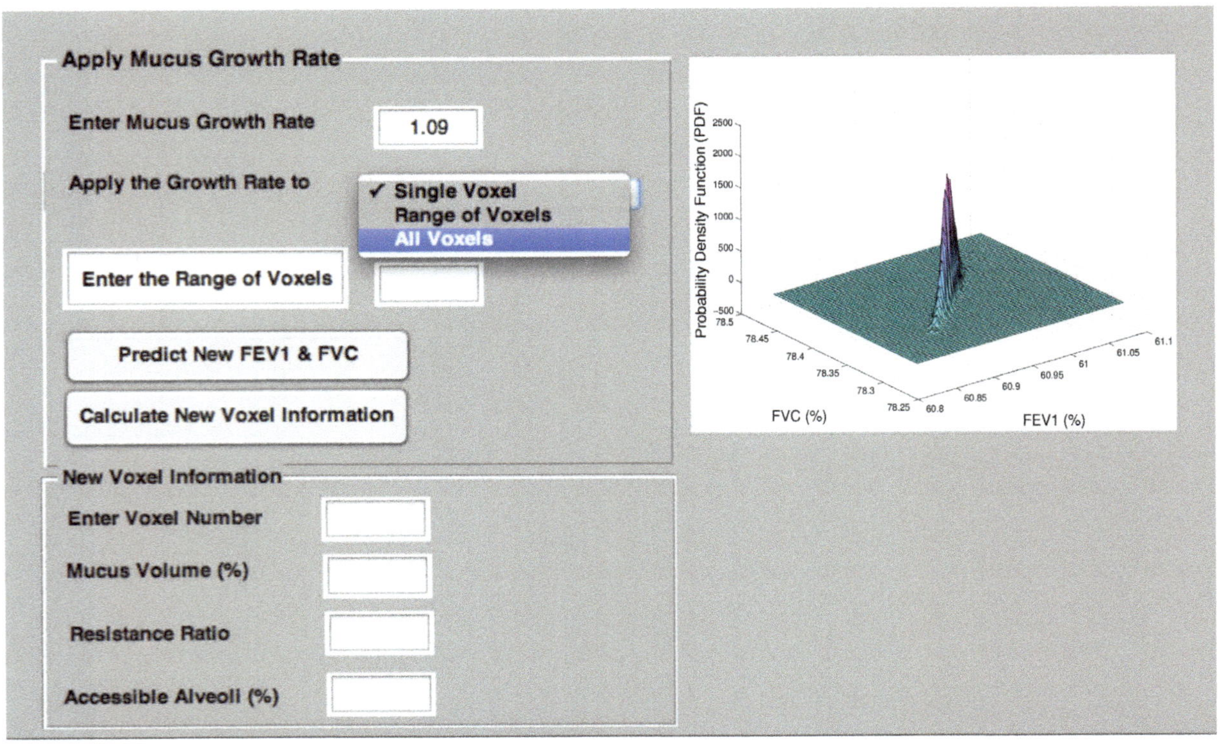

Figure 9. This window provides the user with a probability density function of the predicted FEV_1 and FVC. User can enter a specific mucus growth rate for different voxels and the new FEV_1 and FVC will be calculated.

Supporting Information

File S1 The supporting file Psudo.pdf contains the psudo code of the algorithms and models mentioned in this manuscript.

Acknowledgments

This material is based upon work supported by the National Institutes of Health under Grant no. 56586B.

The funders had no role in study design, data collection and analysis, decision to publish, or preparation of the manuscript.

Author Contributions

Conceived and designed the experiments: SZ AM FR PS. Performed the experiments: SZ AM FR PS. Analyzed the data: SZ AM FR PS. Contributed reagents/materials/analysis tools: SZ AM FR PS. Wrote the paper: SZ AM FR PS.

References

1. Tirouvanziam R (2006) Neutrophilic inflammation as a major determinant in the progression of cystic fibrosis. Drug News Perspect 19: 609–614.
2. Koehler DR, Downey GP, Sweezey NB, Tanswell AK, Hu J (2004) Lung inflammation as a therapeutic target in cystic fibrosis. Amer J of Resp Cell and Mol Biol 31: 377–381.
3. Eichinger M, Puderbach M, Heussel CP, Kauczor HU (2006) Mri in mucoviscidosis (cystic fibrosis). Radiologe, German 46 (4): 275–276.
4. Hopkins SR, Levin DL, Emami K, Kadlecek S, Yu J, et al. (2007) Advances in magnetic resonance imaging of lung physiology. J of App Physiol 102 (3): 1244–1254.
5. Fiel SB, Friedman AC, Caroline DF, Radecki PD, Faerber E, et al. (1987) Magnetic resonance imaging in young adults with cystic fibrosis. Chest 91: 181–184.
6. Theilmann RJ, Arai TJ, Samiee A, Dubowitz DJ, Hopkins SR, et al. (2009) Quantitative mri measurement of lung density must account for the change in t(2) (*) with lung inflation. J of MRI 30: 527–534.
7. Voit EO (2014) Mesoscopic modeling as a starting point for computational analyses of cystic fibrosis as a systemic disease. Biochim et Biophy Acta 1844 (1): 258–270.
8. Zarei S, Mirtar A, Andresen B, Salamon P (2013) Modeling the airflow in a lung with cystic fibrosis. J of Non-Equil Thermodyn 38 (2): 119–140.
9. Zarei S, Mirtar A, Rohwer F, Conrad DJ, Theilmann RJ, et al. (2012) Mucus distribution model in a lung with cystic fibrosis. J of Comp and Math Meth in Med.
10. Weibel ER (1991) Design of airways and blood vessels considered as branching trees. Lung: Sci Found 1: 1061–1071.
11. Altemeier WA, McKinney S, Glenny RW (2005) A fractal analysis of the radial distribution of bronchial capillaries around large airways. J of App Physiol 98: 850–855.
12. Glenny RW, Bernard SL, Robertson HT (2000) Pulmonary blood flow remains fractal down to the level of gas exchange. J of App Physiol 89: 742–748.
13. West BJ (1990) Physiology in fractal dimensions: error tolerance. Anna of Biomed Engi 18 (2): 135–149.
14. Richey M (2010) The evolution of markov chain monte carlo methods. Amer Math Mon 117 (5): 383–413.
15. Saeta PN (2004). The metropolis algorithm: Statistical systems and simulated annealing. URL http://saeta.physics.hmc.edu/courses/p170/Metropolis.pdf.
16. Salamon P, Sibani P, Frost R (2002) Facts, Conjecture, and Improvements for Simulated Annealing. Philadelphia: Society for Industrial and Applied Mathematics.
17. Marieb E, Hoehn K (2010) Human Anatomy and Physiology. Prentice Hall PTR. 8th ED.
18. Kitaoka H, Suk B (1997) Branching design of the bronchial tree based on a diameter-flow relationship. J of App Physiol 82: 968–976.
19. Willner D, Furlan M, Haynes M, Schmieder R, Angly FE, et al. (2009) Metagenomic analysis of respiratory tract dna viral communities in cystic fibrosis and non-cystic fibrosis individuals. PLoS One 4 (10): e7370.
20. Lim YW, Evangelista JS, Schmieder R, Bailey B, Haynes M, et al. (2014) Clinical insights from metagenomic analysis of sputum samples from patients with cystic fibrosis. J of Clin Microbi 52 (2): 425–437.
21. Lim YW, Schmieder R, Haynes M, Furlan M, Matthews TD, et al. (2013) Mechanistic model of rothia mucilaginosa adaptation toward persistence in the cf lung, based on a genome reconstructed from metagenomic data. PloS one 8 (5): e64285.
22. Lim YW, Schmiederb R, Haynesa M, Willnerd D, Furlana M, et al. (2013) Metagenomics and metatranscriptomics: Windows on cf-associated viral and microbial communities. J of Cystic Fibrosis 12 (2): 154–164.
23. Whiteson KL, Meinardi S, Lim YW, Schmieder R, Maughan H, et al. (2014) Breath gas metabolites and bacterial metagenomes from cystic fibrosis airways indicate active ph neutral 2, 3-butanedione fermentation. ISME J.
24. McPhail G, Clancy J (2013) Ivacaftor: The first therapy acting on the primary cause of cystic fibrosis. Drugs of today 49: 253–260.
25. Willner D, Furlan M, Haynes M, Schmieder R, Lim YW, et al. (2011) Spatial distribution of microbial communities in the cystic fibrosis lung. ISME J 6: 471–747.

Cystic Fibrosis Transmembrane Conductance Regulator (CFTR) Allelic Variants Relate to Shifts in Faecal Microbiota of Cystic Fibrosis Patients

Serena Schippa[1]ᵍ, Valerio Iebba[1*]ᵍ, Floriana Santangelo[1], Antonella Gagliardi[1], Riccardo Valerio De Biase[2], Antonella Stamato[2], Serenella Bertasi[2], Marco Lucarelli[3], Maria Pia Conte[1¶], Serena Quattrucci[2¶]

1 Public Health and Infectious Diseases Department, Microbiology Unit, 'Sapienza' University of Rome, Rome, Italy, **2** Regional Cystic Fibrosis Centre, Paediatrics and Infant Neuropsychiatry Department, 'Sapienza' University of Rome, Rome, Italy, **3** Department of Haematology and Cellular Biotechnologies, Sapienza University of Rome, Rome, Italy

Abstract

Introduction: In this study we investigated the effects of the Cystic Fibrosis Transmembrane conductance Regulator (*CFTR*) gene variants on the composition of faecal microbiota, in patients affected by Cystic Fibrosis (CF). *CFTR* mutations (F508del is the most common) lead to a decreased secretion of chloride/water, and to mucus sticky secretions, in pancreas, respiratory and gastrointestinal tracts. Intestinal manifestations are underestimated in CF, leading to ileum meconium at birth, or small bowel bacterial overgrowth in adult age.

Methods: Thirty-six CF patients, fasting and under no-antibiotic treatment, were *CFTR* genotyped on both alleles. Faecal samples were subjected to molecular microbial profiling through Temporal Temperature Gradient Electrophoresis and species-specific PCR. Ecological parameters and multivariate algorithms were employed to find out if *CFTR* variants could be related to the microbiota structure.

Results: Patients were classified by two different criteria: 1) presence/absence of F508del mutation; 2) disease severity in heterozygous and homozygous F508del patients. We found that homozygous-F508del and severe CF patients exhibited an enhanced dysbiotic faecal microbiota composition, even within the CF cohort itself, with higher biodiversity and evenness. We also found, by species-specific PCR, that potentially harmful species (*Escherichia coli* and *Eubacterium biforme*) were abundant in homozygous-F508del and severe CF patients, while beneficial species (*Faecalibacterium prausnitzii*, *Bifidobacterium spp.*, and *Eubacterium limosum*) were reduced.

Conclusions: This is the first report that establishes a link among *CFTR* variants and shifts in faecal microbiota, opening the way to studies that perceive CF as a 'systemic disease', linking the lung and the gut in a joined axis.

Editor: Neeraj Vij, Johns Hopkins School of Medicine, United States of America

Funding: This study was funded by Cystic Fibrosis Lazio Regional Center, Italy, and MIUR Italian Minister for Research. The funders had no role in study design, data collection and analysis, decision to publish, or preparation of the manuscript.

Competing Interests: The authors have declared that no competing interests exist.

* E-mail: valerio.iebba@uniroma1.it

ᵍ These authors contributed equally to this work.

¶ These authors also contributed equally to this work.

Introduction

Cystic fibrosis (CF; OMIM 219700) is an autosomal recessive disorder affecting the exocrine glands of the respiratory, digestive and reproductive systems. The clinical manifestations of CF in affected individuals vary widely, with both age at diagnosis and lethality ranging from the first year of life to the third (and later) decade [1]. In CF, the chronic infection of respiratory tract leads to progressive respiratory deficiency [2]. Mutations in the cystic fibrosis transmembrane conductance regulator (*CFTR*) gene lead to the accumulation of mucus on epithelial surfaces mainly in pancreas, respiratory and gastrointestinal tracts [3,4]. The *CFTR* gene (OMIM 602421) functions as a chloride channel that regulates ions and water transport across epithelial cell membranes. Around 1500 mutations and 300 polymorphisms in the *CFTR* gene are known (Cystic Fibrosis Mutation Database; http://www.genet.sickkids.on.ca/cftr/), usually grouped in five classes representative of all the possible alterations in the maturation process and/or transfer of the CFTR protein [1,5]. In this five-class system, mutations belonging to classes I, II, and III are predicted to have severe functional consequences on CFTR function via different molecular mechanisms. Mutations belonging to classes IV and V, on the other hand, are expected to confer some residual function to CFTR channel, and thus to give milder symptoms. Based on the residual functionality of the protein, mutations are classified as mild or severe, even if a direct

Table 1. Patients' genetics and demographics.

Patient	Sex	Age (years)	CFTR allele, ♂	CFTR allele, ♀	Criterion I[(a)]	Criterion II (1 = severe, 0 = mild)[(b)]	Pancreatic status[(d)]	FEV1%	BMI
1	M	17	F508del	M1V	2	(1)	1	65	17.91
2	F	23	F508del	Y569D	2	(1)	0	97	18.66
3 (s1)[(c)]	F	20	P1013L	F508del	2	(0)	0	87	18.67
4	M	11	F508del	L997F (without R117L)	2	0	0	110	21.33
5 (s1)[(c)]	M	11	P1013L	F508del	2	(0)	0	100	23.14
6	M	8	R553X	F508del	2	1	0	80	15.87
7	M	3	F508del	unknown	2	(0)	0	nd	nd
8	F	33	F508del	F508del	1	1	1	73	18.61
9	M	10	F508del	L1077P	2	1	0	94	19.79
10	M	9	F508del	G542X	2	1	1	100	16.00
11	F	9	4167delCTAAGCC	L1065P	3	nd	1	76	14.57
12	F	14	R117C (without $(TG)_{12}T_5$)	F508del	2	0	0	94	18.44
13	F	11	F508del	991del5	2	1	1	109	17.80
14	M	42	$(TG)_{12}T_5$	F508del	2	0	0	106	23.78
15 (s2)[(c)]	M	9	F508del	F508del	1	1	1	82	15.45
16	M	10	F508del	R347P	2	(0)	0	89	15.91
17 (s2)[(c)]	F	6	F508del	F508del	1	1	1	110	15.20
18 (s3)[(c)]	M	39	2789+5G>A	N1303K	3	nd	0	105	19.33
19 (s3)[(c)]	F	41	2789+5G>A	N1303K	3	nd	0	80	19.47
20	F	26	N1303K	W1282X	3	nd	1	90	19.57
21	M	7	*CFTR*dele2,3 (21 kb)	N1303K	3	nd	1	107	12.85
22	F	9	F508del	L997F (without R117L)	2	0	0	113	25.21
23	M	7	P5L	W1282X	3	nd	0	89	22.31
24	M	9	2789+5G>A	F508del	2	(1)	1	97	15.60
25	F	2	F508del	F508del	1	1	1	nd	nd
26	F	32	N1303K	N1303K	3	nd	1	107	21.22
27	M	14	L1065R	T338I	3	nd	0	116	21.50
28	M	12	711+3A>G	S549R(A>C)	3	nd	0	97	20.00
29	M	13	unknown	R117H (without $(TG)_{12}T_5$)	3	nd	0	104	19.36
30	M	14	F508del	G542X	2	1	1	84	21.87
31	F	13	F508del	F508del	1	1	1	85	18.00
32	F	41	2789+5G>A	N1303K	3	nd	1	84	21.08
33	F	21	L1065P	F508del	2	(0)	0	62	18.29
34	F	50	D1152H	F508del	2	(0)	0	63	23.74
35	M	29	F508del	2790-2A>G	2	(1)	0	92	24.46
36	F	45	unknown	W1282X	3	nd	0	69	23.42

[a](Hm = 1; Ht = 2; N = 3).
[b]when the value is indicated in parenthesis tentative data are available.
[c]s1, s2 a s3 denote a sibling relationship for these three couples of patients.
[d]1 = pancreas insufficiency, 0 = pancreas sufficiency.

correlation among *CFTR* genotype and severity of clinical manifestations is known only for the pancreatic status, not for the lung status [4]. In the gastrointestinal (GI) tract, the loss of the CFTR function results in a dehydrated state of the lumen that is believed to contribute to the insolubility of secreted mucus and glycoproteins. The GI tract represents an additional site where the CF pathology is early manifested, with severe consequences [4,6]. In CF patients many factors predispose to the onset of the small bowel bacterial overgrowth (SBBO) condition, characterized by a high bacterial load in the small intestine [7]. Such a condition could lead to impairment of quality of life at an early stage and also later in the lifespan of an individual. Among the many factors influencing the microbiota composition, the genetic background could act a specific role, as already assessed in other studies [8,9]. Under this hypothesis, the present study aimed to find out a correlation between faecal microbiota composition and the *CFTR* gene mutations in a cohort of CF patients. To this end, the presence of a control cohort was not necessary, because we aimed to depict the variability in microbiota composition mainly driven by different *CFTR* alleles, related to different clinical forms of CF disease. To this purpose, we selected a cohort of 36 CF patients and classified them by means of two different criteria: 1) presence/ absence of F508del mutation; 2) disease severity in heterozygous and homozygous F508del patients. Dominant microbiota of faecal samples was characterized by Temporal Temperature Gradient Gel Electrophoresis (TTGE), a semi-quantitative technique useful for comparative purposes, and by species-specific PCR of cultivable bacterial species usually found in faeces. The results obtained were correlated to the two CF patients classifications, through statistical analysis, in order to find out if mutations in the *CFTR* gene could be related to the microbiota population structure. We also described shifts in faecal microbiota composition driven by *CFTR* genetic background in terms of ecological structure.

Materials and Methods

Ethics Statement

Faecal samples were obtained from hospitalized patients and external controls within the 'Cystic Fibrosis Centre' of the Department of Paediatrics at Hospital 'Policlinico Umberto I' of Rome. Ethics approval for this study was granted by the Ethics Committees of the 'Sapienza' University and 'Policlinico Umberto I' Hospital, Italy. Written informed consent was obtained from parents of all subjects enrolled in this study who were under 18 years of age, while the written informed consent was given autonomously by subjects over (or equal to) 18 years. In any case, written informed consent was obtained upon instructions on ethics, aims, and methodologies employed in the study.

Patients and Classification Criteria

Thirty-six CF patients referred to the 'Regional Cystic Fibrosis Centre' of the Department of Paediatrics at Hospital 'Policlinico Umberto I' of Rome, were enrolled after written informed consent (Table 1). The study protocol was approved by the Committee on Ethical Practice of the 'Policlinico Umberto I' hospital. All patients enrolled did not received antibiotics during 2 month prior to the beginning of the study: this was a rigorous selection criterion, due to the difficulties in not providing antibiotics to CF patients, who usually undergo such a therapy. All patients underwent the same antibiotic treatment (200 mg of ciprofloxacin every 12 hours), suspended 2 months before faecal sampling. All patients enrolled did not suffer from ileum meconium in early stage of life. Furthermore, all patients were fasting one day prior the faecal sampling. All these criteria were chosen to homogenise and reduce the internal variability of microbiota response, in order to have a 'common background' to investigate the role of CFTR genetics on microbiota composition itself. The diagnostic work up of CF was according to international protocols.

Genetic, Biochemical and Clinical Characterization of CF Patients

For all patients a mutational analysis was performed. A first-level genetic investigation was achieved by an ABI PRISM 3100 Avant genetic analyser (Applied Biosystems), through the multiplex DNA test 'PCR/OLA/SCS' (Brinson et al., 1997; Grossman et al., 1994), encompassing the 32 most frequent mutations of the CFTR gene. All patients who had not been characterized by PCR/OLA/SCS were subjected to a second-level genetic investigation, by an ABI PRISM 3130 xl genetic analyser (Applied Biosystems), with direct sequencing of the CFTR gene [10]. The effect of CFTR mutations found and, whenever possible, the functional class, were deduced from literature data [1]. In order to classify the patients we used as criteria of severity: 1) patients characterized by the presence of severe mutations (if known, of class I, II, III) in homozygous or compound heterozygous state and pancreas insufficiency (severe, annotated as 1 in Table 1); 2) patients characterized by the presence of mild mutations (if known, of class IV and V) in homozygous or compound heterozygous state and pancreatic sufficiency (mild, annotated as 0 in Table 1). The mutations found within this case series may be classified as follows. Class I, II or III: G542X, W1282X, F508del, N1303K, L1065P, L1077P, Y569D, S549R(A>C). Class IV or V: R117H, 2789+5G>A, TG12T5, R347P, D1152H, R117C. For the growth evaluation, for patients from birth to 20 years, the weight and height percentiles, the IBW (weigh for height index), and the Body Mass Index (BMI) were assessed, as valid criteria to give assessment of patients nutritional status for all patients age [11]. The assessment of body weight is easy to perform and very useful because the weight gain may be compromised in patients with CF. The height is generally less frequently compromised than the body weight, so its deficit is indicative of a serious and persistent malnutrition. Lung function was assessed by the quantity of air exhaled in one second during a forced breath (FEV1), expressed as a percentage of the theoretical value [12]. As a tool for assessing spirometry was used the Sensor Medics Vmax229. The sweat test was performed with the method of Gibson and Cooke pilocarpine iontophoresis [13], by using Macroduct Collection System and Chloride Meter Jenway System for lecture. The test is considered positive for Cl concentrations above 60 mmol/L, considered negative with values below 40 mmol/L (30 mmol/L for infants). The sweat test with values ranging between 40–60 mmol/L (30–60 mmol/L for infants) were considered borderline. The faecal elastase assay, ELISA stool test Schebo Pancreatic Elastase 1, was used to evaluate the pancreatic exocrine function. Faecal elastase values were considered normal in the range 200–500 mg/g of faeces, borderline between 100–200 mg/g, pathological if less than 100 mg/g of faeces.

Faecal DNA Extraction

Faecal samples were taken from fasting CF patients in a sterile environment placed into the 'Policlinico Umberto I' hospital, directly collected in a 500 mL sterile bottle with large neck, transferred to a 50 mL sterile tube, and immediately frozen at −80°C. Total DNA was extracted within 1 hour from sampling by QIAmp Stool Mini Kit (QIAGEN, Hilden, Germany) following manufacturer's instructions. Starting faecal amount was set at 500 mg, picked up from different chunks within the sample itself, in order to minimize the sampling error. Upon extraction, total DNA concentration was quantified by a NanoDrop spectrophotometer (Thermo Fisher Scientific, Wilmington, Delaware, U.S.A.) at 260 nm, along with the 260/280 ratio, and integrity checked through 1% agarose gel electrophoresis containing EtBr 0.5 µg/ml. We obtained similar DNA concentrations after kit extraction from all CF patients, as assessed by Mann-Whitney U test ($P = 0.348$).

PCR Amplification of Bacterial Gene Coding for 16S rRNA

Universal primers GCclamp-U968 (5′-CGC CCG GGG CGC GCC CCG GGC GGG GCG GGG GCA CGG GGG GAA CGC GAA GAA CCT TAC-3′) and L1401 (5′-GCG TGT GTA CAA GAC CC-3′) were used to amplify the V6–V8 region of bacterial gene coding for 16S rRNA [14]. PCR was performed with Taq DNA-polymerase (Hot Star Taq Plus, QIAGEN). PCR reaction (25 µL) contained 1× buffer per PCR, 2.5 mM $MgCl_2$, 200 µM for each dNTP, 0.5 µM of GCclamp-U968 and L1401 primers, 1.25 U of Taq polymerase and 100 ng of total DNA. The samples were amplified under the following conditions: 95°C for

5 min, cycles at 94°C for 45″, 53°C for 45″, 72°C for one min and 10″, and a final step of 72°C for 30 min. This final elongation step was employed to minimize artefactual 'double bands', which could lead to an overestimation of the actual bacterial diversity. To rule out unspecific products a 'touchdown PCR' was performed with a starting annealing temperature of 58°C and decreasing it by 0.5°C each cycle to reach 53°C, followed by 30 cycles at 53°C. In order to minimize the PCR bias, three 'touchdown PCR' reactions were performed for each sample and subsequently pooled. To minimize hetero-duplex formation and single-stranded DNA (ssDNA) contamination during PCR amplification, that might cause sequence heterogeneity in a single TTGE band, 5 additional cycles of 'reconditioning PCR' were performed, taking 1/10 of the previous pooled PCR volume as template in a new reaction. In order to minimize the PCR bias, three 'reconditioning PCR' reaction were done for each sample and subsequently pooled for TTGE experiments. Successful reaction and DNA concentration was quantified by spectrophotometer measurements at 260 nm and DNA integrity checked through 1% agarose gel electrophoresis containing EtBr 0.5 µg/ml. 500 ng of DNA of PCR product from each sample was used to perform the subsequent TTGE experiments.

TTGE Analysis of Amplified 16S rRNA V6-V8 Region

The DCode Universal Mutation Detection System was used for sequence-specific separation of PCR products. Electrophoresis was performed through a 1 mm thick, 16×16 cm 8% polyacrylamide gel, 7 M urea, 1.25×TAE (Tris-Acetic acid-EDTA, ethylenediaminetetraacetic acid), and, respectively, 40 µL and 400 µL of TEMED (Tetramethylethylenediamine) and 10% ammonium persulfate, using 7 litres of 1.25×TAE as the electrophoresis buffer. Electrophoresis was run at 69 V for 18 hours with an initial temperature of 66°C and a ramp rate of 0.2°C/h. For better resolution, a pre-run of 20 V for 15 minutes were held at the beginning of electrophoresis. Each well was loaded with 500 ng of amplified DNA plus a 2X gel loading dye (0.05% bromophenol blue, 0.05% xylene cyanol, and 70% glycerol). Gels were stained in the dark by immersion for 30 minutes in a solution of 6 µg/ml of EtBr in TAE 1X, de-stained in fresh TAE buffer 1.25X for 30 minutes, and photographed with DigiDoc-It system (UVP, Cambridge, UK). In order to minimize the inter-run variance, TGGE runs were conducted in triplicate.

Species-specific PCR of Bacterial 16S rRNA

We choose to detect, by species-specific PCR, a panel of bacterial species particularly present in human faeces as reported by different authors [15,16]. 16S rRNA gene-targeted primers were utilized to detect them (Table 2). The PCR experiments were performed as previously described [17], with some modifications. Briefly, the PCR was done in triplicate, the starting amount of DNA was 100 ng, and the total number of cycles was 25. The three PCR amplifications for each sample were subsequently pooled, concentrated with Speed Vac (Savant, Holbrook, NY, USA) to reach a final volume approximately equal to 1/3 of the original. The unified PCR reactions were titrated using two different methods: firstly, twenty-five microliters of each concentrated PCR were loaded on a 1% agarose gel containing EtBr 0.5 µg/ml, run for 1 hour at 80 V, photographed with DigiDoc-It system (UVP, Cambridge, UK), and analysed for densitometry with Phoretix 1D software (TotalLab, Newcastle upon Tyne, United Kingdom); secondly, measure of DNA concentration was performed with NanoDrop spectrophotometer (Thermo Fisher Scientific, Wilmington, Delaware, U.S.A.) at 260 nm, using one microliter of unified PCR. DNA titration values obtained from both methods were expressed as nanograms of DNA amount per microliter of PCR. A correction for number of 16S rRNA operons within each bacterial species was done, in order to ensure a suitable inter-species data normalization and interpretation. Mann-Whitney U test was employed to assess differences in relative abundances of bacterial species. A *P* value equal or less to 0.05 was considered statistically significant.

Statistical Methods

Multivariate analysis. Two supervised classification methods, Partial Least Square Discriminant Analysis (PLS-DA) and Orthogonal Projection on Latent Structure Discriminant Analysis (OPLS-DA), were performed on a presence/absence matrix of TTGE bands, derived from the overall 36 TTGE profiles. These multivariate statistical analyses were employed to test the grouping behaviour of the TTGE profiles from CF patients, accordingly to two particular classification criteria: i) F508del homozygous/heterozygous/absence, ii) disease severity upon the non-F508del allele. Three-dimensional score plots were generated on a presence/absence TTGE matrix data by means of PLS-DA/OPLS-DA algorithms implemented in Simca-P+ software (Umetrics, Umeå, Sweden), taking into account two principal components and one orthogonal component. The number of useful components was determined by five-fold cross-validation. Data were automatically mean-centred and unit-variance (UV) scaled by the statistical software. These analyses correlated a number of X variables (TTGE bands) to a set of Y variables (CF patients' category), obtaining the covariance between X and Y. PLS-DA/OPLS-DA approaches created a predictive model, validated through Fisher's test, useful to classify CF patients according to their faecal microbiota composition, as assessed through TTGE and species-specific PCR. A *P* value less than or equal to 0.05 was considered statistically significant. *Clustered Image Mapping (CIM)*. A resuming heatmap figure, to figure out the putative *CFTR* action in shaping faecal bacterial community, was obtained by the on-line software 'CIMminer' (http://discover.nci.nih.gov/cimminer) based on a scaled and centred dataset of TTGE bands and their OPLS-DA coefficient loadings. Weight coefficients were computed by PLS-DA/OPLS-DA algorithm with Simca-P+ software (Umetrics) for each TTGE band (87 X-variables) on each CF patients' classification group. X and Y variables were 2D clustered, based on Euclidean distance dissimilarity matrix and agglomeration method of Ward.

Ecological Features

Five ecological parameters were computed for each faecal TTGE profile, taking into account the number of bands, their relative position, and their volume (in pixels): Simpson biodiversity (H_{si}), Simpson evenness (E_{si}), carrying capacity (Rr), Gini coefficient of concentration (C), and normalized area under Pareto-Lorenz curves ($PL0.5$). Simpson biodiversity index (H_{si}), reflecting the number and relative abundances of the bacterial species within a sample, was calculated for each TTGE lane by the equation $H_{si}=1-\sum_{i=1}^{S} p_i^2$, where $p_i=n_i/N$, n_i= volume (in pixels) of ith TTGE band, N= sum of total TTGE bands pixel volumes, and S= number of TTGE bands. Simpson evenness index (E_{si}), reflecting the distribution of species density within a sample, was calculated by the formula $E_{si}=(1-\sum_{i=1}^{S} p_i^2)\Big/(1-1/S)$, where symbols were the same as above.

The range-weighted richness (Rr), reflecting the carrying capacity of the faecal habitat and richness of microbial commu-

Table 2. Group- and species-specific primers based on 16S rRNA sequences.

Target bacteria	Primer	Sequence (5′ to 3′)	Product size (bp)
Bacteroides fragilis group	g-Bfra-F	ATAGCCTTTCGAAAGRAAGAT	501
	g-Bfra-R	CCAGTATCAACTGCAATTTTA	
Prevotella group	g-Prevo-F	CACRGTAAACGATGGATGCC	529
	g-Prevo-R	GGTCGGGTTGCAGACC	
Bifidobacterium group	g-Bifid-F	CTCCTGGAAACGGGTGG	563
	g-Bifid-R	GGTGTTCTTCCCGATATCTACA	
Clostridium coccoides group	g-Ccoc-F	AAATGACGGTACCTGACTAA	441
	g-Ccoc-R	CTTTGAGTTTCATTCTTGCGAA	
Bifidobacterium adolescentis	BIA-1	GGAAAGATTCTATCGGTATGG	244
	BIA-2	CTCCCAGTCAAAAGCGGTT	
Bifidobacterium longum	BIL-1	GTTCCCGACGGTCGTAGAG	153
	BIL-2	GTGAGTTCCCGGCATAATCC	
Eubacterium biforme	EBI-1	GCTAAGGCCATGAACATGGA	463
	EBI-2	GCCGTCCTCTTCTGTTCTC	
Eubacterium limosum	ELI-1	GGCTTGCTGGACAAATACTG	274
	ELI-2	CTAGGCTCGTCAGAAGGATG	
Fusobacterium prausnitzii	FPR-1	AGATGGCCTCGCGTCCGA	199
	FPR-2	CCGAAGACCTTCTTCCTCC	
Peptostreptococcus productus	PSP-1	AACTCCGGTGGTATCAGATG	268
	PSP-2	GGGGCTTCTGAGTCAGGTA	
Lactobacillus acidophilus	LAA-1	CATCCAGTGCAAACCTAAGAG	286
	LAA-2	GATCCGCTTGCCTTCGCA	
Escherichia coli	ECO-1	GACCTCGGTTTAGTTCACAGA	585
	ECO-2	CACACGCTGACGCTGACCA	
Bacteroides thetaiotaomicron	BT-1	GGCAGCATTTCAGTTTGCTTG	423
	BT-2	GGTACATACAAAATTCCACACGT	
Bacteroides vulgatus	BV-1	GCATCATGAGTCCGCATGTTC	287
	BV-2	TCCATACCCGACTTTATTCCTT	
Bacteroides distasonis	BD-1	GTCGGACTAATACCGCATGAA	273
	BD-2	TTACGATCCATAGAACCTTCAT	
Clostridium clostridiiforme	CC-1	CCGCATGGCAGTGTGTGAAA	255
	CC-2	CTGCTGATAGAGCTTTACATA	

nity, was computed by the equation $Rr = S^2 * Tg$, where S is the total number of TTGE bands in a profile and Tg the temperature gradient comprised between the first and the last band of the same pattern [18]. Rr index was subsequently normalized (Rr_{norm}) to the value of 400, the maximum Rr value achievable for a faecal bacterial habitat, as found in this study and in literature [18]. Gini coefficient of concentration (C), reflecting the inequality of the bacterial population structure was computed by the formula $C = \frac{S}{S-1}\left\{\left(\frac{2}{S^2\bar{n}}\right) * \sum_{i=1}^{S}\left[\left(i^{th} - \frac{S+1}{2}\right)n_i\right]\right\}$, where the portion within curly braces is the Gini coefficient (G), S is the number of TTGE bands, $\bar{n} = \sum_{i=1}^{S} n_i \Big/ S$, n_i is the volume (in pixels) of ith TTGE band, and i^{th} is the number of ith band ($i^{th} = 1,2,\ldots S$) found in a TTGE profile. Surface area between the diagonal and the Pareto-Lorenz curve ($PL0.5$), that measures the structure of the community in terms of its evenness, or the dominance of particular bacterial species, was calculated for each TTGE profile in two step. Firstly, Pareto-Lorenz curve was graphed putting on x-axis the cumulative normalized number of TTGE bands and on y-axis their cumulative normalized volume-intensities (in pixels). Secondly, aforementioned surface area was computed using the macro 'area under curve' employed in SigmaPlot 9.0 (SigmaStat), and subsequently normalized to 0.5 value (the surface area under the diagonal itself): values so obtained are comparable to the Fo functional organization parameter previously proposed [18]. The Mann-Whitney U test was used to assess putative differences among the ecological parameters, and a P value less than or equal to 0.05 was considered significant.

Results

Patients and CFTR Genotyping

A cohort of 36 CF patients was enrolled and underwent to *CFTR* genotyping, as described in Materials and Methods. Both maternal and paternal *CFTR* alleles were sequenced (Table 1), and prevalence of each allele in the entire CF cohort was assessed

(Figure S1). The enrolled 36 CF patients had an overall of 26 different *CFTR* alleles, with a major prevalence of the mutation F508del (24/36, 66.7%), and, at a lesser extent, N1303K (6/36, 16.7%), 2789+5G>A (5/36, 13.9%) and W1282X (3/36, 8.3%), accordingly with literature (Table 1) [1,5]. The other mutations were found in our case series to an allele frequency below 5.6%. Some of them are characteristic of certain ethnic groups, such as W1282X in the original Jews of Central Europe, 3659delC in Sweden and, to come to the Italian reality, T338I in Sardinia, 2183AA>G and R1162X in Northern Italy [1,5]. In order to assess the influence of *CFTR* genotype on faecal microbiota, the unique cohort of patients was divided by two specific classification criteria. Following the first criterion, all the 36 CF patients were divided in three classes: Hom-F508del (homozygous F508del) (n = 5), Het-F508del (heterozygous F508del) (n = 19), and Non-F508del (absence of F508del) (n = 12). Following the second criterion, only patients with homozygosis (n = 5) or heterozygosis (n = 19) for F508del mutation were taken into account. For this second criterion, a combination of the two *CFTR* alleles plus a clinical evaluation (Forced expiratory volume - FEV1%, exocrine pancreas function, and Body mass index - BMI) were taken into account, and a final score of 'mild' (n = 10) and 'severe' (n = 14) was given to each patient (Table 1). The first criterion encompassed all 36 CF patients, whilst the second one comprehended 24 CF patients harbouring at least one F508del allele.

F508del Mutation Drives a Different Faecal Microbiota Composition

Our cohort consisted of 26 *CFTR* genotypes (Table 1, Figure S1), allowing the examination of putative relationships existing among *CFTR* alleles and faecal bacterial community composition. Due to the high prevalence of F508del mutation (Figure S1), we choose to divide patients in 3 classes: homozygous-F508del (n = 5), heterozygous-F508del (n = 19) or non-F508del mutation (n = 12). Their TTGE profiles of faecal microbiota were regressed against this first criterion by means of PLS-DA algorithm, to assess if F508del mutation could affect the faecal microbiota structure in a particular way. We reported representative mean TTGE profiles for each of the three classes, along with a heatmap based on Euclidean distance generated by means of the online tool CIMminer (Figure 1, panel A). In this latter, the red areas correspond to the TTGE bands with higher importance in dividing the three classes, showing how the different genetic background, due to the homozygous-F508del, heterozygous-F508del and non-F508del, arise different faecal microbiota compositions in CF patients. A score plot obtained by the PLS-DA analysis was also depicted (Figure 1, panel B), showing a significant separation among the three classes of CF patients (Total error = 0%, Fisher's $P = 3.1*10^{-14}$).

Faecal Microbiota Composition is Shaped by CF Disease Severity

CFTR gene mutations are commonly divided in 5 classes, upon their phenotypic/clinical severity [1,5]. In order to assess if the faecal microbiota structure would be affected by CF disease severity, we choose all the CF patients harbouring at least one F508del mutation. Once established that F508del drives a different faecal microbiota composition (see above), we focused our attention on homozygous-F508del (n = 5) and heterozigous-F508del (n = 19) patients, dividing them into two distinct classes: mild (n = 10) and severe (n = 14). Their TTGE profiles of faecal microbiota were regressed against this second criterion by means of OPLS-DA algorithm: this criterion was chosen because F508del mutation was found in 24/36 (66.7%) of CF patients, thus allowing a common background to investigate the role of the other *CFTR* allele on faecal microbiota composition. We reported representative mean TTGE profiles for each of the two classes, along with a heatmap based on Euclidean distance generated by means of the online tool CIMminer (Figure 2, panel A). In the heatmap, red areas correspond to the TTGE bands with higher importance in dividing the severe and mild classes, showing how the different genetic background, due to the other non-F508del allele, could shape a different faecal microbiota compositions in CF patients. A score plot obtained by the OPLS-DA analysis was also drawn (Figure 2, panel B), showing a significant separation among the two classes of CF patients (Total error = 0%, Fisher's $P = 1.2*10^{-6}$). Thus, CFTR mutations, driving a mild or severe clinical phenotype in CF patients, could also drive, in some measure, the faecal microbiota composition.

Ecological Parameters Describe the Faecal Microbiota Structure in CF Patients

To determine which aspects of community composition were most related to CFTR mutation, specific ecological parameters were computed for each TTGE profile: Simpson biodiversity (*Hsi*), Simpson equiripartition index (*Esi*), normalized carrying capacity (Rr_{norm}), Gini coefficient of inequality (*C*), and normalized Pareto-Lorenz curves (*PL*0.5). Even if the TTGE is considered a semi-quantitative technique, it can describe bacteria that constitute up to 1% of the total bacterial community [19,20]: thus, due to this resolution power, it can properly describe changes in bacterial community structure. Taking into account all CF patients, without any classification, we found linear correlations among the ecological parameters: *Esi* and *Hsi* ($R^2 = 0.925$), *C* and *PL*0.5 ($R^2 = 0.926$) were linearly and positive correlated, whilst *Esi* and *C*, *Hsi* and *C* were linearly correlated with a negative slope (Figure 3). Rr_{norm} parameter showed no correlation with *Esi*, *Hsi*, *C*, or *PL*0.5 (results not shown). Mann-Whitney U test was used to calculate putative ecological differences among faecal microbiota of homozygous-F508del, heterozygous-F508del and non-F508del groups (criterion I). The same test was used to quantify differences in ecological parameters among severe and mild CF patients (criterion II). In Table 3 are the results. Homozygous F508del mutation led the faecal microbiota to higher evenness (*Esi*) ($P = 0.027$) and higher biodiversity (*Hsi*), compared to heterozygous-F508del and non-F508del. Severe CF patients showed a faecal microbiota with lesser inequality of the bacterial population structure (*C*) and lesser dominance of particular bacterial species (*PL*0.5), compared to the mild one ($P = 0.024$). At a microbial community level, these results could explain why F508del mutation led to a different faecal microbiota composition, as well as the CF disease severity did.

Particular Bacterial Species are Related to the CF Disease Phenotype

Once established that F508del mutation and CF disease severity drive a particular faecal microbiota composition, showing different values of ecological parameters, we shifted our attention from the microbiota to some of its constituting bacterial species. Species-specific PCR assays were performed to achieve a presence/absence and a relative quantification of some cultivable bacterial species usually found in faeces, as reported in literature [15,16]. After an accurate correction for the intra-species number of 16S rDNA operons, a matrix of relative quantification based on 1% agarose gel densitometry was built, combined with species-specific

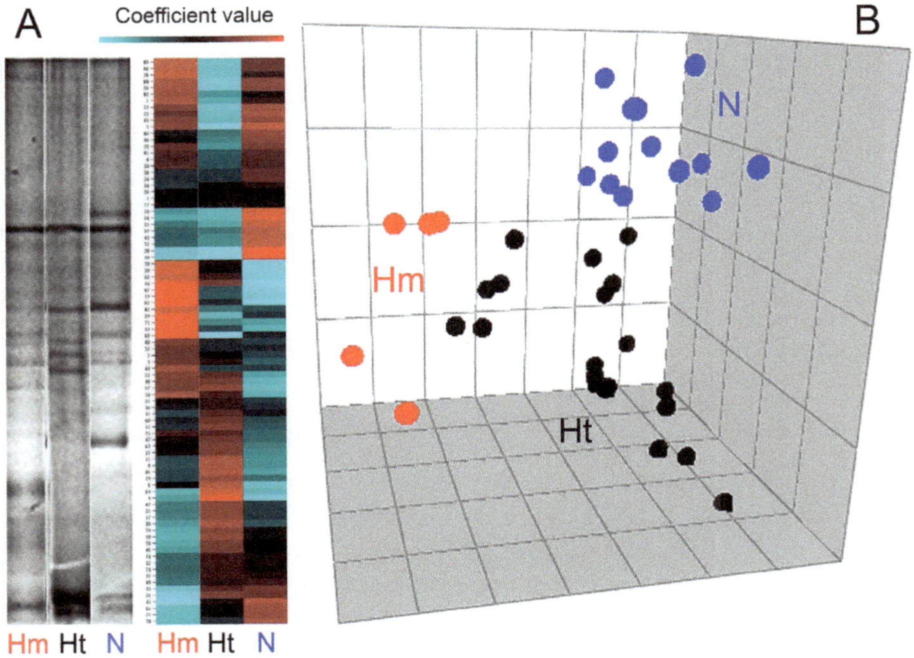

Figure 1. PLS-DA analysis of TTGE profiles, according to F508del mutation. Panel A) On the left are reported representative TTGE profiles from homozygous-F508del (Hm), heterozygous-F508del (Ht) and non-F508del (N) patients. Simca-P+ software was used to compute weight coefficients for each TTGE band (87 *x* variables) on the three different sub-groups of CF patients (3 *y* variables, Hm-Ht-N), with a scaled and centred data set. These coefficients were useful to interpret the influence of the x variables on the y ones. A clustered image heatmap was generated with CIMminer online software (panel A, right). As depicted in the color-coded legend, the higher that the coefficient value is, the higher the weight (red), while the lower that the value is, the lower the weight (turquoise). Panel B) Faecal TTGE profiles of all 36 CF patients were analysed by PLS-DA, and the resulting 3D score plot model gave a significant separation between the three sub-groups: homozygous-F508del (Hm, red circles); heterozygous-F508del (Ht, black circles), and non-F508del (N, blue circles).

prevalence data, and processed with Mann-Whitney U test to assess putative differences in bacterial relative abundances. Among sixteen bacterial species or groups examined (Table 2), only five were found to be differentially distributed, in terms of relative abundance, in faecal samples of CF patients divided by the two classification criteria: *Escherichia coli*, *Faecalibacterium prausnitzii*, *Bifidobacterium* group, *Eubacterium limosum*, *Eubacterium biforme*. We found higher levels of *E. coli* and *E. biforme* in homozygous-F508del patients, and, at the same time, higher levels of *F. prausnitzii*, *Bifidobacterium*, and *E. limosum* in non-F508del patients (Figure 4). Taking into account the criterion II, we found that severe CF patients harboured more *E. coli* and *E. biforme* than mild one, which, in turn, had higher levels of *F. prausnitzii*, *Bifidobacterium*, and *E. limosum* in their faecal samples (Figure 5).

Discussion

Recently, the intricate molecular mechanisms underpinning the host-microbe cross-talk has begun to emerge. Gut microbiota, the biggest bacterial community in our body, exerts many beneficial effects on our health, acting like an 'organ' with peculiar characteristics in its composition and function [21]. Many features can shape the gut microbiota structure: sex [22], diet [23], birth delivery [24], feeding mode [25], and disease status [26]. Up to date, only two studies focused on the role of human genetics as a modifier agent of gut microbiota composition: the first, in Inflammatory Bowel Diseases (IBD) [9], and the second, in Familiar Mediterranean Fever (FMF) [8]. Like FMF, Cystic fibrosis is a good candidate to assess how the genetic background could shape the gut microbiota, due to its monogenic nature (unlike IBD, where 99 loci are known to play a role [27]). During development, intestine is the first district in which high levels of CFTR mRNA are expressed, and are constitutively maintained during all the lifetime [28]. The intestine usually presents high protein or mucous loads, together with low flow rates, and CFTR defects lead to abnormalities in: gastrointestinal tissue morphology, electrolytes secretion, mucus secretion, protein concentration, and protein folding [28]. For this reason, a loss of function of CFTR protein can lead to intestinal obstruction (called ileum meconium) as the earliest clinical phenotype of CF, and to intestinal complications in paediatric/adult age as a secondary site of CF manifestations (after the lung) [28]. Recently, it was found how a diminished pH in airway epithelia from $CFTR^{-/-}$ pigs impaired bacterial killing [29], and it could be speculated a similar event also in the gastrointestinal tract, where a particular microbiota could arise [30].

Our study hypothesis was that *CFTR* genetic background could act as a selective force, able to drive a different gut microbiota, as well as the faecal one, in CF patients. Gut microbiota encompasses mucosa-associated and luminal microbiota, while faeces mainly harbor the luminal part of the gut microbiota. Therefore, we showed here how *CFTR* gene variants were related to shifts in faecal microbiota profiles of CF patients. Particularly, we found that the most common *CFTR* mutation, F508del, found in 66.7% of our patients, led to a peculiar composition of faecal microbiota, especially in the homozygous state (Fig. 1), in which *E. coli* and *E. biforme* species prevailed (Fig. 4). The potential effect that differences in sample size could have on data interpretation, e.g. in the case of the five homozygous F508del patients, was considered and taken into account in the multivariate statistical

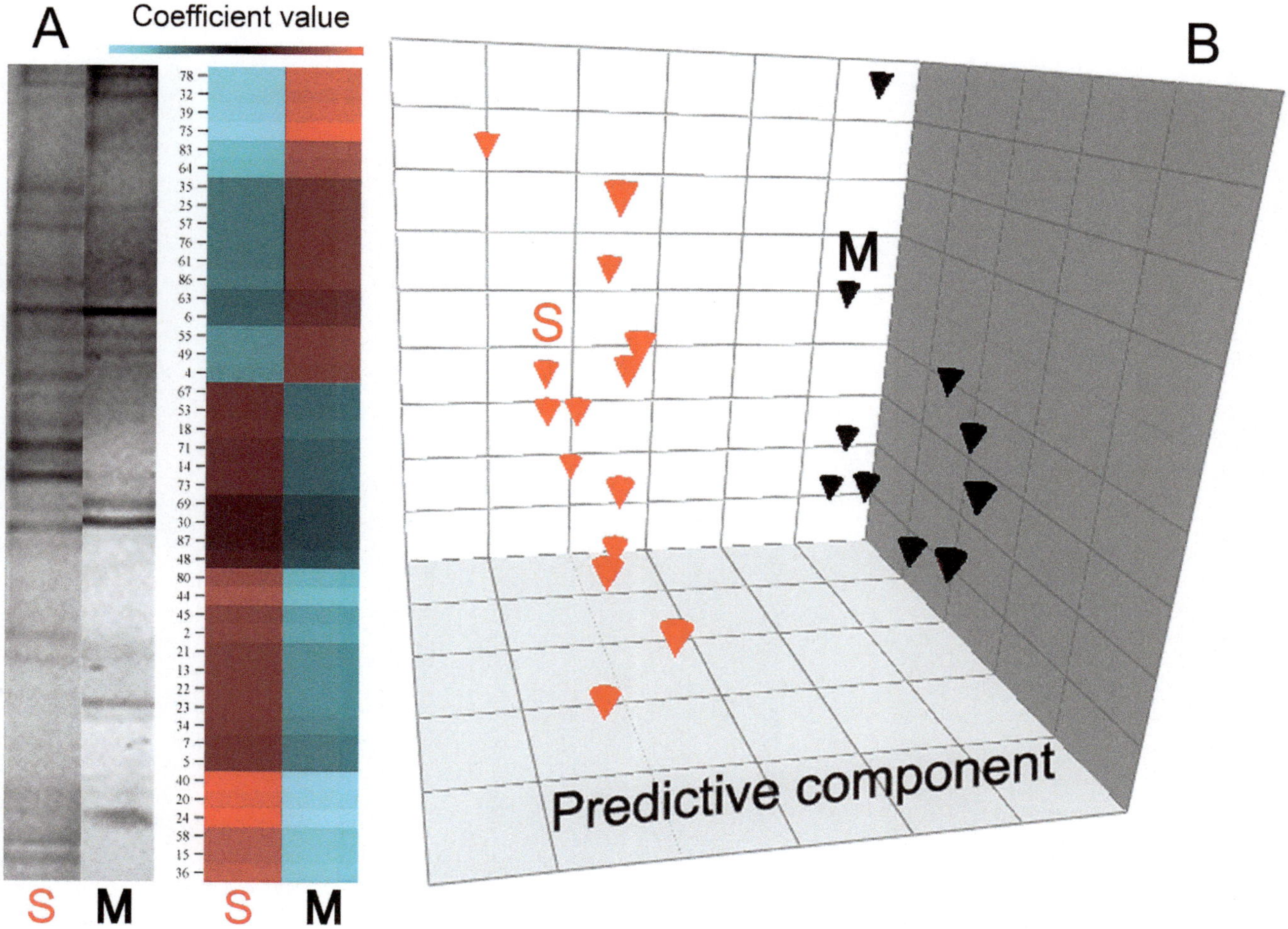

Figure 2. OPLS-DA analysis of TTGE profiles, according to disease severity. Panel A) On the left are reported representative TTGE profiles from severe and mild CF patients. Simca-P+ software was used to compute weight coefficients for each TTGE band (87 *x* variables) on the two subgroups of CF patients (2 *y* variables) harbouring at least one F508del mutation in one allele: severe (S) and mild (M), with a scaled a centred data set. A clustered image heatmap was generated with CIMminer online software (panel A, right). As depicted in the color-coded legend, the higher that the coefficient value is, the higher the weight (red), while the lower that the value is, the lower the weight (turquoise). Panel B) Faecal TTGE profiles of all 24 CF patients harbouring at least one F508del allele were analysed by OPLS-DA, and the resulting 3D score plot model gave a significant separation among the two sub-groups: severe (S, black diamonds) and mild (M, red diamonds).

analysis by intra-variance correction. Such results are to be considered indicative for future studies addressed to investigate the role of homozygous F508del state in human subjects more deeply. F508del mutation arose around 11000 years ago, spreading out during the Neolithic human expansion, due to a putative selective advantage of heterozygous F508del state [31]. Following literature data, F508del mutation belongs to the second class of *CFTR* mutations, in which loss of function of the resulting CFTR protein heavily impairs chloride secretion, leading to a higher thickness and viscosity of the mucus layer [1,5]. It could be arguable that such a peculiar intestinal habitat, along with an inflamed mucosal state, could enhance the adhesion capability of particular bacterial species, such as *E. coli* and *E. biforme*, leading to higher counts in their populations, as already established for *E. coli* strains in Inflammatory Bowel Diseases [32]. Indeed, we found these two bacterial species to be prevalent also in faecal samples from severe CF patients, not from mild (Fig. 5). The mean percentages of *E. coli* and *E. biforme* in faecal samples are usually 1.21% [33] and 1.00% [34], respectively. Thus, the expected *E. coli*/*E. biforme* ratio of the mean relative abundances in a faecal sample from healthy subjects should be around 1.2. Actually, in a parallel on-going study, we found that *E. coli*/*E. biforme* mean ratio within our cohort of healthy subjects was 1.6, and this ratio grew up to 50.4 in an age- and sex-matched CF cohort (unpublished data, not shown here). Notably, *E. coli* differs from *E. biforme* not only for the cell wall properties (the former is Gram-negative, the latter is Gram-positive), but also for antibiotic susceptibility [35].

E. coli was found to be highly prevalent in homozygous-F508del and severe CF patients, which also harboured a different faecal microbiota (Fig. 1 and 2). The high prevalence of *E. coli* found could be due to its enhanced fitness in the CF intestinal habitat as already observed in Celiac disease [36] and IBD [32,37]. We could hypothesize that high levels of *E. coli* in homozygous F508del and severe CF patients would be related to a 'pathobiont' sub-population. Since there is an increasing evidence of intestinal inflammation in CF [38], this habitat could be at the origin of a positive selection for inflammation-adapted *E. coli* 'pathobionts', as well as it happens in other disorders. In IBD patients with underlying genetic mutations, inflammation is targeted to specific members of the microbiota and not to infectious pathogens [39]. Moreover, other authors found that *Escherichia* genus, as well as *Clostridium* and *Enterococcus*, that reside in all people, are usually

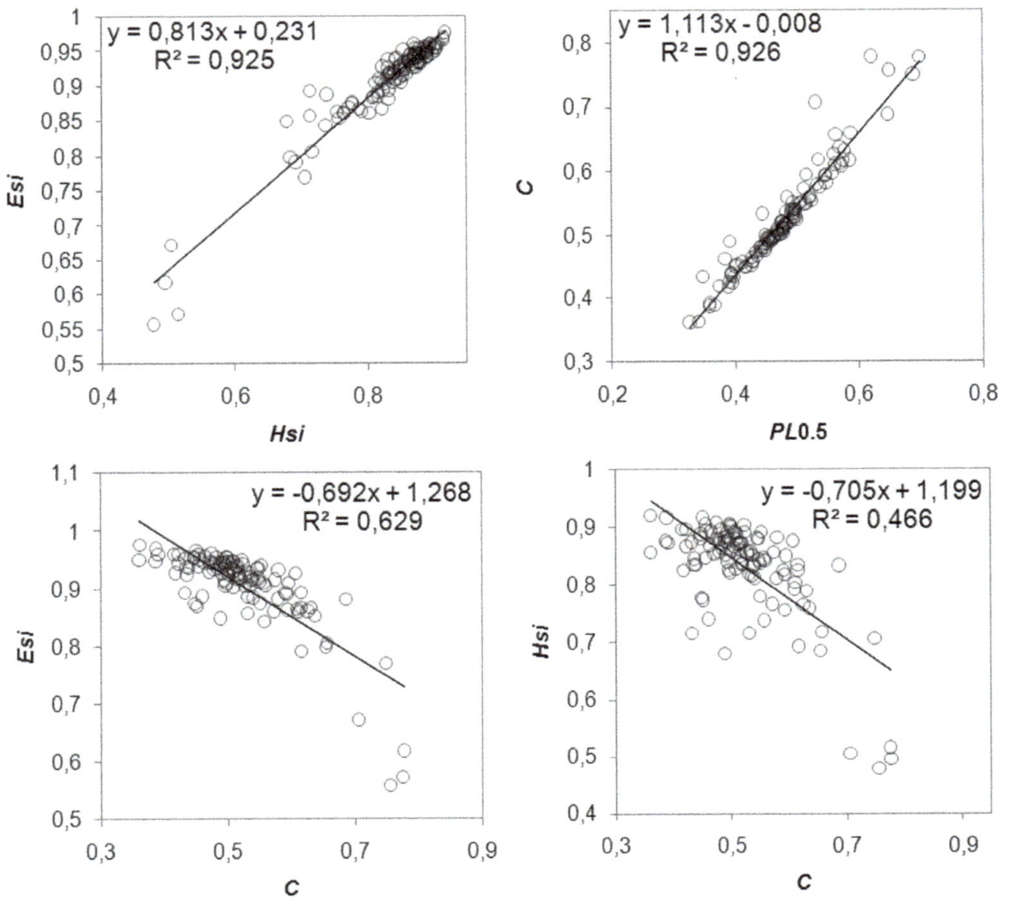

Figure 3. Correlations among ecological features. Faecal TTGE profiles were used to compute five ecological parameters: Simpson biodiversity (*Hsi*), Simpson equiripartition index (*Esi*), normalized carrying capacity (Rr_{norm}), Gini coefficient of inequality (*C*), and normalized Pareto-Lorenz curves (*PL0.5*). Each panel reports the linear equation y = mx+q and the R^2 value, to assess a positive or negative correlation and the goodness of linear fit. Rr_{norm} gave no correlation with any of the other ecological parameters (correlation not shown).

targeted by T cell response in an inflamed intestinal habitat, leading to the 'pathobiont' hypothesis [40,41]. *E. biforme* resulted to be significantly present in homozygous-F508del (Fig. 4) and severe CF patients (Fig. 5). This bacterial species was isolated from human faeces, rumen, sewage and soil, but it was occasionally isolated from wounds, abscesses and periodontitis, thus it may be considered an opportunistic pathogen [34,42]. At the same time, both in homozygous-F508del and severe CF patients, we also found a marked reduction in beneficial bacterial species, as stated in literature, such as *Faecalibacterium prausnitzii* [43], *Bifidobacterium spp.*, and *Eubacterium limosum* [44] (Fig. 4 and 5). Interestingly, it is conceivable that *E. biforme* doesn't belong to the same genus of *E. limosum*, because the former belongs to Erysipelotrichi class, while the latter belongs to Clostridia class, both within the Firmicutes phylum. Thus, a within-the-genus different bacterial habit should be taken unambiguously, albeit *E. biforme* and *E. limosum* apparently have the same 'genus' designation. From the aforementioned results, one could realize that *CFTR* genetic back-

Table 3. Ecological parameters.

Parameter	Homozygous F508del	Heterozygous F508del	Non-F508del	*P* value[a]	Severe	Mild	*P* value
Hsi	0.863±0.008	0.820±0.011	0.829±0.016	**0.048** (Hm-Ht)	0.840±0.009	0.813±0.019	0.398
Esi	0.933±0.005	0.897±0.010	0.905±0.012	**0.027** (Hm-Ht)	0.917±0.007	0.888±0.017	0.112
Rr_{norm}	0.503±0.071	0.370±0.028	0.407±0.040	**0.019** (Hm-Ht)	0.398±0.038	0.398±0.039	0.936
C	0.492±0.015	0.525±0.011	0.538±0.013	0.142 (Hm-N)	0.502±0.013	0.539±0.014	**0.024**
PL0.5	0.456±0.015	0.478±0.011	0.489±0.010	0.179 (Hm-N)	0.460±0.012	0.493±0.013	**0.024**

[a]Hm, homozygous F508del; Ht, heterozygous F508del; N, non-F508del. The lowest *P* value was reported for all comparisons (within round brackets is reported the corresponding match). In bold are the significant *P* values.

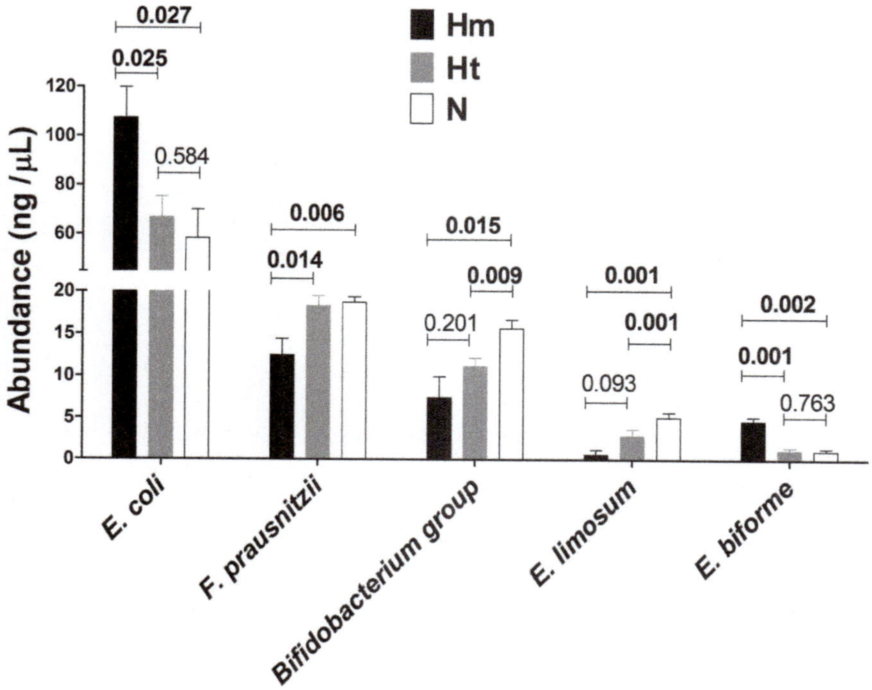

Figure 4. Species-specific PCR, according to F508del mutation. Species-specific PCR were performed on 16 bacterial species or groups, and a Mann-Whitney U test was employed to assess putative differences in their relative abundances (expressed as ng/µL) among homozygous-F508del (Hm, black bars), heterozygous-F508del (Ht, grey bars) and non-F508del (N, white bars) patients. In figure were reported the five bacterial species (or groups) with significant *P* values (in bold) among sub-groups.

ground in homozygous-F508del and severe patients led to an enhanced dysbiosis, with the prevalence of *E. coli* and *E. biforme* species, even within the CF cohort itself. Indeed, we found that biodiversity (*Hsi*), evenness (*Esi*), and carrying capacity (Rr_{norm})

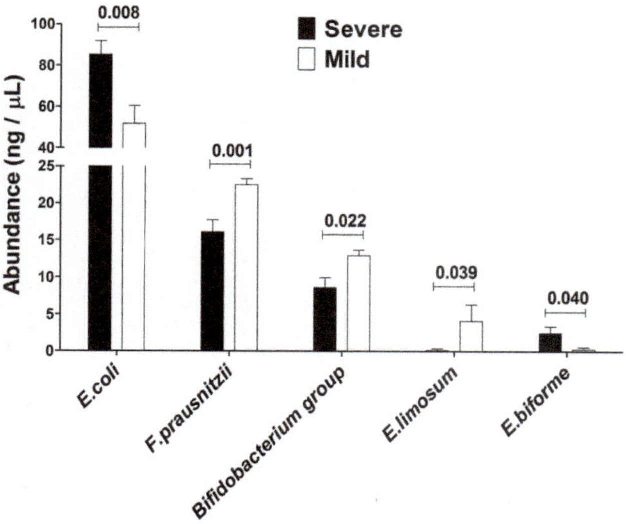

Figure 5. Species-specific PCR, according to disease severity. Species-specific PCR were performed on 16 bacterial species or groups, and a Mann-Whitney U test was employed to assess putative differences in their relative abundances (expressed as ng/µL) among severe (black bars) and mild (white bars) CF patients. In figure were reported the five bacterial species (or groups) with significant *P* values (in bold) among sub-groups.

were significantly higher in homozygous-F508del patients, while inequality (C) and community dominance (*PL*0.5) were lower in severe CF patients (Table 3). These results are in agreement with the hypothesis of an enhanced SBBO in the gut of CF patients [7], eventually leading to a major load of bacterial counts and by-products that could stimulate an exaggerated mucosal response in the gut. Owing to faeces that mainly represent the luminal bacteria, in order to properly assess an *in situ* dysbiotic event, further experiments should be done on intestinal biopsies from CF patients, similarly to what has recently been done on samples from transplanted lungs [45]. Such a requirement could be difficult to be achieved, because CF patients usually don't undergo gastro-duodenoscopy or endoscopy in their clinical follow-up, and, most importantly, intestinal symptoms are commonly underestimated [2,6,28]. It is noteworthy that our cohort was not under antibiotic treatment for two months before faecal sampling, nor the patients underwent a probiotic usage: thus, the role of the *CFTR* gene on shaping the faecal microbiota was not influenced by such treatments. Previously, it was demonstrated a relation among *CFTR* gene mutations and modifications induced in the airway microbiota in 51 CF patients [46], thus, the common genetic background could establish a link among the two main body districts in which CFTR mRNA is expressed: the lung and the gut [28]. Recent studies evidenced an emerging view of an intimate cross-talk [47] existing among the lung and the gut, especially in CF [48]. Thus, CF disease could be perceived as a 'systemic disease', in which pulmonary and intestinal habitats are inter-connected in a 'lung-gut axis' by immunological system, common genetic background (like *CFTR*), and, ultimately, some bacterial or viral species, or they by-products [47]. Clinical studies should be pointed towards a holistic view of the comorbidities existing within a disease: such an effort should also ameliorate the CF treatment regimens. The present study was only on an observational basis: further experiments with mice, or pigs, carrying mutated *CFTR* variants, would shed light on the actual microbiota-modulating properties of *CFTR* gene. This kind of study would improve the knowledge on the refined interactions existing among host and microbiota, important step to set up new therapy strategies aimed at restoring and maintaining an healthy intestinal microbiota in CF patients, and to ameliorate their clinical conditions.

Supporting Information

Figure S1 CFTR alleles prevalence. All *CFTR* mutations found in this study are reported in descending order of prevalence. On *x*-axis is shown the percentage of patients (n = 36, black bars), or the percentage of *CFTR* alleles (n = 72, white bars), harbouring almost one copy of the mutation depicted on *y*-axis.

Author Contributions

Conceived and designed the experiments: VI SS. Performed the experiments: VI FS AG. Analyzed the data: VI. Contributed reagents/materials/analysis tools: RDB AS SB ML MPC SQ. Wrote the paper: VI SS.

References

1. Castellani C, Cuppens H, Macek M Jr, Cassiman JJ, Kerem E, et al. (2008) Consensus on the use and interpretation of cystic fibrosis mutation analysis in clinical practice. J Cyst Fibros 7: 179–196.
2. Davis PB, Drumm M, Konstan MW (1996) Cystic fibrosis. Am J Respir Crit Care Med 154: 1229–1256.
3. Boucher RC (2002) An overview of the pathogenesis of cystic fibrosis lung disease. Adv Drug Deliv Rev 54: 1359–1371.
4. Ahmed N, Corey M, Forstner G, Zielenski J, Tsui LC, et al. (2003) Molecular consequences of cystic fibrosis transmembrane regulator (CFTR) gene mutations in the exocrine pancreas. Gut 52: 1159–1164.
5. Rowntree RK, Harris A (2003) The phenotypic consequences of CFTR mutations. Ann Hum Genet 67: 471–485.
6. Casaccia G, Trucchi A, Nahom A, Aite L, Lucidi V, et al. (2003) The impact of cystic fibrosis on neonatal intestinal obstruction: the need for prenatal/neonatal screening. Pediatr Surg Int 19: 75–78.
7. Fridge JL, Conrad C, Gerson L, Castillo RO, Cox K (2007) Risk factors for small bowel bacterial overgrowth in cystic fibrosis. J Pediatr Gastroenterol Nutr 44: 212–218.
8. Khachatryan ZA, Ktsoyan ZA, Manukyan GP, Kelly D, Ghazaryan KA, et al. (2008) Predominant role of host genetics in controlling the composition of gut microbiota. PloS one 3: e3064.
9. Frank DN, Robertson CE, Hamm CM, Kpadeh Z, Zhang T, et al. (2011) Disease phenotype and genotype are associated with shifts in intestinal-associated microbiota in inflammatory bowel diseases. Inflamm Bowel Dis 17: 179–184.
10. Lucarelli M, Narzi L, Piergentili R, Ferraguti G, Grandoni F, et al. (2006) A 96-well formatted method for exon and exon/intron boundary full sequencing of the CFTR gene. Anal Biochem 353: 226–235.
11. Borowitz D, Baker RD, Stallings V (2002) Consensus report on nutrition for pediatric patients with cystic fibrosis. J Pediatr Gastroenterol Nutr 35: 246–259.
12. Lewiston N, Moss R, Hindi R, Rubinstein S, Sullivan M (1987) Interobserver variance in clinical scoring for cystic fibrosis. Chest 91: 878–882.
13. Gibson LE, Cooke RE (1959) A test for concentration of electrolytes in sweat in cystic fibrosis of the pancreas utilizing pilocarpine by iontophoresis. Pediatrics 23: 545–549.
14. Nubel U, Engelen B, Felske A, Snaidr J, Wieshuber A, et al. (1996) Sequence heterogeneities of genes encoding 16S rRNAs in *Paenibacillus polymyxa* detected by temperature gradient gel electrophoresis. J Bacteriol 178: 5636–5643.
15. Wang RF, Cao WW, Cerniglia CE (1996) PCR detection and quantitation of predominant anaerobic bacteria in human and animal fecal samples. Appl Environ Microbiol 62: 1242–1247.
16. Matsuki T, Watanabe K, Fujimoto J, Miyamoto Y, Takada T, et al. (2002) Development of 16S rRNA-gene-targeted group-specific primers for the detection and identification of predominant bacteria in human feces. Appl Environ Microbiol 68: 5445–5451.
17. Conte MP, Schippa S, Zamboni I, Penta M, Chiarini F, et al. (2006) Gut-associated bacterial microbiota in paediatric patients with inflammatory bowel disease. Gut 55: 1760–1767.
18. Marzorati M, Wittebolle L, Boon N, Daffonchio D, Verstraete W (2008) How to get more out of molecular fingerprints: practical tools for microbial ecology. Environ Microbiol 10: 1571–1581.
19. Zoetendal EG, Akkermans AD, De Vos WM (1998) Temperature gradient gel electrophoresis analysis of 16S rRNA from human fecal samples reveals stable and host-specific communities of active bacteria. Appl Environ Microbiol 64: 3854–3859.
20. Zoetendal EG, Cheng B, Koike S, Mackie RI (2004) Molecular microbial ecology of the gastrointestinal tract: from phylogeny to function. Curr Issues Intest Microbiol 5: 31–47.
21. Ley RE, Peterson DA, Gordon JI (2006) Ecological and evolutionary forces shaping microbial diversity in the human intestine. Cell 124: 837–848.
22. Li M, Wang B, Zhang M, Rantalainen M, Wang S, et al. (2008) Symbiotic gut microbes modulate human metabolic phenotypes. Proc Natl Acad Sci U S A 105: 2117–2122.
23. De Filippo C, Cavalieri D, Di Paola M, Ramazzotti M, Poullet JB, et al. (2010) Impact of diet in shaping gut microbiota revealed by a comparative study in children from Europe and rural Africa. Proc Natl Acad Sci U S A 107: 14691–14696.
24. Biasucci G, Rubini M, Riboni S, Morelli L, Bessi E, et al. (2010) Mode of delivery affects the bacterial community in the newborn gut. Early Hum Dev 86 Suppl 1: 13–15.
25. Adlerberth I (2008) Factors influencing the establishment of the intestinal microbiota in infancy. Nestle Nutr Workshop Ser Pediatr Program 62: 13–29; discussion 29–33.
26. Iebba V, Aloi M, Civitelli F, Cucchiara S (2011) Gut microbiota and pediatric disease. Dig Dis 29: 531–539.
27. Lees CW, Barrett JC, Parkes M, Satsangi J (2011) New IBD genetics: common pathways with other diseases. Gut 60: 1739–1753.
28. Tizzano EF, Buchwald M (1995) CFTR expression and organ damage in cystic fibrosis. Ann Intern Med 123: 305–308.
29. Pezzulo AA, Tang XX, Hoegger MJ, Alaiwa MH, Ramachandran S, et al. (2012) Reduced airway surface pH impairs bacterial killing in the porcine cystic fibrosis lung. Nature 487: 109–113.
30. Duytschaever G, Huys G, Bekaert M, Boulanger L, De Boeck K, et al. (2011) Cross-sectional and longitudinal comparisons of the predominant fecal microbiota compositions of a group of pediatric patients with cystic fibrosis and their healthy siblings. Appl Environ Microbiol 77: 8015–8024.
31. Wiuf C (2001) Do delta F508 heterozygotes have a selective advantage? Genet Res 78: 41–47.
32. Iebba V, Conte MP, Lepanto MS, Di Nardo G, Santangelo F, et al. (2012) Microevolution in *fimH* gene of mucosa-associated *Escherichia coli* strains isolated from pediatric patients with inflammatory bowel disease. Infect Immun 80: 1408–1417.
33. Moore WE, Moore LH (1995) Intestinal floras of populations that have a high risk of colon cancer. Appl Environ Microbiol 61: 3202–3207.
34. Schwiertz A, Le Blay G, Blaut M (2000) Quantification of different *Eubacterium* spp. in human fecal samples with species-specific 16S rRNA-targeted oligonucleotide probes. Appl Environ Microbiol 66: 375–382.
35. Le Blay G, Lacroix C, Zihler A, Fliss I (2007) In vitro inhibition activity of nisin A, nisin Z, pediocin PA-1 and antibiotics against common intestinal bacteria. Lett Appl Microbiol 45: 252–257.
36. Schippa S, Iebba V, Barbato M, Di Nardo G, Totino V, et al. (2010) A distinctive 'microbial signature' in celiac pediatric patients. BMC Microbiol 10: 175.
37. Schippa S, Iebba V, Totino V, Santangelo F, Lepanto M, et al. (2012) A potential role of *Escherichia coli* pathobionts in the pathogenesis of pediatric inflammatory bowel disease. Can J Microbiol 58: 426–432.
38. Lee JM, Leach ST, Katz T, Day AS, Jaffe A, et al. (2012) Update of faecal markers of inflammation in children with cystic fibrosis. Mediators Inflamm 2012: 948367.
39. Packey CD, Sartor RB (2009) Commensal bacteria, traditional and opportunistic pathogens, dysbiosis and bacterial killing in inflammatory bowel diseases. Curr Opin Infect Dis 22: 292–301.
40. Chow J, Mazmanian SK (2010) A pathobiont of the microbiota balances host colonization and intestinal inflammation. Cell Host Microbe 7: 265–276.
41. Chow J, Lee SM, Shen Y, Khosravi A, Mazmanian SK (2010) Host-bacterial symbiosis in health and disease. Advances in immunology 107: 243–274.
42. Harper-Owen R, Dymock D, Booth V, Weightman AJ, Wade WG (1999) Detection of unculturable bacteria in periodontal health and disease by PCR. J Clin Microbiol 37: 1469–1473.
43. Sokol H, Pigneur B, Watterlot L, Lakhdari O, Bermudez-Humaran LG, et al. (2008) *Faecalibacterium prausnitzii* is an anti-inflammatory commensal bacterium identified by gut microbiota analysis of Crohn disease patients. Proc Natl Acad Sci U S A 105: 16731–16736.
44. Roh H, Ko HJ, Kim D, Choi DG, Park S, et al. (2011) Complete genome sequence of a carbon monoxide-utilizing acetogen, *Eubacterium limosum* KIST612. J Bacteriol 193: 307–308.

45. Goddard AF, Staudinger BJ, Dowd SE, Joshi-Datar A, Wolcott RD, et al. (2012) Direct sampling of cystic fibrosis lungs indicates that DNA-based analyses of upper-airway specimens can misrepresent lung microbiota. Proc Natl Acad Sci U S A 109: 13769–13774.
46. Cox MJ, Allgaier M, Taylor B, Baek MS, Huang YJ, et al. (2010) Airway microbiota and pathogen abundance in age-stratified cystic fibrosis patients. PloS one 5: e11044.
47. Keely S, Talley NJ, Hansbro PM (2012) Pulmonary-intestinal cross-talk in mucosal inflammatory disease. Mucosal Immunol 5: 7–18.
48. Rogers GB, Carroll MP, Hoffman LR, Walker AW, Fine DA, et al. (2010) Comparing the microbiota of the cystic fibrosis lung and human gut. Gut Microbes 1: 85–93.

23

Hemoglobin Oxygen Affinity in Patients with Cystic Fibrosis

Dieter Böning[1]*, Angela Littschwager[1], Matthias Hütler[1], Ralph Beneke[1], Doris Staab[2]

1 Institut für Sportmedizin, Charité - Universitätsmedizin Berlin, Berlin, Germany, **2** Klinik für Pädiatrische Pneumologie und Immunologie, Charité - Universitätsmedizin Berlin, Berlin, Germany

Abstract

In patients with cystic fibrosis lung damages cause arterial hypoxia. As a typical compensatory reaction one might expect changes in oxygen affinity of hemoglobin. Therefore position (standard half saturation pressure P_{50}st) and slope (Hill's n) of the O_2 dissociation curve as well as the Bohr coefficients (BC) for CO_2 and lactic acid were determined in blood of 14 adult patients (8 males, 6 females) and 14 healthy controls (6 males, 8 females). While Hill's n amounted to approximately 2.6 in all subjects, P_{50}st was slightly increased by 1mmHg in both patient groups (controls male 26.7±0.2, controls female 27.0±0.1, patients male 27.7±0.5, patients female 28.0±0.3 mmHg; mean and standard error, overall $p<0.01$). Main cause was a rise of 1–2 µmol/g hemoglobin in erythrocytic 2,3-biphosphoglycerate concentration. One patient only, clearly identified as an outlier and with the mutation G551D, showed a reduction of both P_{50}st (24.5 mmHg) and [2,3-biphosphoglycerate] (9.8 µmol/g hemoglobin). There were no differences in $BCCO_2$, but small sex differences in the BC for lactic acid in the controls which were not detectable in the patients. Causes for the right shift of the O_2 dissociation curve might be hypoxic stimulation of erythrocytic glycolysis and an increased red cell turnover both causing increased [2,3-biphosphoglycerate]. However, for situations with additional hypercapnia as observed in exercising patients a left shift seems to be a more favourable adaptation in cystic fibrosis. Additionally when in vivo PO_2 values were corrected to the standard conditions they mostly lay left of the in vitro O_2 dissociation curve in both patients and controls. This hints to unknown fugitive factors influencing oxygen affinity.

Editor: Shree Ram Singh, National Cancer Institute, United States of America

Funding: Funding provided by the following Foundation: Christiane Herzog Stiftung für Mukoviszidose-Kranke, http://www.christianeherzogstiftung.de/. The funders had no role in study design, data collection and analysis, decision to publish, or preparation of the manuscript.

Competing Interests: The authors have declared that no competing interests exist.

* E-mail: dieter.boening@charite.de

Introduction

Cystic fibrosis (CF) is the most frequent genetic disease in Caucasians [1–3]. Mutations on chromosome 7 (location 7q31.2) reduce the effectiveness of the cystic fibrosis transmembrane conductance regulator (CFTR), which is essential for the secretion of chloride (Cl^-) and consequently water in many glands. The clinical manifestation with heaviest impact is the progressive pulmonary disease. Because of the resulting deteriorated lung function in patients with cystic fibrosis causing hypoxia and partly also hypercapnia one might expect compensatory reactions in concentration and oxygen affinity of hemoglobin (Hb) to secure oxygen loading in spite of the reduced oxygen pressure (PO_2) in pulmonary capillaries.

There are various strategies of defense against arterial hypoxia [4–8]. In addition to hyperventilation most healthy humans, except partly Tibetans and Ethiopeans [9–11], react to hypoxia with an increase in Hb concentration ([Hb]) which facilitates sufficient binding of oxygen at lowered PO_2 in the lungs. Furthermore a right shift of the oxygen dissociation curve (ODC) under standard conditions (pH 7.4, PCO_2 40 mmHg, 37°C) partly compensates for the reduced diffusion pressure in the tissues because of the low oxygen saturation (SO_2) in the capillaries; the shift is caused by more 2,3-biphosphoglyrate (BPG) in the red cells. In contrast typical altitude animals like llamas, guinea pigs and partly birds possess left-shifted ODCs securing oxygen loading in the lungs and rather low [Hb] reducing circulatory resistance. In addition small red blood cells and a dense capillary net in the tissues diminish the diffusion distance and thus compensate for the decreased capillary PO_2 [12]. The human fetus exists also at very low arterial PO_2 but the concentration of the high affinity fetal Hb (HbF) is increased. Recent in vivo determinations of the ODC in adults point to a possible left shift of its upper part at altitude [13,14].

Astonishingly few studies investigated the combined effect of hypoxia and hypercapnia. The fetal conditions with higher arterial PCO_2 than in maternal blood point to an advantage of a left shifted ODC. Moles living in earth holes with reduced air exchange inspire hypoxic/hypercapnic gas and possess also Hb with increased oxygen affinity [15]. Huckauf et al ([16]) describe a left shifted ODC in patients with chronic obstructive lung disease and in a review Morgan [17] mentions that [BPG] is often reduced in critically ill patients.

Patients with cystic fibrosis often show normal or even anemic [Hb] (e. g. [18–20]. Interestingly, however, they may possess an increased red cell volume masked by a concomitant rise in plasma volume [21,22]. Compensatory reactions of oxygen affinity in cystic fibrosis have been investigated rarely. Slight right shifts of the standard ODC, characterized by a rise of P_{50}st and caused by increased [BPG], were detected by some authors [18,23], while others found unchanged [BPG] or P_{50}st [19,24].

However, there are various additional mechanisms for the regulation of oxygen affinity. Besides phosphates other anions like lactate, chloride and glutathione (e. g. [25,26]) bind to Hb. Depending on the binding site these substances also influence the cooperativity of the subunits visible as change in the slope of the ODC (Hill's n); additionally they may modify the intraerythrocytic pH. The Bohr effect, which in the physiological pH range causes an increase of PO_2 at constant saturation by acidification (essential in working muscles), may vary depending on various factors like oxygen saturation [27,28], type of acid [27,28], substance concentrations and age of the erythrocytes (e. g. [29]); in altitude residents a tendency to lowered Bohr coefficients ($BC = \Delta logPO_2/\Delta pH$) has been observed [30,31]. Also sex differences in oxygen binding properties have been described: women [32–34] as well as children [35] tend to higher P_{50}st than men. Finally in vivo variations of the ODC in venous blood of anemic patients as well as of trained subjects have been observed during exercise which were no more detectable after in vitro equilibration of blood [36–38]. The underlying mechanisms are not yet clarified.

Previous studies on oxygen affinity in cystic fibrosis were performed on rather heterogeneous groups of patients. Differences in the severity of the illness are almost inevitable but possible effects of age and sex were not considered. Also control groups were small or not clearly defined or even lacking. To our knowledge neither cooperativity (Hill's n) nor the Bohr effect have ever been studied in cystic fibrosis.

Considering all these factors it seemed worthwhile to perform a systematic study of mechanisms influencing blood O_2 affinity as possible facilitation of oxygen uptake in cystic fibrosis.

Methods

Study Participants

Measurements were performed in 14 adult patients and 14 controls; anthropometric data are presented in Table 1. The patients (8 males, 6 females) showed severely reduced lung function but were in a stable clinical condition. One male subject was bearer of the Class III G551D mutation which is one of five mutations with a frequency >0.1% accounting for 2 to 3% mutations worldwide. It impairs CFTR-mediated Cl^- transport by limiting channel gating at the cell surface [3,39].

The patients were the members of a group with exercise therapy. They usually lived at home but were under continuous supervision by physicians of the pediatric clinic of the faculty. Twice a week they performed a disease status tailored exercise program addressing endurance, strength, coordination and flexibility supervised by staff of the Institute of Sports Medicine and received individual advice for additional daily exercises at home. Occasionally some patients used short term oxygen supplementation, but not on the test day. The nonsmoking controls (6 males, 8 females) were physically active but not specifically or regularly training staff members and students. One female was slightly anemic ([Hb] 11.2 g/dl), but all other measurements yielded clinically normal values within the range of the group. The study protocol was approved by the ethics committee of the faculty (Ethikkommission, Charité – Universitätsmedizin Berlin, Ethikausschuss CBF, No. ek.185-13b) and written informed consent was obtained from all participants.

Study Procedure

The subjects arrived at the laboratory between 9.00 and 10.00 a.m. Lung function (forced vital capacity FVC, forced expiratory

Table 1. Subjects.

	n	Age	Body mass	Height	BMI	FVC	FEV1	PEF
		years	kg	cm	kg/m²	%	%	%
Controls male	6	28±3	80.4±3.2	185±4	24.2±1.2	93±2	92±3	102±8
Controls female	8	27±2	62.8±3.0	171±3	21.5±0.8	117±4	104±5	98±10
Patients male	8	28±2	59.0±3.0	177±4	18.8±0.6	59±7	38±6	57±5
Patients female	6	29±1	48.8±1.7	162±2	18.6±0.5	56±8	37±6	51±12

Means and standard errors (SE). BMI body mass index, FVC forced vital capacity, FEV1 forced expiratory volume during 1 s; PEF peak expiratory flow. % of expected values for age and sex [40] or of individual FVC. All anthropometrical and lung function values are significantly (P<0.001) reduced in the patients.

volume during 1 s FEV1, peak expiratory flow PEF) was measured with a spirometer system (Oxycon gamma, Mijnhardt, Bunnik, The Netherlands). Percent of expected values for age and sex [40] or of individual FVC are presented in Table 1. Blood was sampled in supine position. Acid base status at 37°C (ABL 500 or 510 with no systematic difference between apparatus, Radiometer Copenhagen, Denmark), oxygenation status (PO_2, SO_2, COHb, MetHb) and [Hb] (OSM 3; Radiometer Copenhagen, Denmark) were measured in heparinized blood samples taken from hyperemized ear-lobes. Values for PO_2 are slightly lower than in arterial blood [41], but this is of negligible importance for saturations above 90% in the flat part of the ODC. Fifty ml of venous blood were drawn without stasis using heparinized vaccutainers and stored in an ice-water mixture. Oxygenation status, [Hb], hematocrit (Hct, microhematocrit method) and [Cl^-] in plasma (EML 100, Radiometer Copenhagen) were determined immediately. Aliquots were deproteinized and stored at −20°C for duplicate measurements of ATP and BPG concentrations (enzymatic kits, Sigma Diagnostics) on the next day.

Five ml each were equilibrated 20 min in sphere tonometers at 37°C with air/CO_2 or nitrogen/CO_2 mixtures (3, 6 or 10% CO_2). Lactic acid (13.5 mmol/l blood) was added to an additional sample equilibrated thereafter with 6% CO_2 in air or N_2. After taking aliquots for additional ATP and BPG measurements 0.2 ml of oxygenated blood were successively added 8 to 10 times to 1 ml deoxygenated blood using 2 connected syringes and mixed. After measurement of SO_2, COHb, MetHb, [Hb], pH, PCO_2 and PO_2, ODCs were drawn in the Hill plot (log SO_2/100-SO_2) versus log PO_2).

Samples of native blood as well as of blood equilibrated with N_2/6% CO_2 and with air/6% CO_2 were centrifuged for 10 min (3500 rpm, 4°C). Part of the red cell sediment was hemolyzed by repeated freezing and thawing and used for measurement of pH and [Cl^-] in the erythrocytes.

Twelve patients (7 males, 5 females) performed an incremental test (initially 0.3 W/kg, plus 0.3 W/kg every 2 min) until exhaustion on a cycle ergometer (Lode Excalibur, The Netherlands) during exercise therapy. Blood gases and lactate concentration (Ebio plus, Eppendorf, Germany) were measured in ear lobe blood and used to calculate P_{50} at exhaustion.

Calculations

The slope n of the oxygen dissociation curves linearized in the Hill plot served as measure of cooperativity. For 5% steps of SO_2 between 15 and 90% logPO_2 values were calculated from the regression equations and the corresponding pH values obtained by interpolation. Comparison of the ODCs for 3 and 10% CO_2 yielded Bohr coefficients for CO_2 ($BCCO_2$), comparison of the 6% CO_2 and the 13.5 mmol/l lactic acid curves yielded Bohr coefficients for fixed acid (BCLa) at each saturation step. P_{50}st were calculated from the curves of blood equilibrated with 6% CO_2 by use of the corresponding individual $BCCO_2$. Mean cellular hemoglobin concentrations (MCHC) calculated from [Hb] and Hct were corrected for 2% trapped plasma. $[Cl^-]_{ery}$ were corrected for 10% in the sediment after centrifugation with 3500 rpm; because of the large buffer capacity of red cells this is not necessary for pH_{ery}. Electrodes in the electrolyte analyser measure concentrations in water [42]; therefore $[Cl^-]_{ery}$ is given per l cell water. Values for the control subjects coincide with titrimetric measurements [43]. In vitro blood buffer capacities ($-\Delta$[acid]/ΔpH) for CO_2 and lactic acid were calculated from the measurements in the corresponding equilibrated samples.

Statistics

All data are presented as means±standard errors (SE). Dependent on the number of comparisons, t-tests or analysis of variance (ANOVA) were used for significance calculations. The probability that an outlier does not belong to a sample was tested eventually [44]. Differences with $P<0.05$ were considered as significant.

Results

Anthropometry and Pathology

Table 1 shows marked reduction in both body height and body mass in the patients compared to healthy subjects. Their lung function was substantially impeded by restrictive as well as obstructive damage visible from low vital capacity and expiratory flow (FEV1, PEV); FEV1 ranged between 22 and 74%.

Blood Gases and Acid Base Status

The impaired lung function of the patients caused a reduction of ear-lobe PO_2 and SO_2 (Table 2). Generally these values were also slightly lower in males than in females. Correspondingly, PCO_2 tended to higher values in males and in patients. However, the pH was equal in all subgroups because of non-respiratory compensation visible as increased base excess in males and in patients. Venous blood pH scattered more, but there were also no systematic differences among groups (means between 7.35 and 7.38); red cell pH showed no influence of sex or illness as well (means about 7.16). In vitro buffer capacities of blood tended to higher values in all males; this was significant for acidification with CO_2 as well as lactic acid (both $P<0.05$; latter not shown in Table 2) in oxygenated blood. Concentrations of COHb (controls male 0.6±0.1%, controls female 0.4±0.1%, patients male 0.6±0.2%, patients female 0.7±0.1%) and MetHb (controls male 0.5±0.1%, controls female 0.6±0.1%, patients male 0.5±0.1%, patients female 0.5±0.1%) were low and not different among groups.

Blood Composition

[Hb] and Hct were higher in males than females, but there were no significant differences between controls and patients (Table 3). In the male patients [Hb] was negatively correlated with FEV1 ($r=-0.762$, $P<0.05$). MCHC, however, was slightly but significantly lowered in patients. They showed also slightly decreased [Cl^-] in plasma and red cells. [BPG] and [ATP] were significantly increased in the patients inspite of very low [BPG] (9.8 μmol/gHb) in the subject with the G551D mutation. Additionally there was a sex difference for [BPG] with higher concentrations in females. After equilibration [BPG] and [ATP] tended to slightly higher values (0.9 and 0.2 μmol/gHb on average, respectively, not significant) compared to native blood.

Oxygen Dissociation Curves

In the Hill plot (Fig. 1) all curves were linear (correlation coefficients better than 0.98, not corrected for the slightly decreasing pH with rising saturation) and the slopes amounted to approximately 2.6 with very little scattering in all groups (Table 4).

The standard half saturation pressures (Table 4) corresponded to known normal values in the controls. In patients P_{50}st was significantly increased by 1 mmHg (with slightly but not significantly higher values for females). When corrected to arterialized pH and PCO_2, all means were 0.8 mmHg lower. The patient with the G551D mutation presented a markedly lowered P_{50}st of 24.5 mmHg (arterialized blood 23.3 mmHg) clearly identified as

Table 2. Blood gases and acid-base status.

		PO_{2art}	SO_{2art}	PCO_{2art}	pH_{art}	SBE	Buffer Cap
	n	mmHg	%	mmHg		mmol/l	mmol/l
Controls male	6	91.4±3.0	95.9±0.3	38.0±1.6	7.430±0.006	1.3±0.7	29.9±1.2
Controlsfemale	8	99.3±1.2	96.8±0.2	34.4±1.6	7.430±0.008	−0.9±0.7	25.2±1.0
Patients male	8	64.9±3.5	91.2±1.5	41.7±1.8	7.423±0.008	3.4±0.5	28.9±0.7
Patients female	6	70.5±2.7	93.3±0.7	37.2±2.0	7.427±0.012	1.4±0.7	26.8±1.0
Anova	sex	a		a		b	a
	illness	c	d			d	

Means ± SE. art measurements in ear lobe blood. Standard base excess (SBE, 100% SO_2, standardized [Hb] of 5 g/dl, [71]) measured in venous blood. Buffer Cap: in vitro buffer capacity for CO_2 in oxygenated blood ($-\Delta[HCO_3^-]_{plasma}/\Delta$ pH). ANOVA: a P<0.05, b P<0.01 or better for differences between males and females, c P<0.05, d P<0.01 or better for differences between controls and patients.

Table 3. Substance concentrations in venous blood.

		[Hb]	Hct	MCHC	$[Cl^-]_{plasma}$	$[Cl^-]_{ery}$	$[BPG]_{ery}$	$[ATP]_{ery}$
	n	g/dl	%	g/dl	mmol/l	mmol/l H_2O	μmol/gHb	μmol/gHb
Controls male	6	15.4±0.4	45.7±0.8	33.8±0.5	103.3±0.5	73.9±1.1	13.3±1.2	4.1±0.3
Controls female	8	12.8±0.4	39.6±0.2	32.8±0.3	103.2±0.4	76.0±1.5	14.6±0.8	4.2±0.2
Patients male	8	14.7±0.4	46.5±1.5	31.9±0.4	99.6±0.5	71.9±1.9	14.1±0.8*	4.6±0.1
Patients female	6	12.9±0.4	42.0±1.3	31.8±0.6	100.3±1.2	73.0±1.3	16.7±1.5	4.3±0.3
Anova	sex	a	a				a	
	illness			c	d	c	c	d

Means ± SE. Significance levels indicated like for Table 2. MCHC and $[Cl^-]_{ery}$ corrected for 2% and 10% trapped plasma, respectively. *14.8±0.5 without the patient with the G551D mutation.

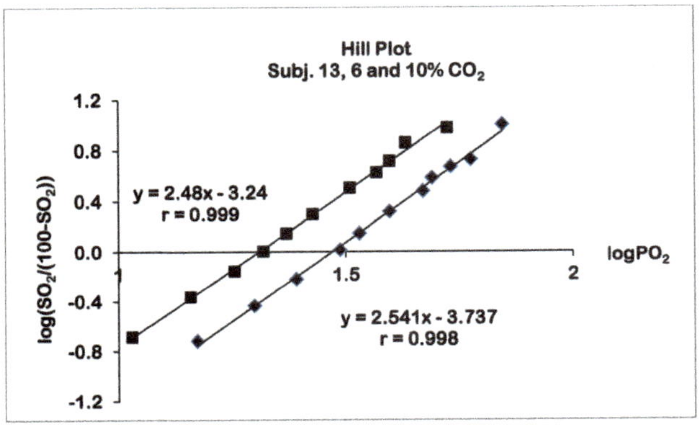

Figure 1. Two oxygen dissociation curves of one subject in the Hill plot.

an outlier ($P<0.02$). Without the latter value mean P_{50}st for the male patients rose by 0.4 mmHg.

Regression analysis including all subjects yielded a significant relation between [BPG] in the equilibrated samples and P_{50}st (Fig. 2). The male patient with the extremely low P_{50}st value fell, however, far outside of his group with a correspondingly low [BPG].

Bohr Coefficients

The Bohr coefficients (Fig. 3) for CO_2 corresponded to published data: The value was about −0.5 and decreased numerically with higher saturations ($P<0.01$ for all subjects); there was also a tendency to lower values in women. No influence of the disease was visible. The Bohr coefficients for lactic acid (Fig. 4) were generally lower numerically than for CO_2 in all groups up to 45% saturation (−0.40 to −0.45). Differences between males and females at higher SO_2 disappeared in the patients (interaction sex-illness $P<0.01$). Among the patients the subject with the G551D mutation presented the highest BC for both acids between 70 and 90% SO_2 (approx. −0.54).

Exercise Tests in Patients

At exhaustion SO_2 dropped in all patients resulting from reduced PO_2 and both respiratory and non-respiratory acidosis which caused a rise of P_{50} (Table 5). Again the subject with the G551D mutation showed the lowest P_{50} value (29.6 mmHg).

In vivo Effects

When the PO_2 values in non-equilibrated venous blood (fresh or stored in ice until measurement) were corrected with the corresponding Bohr coefficients ($BCCO_2$) to pH 7.4, they should have fallen on the individual standard ODC. However, in the range between 45 and 90% SO_2 there was a tendency for a deviation to the left (Fig. 5) in controls (−1.8±0.4 mmHg, $P<0.05$) as well as in patients (−2.2±0.4 mmHg, $P<0.001$). Some samples with higher values of SO_2 were not considered, because the BCs were not measured for SO_2>90%. In addition there is large scattering of PO_2 in the flat part of the ODC. There was no correlation between PO_2 differences and [BPG] differences for native and equilibrated blood.

Discussion

Synopsis of Results

Our results confirm former investigations that there is a small right shift of the standard ODC in most patients with cystic fibrosis probably caused by slightly increased intraerythrocytic concentrations of organic phosphates [18,23]. This is accompanied by a constant slope of the ODC and only small changes of the Bohr coefficients. In spite of the lacking hypocapnia this reaction is similar to the typical human acclimatization to altitude but seems to be attenuated. During exercise the right shift of the ODC is enforced by hypercapnia in CF patients and a clear drawback for arterial oxygen loading. Interestingly there seems to exist an additional mechanism in controls as well as in patients: The in vivo standard ODC falls slightly left of the in vitro curve.

Blood Gases and Acid Base Status

The deterioration of lung function in the patients results in hypoxia visible in arterialized blood; a tendency to a slightly higher PCO_2 than in the controls is not significant probably because of the low number of measurements and the resting situation; when exercising the increase in PCO_2 is more marked. Measurements in 69 patients in our laboratory showed corresponding results; $PaCO_2$ increased with the severity of the illness at rest as well as during exercise [45]. This is different to healthy subjects who always show a decrease of $PaCO_2$ at high work load. The arterial oxygen saturation in patients at rest is as low as in highlanders [46,47] living 2600 m above sea level (inspiratory PO_2 approx. 120 mmHg). But in spite of a similar reduction of spirometric values the female patients show higher PO_2 and lower PCO_2 than the male patients like their healthy counterparts. Probably the long-known stimulation of respiratory brain centres by female

Table 4. Characteristics of the oxygen dissociation curves.

		P_{50}standard	Hill's n
	n	mmHg	6% CO_2
Controls male	6	26.7±0.2	2.63±0.02
Controls female	8	27.0±0.1	2.56±0.02
Patients male	8	27.7±0.5*	2.57±0.03
Patients female	6	28.0±0.3	2.61±0.03
Anova	sex		
	illness	d	

Means ± SE. Significance levels indicated as for Table 2. P_{50}standard: standard half saturation pressure calculated from the curves of blood equilibrated with 6% CO_2.*28.1±0.3 mmHg without the patient with the G551D mutation.

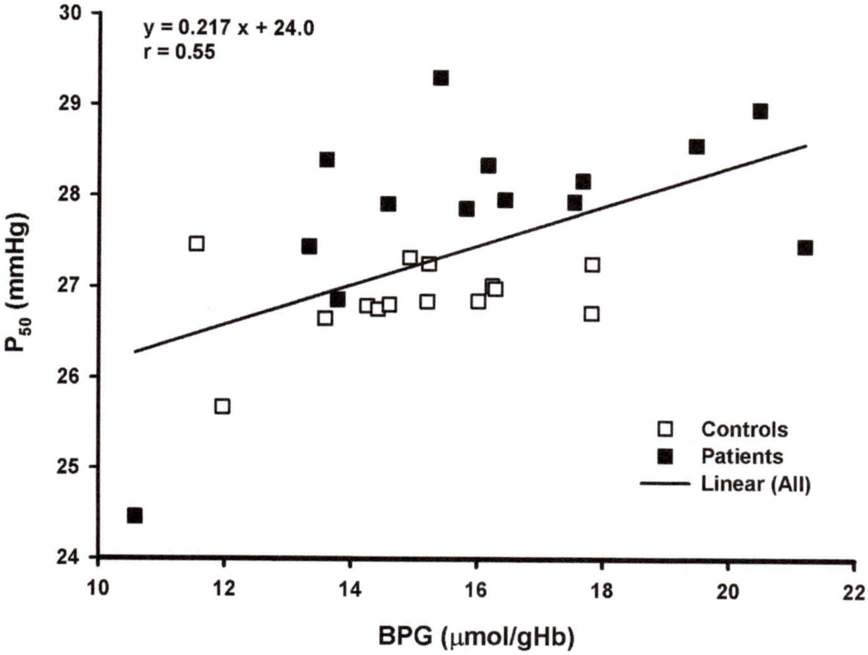

Figure 2. Dependence of P_{50}st on BPG concentration (means of equilibrated samples). Regression line for all values, correlation coefficient r different from zero ($P<0.01$).

hormones important for fetal oxygen supply is the cause (reviewed in [47]). The fact that arterialized pH is equal in all subgroups in spite of differences in PCO_2 demonstrates the importance of acid-base homeostasis for physiological functions. Non-respiratory compensation is mainly done by renal excretion/reabsorption of bicarbonate. In the patients the osmotic effect of the rise of $[HCO_3^-]$ is counteracted by a decrease of $[Cl^-]$. Also the loss of chloride via sweat glands might play a role. The slightly increased in vitro buffer capacity in both male groups is obviously caused by the higher Hb concentration. In cystic fibrosis the slight rise in bicarbonate concentration as well as the possibly increased Hb mass [21,22] help to attenuate the extracellular pH changes during exercise [48] caused by CO_2 retention.

Blood Composition

Hb concentrations showed typical sex differences but no sign of anemia in the patients. The latter might be expected in CF because of frequent problems with iron resorption. However, in

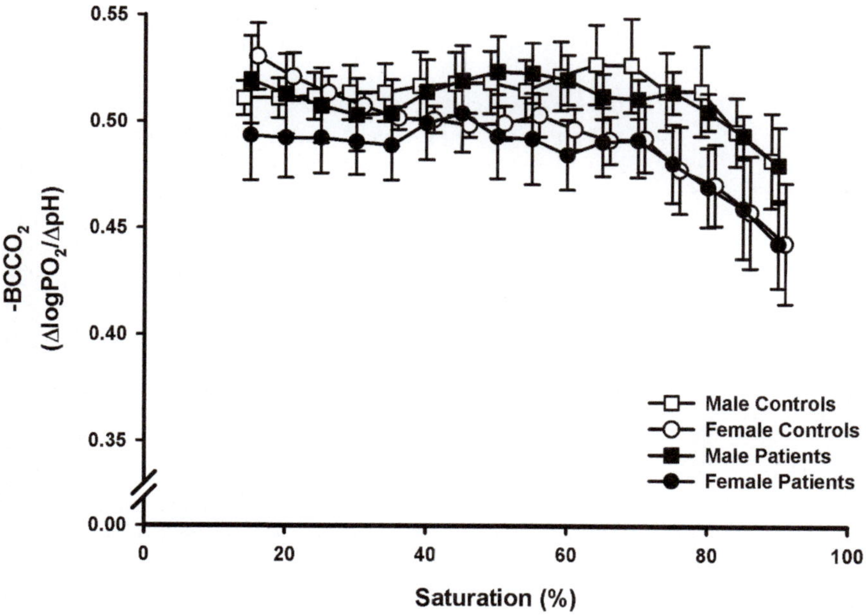

Figure 3. Saturation-dependent Bohr coefficients for acidification with CO_2 ($BCCO_2$). Means and standard errors.

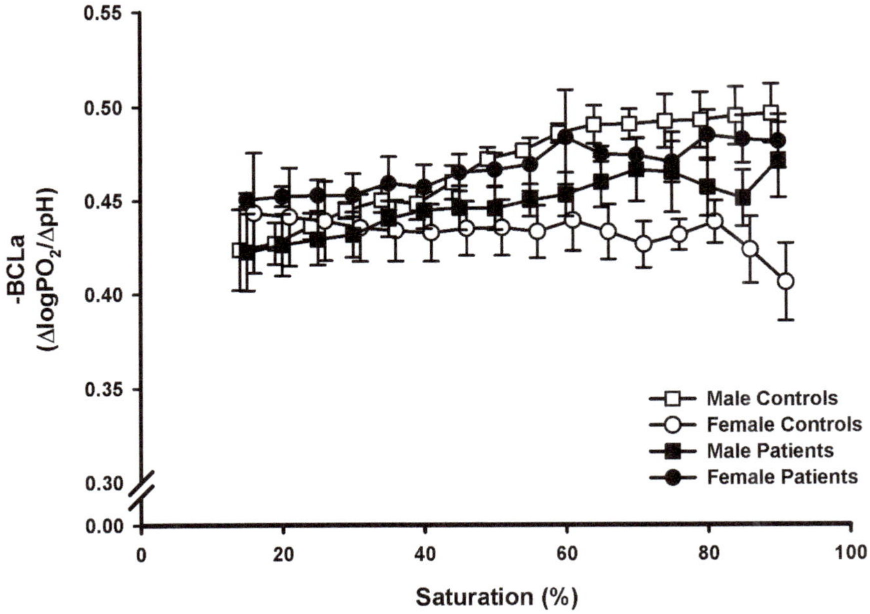

Figure 4. Saturation-dependent Bohr coefficients for acidification with lactic acid (BCLa). Means and standard errors.

our patients iron metabolism was routinely checked and deficiency was treated. One explanation for normal [Hb] in other studies might be the counteracting effects between iron deficiency and hypoxia [49]. Christoforou et al. [19] described a negative correlation of [erythropoietin] with FVC and FEV1. Such a dependency is probably the cause of the correlation between [Hb] and FEV1 in our male patients. Some authors [21,22] have even observed an increase in red cell volume in CF probably stimulated by erythropoietin which might be explained as a typical hypoxia reaction. However, only in a fraction of the corresponding studies [19,20,50,51]http://www.ncbi.nlm.nih.gov/ pubmed?term = McColley%20SA%5BAuthor%5D&cauthor = true&cauthor_uid = 21365780 erythropoietin concentration was increased. Own unpublished measurements support the idea of chronic stimulation of erythropoesis in CF patients based on elevated erythropoietin as well as soluble transferrin receptor concentrations in a cohort of 79 CF patients. Also a low MCHC like in the patients is often related to an increased water content typical for young erythrocytes. Furthermore in patients the high level of the soluble transferrin receptor [20] might be indicative for an increased red cell production and thus a reduced erythrocytic age. However, also a link between CFTR and the function of the hypoxia inducible factor has been put forward [52] which may serve as one potential reason for a lack of increased [Hb] in CF patients.

Factors possibly increasing [BPG] and [ATP] are low SO_2 (reducing product inhibition because of BPG binding to Hb) and alkalosis (stimulating glycolysis and thus BPG synthesis). A probable explanation for the rather small increase of [BPG] and P_{50}st in CF compared to highlanders with similarly lowered arterial SO_2 and equal pH at rest (e. g. 18 µmol/g Hb in [30]) might be the different effect of physical activity: CO_2 retention causes respiratory acidosis already during moderate physical activity in the patients while highlanders effectively hyperventilate at each exercise level. In the present patient group with normal daily life and exercise therapy physical activity was obviously a factor of some importance. Additionally a low red cell age as suggested above might lead to elevated [BPG] as well as [ATP] because of high enzymatic activity [29]. The low [BPG] in the patient with the G551D mutation possibly results from changed enzyme activities because no differences in erythrocyte physiology were detectable. CFTR is incorporated into the red cell membrane (e. g. [53]), but a relation to BPG metabolism remains speculative.

[Cl^-] in red cells in part follows passively changes in plasma [Cl^-] and therefore is lowered in patients. Generally the marked concentration difference results from the high erythrocytic content of non-diffusible anions (Hb^- and organic phosphates) causing a Donnan equilibrium. Cl^- crosses the cell membrane mainly through band 3 channels. The reduction of the number of CFTR molecules in patients (e. g. [53]) does not affect this exchange [24]. Cl^- concurs with BPG for the same binding sites on Hb [54] but its affinity is lower and the small decrease of its concentration in CF is compensated for by increased [BPG].

Oxygen Dissociation Curves

The P_{50}st values of controls scatter around the normal mean value (approximately 27 mmHg) without significant sex differences. The generally higher P_{50}st in patients results from the increased [BPG] (change approx. 0.6 mmHg per µmole BPG/gHb according to [55]) while ATP plays only a minor role because of complexing with Mg^{++}. This corresponds to the typical chronic hypoxic reaction of most humans. It allows to extract more oxygen in the tissue capillaries without lowering the diffusion pressure, but it is not helpful for oxygen loading in pulmonary capillaries. In highlanders with similar reduction of arterial SO_2 P_{50}st scatters around 30 mmHg [30]. In both healthy subjects and patients the reaction (affinity change, increased ventilation and partly stimulated erythropoesis) is a sufficient compensation of moderate hypoxia at rest but maximal performance capacity is reduced. The left shift of the ODC in moles [15] living and working under comparable conditions (inspiring air with reduced O_2 and increased CO_2 content) as the patients is more reasonable but is rare in humans. Under extreme acute conditions (above 6000 m of altitude) healthy mountaineers lower their P_{50} by extreme hyperventilation [56] which is not a sustainable option for CF-

Table 5. Blood gases, acid-base status and P_{50} of patients at maximal exercise.

	n	Powermax Watt/kg	PO_{2art} mmHg	SO_{2art} %	PCO_{2art} mmHg	pH_{art}	[Lactate] mmol/l	P_{50} mmHg
Patients male	7	2.2±0.3	58.9±5.4	80.1±3.1	48.3±4.0	7.240±0.018	7.9±1.1	33.1±0.9
Patients female	5	1.8±0.1	55.6±2.1	82.6±4.0	51.2±3.6	7.227±0.031	8.8±0.6	33.7±0.9

Means ± SE. Measurements in ear lobe blood. P_{50} for actual pH. All differences to rest significant for all patients as well as subgroups except SO_2 for subgroup patients female ($P<0.054$).

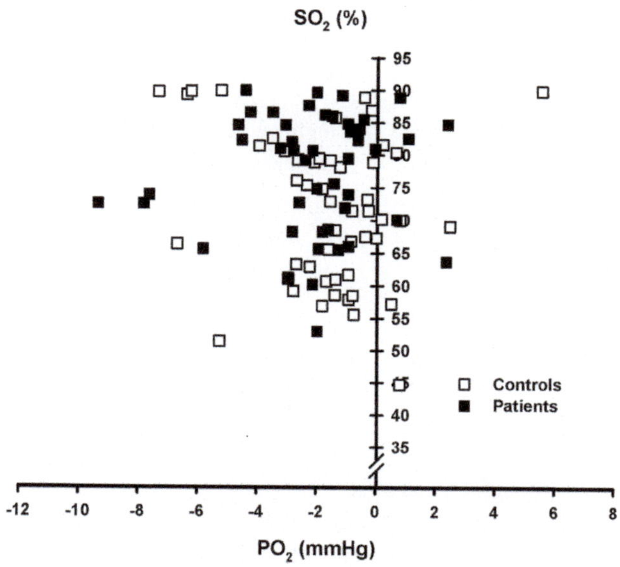

Figure 5. Deviation of in vivo PO_2 corrected to pH 7.4 from the corresponding individual standard ODC between 40 and 90% in controls and patients.

patients. For chronic acclimatization a reduction of [BPG] would be more appropriate. Surprisingly the male patient with the G551D mutation showed such an effect. One can estimate that a reduction of P_{50}st like in his blood would raise the arterial SO_2 at exhaustion in the male patients by 4%.

Interestingly in the 3 papers with P_{50}st measurements in CF patients single low P_{50}st values between 23.5 and 25.5 mmHg can be found [18,19,23]. This points to a special form of hypoxia acclimatization in some patients similar to that in moles.

The magnitude of a change in P_{50}st may reflect further compensating mechanisms. Rosenthal et al [18] showed that P_{50}st is negatively correlated with systemic oxygen delivery which depends on arterial SO_2, [Hb] and cardiac output. This means that low [Hb] or cardiac output favor a rise of P_{50}st. Indeed Arturson [57] described a P_{50}st increase with falling [Hb] in chronic pulmonary insufficiency. The present CF patients were not anemic. This might also explain why we observed a small tendency rather than a substantial change in P_{50}st.

Hill's n did not deviate much from the usually expected value of 2.7 for HbA (e.g. [55]). BPG binds to Deoxy-Hb only which may therefore increase Hill's n with rising concentration. A sligtly higher n in highlanders [30] and anemic patients [58] might be explained by this mechanism. However, the [BPG] differences between controls and patients in this study are too small to cause measurable effects.

Bohr Effect and Exercise

Similar like in altitude inhabitants [30,31] the Bohr coefficients are little changed in patients with cystic fibrosis. The coefficients for CO_2 correspond to published values [27,28,33]. They are large (numerically) at low saturation because of oxygenation dependent binding of carbamate in addition to H^+ effects during acidification with CO_2. They are lower at very high saturation; the Bohr effect disappears when all Hb molecules are in the R (relaxed) state. Anions (Cl^-, La^- and BPG) compete with CO_2 at the terminal valines (e. g. [25]). Therefore $BCCO_2$ increases at low [BPG]; this might be the cause for the rather high value in the patient with mutation G 551D. The fixed acid Bohr coefficients are small especially at low saturation compared to $BCCO_2$. The slight unexplained influence of CF on BCLa plays only a very modest role, because the peak lactic acid concentration during exercise is rather low in the patients (Table 5) compared to healthy subjects (e. g. [59]). In the lungs the Bohr effect of CO_2 is helpful for oxygen loading, when CO_2 leaves the blood, especially during hyperventilation with resulting hypocapnia during heavy exercise. In the patients with exercise hypercapnia and mostly high $P_{50}st$, however, an increase of $BCCO_2$ would be detrimental in this situation.

In vivo Effects

The left shift of the in vivo PO_2/SO_2 pairs relative to the in vitro standard ODCs is on an average modest (approx. 2 mmHg) but 17 differences amount to more than 4 mmHg. Differences in ODCs as well as BCs between fresh blood immediately after sampling and blood after equilibration in tonometers have occasionally been observed (e. g. [38,60]). Concentration changes of BPG, ATP, Cl^-, nitrocompounds or glutathione are possible causes. The means of [BPG] and [ATP] increase slightly but not significantly after equilibration compared to fresh venous samples explaining only 0.7 mmHg of the difference at 50% SO_2. Intraerythrocytic [Cl^-] changes are larger for a given ΔpH in vivo than in vitro resulting from exchange with the interstitial fluid [59]. Because of the opposite effects of SNO-Hb and Hb[FENO] on oxygen affinity [61] NO usually exerts no measurable influence on the ODC neither in vitro nor in vivo if no methemoglobin is formed [62–65]. In our experiments MetHb was stable. For an allosteric effect intraerythrocytic [NO] is by far too low even in Tibetans who present very high values [66]. In contrast to NO glutathione is present in millimolar concentrations in the red cells [67] and binds to oxy-Hb thus shifting the curve to the left and reducing the Bohr effect [26,68]. But a marked deficiency of extra- and intracellular glutathione possibly including erythrocytes in CF patients has been suggested [69] which might be related to the disturbed function of CFTR as glutathione transporter [52]. Very recently also an effect of glutamate on P50 was observed [70]; this substance binds to Ca^{++} channel proteins in the cell membrane and may be interchanged with muscle fibres. Thus at the moment a clear cause for the in vivo – in vitro difference of PO_2 remains unknown, but apparently it rises with SO_2. This produces a left shift of the in vivo ODC between 50 and 90% SO_2, which is an advantage for oxygen loading. Recently similar results were found at 3600 m of altitude [13,14]. Interestingly at low saturations "standardized" in vivo PO_2/SO_2 pairs tend to lie right of the in vitro curve, especially in venous blood returning from exercising muscles [36–38,55,60]. The result of this opposite changes is a markedly steepened complete in vivo oxygen dissociation curve probably in healthy subjects as well as in CF patients. Such a property is favorable for both loading and unloading of O_2 in lungs and consuming tissues.

Conclusions

The majority of the patients with cystic fibrosis in our study react to the problem of pulmonary oxygen uptake like man at altitude with a small right shift of the in vitro ODC caused by increased organic phosphate concentrations in the red cells. This improves oxygen diffusion into the consuming tissues, but is a drawback for arterialization. Healthy subjects can compensate this by hyperventilation thus reducing arterial PCO_2 with resulting left shift of the ODC during oxygenation. This is not possible for CF patients especially when CO_2 production is increased during exercise. A probably more appropriate left shift by reduction of [BPG] was observed in one patient with the G551D mutation. Also in other papers occasional left shifts can be detected. Whether this is a genetic effect, remains an intriguing question. The slope of the in vitro ODC and the Bohr coefficients were not markedly affected by the disease. Under in vivo conditions, there is a tendency for a left shift of the upper part of the ODC in both healthy controls and patients pointing to unknown affinity modifying factors which improve oxygen loading in the lungs.

Acknowledgments

The authors thank all subjects for their willing cooperation and B. Himmelsbach-Wegner for technical assistance.

Author Contributions

Conceived and designed the experiments: DB MH RB DS. Performed the experiments: AL MH RB. Analyzed the data: DB AL MH RB DS. Wrote the paper: DB AL MH RB DS. Designed the methods used for measurement and evaluation of oxygen dissociation curves: DB MH.

References

1. Cohen TS, Prince A (2012) Cystic fibrosis: a mucosal immunodeficiency syndrome. Nat Med 18: 509–519.
2. Zielenski J (2000) Genotype and phenotype in cystic fibrosis. Respiration 67: 117–133.
3. Derichs N (2013) Targeting a genetic defect: cystic fibrosis transmembrane conductance regulator modulators in cystic fibrosis. Eur Respir Rev 22: 58–65.
4. Baumann R, Bartels H, Bauer C (1987) Blood oxygen transport. In: Fishman AP, Cherniak NS, Widdicombe JG, Geiger SR, editors. Handbook of Physiology Sect. 3. Washington DC: Am. Physiol. Soc. 147–172.
5. Samaja M, Crespi T, Guazzi M, Vandegriff KD (2003) Oxygen transport in blood at high altitude: role of the hemoglobin-oxygen affinity and impact of the phenomena related to hemoglobin allosterism and red cell function. Eur J Appl Physiol 90: 351–359.
6. Weber RE (2007) High-altitude adaptations in vertebrate hemoglobins. Respir Physiol Neurobiol 158: 132–142.
7. Storz JF, Moriyama H (2008) Mechanisms of hemoglobin adaptation to high altitude hypoxia. High Alt Med Biol 9: 148–157.
8. Winslow RM (2007) The role of hemoglobin oxygen affinity in oxygen transport at high altitude. Respir Physiol Neurobiol 158: 121–127.
9. Morpurgo G, Arese P, Bosia A, Pescarmona GP, Luzzana M, et al. (1976) Sherpas living permanently at high altitude: a new pattern of adaptation. Proc Nat Acad Sci USA 73: 747–751.
10. Beall CM, Decker MJ, Brittenham GM, Kushner I, Gebremedhin A, et al. (2002) An Ethiopian pattern of human adaptation to high-altitude hypoxia. Proc Natl Acad Sci U S A 99: 17215–17218.
11. Beall CM (2007) Two routes to functional adaptation: Tibetan and Andean high-altitude natives. Proc Natl Acad Sci U S A 104 Suppl 1: 8655–8660.
12. Jürgens KD, Pietschmann M, Yamaguchi K, Kleinschmidt T (1988) Oxygen binding properties, capillary densities and heart weights in high altitude camelids. J Comp Physiol B 158: 469–477.
13. Balaban DY, Duffin J, Preiss D, Mardimae A, Vesely A, et al. (2013) The in-vivo oxyhaemoglobin dissociation curve at sea level and high altitude. Respir Physiol Neurobiol 186: 45–52.
14. Böning D, Pries AR (2013) Unknown in vivo factors influencing the oxygen dissociation curve? Respir Physiol Neurobiol 188: 79–80.
15. Campbell KL, Storz JF, Signore AV, Moriyama H, Catania KC, et al. (2010) Molecular basis of a novel adaptation to hypoxic-hypercapnia in a strictly fossorial mole. BMC Evol Biol 10: 214.
16. Huckauf H, Schäfer JH, Kollo D (1976) Oxygen affinity of haemoglobin and red cell acid-base status in patients with severe chronic obstructive lung disease. Bull Europ Physiopath Resp 12: 129–142.
17. Morgan TJ (1999) The oxyhaemoglobin dissociation curve in critical illness. Crit Care Resusc 1: 93–100.
18. Rosenthal A, Khaw KT, Shwachman H (1977) Hemoglobin-oxygen equilibrium in cystic fibrosis. Pediatrics 59: 919–926.
19. Christoforou E, Papassotiriou I, Skarmoutsou C, Doudounakis S, Stamoulakatou A, et al. (2005) Soluble transferrin receptors and tissue oxygenation in non-anaemic cystic fibrosis patients. J Cyst Fibros 4: 151–156.
20. Vichinsky EP, Pennathur-Das R, Nickerson B, Minor M, Kleman K, et al. (1984) Inadequate erythroid response to hypoxia in cystic fibrosis. J Pediatr 105: 15–21.
21. Rosenthal A, Button LN, Khaw KT (1977) Blood volume changes in patients with cystic fibrosis. Pediatrics 59: 588–594.

22. Wagener JS, McNeill GC, Taussig LM, Corrigan JJ, Lemen R (1983) Ferrokinetic and hematologic studies in cystic fibrosis patients. Am J Pediatr Hematol Oncol 5: 153–160.
23. Orzalesi MM, Motoyama EK (1973) Blood oxygen affinity in children with cystic fibrosis. Am Rev Respir Dis 107: 928–931.
24. Berghout AG, Bender SW (1984) Anion transport and 2,3-diphosphoglycerate in cystic fibrosis red blood cells. Pediatr Res 18: 1017–1020.
25. Böning D, Schünemann HJ, Maassen N, Busse MW (1993) Reduction of oxylabile CO_2 in human blood by lactate. J Appl Physiol 74: 710–714.
26. Craescu CT, Poyart C, Schaeffer C, Garel MC, Kister J, et al. (1986) Covalent binding of glutathione to hemoglobin. II. Functional consequences and structural changes reflected in NMR spectra. J Biol Chem 261 (31): 14710–14716.
27. Garby L, Robert M, Zaar B (1972) Proton- and carbamino-linked oxygen affinity of normal human blood. Acta Physiol Scand 84: 482–492.
28. Meier U, Böning D, Rubenstein HJ (1974) Oxygenation dependent variations of the Bohr coefficient related to whole blood and erythrocyte pH. Pflügers Arch 349: 203–213.
29. Schmidt W, Böning D, Braumann KM (1987) Red cell age effects on metabolism and oxygen affinity in humans. Respir Physiol 68: 215–225.
30. Schmidt W, Dahners HW, Correa R, Ramirez R, Rojas J, et al. (1990) Blood gas transport properties in endurance-trained athletes living at different altitudes. Int J Sports Medicine 11: 15–21.
31. Morpurgo G, Battaglia P, Bernini L (1970) Higher Bohr effect in Indian natives of Peruvian Highlands as compared with Europeans. Nature (Lond) 227: 387–388.
32. Humpeler E, Vogel S (1977) Oxygen affinity of hemoglobin in postmenopausal women. Pflügers Arch 372: 287–290.
33. Böning D, Draude W, Trost F, Meier U (1978) Interrelation between Bohr and temperature effects on the oxygen dissociation curve in men and women. Respir Physiol 34: 195–207.
34. Humpeler E, Amor H (1973) Sex differences in the oxygen affinity of hemoglobin. Pflügers Arch 343: 151–156.
35. Morse M, Cassels DE, Holder M, O'Connell E, Swanson A (1950) The position of the oxygen dissociation curve of the blood in normal children and adults. J Clin Invest 29: 1091–1097.
36. Rasmussen B, Klausen K, Clausen JP, Trap-Jensen J (1975) Pulmonary ventilation, blood gases and blood pH after training of the arms or the legs. J Appl Physiol 38: 250–256.
37. Sproule BJ, Mitchell JH, Miller WF (1960) Cardiopulmonary physiological responses to heavy exercise in patients with anemia. J Clin Invest 39: 378–388.
38. Böning D, Schweigart U, Tibes U, Hemmer B (1975) Influences of exercise and endurance training on the oxygen dissociation curve of blood unter in vivo and in vitro conditions. Eur J Appl Physiol 34: 1–10.
39. Barrett PM, Alagely A, Topol EJ (2012) Cystic fibrosis in an era of genomically guided therapy. Hum Mol Genet 21: R66-R71.
40. Quanjer PH, Tammeling GJ, Cotes JE, Fabbri LM, Matthys H, et al. (1993) Symbols, abbreviations and units. Working Party Standardization of Lung Function Tests, European Community for Steel and Coal. Eur Respir J Suppl 16: 85–100.
41. Hughes JM (1996) Blood gas estimations from arterialized capillary blood versus arterial puncture: are they different? Eur Respir J 9: 184–185.
42. Ben Rayana MC, Burnett RW, Covington AK, D'Orazio P, Fogh-Andersen N, et al. (2008) IFCC guideline for sampling, measuring and reporting ionized magnesium in plasma. Clin Chem Lab Med 46: 21–26.
43. Böning D, Tibes U, Schweigart U (1976) Red cell hemoglobin, hydrogen ion and electrolyte concentrations during exercise in trained and untrained subjects. Eur J Appl Physiol 35: 243–249.
44. Diem K, Lentner C (1969) Wissenschaftliche Tabellen. Geigy, AG, Basel.
45. Uhle MJ (2004) Zur Nutzbarkeit ventilatorischer Messverfahren in der Diagnostik der submaximalen Leistungsfähigkeit bei Patienten mit Zystischer Fibrose (About the usability of ventilatory measuring methods in diagnosis of submaximal exercise performance capacity in patients with cystic fibrosis) [dissertation]. Charité - Universitätsmedizin Berlin.
46. Böning D, Rojas J, Serrato M, Ulloa C, Coy L, et al. (2001) Hemoglobin mass and peak oxygen uptake in untrained and trained residents of moderate altitude. Int J Sports Med 22: 572–578.
47. Cristancho E, Reyes O, Serrato M, Mora MM, Rojas JA, et al. (2007) Arterial oxygen saturation and hemoglobin mass in postmenopausal untrained and trained altitude residents. High Alt Med Biol 8: 296–306.
48. Böning D, Rojas J, Serrato M, Reyes O, Coy L, et al. (2008) Extracellular pH defense against lactic acid in untrained and trained altitude residents. Eur J Appl Physiol 103: 127–137.
49. O'Connor TM, McGrath DS, Short C, O'Donnell MJ, Sheehy M, et al. (2002) Subclinical anaemia of chronic disease in adult patients with cystic fibrosis. J Cyst Fibros 1: 31–34.
50. Fischer R, Simmerlein R, Huber RM, Schiffl H, Lang SM (2007) Lung disease severity, chronic inflammation, iron deficiency, and erythropoietin response in adults with cystic fibrosis. Pediatr Pulmonol 42: 1193–1197.
51. Watts KD, McColley SA (2011) Elevated vascular endothelial growth factor is correlated with elevated erythropoietin in stable, young cystic fibrosis patients. Pediatr Pulmonol 46: 683–687.
52. Duranton C, Rubera I, Cougnon M, Melis N, Chargui A, et al. (2012) CFTR is involved in the fine tuning of intracellular redox status: physiological implications in cystic fibrosis. Am J Pathol 181: 1367–1377.
53. Schillers H (2008) Imaging CFTR in its native environment. Pflügers Arch 456: 163–177.
54. Rollema HS, De Bruin SA, Janssen LHM, Van Os GAJ (1975) Effect of potassium chloride on Bohr effect of human hemoglobin. J Biol Chem 250: 1333–1339.
55. Braumann KM, Böning D, Trost F (1979) Oxygen dissociation curves in trained and untrained subjects. Eur J Appl Physiol 42: 51–60.
56. West JB, Schoene RB, Milledge JS (2007) High Altitude Medicine and Physiology. London: Hodder Arnold.
57. Arturson G (1971) Changes in blood oxygen affinity during anaemia and cardiac and pulmonary insufficiency. Acta Anaesth Scand 45: 39–44.
58. Böning D, Enciso G (1987) Hemoglobin-oxygen affinity in anemia. Blut 54: 361–368.
59. Böning D, Klarholz C, Himmelsbach B, Hütler M, Maassen N (2007) Causes of differences in exercise-induced changes of base excess and blood lactate. Eur J Appl Physiol 99: 163–171.
60. Braumann KM, Böning D, Trost F (1982) Bohr effect and slope of the oxygen dissociation curve after physical training. J Appl Physiol Respir Environ Exerc Physiol 52: 1524–1529.
61. Mairbäurl H, Weber RE (2013) Oxygen transport by hemoglobin. Compr Physiol 2 : 1463–1489.
62. Head CA, Brugnara C, Martinez-Ruiz R, Kacmarek RM, Bridges KR, et al. (1997) Low concentrations of nitric oxide increase oxygen affinity of sickle erythrocytes in vitro and in vivo. J Clin Invest 100: 1193–1198.
63. Hrinczenko BW, Alayash AI, Wink DA, Gladwin MT, Rodgers GP, et al. (2000) Effect of nitric oxide and nitric oxide donors on red blood cell oxygen transport. Br J Haematol 110: 412–419.
64. von Pickardt B (2003) Wirkung NO-freisetzender Verbindungen auf die Sauerstoffbindungskurve (Effect of NO liberating substances on the oxygen dissociation curve) [dissertation]. Freie Universität Berlin.
65. Gladwin MT, Schechter AN, Shelhamer JH, Pannell LK, Conway DA, et al. (1999) Inhaled nitric oxide augments nitric oxide transport on sickle cell hemoglobin without affecting oxygen affinity. J Clin Invest 104: 937–945.
66. Erzurum SC, Ghosh S, Janocha AJ, Xu W, Bauer S, et al. (2007) Higher blood flow and circulating NO products offset high-altitude hypoxia among Tibetans. Proc Natl Acad Sci U S A 104: 17593–17598.
67. Hütler M, Pollmann C, Beneke R, Leithauser R, Böning D (2000) Measurable amount of glutathione in blood is influenced by oxygen saturation of hemoglobin. Clin Chim Acta 301: 213–217.
68. Smith JE, Lee M, Agar S, Du D (1976) Oxygen-hemoglobin equilibrium of normal and glutathione- deficient sheep. Am J Vet Res 37: 1135–1137.
69. Hudson VM (2001) Rethinking cystic fibrosis pathology: the critical role of abnormal reduced glutathione (GSH) transport caused by CFTR mutation. Free Radic Biol Med 30: 1440–1461.
70. Makhro A, Hanggi P, Goede JS, Wang J, Bruggemann A, et al. (2013) N-methyl-D-aspartate receptors in human erythroid precursor cells and in circulating red blood cells contribute to the intracellular calcium regulation. Am J Physiol Cell Physiol 305: C1123-C1138.
71. Christiansen TF (1981) An algorithm for calculating the concentration of the base excess of blood. In: Siggaard-Andersen O, editors. Proceedings of the IFCC Expert Panel on pH and blood gases held at Herved Hospital 1980. Copenhagen: Radiometer A/S. 77–81.

Insulin-Like Growth Factor 1 (IGF-1) Enhances the Protein Expression of CFTR

Ha Won Lee[1], Jie Cheng[1], Olga Kovbasnjuk[2], Mark Donowitz[1], William B. Guggino[1]*

1 Department of Physiology, Johns Hopkins University, School of Medicine, Baltimore, Maryland, United States of America, **2** Department of Medicine, Johns Hopkins University, School of Medicine, Baltimore, Maryland, United States of America

Abstract

Low levels of insulin-like growth factor 1 (IGF-1) have been observed in the serum of cystic fibrosis (CF) patients. However, the effects of low serum IGF-1 on the cystic fibrosis transmembrane conductance regulator (CFTR), whose defective function is the primary cause of cystic fibrosis, have not been studied. Here, we show in human cells that IGF-1 increases the steady-state levels of mature wildtype CFTR in a CFTR-associated ligand (CAL)- and TC10-dependent manner; moreover, IGF-1 increases CFTR-mediated chloride transport. Using an acceptor photobleaching fluorescence resonance energy transfer (FRET) assay, we have confirmed the binding of CAL and CFTR in the Golgi. We also show that CAL overexpression inhibits forskolin-induced increases in the cell-surface expression of CFTR. We found that IGF-1 activates TC10, and active TC10 alters the functional association between CAL and CFTR. Furthermore, IGF-1 and active TC10 can reverse the CAL-mediated reduction in the cell-surface expression of CFTR. IGF-1 does not increase the expression of ΔF508 CFTR, whose processing is arrested in the ER. This finding is consistent with our observation that IGF-1 alters the functional interaction of CAL and CFTR in the Golgi. However, when ΔF508 CFTR is rescued with low temperature or the corrector VRT-325 and proceeds to the Golgi, IGF-1 can increase the expression of the rescued ΔF508 CFTR. Our data support a model indicating that CAL-CFTR binding in the Golgi inhibits CFTR trafficking to the cell surface, leading CFTR to the degradation pathway instead. IGF-1-activated TC10 changes the interaction of CFTR and CAL, allowing CFTR to progress to the plasma membrane. These findings offer a potential strategy using a combinational treatment of IGF-1 and correctors to increase the post-Golgi expression of CFTR in cystic fibrosis patients bearing the ΔF508 mutation.

Editor: Effie C. Tsilibary, National Center for Scientific Research Demokritos, Greece

Funding: This work was supported by the Cystic Fibrosis Foundation GUGGINO5X0, Korea Science and Engineering Foundation (KOSEF), and the National Institutes of Health (NHLBI PO1 HL51811 to WBG, NIDDK PO1 DK072084 to WBG, MD, OK; and RO1 DK 58928 to OK). The funders had no role in study design, data collection and analysis, decision to publish, or preparation of the manuscript.

Competing Interests: The authors declare that there are no completing interests.

* E-mail: wguggino@jhmi.edu

Introduction

Cystic fibrosis is a genetic disease caused by mutations in CFTR [1]. CFTR's primary function is to move chloride ions across the plasma membrane of epithelial cells; this is a key function in the normal operation of several organs, including the airways, the intestinal tract, the pancreas, the epididymis, and the sweat duct (see [2] for a review). Dysfunctional chloride transport of mutant CFTRs leads to pathologically low levels of fluid, accompanied by altered composition in the airways, pancreatic duct, and intestinal tract, and it causes symptoms such as bacterial airway infections, chronic inflammation, growth retardation, male infertility, and obstruction of pancreatic ducts and the gastrointestinal tract. Failure to absorb fluid in the sweat ducts leads to high sweat chloride in patients, a symptom that has been used as a defining factor prior to the identification of the CF gene [3].

Because CFTR is localized at the cell surface to transport chloride ions, CFTR mutations resulting in improper localization (e.g., the most common mutation, ΔF508 CFTR) are particularly severe [4,5]. Therefore, the processes involved in the trafficking of both wildtype and ΔF508 CFTR have been studied extensively (see [6] for a review). It is now well known that CFTR trafficking to the cell surface is regulated by PDZ proteins (the Golgi reassembly stacking protein [GRASP], CFTR-associated ligand [CAL], Na^+/H^+ exchanger regulatory factor [NHERF1/2], and CFTR-associated protein 70 [CAP70]), which bind to CFTR [7–10]. These proteins assemble CFTR into protein complexes in the ER, Golgi, or plasma membrane in polarized epithelial cells [8,10] and ultimately regulate CFTR localization at the apical membrane by allowing CFTR to reach the plasma membrane, sequestering it within the cell, or targeting it for degradation (see [11] for review). For example, GRASP is localized to the Golgi [12]. When ER stress occurs, GRASP is phosphorylated and then binds to CFTR, leading to CFTR trafficking from the ER to the cell surface through a unique trafficking pathway [9]. CAL regulates the total and cell-surface expression of CFTR, either by enhancing the lysosomal degradation of CFTR [7] or allowing it to traffic to the plasma membrane, depending on which secondary proteins are bound to CAL [13]. At the plasma membrane, NHERF and CAP70 stabilize CFTR and allow CFTR to form an efficient functional complex [8,14,15].

As previously mentioned, CAL and its associated binding proteins regulate the lysosomal degradation and surface expression of CFTR [13,16]. CAL is an adaptor protein that has multiple protein-interacting domains, including a PDZ domain that binds CFTR and two coiled-coil domains that are responsible for its

Golgi localization. Syntaxin 6 (STX6), a soluble N-ethylmaleimide-sensitive factor-activating protein receptor protein (SNARE) protein, and TC10, a small GTPase of the Rho family, are known to bind to CAL in the region of the coiled-coil domains [17,18].

STX6 is involved in intracellular vesicle trafficking [16,18,19]. Binding of STX6 to CAL reduces CFTR protein expression by increasing the transport of CFTR to the lysosome and thus promoting the lysosomal degradation of CFTR. Therefore, when bound to STX6, CAL is a negative regulator of both the total and cell surface expression of CFTR. In contrast, TC10 is a positive regulator of CFTR surface expression: By binding to CAL, it promotes the trafficking of CFTR to the plasma membrane and increases the total and cell-surface expression of CFTR [13]. Although the interaction of CFTR with CAL, TC10, and STX6 has been studied, how these pathways are regulated is not known. Information on how this regulation occurs certainly has implications for our understanding of both wildtype CFTR and the mutant ΔF508 CFTR.

Given that active TC10 promotes the trafficking of CFTR to the cell surface [13], the question to be asked is how TC10 is activated to increase the surface expression of CFTR.? IGF-1 and insulin activate TC10 through a GTP exchange factor in neurons and adipocytes [20,21]. IGF-1 activates TC10 in neurons for neuronal growth, and insulin increases GLUT4 vesicle translocation in adipocytes for glucose uptake by activating TC10 [21–23]. Thus, it is likely that IGF-1 and/or insulin is(are) the upstream activator(s) of TC10 that ultimately regulate(s) CFTR protein expression. CF patients as well as CF pig models have low IGF-1 levels in their serum [24–27], an observation that also has implications for the pathophysiology of CF. Therefore, in this report, we tested whether IGF-1 alters CFTR expression. Dominant-negative TC10 was used to determine whether TC10 activation is required for any of the IGF-1-induced changes in CFTR protein expression. Our results showed that TC10, activated via IGF-1, does indeed alter the functional interaction between CFTR and CAL, ultimately increasing CFTR surface expression. We also suggest that IGF-1 may have therapeutic value in patients bearing the ΔF508 CFTR mutation.

Materials and Methods

Reagents and Antibodies

IGF-1, forskolin, and brefeldin A were obtained from Sigma. cDNAs encoding EYFP-tagged wildtype or mutant CFTR were subcloned with the pEYFP-C1 plasmid (Clontech), and cDNA encoding ECFP-tagged CAL was subcloned with the pECFP-C1 plasmid (Clontech), in the same manner that GFP was tagged to CFTR and CAL in previous studies [7,28]. Anti-CFTR antibodies were obtained from the University of North Carolina (217) and Upstate (M3A7). Anti-GFP antibody (ab290) and anti-Na,K-ATPase antibody (464.6) were purchased from Abcam, anti-HA antibody (12CA5) from Roche, and anti-HA antibody conjugated with HRP from Sigma. Anti-GM130 antibody (35/GM130) was obtained from BD Bioscience and Alexa-647 goat anti-mouse IgG from Invitrogen.

Cell Culture and Transfection

HeLa cells were cultured in Dulbecco's modified Eagle's medium (DMEM, Invitrogen) supplemented with 10% fetal bovine serum (FBS, Invitrogen) and penicillin/streptomycin (Invitrogen) in a humidified 37°C CO_2 incubator. CFBE41o- cells (a cell line from bronchial epithelial cells of a cystic fibrosis patient [29,30], kindly provided by Dr. Gruenert) were cultured in minimum essential medium Eagle (MEM, Invitrogen) with 10% FBS and penicillin/streptomycin, and CFBE-WTCFTR cells (CFBE41o- cells stably transfected with wildtype CFTR [30], kindly provided by Dr. Gruenert) were cultured in MEM with 10% FBS, penicillin/streptomycin and 300 μg/ml hygromycin B. For serum starvation, HeLa cells were cultured in DMEM with 0.5% FBS, and CFBE and CFBE-WTCFTR cells were cultured in MEM without FBS. Cells were transiently transfected with Lipofectamine 2000 reagent (Invitrogen) according to the manufacturer's instruction and incubated for 24–48 hours.

Coimmunoprecipitation and Western Blotting

Cells were washed twice with cold Dulbecco's phosphate buffered saline (DPBS, Invitrogen), and then resuspended in lysis buffer (150 mM Tris, 50 mM NaCl, 1% Nonidet P-40, pH 7.4) with protease inhibitor cocktail (Roche). After 20 minutes on ice, the lysates were cleared by centrifugation at 15,000 g for 20 minutes. Pellets were discarded, and supernatants were used for further experiments. Protein G-Sepharose (GE Healthcare) was mixed with cleared lysates and primary antibodies and incubated on a rotary shaker at 4°C overnight. The beads were washed three times with lysis buffer and incubated in Laemmli buffer at 95°C for 5 minutes or at 42°C for 20 minutes. Total cleared lysates were denatured in Laemmli buffer at 42°C for 20 minutes. The protein concentration of each sample was measured with a BCA protein assay kit (Thermo Scientific), and equal amounts of total proteins were loaded on HCl-Tris gels.

Proteins were separated by SDS-PAGE and transferred to PVDF membranes (BioRad). After the transfer, the membranes were blocked with 5% nonfat milk in Tris-buffered saline with 0.05% Tween 20 (TBST) for 1 hour. The membranes were incubated with primary antibodies in 5% milk in TBST at 4°C overnight. The membranes were washed four times with TBST and incubated with Clean-Blot IP Detection Reagent (Thermo Scientific) or appropriate horseradish peroxidase-conjugated secondary antibodies (GE Healthcare).

Cell-surface Biotinylation

After cells were washed four times with cold DPBS containing 1 mM Ca^{2+} and 1 mM Mg^{2+}, they were incubated with 0.5 mg/ml sulfo-NHS-SS-biotin (Thermo Scientific) in DPBS with Ca^{2+} and Mg^{2+} at 4°C for 30 minutes. Free sulfo-NHS-SS-biotin was then quenched by washing with cold 192 mM glycine in DPBS four times. Cells were lysed with lysis buffer, and the lysates were centrifuged at 15,000 g at 4°C for 20 minutes. The supernatants were incubated with NeutrAvidin UltraLink Resin (Thermo Scientific) at 4°C for 5 hours or overnight. The beads were washed twice with lysis buffer, and proteins were eluted with Laemmli buffer at 42°C for 20 minutes. Biotinylated protein samples were analyzed by western blotting as described above.

TC10 Activity Assays

HA-tagged TC10 [13] was transfected into cells. The transfected cells were serum-starved, and after 24 hours, the cells were treated with 0.1 μg/ml IGF-1 for another 24 hours. After a wash with cold DPBS, the cells were scraped in magnesium-containing lysis buffer (Millipore), and the cell lysates were incubated with GST-PAK-1 PBD-conjugated agarose beads (Millipore) for 1 hour and washed with the lysis buffer three times [31,32]. Laemmli buffer was added to the beads and boiled for 5 minutes.

Fluorescence Microscope and Acceptor Photobleaching Fluorescence Resonance Energy Transfer (FRET)

A Zeiss LSM 510 laser scanning system and 40x oil-immersion lens were used. Cells were seeded onto cover glasses or a glass-bottom dish. The following steps were done at room temperature: After a wash with cold DPBS, cells were fixed with 4% paraformaldehyde for 10 minutes. For immunostaining, after the fixation, cells were permeabilized with DPBS containing 0.1% Triton X-100 for 20 minutes and blocked with 1% bovine albumin serum or 5% goat serum (both from Sigma) for 1 hour. After blocking, the cells were incubated with primary antibodies and then with secondary antibodies conjugated to Alexa 647. Cells were mounted using ProLong Gold with DAPI (Invitrogen).

CFP was excited by a 458-nm Argon/2 laser, and the emission was detected with a 465–510 filter; YFP was excited by a 514-nm Argon/2 laser, and the emission was detected with a 520–555 filter. Alexa 647 was excited by a 633-nm HeNe633 and detected with a 646–700 filter. The 16-bit look-up table originally provided with ImageJ was applied to CFP images taken for FRET.

CFP/YFP pairs were used for acceptor photobleaching FRET. Images for CFP and YFP were collected before and after photobleaching with the 514-nm Argon/2 laser at the maximum intensity. From the images, the signal intensity of CFP was measured with ImageJ image software (NIH), and FRET efficiency was calculated using the following formula: $FRET\ efficiency\ (\%) = \left(1 - \frac{I_{Pre}}{I_{Post}}\right) \times 100$, where I_{Pre} and I_{Post} correspond to the CFP signal intensity (background signal was subtracted) before and after photobleaching, respectively.

For quantification of the colocalization, Pearson's correlation coefficients were calculated with an ImageJ plugin, Colocalization Test (Wright Cell Image Facility, Canada).

Short-circuit Current Measurements

Short-circuit current (I_{SC}) measurements were performed in a six-channel Easy-Mount chamber system (Physiologic Instruments, San Diego, CA) that accepts Snapwell filters (Corning Costar, Acton, MA; 3407). I_{SC} was measured with a VCCMC6 multichannel voltage-current clamp amplifier (Physiologic Instruments) in the voltage-clamp mode. Data were acquired on an 1.71-GHz PC running Windows XP (Microsoft, Redmond, WA) and equipped with DI-720 (DATAQ Instruments, Akron, OH), with Acquire and Analyze version 2.3.159 (Physiologic Instruments) software. Cells were cultured to confluence on Snapwell filters before measurement. The cell monolayers were bathed on both sides with solution containing 115 mM NaCl, 25 mM sodium gluconate, 5 mM potassium gluconate, 1.2 mM $MgCl_2$, 1.2 mM $CaCl_2$, 10 mM D-glucose and 10 mM HEPES (pH 7.4 with NaOH). The mucosal side was replaced with a low Cl^- solution containing 139 mM sodium gluconate, 1.2 mM NaCl, 5 mM potassium gluconate, 1.2 mM $MgCl_2$, 1.2 mM $CaCl_2$, 10 mM D-glucose, and 10 mM HEPES (pH 7.4 with NaOH). The solution was constantly circulated, maintained at 37°C, and bubbled gently with air. Amiloride (20 μM) was added to the mucosal solution, and after stabilization, forskolin (10 μM) was added to the serosal chamber, followed by the CFTR channel inhibitor CFTRinh-172 (5 μM).

Statistical Analysis

All quantitative results are given as averages ± standard error (SE). Statistical significance was determined using Student's *t*-test. Values of $p<0.05$ were considered significant.

Results

CAL Binds to CFTR at the Golgi

To find out how CAL regulates CFTR trafficking, we investigated the interaction between CAL and CFTR by using an acceptor photobleaching FRET assay. For the assay, expression vectors of CFP-tagged CAL and YFP-tagged CFTR were constructed. As a first step, the binding of CAL-CFP and YFP-CFTR was confirmed by coimmunoprecipitation in HeLa cells (Fig. 1A). Next, CAL-CFP was transiently transfected into HeLa cells with YFP-CFTR or with YFP-ΔTRL CFTR, which does not bind CAL, and their FRET efficiency was then measured. The FRET results (Fig. 1B-E) confirmed the binding of YFP-CFTR and CAL-CFP, showing that the FRET efficiency of CAL-CFP and YFP-wildtype CFTR was significantly higher than that of the negative controls (CAL-CFP alone or with YFP-ΔTRL CFTR). These results demonstrate that CAL binds CFTR, but not ΔTRL CFTR, *in vivo* and that the detected FRET is specific for the binding of CAL to CFTR.

The cell compartment in which CAL binds CFTR was determined by immunostaining for GM130, a Golgi marker. CAL-CFP and YFP-CFTR were colocalized with GM130 (Fig. 1F). Their colocalization within the Golgi and their binding suggest that CAL-CFP binds to YFP-CFTR in the Golgi. To support this result, we examined the FRET between CAL-CFP and YFP-CFTR after treatment with brefeldin A (BFA), a chemical that disrupts Golgi structure. Following treatment of cells with 10 μg/ml BFA at 37°C for 30 minutes, CAL-CFP was expressed throughout the cells, and the FRET between CAL-CFP and YFP-CFTR was reduced markedly (Fig. 2C,E). Thus, the *in vivo* binding of CAL-CFP and YFP-CFTR appears to depend upon the Golgi being intact, again suggesting that the Golgi apparatus is required for the binding of CAL-CFP and YFP-CFTR.

In order to examine more closely the trafficking of CAL and CFTR after forskolin treatment, we cotransfected 1.5 μg of YFP-CFTR and 0.5 μg of CAL-CFP expression plasmids into HeLa cells. After a 24-hour incubation, we treated the cells with 100 μM forskolin at 37°C for 30 minutes and immunostained the cells with an anti-GM130 antibody. We then used a plugin of ImageJ to calculate Pearson's correlation coefficients to determine the quantitative colocalization of GM130 with CAL-CFP and YFP-CFTR. Interestingly, forskolin did not change the Pearson's correlation coefficient between GM130 and CAL-CFP but reduced the coefficient between GM130 and YFP-CFTR (Fig. 3). Thus, following forskolin treatment, less CFTR was localized to the Golgi. Surprisingly, forskolin did not change the localization of CAL (Fig. 3), suggesting that the binding of CAL to CFTR occurs in the Golgi as shown above, but CAL does not move with CFTR out of the Golgi.

To verify that CFTR and CAL were not moving together to the plasma membrane in response to forskolin treatment, we examined the interaction between CFTR and CAL by the acceptor photobleaching FRET assay, utilizing the experimental conditions described above. More CFTR was present at the cell surface after forskolin treatment (Fig. 2D, Fig. 3, and CFTR-only sample results of Fig. 4), whereas CAL-CFP was still located in the cytosol (Fig. 2D and Fig. 3). Moreover, the treatment of forskolin reduced the FRET of CAL-CFP and YFP-CFTR (Fig. 2D, E), suggesting that forskolin reduces the association of CAL-CFP with YFP-CFTR and enhances CFTR movement to the cell surface, while CAL remains in the Golgi.

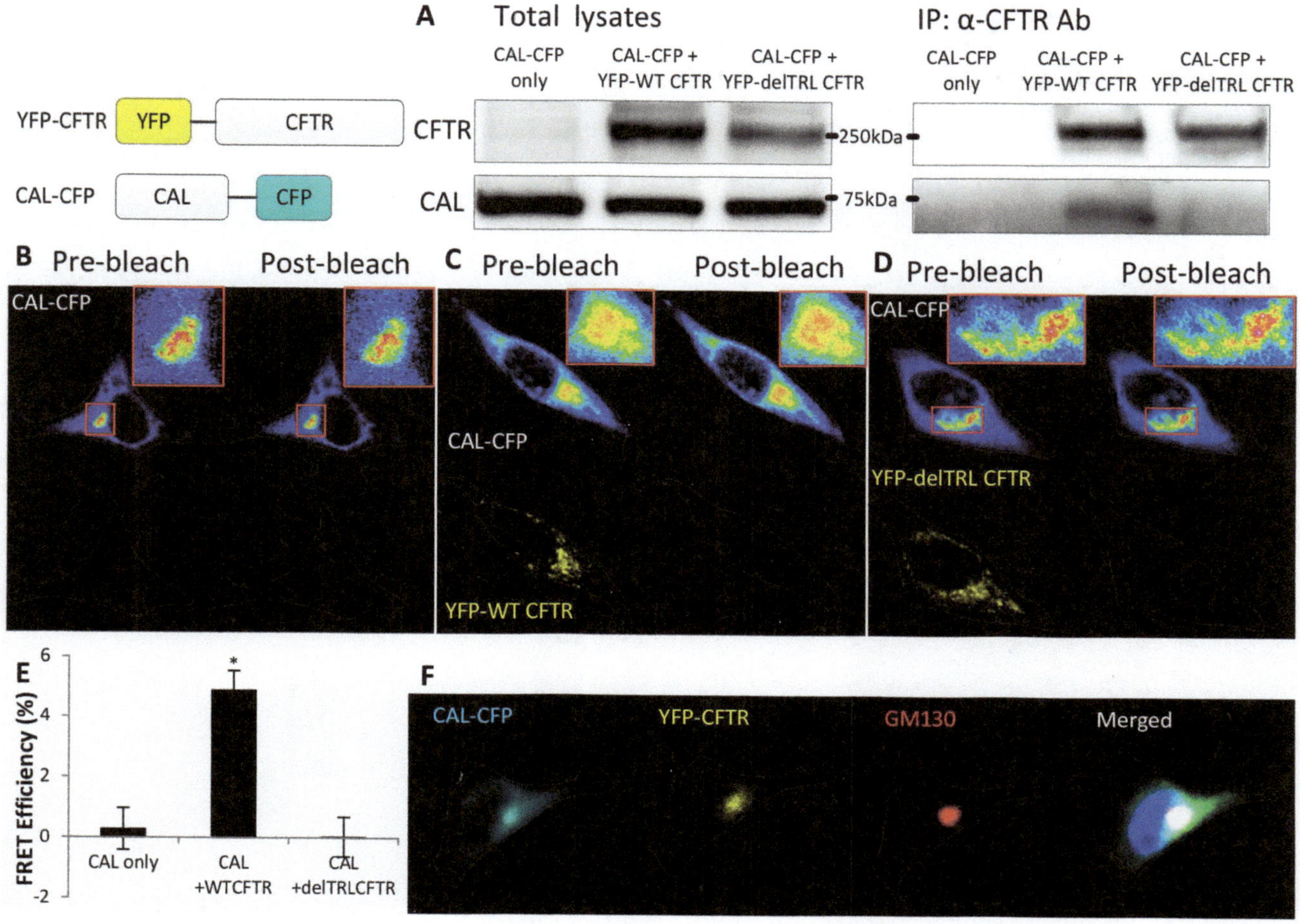

Figure 1. CAL-CFP binds YFP-CFTR in vivo, and CAL and CFTR are colocalized in the Golgi in HeLa cells. The N terminus of CFTR was tagged with YFP, and CFP was tagged to the C terminus of CAL was tagged with CFP. In HeLa cells, CAL-CFP was transiently expressed alone (A,B), with YFP-wildtype CFTR (A,C), or with YFP-delTRL CFTR (A,D). (A) Left panel: CAL-CFP, YFP-wildtype CFTR, and YFP-delTRL CFTR from total lysates were immunoblotted with anti-GFP antibody. Right panel: The cell lysates were immunoprecipitated with anti-CFTR antibody. (B-D) The left columns are the images before photobleaching with a 514-nm laser, and the right columns are the images after photobleaching. CFP and YFP are pseudocolored with a 16-bit lookup table (provided with ImageJ) and yellow, respectively. E shows the statistical analysis of the FRET efficiency obtained from the images. Results are means ±SE. (n = 11–13) *p<0.001. (F) YFP-CFTR and CAL-CFP were colocalized with GM130. HeLa cells that had been transfected with YFP-CFTR and CAL-CFP were immunostained with anti-GM130 antibody. The right-most panel shows the merged image of CAL-CFP, YFP-CFTR, GM130, and DAPI. (B–D, F). Cell outlines are drawn with gray lines.

Overexpression of CAL Inhibits the Forskolin-induced Promotion of CFTR Trafficking to the Cell Surface

To study the effect of CAL on the cell-surface expression of CFTR, we varied the doses of the CAL-CFP *versus* YFP-CFTR cDNA cotransfected into HeLa cells. We also performed a cell-surface biotinylation assay to measure the forskolin-induced changes in the cell-surface expression of CFTR. Fig. 4 shows that when YFP-CFTR was expressed alone, the 30-minute treatment with forskolin enhanced the CFTR expression at the cell surface, as previously shown [33,34]. When the ratio of the transfected amount of CAL-CFP cDNA to YFP-CFTR cDNA was 1:3, the same ratio we used in both the FRET assay and cell imaging studies, forskolin still increased the cell-surface expression of CFTR. However, when we transfected three times more CAL-CFP than YFP-CFTR cDNA (3:1), forskolin no longer increased the surface expression of CFTR (Fig. 4). In all cases, forskolin did not change the total expression of CFTR (Fig. 4). Therefore, changes in CAL expression levels regulate CFTR's progress to the cell surface.

Active TC10 Alters CAL-CFTR Binding and Increases the Steady-state Levels of CFTR at the Cell Surface, Even with Highly Overexpressed CAL

Previously, we showed that the constitutively active form of TC10 increases the surface expression of CFTR by binding to CAL [13]. We were curious to see whether active TC10 would also alter the CAL-CFTR interaction. The FRET assay showed that a constitutively active TC10 mutant, Q75L TC10, which remains in the GTP-bound form, does indeed reduce the FRET between CAL-CFP and YFP-CFTR. Importantly, the dominant-negative mutant T31N TC10, which remains in the GDP form, did not affect the FRET (Fig. 5A). These results indicate that active TC10 does indeed alter the binding of CFTR and CAL.

To test this possibility further, we cotransfected 1.5 µg of CAL-CFP cDNA with 1.5 µg of YFP-CFTR cDNA. This ratio inhibited the effects of forskolin on CFTR surface expression (Fig. 5B), as in Fig. 4. However, when the same amounts of CAL-CFP and YFP-CFTR cDNAs were cotransfected along with the active form of TC10 (Q75L TC10), forskolin was able to increase the surface

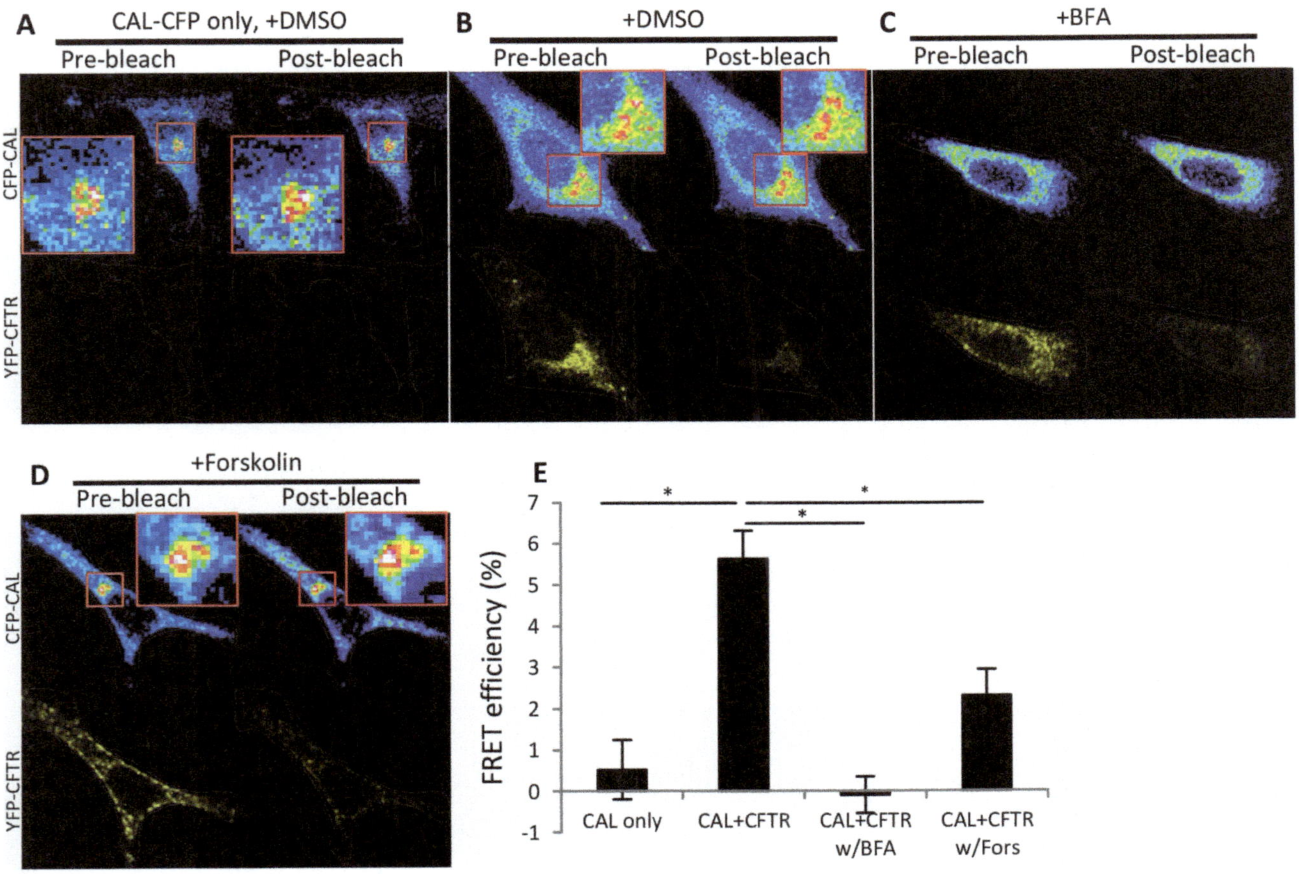

Figure 2. Disrupting the Golgi structure with brefeldin A and increasing the cell-surface expression of CFTR with forskolin diminish the FRET of CAL and CFTR. HeLa cells were transfected with CAL-CFP (0.5 μg) only (A) or with CAL-CFP (0.5 μg) and YFP-CFTR (1.5 μg) (B–D). DMSO (A, B), 10 μg/ml brefeldin A (BFA) (C), or 100 μM forskolin (D) was added at 37°C for 30 minutes. Images before (left columns) and after (right columns) photobleaching with a 514-nm laser are shown. CFP and YFP are pseudocolored with a 16-bit lookup table and yellow, respectively. Cell outlines are drawn with gray lines. (E) is the statistical analysis of the FRET efficiency of CAL and CFTR. The FRET efficiency of CAL and CFTR was reduced when BFA or forskolin was added. Results are means ±SE. (n = 44–68) *$p < 0.001$.

expression of CFTR. Note that co-transfection of the dominant-negative form of TC10, T31N TC10, did not counter the effects of CAL overexpression, and in that case, forskolin did not increase CFTR surface expression (Fig. 5B). These data suggest that active TC10 enhances CFTR expression at the cell surface, even when CAL is overexpressed.

IGF-1 increases the Steady State Levels of CFTR via TC10 and CAL

To determine whether the effects of TC10 are physiological, we utilized IGF-1, which is known to activate TC10 in neurons [21]. HeLa cells were transfected with YFP or YFP-CFTR, and after a 24-hour serum starvation, 0.1 μg/ml IGF-1 was applied for an additional 24 hours. IGF-1 increased the protein expression of YFP-CFTR but not of YFP alone (Fig. 6A); moreover, IGF-1 increased the CFTR expression level at the cell surface in HeLa cells (Fig. 6B). Because the two vector constructs share the same CMV promoter in the same backbone vector, the effects of IGF-1 on YFP-CFTR must be the result of post-transcriptional regulation. Furthermore, our results support the specificity of IGF-1′s effects on CFTR, in that IGF-1 treatment of HeLa cells did not change the protein expression of an endogenous plasma membrane protein, Na,K-ATPase (Fig. 6A).

To determine whether this regulation occurs in bronchial epithelial cells from cystic fibrosis patients (CFBE41o-, referred to as CFBE), we treated CFBE-WTCFTR cells (CFBE cells stably transfected with CFTR) with IGF-1. The effect was identical to that observed in the HeLa cells; IGF-1 increased the protein expression of CFTR but not of Na,K-ATPase (Fig. 6A). These data demonstrate that the effects of IGF-1 are not general, but specific for CFTR, and perhaps other proteins that share the same IGF-1-specific trafficking pathway.

To assess the function of CFTR in CFBE-WTCFTR cells, we measured CFTR-mediated Cl^- transport activity in IGF-1-treated cells. CFBE-WTCFTR cells grown on permeable supports were serum-starved for 24 hours, then treated with 0.1 μg/ml IGF-1 for 24 hours. High-resistance epithelial layers of CFBE-WTCFTR cells (whose average resistance was >1,200 $\Omega \cdot cm^2$ for both control and IGF-1-treated cells) were mounted in Ussing chambers to measure the short-circuit current (I_{SC}). As shown in Fig. 6C and D, the forskolin-activated I_{SC} in IGF-1 treated cells was significantly higher than the control cells. I_{SC} was completely inhibited by the CFTR inhibitor CFTRinh-172, showing that the currents were indeed CFTR-dependent.

To determine whether IGF-1 activates TC10 in CFBE and HeLa cells, we used a peptide (PAK-1 PBD) that binds selectively to activated TC10 [31,32]. Treatment with IGF-1 increased the

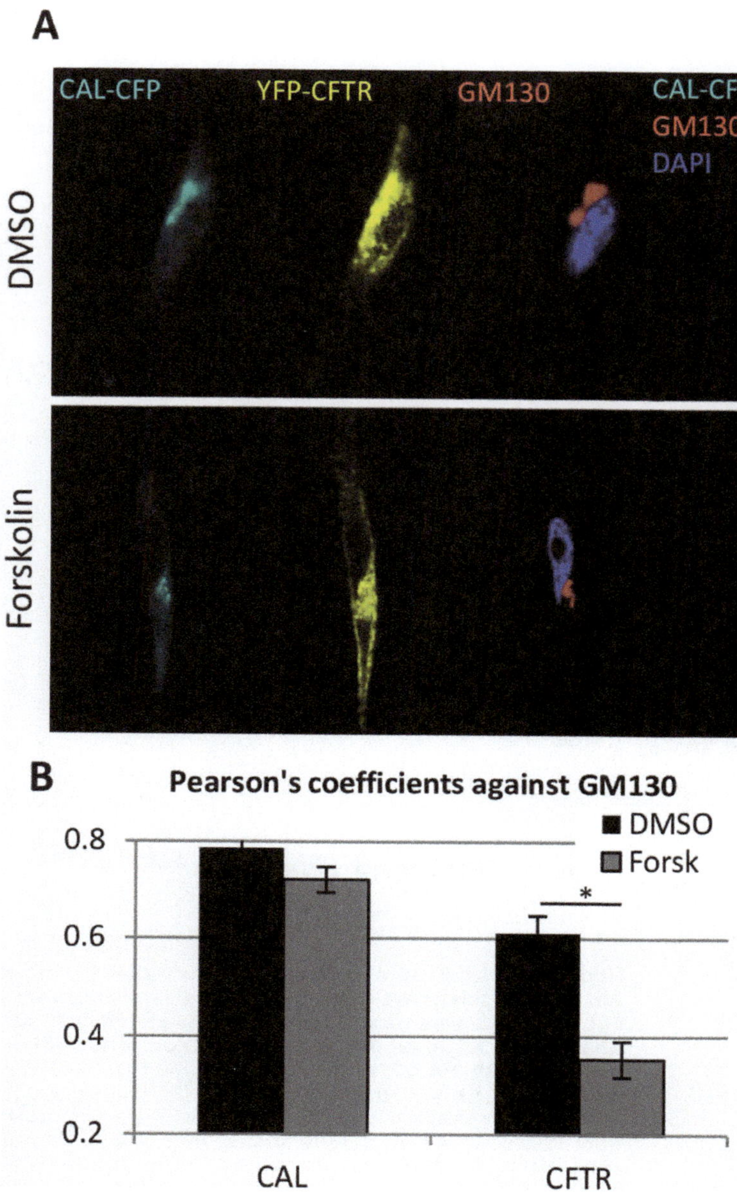

Figure 3. Forskolin treatment relocates CFTR, but not CAL, out of the Golgi in HeLa cells. HeLa cells were transfected with CAL-CFP (0.5 μg) and YFP-CFTR (1.5 μg). GM130 was immunostained with anti-GM130 antibody, followed by secondary antibody conjugated with Alexa-647. DMSO (A, upper panel) or 100 μM forskolin (A, lower panel) was added at 37°C for 30 minutes. (B) The graph shows Pearson's correlation coefficients of GM130 and CAL or of GM130 and CFTR. The coefficients were calculated using an ImageJ plugin, the Colocalization Test. Pearson's correlation coefficients of GM130 and CAL-CFP were not altered in the presence of forskolin, but those of GM130 and YFP-CFTR were reduced by forskolin treatment. Results are means ±SE. (n = 6–9) *$p<0.01$.

level of activated TC10 in HeLa cells and in CFBE cells transfected with HA-tagged TC10 (Fig. 7A). When T31N TC10 was coexpressed with CFTR to suppress the endogenous activity of TC10, the IGF-1-induced increase of YFP-CFTR expression was abolished (Fig. 7B). Thus, activation of TC10 is required for IGF-1 to increase CFTR expression.

Given our observation that active TC10 reduced the FRET of CAL and CFTR, we reasoned that a similar mechanism might be involved in the IGF-1-mediated regulation of the steady-state levels of CFTR. Indeed, CAL-CFTR FRET was also reduced by IGF-1 (Fig. 7C). Therefore, we surmised that if IGF-1 increases the expression of CFTR by suppressing CAL, overexpression of CAL would reduce the effects of IGF-1. As expected, over-expression of CAL reduced the increase in CFTR expression induced by IGF-1 in HeLa cells (Fig. 7D). The effect of CAL overexpression could be reversed by the co-overexpression of TC10. In this case, IGF-1 still increased the steady-state levels of CFTR even when CAL was overexpressed (Fig. 7D). This result demonstrates that TC10, activated by IGF-1, can increase the steady-state levels of CFTR in a dominant fashion over CAL.

As shown in HeLa cells and also in CFBE-WTCFTR cells, IGF-1 increased CFTR protein expression via TC10 (Fig. 6A, Fig. 7B). This increase by IGF-1 was inhibited by CAL overexpression. However, CAL's inhibition of IGF-1 was overcome by co-overexpression of TC10, again showing the dominance of TC10 in this process (Fig. 7E).

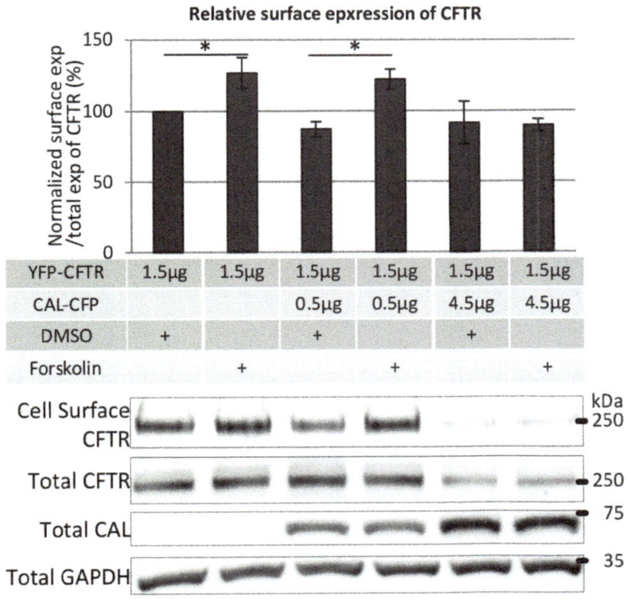

Figure 4. Forskolin fails to increase the cell-surface expression of CFTR with highly overexpressed CAL. HeLa cells were transfected with YFP-CFTR and CAL-CFP as indicated in the table. At 48 hours after transfection, cells were treated with DMSO or 100 μM forskolin at 37°C for 30 minutes. CFTR at the cell surface was then biotinylated. Cell surface-biotinylated CFTR, total CFTR, and total CAL were immunoblotted with anti-GFP antibody, and GAPDH was immunoblotted with anti-GAPDH antibody. The graph shows the ratio of the cell surface-biontinylated CFTR expression level to the total CFTR expression level, normalized by the ratio of the YFP-CFTR-alone samples with the DMSO treatment (%). When CAL was not overexpressed or 0.5 μg of CAL was transfected, forskolin increased the cell-surface expression of CFTR. However, when 4.5 μg of CAL was transfected, forskolin did not increase the cell-surface expression of CFTR. The total expression of CFTR was not altered by the forskolin treatment in all cases. Results are means ±SE. (n = 4) *$p<0.05$.

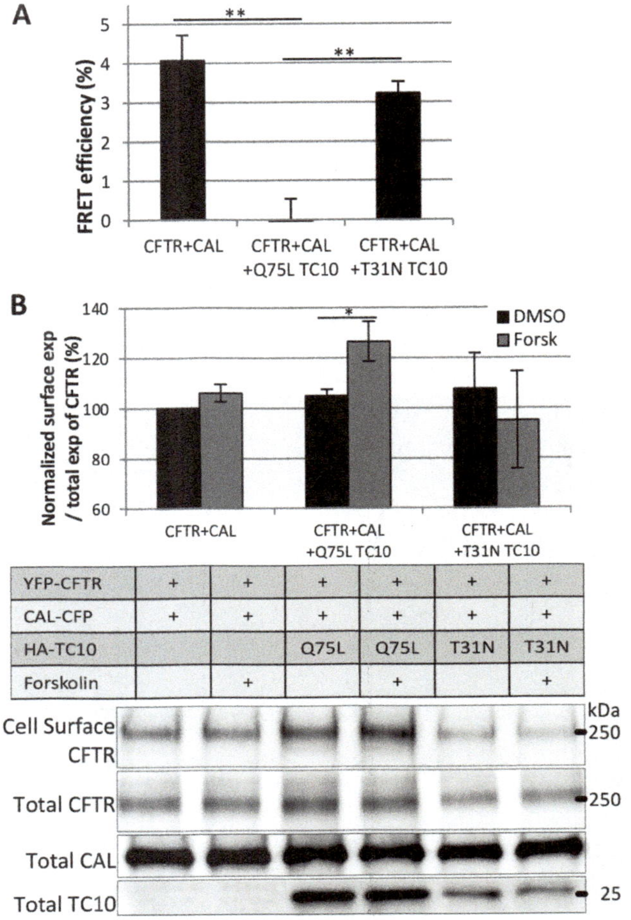

Figure 5. Active TC10 enhances CFTR expression at the cell surface, and this effect is impeded by highly overexpressed CAL HeLa cells were transfected with 1.5 μg of YFP-CFTR plus 0.5 μg (A) or 1.5 μg (B) of CAL-CFP expression vector without HA-TC10, with HA-Q75L TC10, or with HA-T31N TC10, as indicated. (A) The FRET efficiency of CAL and CFTR was reduced by a constitutively active mutant of TC10 (Q75L TC10) but not by a dominant-negative mutant, T31N TC10. (B) HeLa cells were treated with DMSO or 100 μM forskolin at 37°C for 30 minutes as described in the table. CFTR at the cell surface was biotinylated. The graph shows the ratio of cell surface-biontinylated CFTR to total CFTR, normalized by the ratio of the samples with YFP-CFTR and CAL-CFP treated with DMSO (%). Results are means ±SE. (In A, n = 7–13; B, n = 4) *$p<0.05$ and **$p<0.005$.

IGF-1 Increases the Expression of Rescued ΔF508 CFTR, but not ΔF508 CFTR

ΔF508 CFTR is misfolded and resides primarily in the ER [4]. Most of the misfolded ΔF508 CFTR is degraded by ER-associated degradation and does not proceed to the Golgi. However, incubating cells at the low temperature [35] or treating with correctors [36–39] allows ΔF508 CFTR to proceed to the Golgi and the cell surface. Because ΔF508 CFTR is only core-glycosylated in the ER, it is detected by western blotting as a lower molecular weight B band, which resides primarily in ER; rescued ΔF508 CFTR, in contrast, is detected as a B band and a higher molecular weight C band, which is the Golgi-processed glycoform. We therefore transfected HeLa cells and CFBE cells with YFP-tagged ΔF508 CFTR and then rescued ΔF508 by incubating the cells at 27°C for 2 days [35] (Fig. 8). ΔF508 CFTR in CFBE cells was also rescued by incubating the cells with a corrector, VRT-325, at 37°C for 2 days [36] (Fig. 8B). IGF-1 did not increase the expression of ΔF508 CFTR; however, it did increase the expression of the C band of rescued ΔF508 CFTR as well as the B band of rescued ΔF508 CFTR (Fig. 8).

Discussion

The question of how CAL regulates the trafficking of CFTR to the lysosome for degradation and, at the same time, to the cell surface remains unanswered. Where CAL molecules bind would be important information for understanding how CAL regulates CFTR. Our data have confirmed that CFTR and CAL are colocalized to the Golgi. We have also developed an acceptor photobleaching FRET assay to assess the binding of CAL and CFTR in the Golgi. Initially, we obtained FRET between CFTR labeled on the N-terminus with YFP and CAL labeled on the C-terminus with CFP and confirmed that the FRET assay showed the *in vivo* binding of CAL and CFTR. We then observed that when the normal structure of the Golgi was chemically disrupted, FRET was reduced, implying that the binding of CAL and CFTR was also disrupted and that the Golgi is required for their binding. When a decreased amount of CFTR was found in the Golgi after treatment with forskolin, which promotes the movement of CFTR from the Golgi to the cell surface, FRET between CAL and CFTR

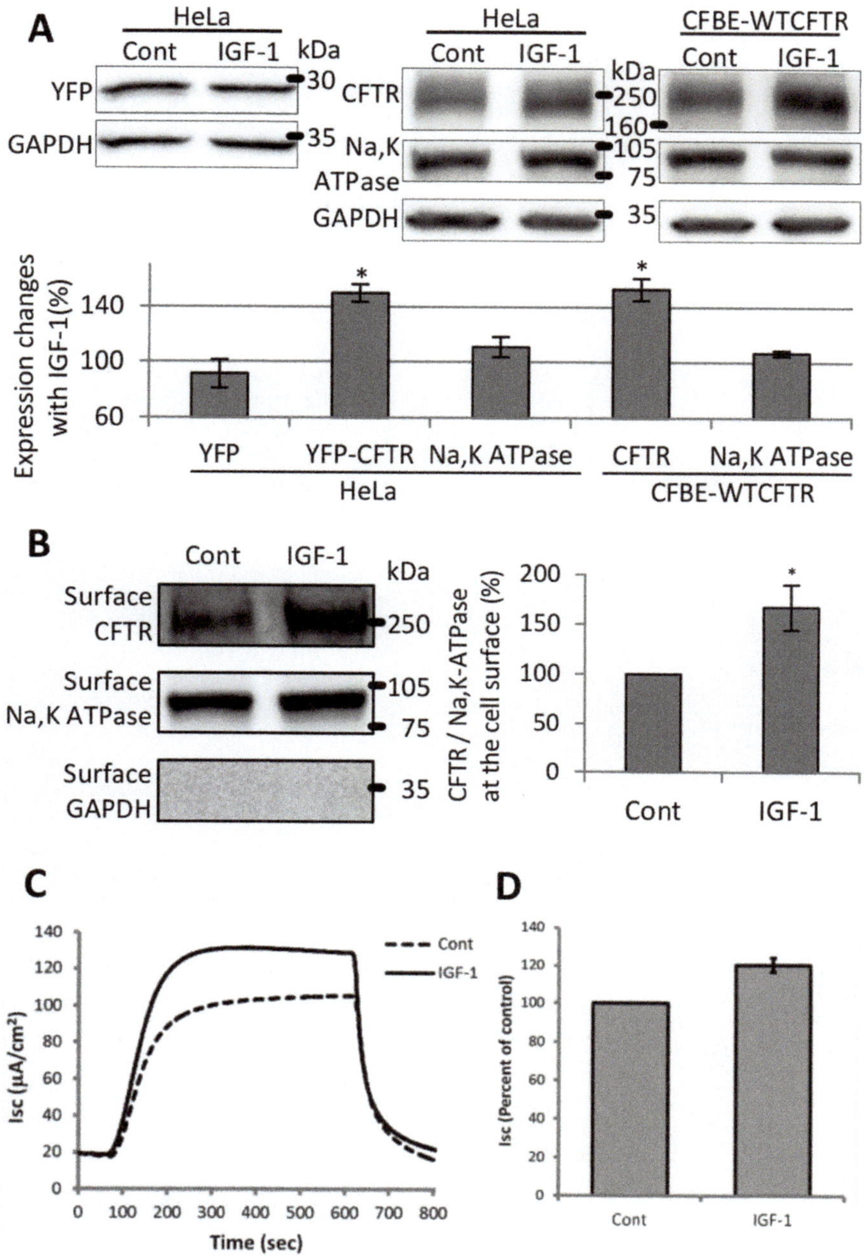

Figure 6. IGF-1 increases the protein expression level of CFTR and increases CFTR-mediated chloride transport in bronchial epithelial cells. (A) IGF-1 specifically increases the expression level of CFTR. HeLa cells were transfected with YFP or YFP-CFTR and incubated for one day, or confluent CFBE-WTCFTR cells were used. The graph in the right lower panel shows the expression of YFP, YFP-CFTR, CFTR, or Na,K-ATPase normalized by the GAPDH expression and normalized again by the corresponding control samples (%). (B) CFTR expression at the cell surface was increased by IGF-1 in HeLa cells. Proteins at the cell surface were cell surface-biotinylated. The graph in the right panel shows the expression of YFP-CFTR at the cell surface normalized by the Na,K-ATPase expression at the cell surface and normalized again by the corresponding control samples (%). (A,B) Cells were starved for 24 hours and then treated with 0.1 µg/ml IGF-1 for the next 24 hours. Results are means ±SE. (n = 3) (C) CFBE-WTCFTR cells grown on permeable supports were starved for 24 hours, then treated with 0.1 µg/ml IGF-1 for 24 hours. Cells were then mounted on the Ussing chamber setup, where short-circuit currents were measured as described in Materials and Methods. In the graph, 10 µM forskolin was added at the first arrow, and 5 µM CFTRinh-172 was added at the second arrow. (D) Ratio of I_{SC} between cells treated with 0.1 µg/ml IGF-1 (IGF-1) and untreated cells (Cont). Error bars represent SE. (n = 5). *p<0.05 and **p<0.005.

was also reduced. This finding supports the hypothesis that CAL binds CFTR and regulates the trafficking of CFTR at the Golgi.

Active TC10 has been shown to enhance CFTR expression [13], and we have found that it promotes the trafficking of CFTR to the cell surface, even in the presence of highly overexpressed CAL, suggesting that the role of TC10 is dominant over CAL. One possible mechanism to explain these findings is that active TC10 disrupts the binding of CAL to CFTR by proceeding with CFTR to the plasma membrane and leaving CAL behind in the Golgi. Alternatively, TC10 could alter the conformation of the CFTR-CAL complex, thereby increasing the distance between the fluorescent tags on the N-terminus of CFTR and on CAL that

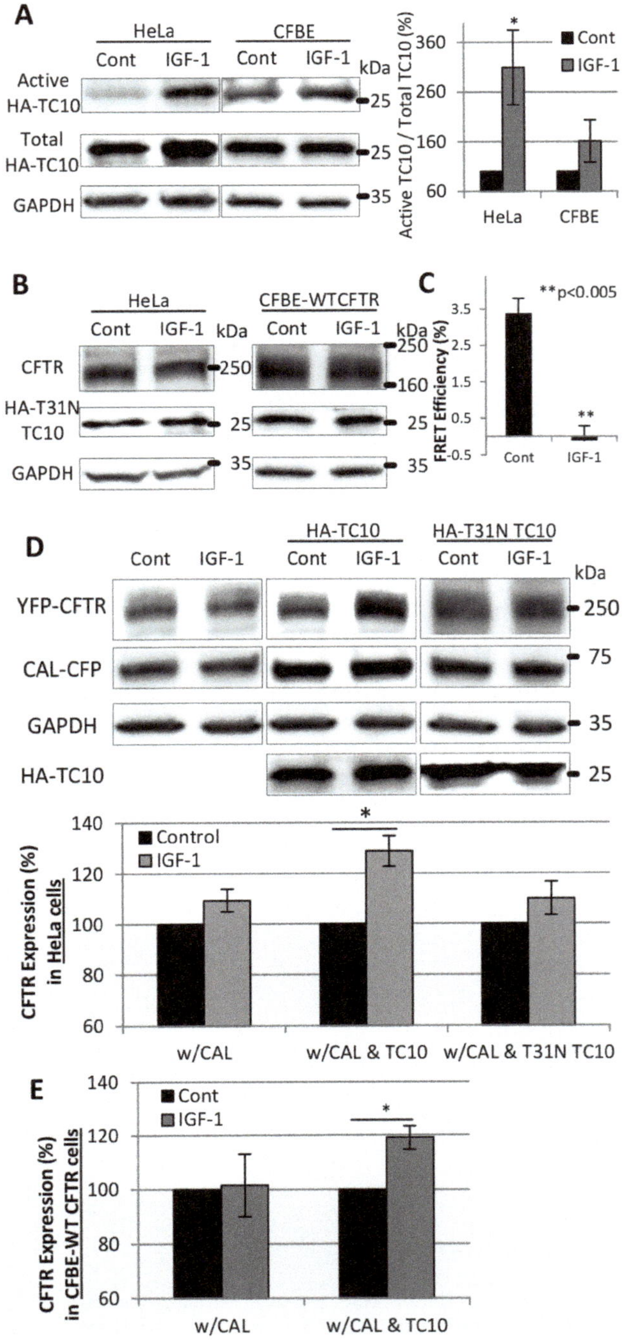

Figure 7. TC10 and CAL are involved in the IGF-1-mediated increase in CFTR expression level. (A) IGF-1 activates TC10. After HeLa cells or CFBE cells were transfected with HA-TC10, active TC10 was pulled down from the cell lysates with GST-PAK1 PBD peptide-conjugated beads. Total TC10 and GAPDH are from total cell lysates. The graph shows the amount of active TC10 normalized by the amount of total TC10 expression (%). (B) Dominant-negative TC10 (T31N TC10) inhibited the effects of IGF-1, increasing the CFTR expression. HeLa cells were cotransfected with YFP-CFTR and HA-T31N TC10, or CFBE-WTCFTR cells were transfected with HA-T31N TC10. Shown are representative images. (C) The FRET efficiency of CAL and CFTR was reduced by IGF-1. HeLa cells transfected with CAL and CFTR were starved for 4 hours and treated with 0.1 μg/ml IGF-1 for 30 minutes. (D,E) The CAL overexpression inhibited effects of IGF-1 increasing the CFTR expression, but the cotransfection with wildtype TC10 recovered the effects of IGF-1 on the CFTR expression in HeLa cells (D) and CFBE-WT CFTR cells (E). HeLa cells were transfected with YFP-CFTR and CAL-CFP without or with TC10 or T31N TC10. CFBE-WT CFTR cells were transfected with CAL-CFP without or with TC10. The CFTR expression level was normalized by the GAPDH expression level and normalized again by the corresponding control samples (%). (A,B,D,E) Cells were starved for 24 hours, and then 0.1 μg/ml IGF-1 was added for the next 24 hours. (A,C–E) Results are means ±SE. (n = 3) *$p<0.05$ and **$p<0.005$.

bind to the C-terminus of CFTR. This alteration in conformation would also reduce the FRET of CAL and CFTR by active TC10, while CAL still binds CFTR. Indeed, our lab has shown in a previous report by coimmunoprecipitation that CAL and CFTR remain associated following active TC10 overexpression [13]. TC10 is known to bind to the N-terminal coiled-coil domain of CAL and not to the PDZ domain where CFTR binds [17]; thus, it is not surprising that CAL can still bind CFTR in the presence of TC10. TC10, by inducing conformational changes, might move the whole CAL-CFTR complex away from the Golgi toward the plasma membrane, since our previous report showed that active TC10 relocates CAL toward the plasma membrane in COS7 cells [13]. At or near the plasma membrane, CFTR would competitively bind to NHERF, which has a higher affinity for the PDZ domain of CFTR than does CAL [40], and thereby enhance the CFTR expression at the plasma membrane by stabilizing CFTR [41].

TC10 has two known mechanisms for regulating membrane trafficking: It recruits excocyst complex proteins (e.g., Exo70, Sec6, and Sec8) to GLUT4 vesicles in adipocytes and to plasmalemmal precursor vesicles in neurons [21–23]. These complexes are involved in the exocytosis of membrane vesicles. Secondly, TC10 uses PI3K-dependent signaling by increasing phosphatidylinositol 3-phosphate (PI3P) [42–44]. The increased PI3P level induces exocytosis of membrane vesicles and raises the intriguing possibility that when present together in cells, GLUT4 and CFTR may traffic together to the plasma membrane in the same TC10 activated pathway. The current study proposes a novel, third mechanism for TC10 regulation whereby active TC10 alters the binding of a cargo molecule, CFTR, to an adaptor protein, CAL, and thereby enhances the trafficking of the cargo (i.e., CFTR) to the plasma membrane.

TC10 is located downstream of the IGF-1 receptor cascade [21–23]. We show here that IGF-1 activates TC10 and increases CFTR expression in CFBE and HeLa cells, but does not increase CFTR expression in the presence of the dominant-negative TC10. Furthermore, we have shown that IGF-1 increases CFTR expression by activating TC10. As we saw in the case of constitutively active TC10, IGF-1 alters the CFTR-CAL interaction and enhances CFTR expression.

In bronchial epithelial cells, adequate expression of the CFTR protein is required to prevent bacterial infection, which is the most common CF symptom [45,46]. The reports that bronchial epithelial cells express the IGF-1 receptor [47] and react to IGF-1 [48,49] suggest that these cells may have IGF-1 signaling. Our results also indicate that that IGF-1 selectively increases CFTR protein expression and CFTR-mediated chloride transport in a cell line model, CFBE cells (the bronchial epithelial cell line from cystic fibrosis patients). Therefore, our results raise the possibility that IGF-1 treatment could increase CFTR expression in vivo.

Serum IGF-1 levels vary physiologically and pathologically in individuals in response to aging, caloric uptake, injury, and other conditions, and they regulate IGF-1 signaling, causing mitogenic effects such as cell proliferation, tissue regeneration, and body growth [50–53]. According to our present results, changes in the level of IGF-1 would be expected to alter CFTR protein expression. CAL also binds other plasma membrane proteins

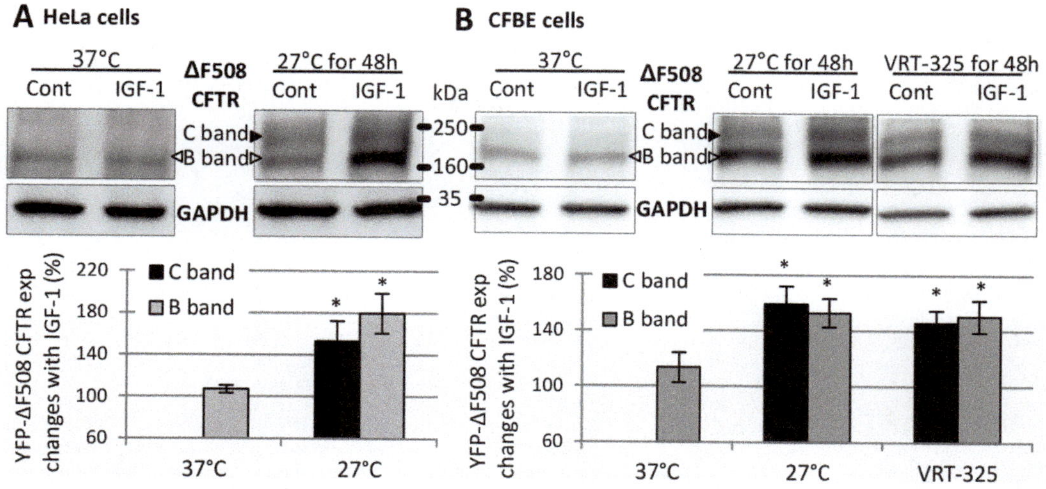

Figure 8. IGF-1 increases the expression level of rescued ΔF508 CFTR but not unrescued ΔF508 CFTR. HeLa cells (A) and CFBE cells (B) were transfected with YFP-ΔF508 CFTR, and after 1 day, plates of both cell lines were incubated at 37°C or at 27°C for 2 days; additional plates of CFBE cells were incubated with 5 μM VRT-325 at 37°C for 2 days. At the same time, 1 day after the transfection, these cells were serum-starved, and on next day, 0.1 μg/ml IGF-1 was added for 1 day. The expression level of ΔF508 CFTR in the cell lysates was assessed by western blotting. When unrescued (incubated at 37°C), ΔF508 CFTR showed one band (the B band), but when rescued (incubated at 27°C or with VRT-325 at 37°C), it showed two bands (B and C). IGF-1 did not increase the expression level of unrescued ΔF508 CFTR but did increase the expression level of rescued ΔF508 CFTR. The ΔF508 CFTR expression level was normalized by the GAPDH expression level, and the ΔF508 CFTR expression change as a result of IGF-1 treatment was then calculated by normalizing again with the non-treated control samples (%). Results are means ±SE. (n = 6 for HeLa at 27°C and CFBE at 37°C, n = 3 for all the others) *$p<0.05$.

such as the β1-adrenergic receptor, ClC-3B, somatostatin receptor subtype 5, and cadherin 23, and enhances their lysosomal degradation [54–57]. If TC10 also regulates the CAL-dependent degradation of these proteins, IGF-1 could also post-translationally regulate the expression levels of these plasma membrane proteins. IGF-1 levels are low in the serum of CF patients and the CF pig model [26,27]; therefore, IGF-1 has been studied and used in a clinical trial to reverse growth retardation in CF patients [25,58].

ΔF508 CFTR, the most common CF mutation, is degraded by ER-associated degradation and does not reach the Golgi or plasma membrane [59]. Our results show that IGF-1 does not change the expression level of ΔF508 CFTR, consistent with our proposal that IGF-1 alters the binding of CAL to CFTR at the Golgi, since almost all of ΔF508 CFTR is sequestered in the ER and does not proceed to the Golgi [60]. However, IGF-1 does increase the expression of rescued ΔF508 CFTR, because when ΔF508 CFTR is rescued by correctors or low temperature, it moves out of the ER to the Golgi and the cell surface [35,38,61]. Interestingly, IGF-1 does not increase the intensity of un-rescued ΔF508 CFTR band B, whose N-glycosylation is initiated in the ER but not finalized in the Golgi; however, it does increase its intensity when ΔF508 CFTR is corrected by low temperature or VRT-325. These data suggest that the rescued immature B band of ΔF508 CFTR may in some instances exit the ER through an unconventional trafficking pathway, perhaps enhanced by TC10 acting through IGF-1, and reach the plasma membrane in an immature form [62]. However, more work is needed to establish this effect conclusively. Correctors have been developed and are currently in clinical trials [37,38]. Thus, it is possible that an additive treatment combining IGF-1 with a corrector would be more effective for cystic fibrosis than a corrector alone.

Acknowledgments

We thank Dr. B. Cha for assistance with setting up the FRET assay and Dr. Deborah McClellan for editorial assistance.

Author Contributions

Conceived and designed the experiments: HWL OK MD WG. Performed the experiments: HWL JC. Analyzed the data: HWL WBG. Contributed reagents/materials/analysis tools: OK. Wrote the paper: HWL WBG.

References

1. Riordan JR, Rommens JM, Kerem B, Alon N, Rozmahel R, et al. (1989) Identification of the cystic fibrosis gene: cloning and characterization of complementary DNA. Science 245: 1066–1073.
2. Rowe SM, Miller S, Sorscher EJ (2005) Cystic Fibrosis. New England Journal of Medicine 352: 1992–2001.
3. Gibson LE, Cooke RE (1959) A test for concentration of electrolytes in sweat in cystic fibrosis of the pancreas utilizing pilocarpine by iontophoresis. Pediatrics 23: 545–549.
4. Cheng SH, Gregory RJ, Marshall J, Paul S, Souza DW, et al. (1990) Defective intracellular transport and processing of CFTR is the molecular basis of most cystic fibrosis. Cell 63: 827–834.
5. Kerem BS, Buchanan JA, Durie P, Corey ML, Levison H, et al. (1989) DNA marker haplotype association with pancreatic sufficiency in cystic fibrosis. Am J Hum Genet 44: 827–834.
6. Bertrand CA, Frizzell RA (2003) The role of regulated CFTR trafficking in epithelial secretion. Am J Physiol Cell Physiol 285: C1–18.
7. Cheng J, Moyer BD, Milewski M, Loffing J, Ikeda M, et al. (2002) A Golgi-associated PDZ Domain Protein Modulates Cystic Fibrosis Transmembrane Regulator Plasma Membrane Expression. Journal of Biological Chemistry 277: 3520–3529.
8. Wang S, Yue H, Derin RB, Guggino WB, Li M (2000) Accessory Protein Facilitated CFTR-CFTR Interaction, a Molecular Mechanism to Potentiate the Chloride Channel Activity. Cell 103: 169–179.
9. Gee Heon Y, Noh Shin H, Tang Bor L, Kim Kyung H, Lee Min G (2011) Rescue of ΔF508-CFTR Trafficking via a GRASP-Dependent Unconventional Secretion Pathway. Cell 146: 746–760.
10. Sun F, Hug MJ, Lewarchik CM, Yun CHC, Bradbury NA, et al. (2000) E3KARP Mediates the Association of Ezrin and Protein Kinase A with the

Cystic Fibrosis Transmembrane Conductance Regulator in Airway Cells. Journal of Biological Chemistry 275: 29539–29546.
11. Guggino WB, Stanton BA (2006) New insights into cystic fibrosis: molecular switches that regulate CFTR. Nat Rev Mol Cell Biol 7: 426–436.
12. Shorter J, Watson R, Giannakou ME, Clarke M, Warren G, et al. (1999) GRASP55, a second mammalian GRASP protein involved in the stacking of Golgi cisternae in a cell-free system. EMBO J 18: 4949–4960.
13. Cheng J, Wang H, Guggino WB (2005) Regulation of cystic fibrosis transmembrane regulator trafficking and protein expression by a Rho family small GTPase TC10. J Biol Chem 280: 3731–3739.
14. Moyer BD, Duhaime M, Shaw C, Denton J, Reynolds D, et al. (2000) The PDZ-interacting Domain of Cystic Fibrosis Transmembrane Conductance Regulator Is Required for Functional Expression in the Apical Plasma Membrane. Journal of Biological Chemistry 275: 27069–27074.
15. Bezprozvanny I, Maximov A (2001) PDZ domains: More than just a glue. Proceedings of the National Academy of Sciences 98: 787–789.
16. Cheng J, Cebotaru V, Cebotaru L, Guggino WB (2010) Syntaxin 6 and CAL Mediate the Degradation of the Cystic Fibrosis Transmembrane Conductance Regulator. Mol Biol Cell 21: 1178–1187.
17. Neudauer CL, Joberty G, Macara IG (2001) PIST: A Novel PDZ/Coiled-Coil Domain Binding Partner for the Rho-Family GTPase TC10. Biochemical and Biophysical Research Communications 280: 541–547.
18. Charest A, Lane K, McMahon K, Housman DE (2001) Association of a Novel PDZ Domain-containing Peripheral Golgi Protein with the Q-SNARE (Q-solubleN-Ethylmaleimide-sensitive Fusion Protein (NSF) Attachment Protein Receptor) Protein Syntaxin 6. Journal of Biological Chemistry 276: 29456–29465.
19. Kuliawat R, Kalinina E, Bock J, Fricker L, McGraw TE, et al. (2004) Syntaxin-6 SNARE Involvement in Secretory and Endocytic Pathways of Cultured Pancreatic {beta}-Cells. Mol Biol Cell 15: 1690–1701.
20. Chiang SH, Baumann CA, Kanzaki M, Thurmond DC, Watson RT, et al. (2001) Insulin-stimulated GLUT4 translocation requires the CAP-dependent activation of TC10. Nature 410: 944–948.
21. Dupraz S, Grassi D, Bernis ME, Sosa L, Bisbal M, et al. (2009) The TC10-Exo70 complex is essential for membrane expansion and axonal specification in developing neurons. J Neurosci 29: 13292–13301.
22. Inoue M, Chang L, Hwang J, Chiang SH, Saltiel AR (2003) The exocyst complex is required for targeting of Glut4 to the plasma membrane by insulin. Nature 422: 629–633.
23. Inoue M, Chiang SH, Chang L, Chen XW, Saltiel AR (2006) Compartmentalization of the Exocyst Complex in Lipid Rafts Controls Glut4 Vesicle Tethering. Molecular Biology of the Cell 17: 2303–2311.
24. Taylor AM, Bush A, Thomson A, Oades PJ, Marchant JL, et al. (1997) Relation between insulin-like growth factor-I, body mass index, and clinical status in cystic fibrosis. Archives of Disease in Childhood 76: 304–309.
25. Taylor AM, Thomson A, Bruce-Morgan C, Ahmed ML, Watts A, et al. (1999) The relationship between insulin, IGF-I and weight gain in cystic fibrosis. Clinical Endocrinology 51: 659–665.
26. Hardin DS, Ferkol T, Ahn C, Dreimane D, Dyson M, et al. (2005) A retrospective study of growth hormone use in adolescents with cystic fibrosis. Clinical Endocrinology 62: 560–566.
27. Rogan MP, Reznikov LR, Pezzulo AA, Gansemer ND, Samuel M, et al. (2010) Pigs and humans with cystic fibrosis have reduced insulin-like growth factor 1 (IGF1) levels at birth. Proceedings of the National Academy of Sciences 107: 20571–20575.
28. Moyer BD, Loffing J, Schwiebert EM, Loffing-Cueni D, Halpin PA, et al. (1998) Membrane Trafficking of the Cystic Fibrosis Gene Product, Cystic Fibrosis Transmembrane Conductance Regulator, Tagged with Green Fluorescent Protein in Madin-Darby Canine Kidney Cells. Journal of Biological Chemistry 273: 21759–21768.
29. Bruscia E, Sangiuolo F, Sinibaldi P, Goncz KK, Novelli G, et al. (2002) Isolation of CF cell lines corrected at DeltaF508-CFTR locus by SFHR-mediated targeting. Gene Ther 9: 683–685.
30. Illek B, Maurisse R, Wahler L, Kunzelmann K, Fischer H, et al. (2008) Cl transport in complemented CF bronchial epithelial cells correlates with CFTR mRNA expression levels. Cell Physiol Biochem 22: 57–68.
31. Taylor SJ, Shalloway D (1996) Cell cycle-dependent activation of Ras. Current Biology 6: 1621–1627.
32. Benard V, Bohl BP, Bokoch GM (1999) Characterization of Rac and Cdc42 Activation in Chemoattractant-stimulated Human Neutrophils Using a Novel Assay for Active GTPases. Journal of Biological Chemistry 274: 13198–13204.
33. Bradbury N, Jilling T, Berta G, Sorscher E, Bridges R, et al. (1992) Regulation of plasma membrane recycling by CFTR. Science 256: 530–532.
34. Denning GM, Ostedgaard LS, Cheng SH, Smith AE, Welsh MJ (1992) Localization of cystic fibrosis transmembrane conductance regulator in chloride secretory epithelia. J Clin Invest 89: 339–349.
35. Denning GM, Anderson MP, Amara JF, Marshall J, Smith AE, et al. (1992) Processing of mutant cystic fibrosis transmembrane conductance regulator is temperature-sensitive. Nature 358: 761–764.
36. Yu GJ, Yoo CL, Yang B, Lodewyk MW, Meng L, et al. (2008) Potent s-cis-Locked Bithiazole Correctors of ΔF508 Cystic Fibrosis Transmembrane Conductance Regulator Cellular Processing for Cystic Fibrosis Therapy. Journal of Medicinal Chemistry 51: 6044–6054.
37. Van Goor F, Hadida S, Grootenhuis PD, Burton B, Stack J, et al. (2009) VX-809, a CFTR corrector, increases the cell surface density of functional F508del-CFTR in pre-clinical models of cystic fibrosis. Pediatric Pulmonology 44: 154–155.
38. Van Goor F, Hadida S, Grootenhuis PDJ, Burton B, Stack JH, et al. (2011) Correction of the F508del-CFTR protein processing defect in vitro by the investigational drug VX-809. Proceedings of the National Academy of Sciences 108: 18843–18848.
39. Pedemonte N, Lukacs GL, Du K, Caci E, Zegarra-Moran O, et al. (2005) Small-molecule correctors of defective Î”F508-CFTR cellular processing identified by high-throughput screening. The Journal of Clinical Investigation 115: 2564–2571.
40. Cushing PR, Fellows A, Villone D, Boisguérin P, Madden DR (2008) The Relative Binding Affinities of PDZ Partners for CFTR: A Biochemical Basis for Efficient Endocytic Recycling. Biochemistry 47: 10084–10098.
41. Moyer BD, Denton J, Karlson KH, Reynolds D, Wang S, et al. (1999) A PDZ-interacting domain in CFTR is an apical membrane polarization signal. The Journal of Clinical Investigation 104: 1353–1361.
42. Maffucci T, Brancaccio A, Piccolo E, Stein RC, Falasca M (2003) Insulin induces phosphatidylinositol-3-phosphate formation through TC10 activation. EMBO J 22: 4178–4189.
43. Lodhi IJ, Bridges D, Chiang SH, Zhang Y, Cheng A, et al. (2008) Insulin Stimulates Phosphatidylinositol 3-Phosphate Production via the Activation of Rab5. Molecular Biology of the Cell 19: 2718–2728.
44. Kelly KL, Ruderman NB (1993) Insulin-stimulated phosphatidylinositol 3-kinase. Association with a 185-kDa tyrosine-phosphorylated protein (IRS-1) and localization in a low density membrane vesicle. Journal of Biological Chemistry 268: 4391–4398.
45. Guggino WB (1999) Cystic Fibrosis and the Salt Controversy. Cell 96: 607–610.
46. Vij N, Mazur S, Zeitlin PL (2009) CFTR Is a Negative Regulator of NFκB Mediated Innate Immune Response. PLoS ONE 4: e4664.
47. Kim WY, Jin Q, Oh SH, Kim ES, Yang YJ, et al. (2009) Elevated Epithelial Insulin-like Growth Factor Expression Is a Risk Factor for Lung Cancer Development. Cancer Research 69: 7439–7448.
48. Siegfried JM, Kasprzyk PG, Treston AM, Mulshine JL, Quinn KA, et al. (1992) A mitogenic peptide amide encoded within the E peptide domain of the insulin-like growth factor IB prohormone. Proceedings of the National Academy of Sciences 89: 8107–8111.
49. Shoji S, Ertl RF, Linder J, Koizumi SI, Duckworth WC, et al. (1990) Bronchial Epithelial Cells Respond to Insulin and Insulin-like Growth Factor-I as a Chemoattractant. Am J Respir Cell Mol Biol 2: 553–557.
50. Thissen JP, Ketelslegers JM, Underwood LE (1994) Nutritional Regulation of the Insulin-Like Growth Factors. Endocrine Reviews 15: 80–101.
51. Corpas E, Harman SM, Blackman MR (1993) Human Growth Hormone and Human Aging. Endocrine Reviews 14: 20–39.
52. Florini JR, Ewton DZ, Coolican SA (1996) Growth Hormone and the Insulin-Like Growth Factor System in Myogenesis. Endocrine Reviews 17: 481–517.
53. Le Roith D, Bondy C, Yakar S, Liu JL, Butler A (2001) The Somatomedin Hypothesis: 2001. Endocrine Reviews 22: 53–74.
54. He J, Bellini M, Xu J, Castleberry AM, Hall RA (2004) Interaction with Cystic Fibrosis Transmembrane Conductance Regulator-associated Ligand (CAL) Inhibits β1-Adrenergic Receptor Surface Expression. Journal of Biological Chemistry 279: 50190–50196.
55. Gentzsch M, Cui L, Mengos A, Chang XB, Chen JH, et al. (2003) The PDZ-binding Chloride Channel ClC-3B Localizes to the Golgi and Associates with Cystic Fibrosis Transmembrane Conductance Regulator-interacting PDZ Proteins. Journal of Biological Chemistry 278: 6440–6449.
56. Wente W, Stroh T, Beaudet A, Richter D, Kreienkamp Jr H (2005) Interactions with PDZ Domain Proteins PIST/GOPC and PDZK1 Regulate Intracellular Sorting of the Somatostatin Receptor Subtype 5. Journal of Biological Chemistry 280: 32419–32425.
57. Xu Z, Oshima K, Heller S (2010) PIST regulates the intracellular trafficking and plasma membrane expression of Cadherin 23. BMC Cell Biology 11: 80.
58. Bucuvalas JC, Chernausek SD, Alfaro MP, Krug SK, Ritschel W, et al. (2001) Effect of Insulinlike Growth Factor-1 Treatment in Children With Cystic Fibrosis. Journal of Pediatric Gastroenterology and Nutrition 33: 576–581.
59. Jensen TJ, Loo MA, Pind S, Williams DB, Goldberg AL, et al. (1995) Multiple proteolytic systems, including the proteasome, contribute to CFTR processing. Cell 83: 129–135.
60. McKone EF, Emerson SS, Edwards KL, Aitken ML (2003) Effect of genotype on phenotype and mortality in cystic fibrosis: a retrospective cohort study. The Lancet 361: 1671–1676.
61. Loo TW, Bartlett MC, Clarke DM (2005) Rescue of ΔF508 and Other Misprocessed CFTR Mutants by a Novel Quinazoline Compound. Molecular Pharmaceutics 2: 407–413.
62. Luo Y, McDonald K, Hanrahan JW (2009) Trafficking of immature DeltaF508-CFTR to the plasma membrane and its detection by biotinylation. Biochem J 419: 211–219.

Impact of Osteopathic Treatment on Pain in Adult Patients with Cystic Fibrosis – A Pilot Randomized Controlled Study

Dominique Hubert[1,2]*, Lucile Soubeiran[3], Fabrice Gourmelon[3], Dominique Grenet[4], Raphaël Serreau[3], Elodie Perrodeau[5], Rafael Zegarra-Parodi[6], Isabelle Boutron[5,2]

1 Adult CF Center and Pulmonology Department, Hôpital Cochin APHP, Paris, France, **2** Université Paris Descartes, Sorbonne Paris Cité, Paris, France, **3** Clinical Research Department, Hôpital Cochin APHP, Paris, France, **4** Adult CF Center and Pulmonology Department, Hôpital Foch, Suresnes, France, **5** Clinical Epidemiology Center, Hôpital Hôtel Dieu APHP, Paris, France, **6** A.T. Still Research Institute, A.T. Still University, Kirksville, Missouri, United States of America

Abstract

Background: Pain is a common complication in patients with cystic fibrosis (CF) and is associated with shorter survival. We evaluated the impact of osteopathic manipulative treatment (OMT) on pain in adults with CF.

Methods: A pilot multicenter randomized controlled trial was conducted with three parallel arms: OMT (group A, 16 patients), sham OMT (sham treatment, group B, 8 patients) and no treatment (group C, 8 patients). Medical investigators and patients were double-blind to treatment for groups A and B, who received OMT or sham OMT monthly for 6 months. Pain was rated as a composite of its intensity and duration over the previous month. The evolution of chest/back pain after 6 months was compared between group A and groups B+C combined (control group). The evolution of cervical pain, headache and quality of life (QOL) were similarly evaluated.

Results: There was no statistically significant difference between the treatment and control groups in the decrease of chest/back pain (difference = −2.20 IC95% [−4.81; 0.42], p = 0.098); also, group A did not differ from group B. However, chest/back pain decreased more in groups A (p = 0.002) and B (p = 0.006) than in group C. Cervical pain, headache and QOL scores did not differ between the treatment and control groups.

Conclusion: This pilot study demonstrated the feasibility of evaluating the efficacy of OMT to treat the pain of patients with CF. The lack of difference between the group treated with OMT and the control group may be due to the small number of patients included in this trial, which also precludes any definitive conclusion about the greater decrease of pain in patients receiving OMT or sham OMT than in those with no intervention.

Trial Registration: ClinicalTrials.gov NCT01293019

Editor: D. William Cameron, University of Ottawa, Canada

Funding: This work was supported by Vaincre la Mucoviscidose and Fondation de France, Paris, France, who had no role in the design of the study, the collection or analysis of the data, or the preparation of the manuscript.

Competing Interests: Another author, Rafael Zegarra-Parodi is an osteopathic practitioner in Paris and works in a private practice: Cabinet Victor Hugo, 7 rue Georges Ville, 75116 Paris (France), without any conflict of interest with this article. He is also a Research Assistant Professor, A.T. Still Research Institute, Kirksville, MO (USA) http://www.atsu.edu/kcom/faculty_staff bios/Zegarra-Parodi-R-Bio.htm, and the authors now give this affiliation for the present publication.

* Email: dominique.hubert@cch.aphp.fr

Introduction

Cystic Fibrosis (CF) is an inherited multi systemic autosomal recessive disease with high morbidity and mortality, involving primarily the lungs and gastrointestinal tract [1]. The daily routine of a CF patient generally requires long-term home care, including oral and inhaled antibiotics, pancreatic enzyme replacement, mucolytic agents, vitamin supplements, and daily physiotherapy. In addition, these patients often require home or in-hospital intravenous antibiotic therapy during pulmonary exacerbations. Significant advances in the management of respiratory infection and pancreatic insufficiency, coupled with better quality of care by specialist multidisciplinary teams, have resulted in a significant improvement in the median survival age, which approaches 40 years [2–3]. Until recently, the majority of patients with CF were paediatric. Today, many reach adulthood and, in many countries there are now as many adults as children, if not more [2–3]. Consequently, greater attention is being paid to patients' quality of life (QOL). CF patients frequently complain of pain, mainly back pain, chest pain and headache [4–11]. Although pain in adults with CF is associated with lower QOL [5–6,11], increased risk of exacerbation [6] and decreased survival [6,12], it is often neglected by the treating physicians [5,8]. In addition to drug treatment,

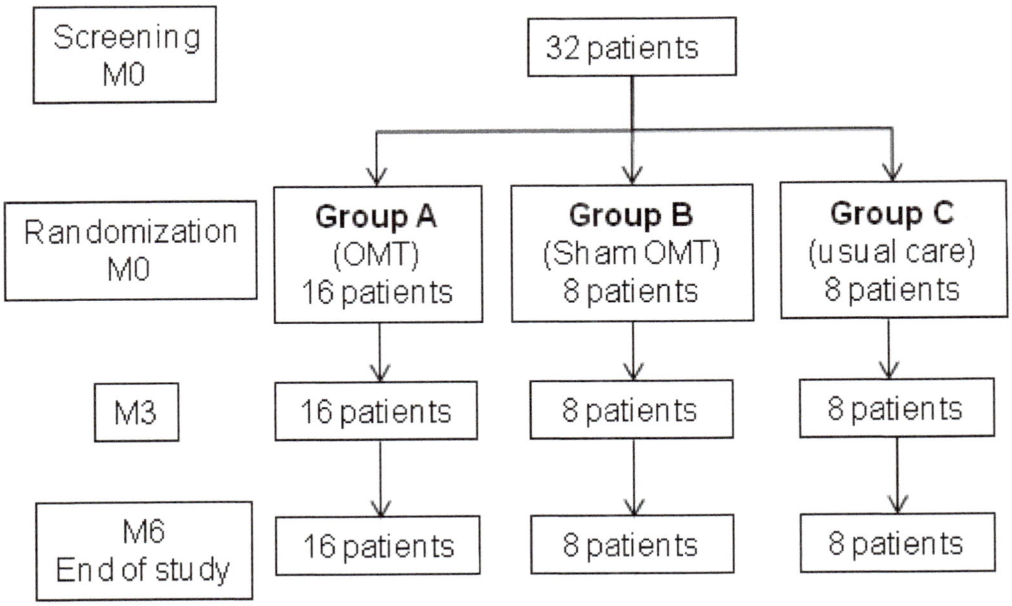

Figure 1. Flow chart.

many patients with CF use non-drug treatments and complementary and alternative medicine (CAM) [5–6,8,13–15] including osteopathic manipulative treatment (OMT). However, this type of treatment has never been evaluated in CF.

The aim of this pilot study was to demonstrate the feasibility of evaluating the efficacy of OMT to treat the pain of adult patients with CF.

Materials and Methods

The protocol for this trial and supporting CONSORT checklist are available as supporting information; see Checklist S1 and Protocol S1.

Ethic Statement

The study was approved by our Institutional Review Committee (Comité de Protection des Personnes "Ile de France II" # 2009-A00359-48) and all subjects provided written informed consent. The study was registered at ClinicalTrials.gov #NCT01293019 on February 9, 2011 (http://clinicaltrials.gov/ct2/show/NCT01293019). The delay in registering the study was due to a change in the statistician responsible for the study. The authors confirm that all ongoing and related trials for this intervention are registered.

Study Design

This pilot study was a three-arm, parallel group, randomized controlled trial.

Setting and Participants

The study was carried out in two adult CF centers: Cochin University Hospital, Paris, France; and Foch Hospital, Suresnes, France.

The inclusion criteria were age 18 or older, diagnosis of CF (positive sweat test and/or two CFTR disease-causing mutations) and cervical, back or chest pain, rated 2 or higher on a 10-point visual analog scale (VAS) [16] or requiring painkillers during the previous month. The exclusion criteria were treatment with OMT or other forms of spinal manipulation in the past three months, pregnancy, lung transplantation, being on a waiting list for lung transplantation, and participation in another clinical trial.

Randomization and Treatment

The patients were randomly assigned to one of the three groups: OMT (experimental treatment) for 16 patients (group A), sham OMT (sham treatment) for 8 patients (group B) and no additional treatment (usual care) for 8 patients (group C). Randomization was performed according to a computer-generated list with blocks of fixed size, stratified by center. In each block of four, there were two arms A, one arm B and one arm C. The list was prepared and maintained by an independent statistician at an independent clinical trial unit. The investigators did not have access to the randomization list, and allocation was concealed through an internet-based system.

For cases receiving experimental treatment or sham OMT, medical investigators, patients and outcome assessors were blinded, and only the osteopathic practitioner knew the allocation to the treatment arm. However, blinding was not feasible for cases receiving usual care without OMT.

Intervention and Comparator

The experimental treatment was OMT. The intervention consisted of six monthly sessions of OMT. All OMT was provided by a single osteopathic practitioner (LS) trained according to international standards [17] and who had four years of experience in treating CF patients.

A standardized treatment plan for diagnosed somatic dysfunction was used [18–20]. Each osteopathic visit lasted 1 hour and consisted of three periods for both groups: (1) interview focusing on pain location, (2) full osteopathic examination [21] (Table S1), (3) intervention consisting of either OMT or light touch sham OMT according to the randomization arm (Table S2, Table S3, Table S4). (See the supplementary Methods section for more details).

The control group was divided into two groups. One group was treated according to usual care and received no OMT. Patients in the sham OMT group received light touch at the skull and at the

Table 1. Baseline characteristics of the study participants.

Characteristics	Osteopathic treatment (Group A) N=16	Sham and usual care (Groups B+C) N=16
Age (yr) – mean ± SD	31±6	37±11
Sex		
Male – n (%)	1 (6.2)	5 (31.2)
Female – n (%)	15 (93.8)	11 (68.8)
FEV1 (% pred) - mean ± SD	53.9±22.6	46.8±18.7
BMI (kg/m²) -mean ± SD	21.6±3.8	22.1±4.0
Chest/Back pain - med, [Q1;Q3]		
VAS (range 0–10)	5.5 [5;7]	5.0 [4;7]
Days in the previous month (range 0–30)	30 [24.2;30]	30 [30;30]
Composite outcome(range 0–10)	7.5 [6.2;8.1]	7.5 [6.9;8.1]
Neck/Trapezius pain - med, [Q1;Q3]		
VAS (range 0–10)	1.5 [0;5]	3.0 [0;5]
Days in the previous month (range 0–30)	2 [0;27]	30 [0;30]
Composite outcome(range 0–10)	1.8 [0;6.6]	6.5 [0;7.5]
Headache - med, [Q1;Q3]		
VAS (range 0–10)	3.0 [0;5.2]	0 [0;4.2]
Days in the previous month (range 0–30)	1.5 [0;30]	0 [0;3]
Composite outcome(range 0–10)	2.5 [0;7.1]	0 [0;1.2]
QOL scores - med, [Q1;Q3] (range 0–100)		
Physical functioning	50 [32;56.2]	40 [21;57.2]
Energy/well-being	50 [23;58]	37.5 [25;52]
Body image	67 [56;78]	67 [44;78]
Respiratory symptoms	52 [51;63.2]	55 [32;76]

sacrum, a sham osteopathic procedure used in previous trials [22–23], to ensure that manual contact time was similar in the experimental and sham OMT groups.

Outcomes

The primary efficacy endpoint was a composite outcome reflecting the intensity of pain and the number of painful days over the previous month evaluated after 6 months. For each patient, we calculated the mean value of the two following variables: (1) chest and back pain over the previous month (VAS from 0 to 10) [15] and (2) [the number of days with chest and back pain in the previous month/number of days in the previous month] ×10 (thus a score from 0 to 10).

Secondary endpoints included:

- Pain involving the neck and trapezius at 6 months evaluated as the mean value of: neck and trapezius pain over the previous month (VAS from 0 to 10) and [the number of days with neck and trapezius pain in the previous month/number of days in the previous month]×10 (score from 0 to 10).
- Headache at 6 months evaluated as the mean value of: headache over the previous month (VAS from 0 to 10) and [the number of days with headache in the previous month/number of days in the previous month]×10 (score from 0 to 10).
- QOL scores at 6 months with validated French-language versions of the questionnaire (Cystic Fibrosis Questionnaire (CFQ) 14+) [24]. Four domains were studied: physical functioning; energy/well-being; body image; and respiratory symptoms.
- The need for analgesics.

At the end of the study, all patients completed a questionnaire to collect data about their interest in the study and their satisfaction with the treatment received.

Data Collection

At the base-line visit, we collected demographic data and information about the characteristics of the patient's CF, including respiratory function evaluated by measuring forced expiratory volume in one second (FEV1), and nutritional status evaluated with the body mass index (BMI). All patients were evaluated at the base-line visit (M0), after 3 months (M3) and after 6 months (M6) at the end of the study. Upon entry into the study, the participants were given a diary in which they recorded their pain symptoms(location and intensity) daily at baseline and during the trial; this diary was kept at home and brought for each study visit, and returned to the investigators at the end of the study. The CF physicians (DH or DG) checked the patient's diary and recorded the patient's pain after the patient had self-reported his pain on a VAS (mean value and number of painful days in the previous month), collected the CFQ 14+, listed concomitant treatment including analgesics, and adverse events. The osteopathic practitioner (LS) performed osteopathic tests for all patients.

Sample Size

We planned to include 32 subjects (16 in the OMT group, 8 in the sham OMT group and 8 in the usual care group). Because this study was a pilot study in a rare disease, there was no formal

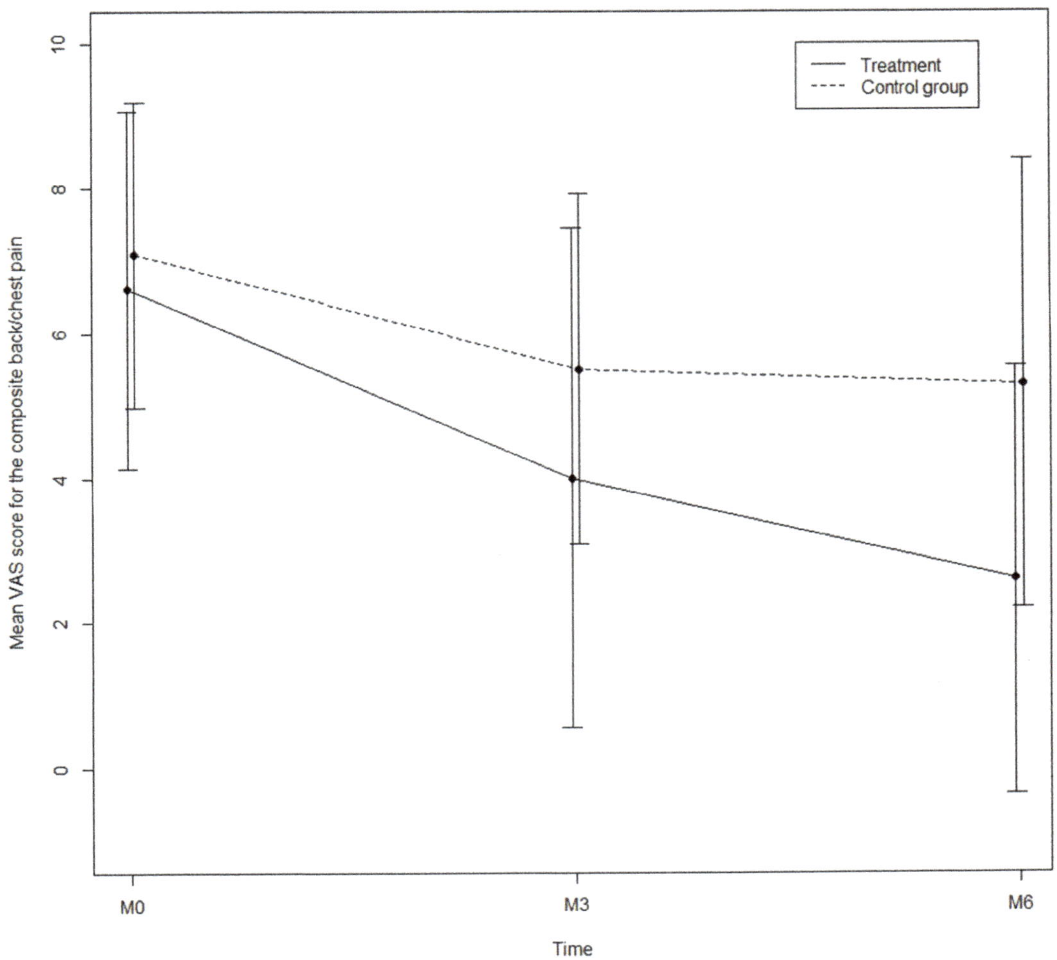

Figure 2. Composite chest/back pain at inclusion (M0), after 3 months (M3) and at the end of the study (M6) in the OMT group (A) and control group (B+C). VAS: visual analog scale.

calculation of sample size; nevertheless, this sample was expected to be sufficient to identify a difference of one standard deviation between the mean VAS for pain in the OMT group versus the two other groups with $1-\beta=80\%$ and $\alpha=5\%$.

Statistical Analyses

All randomized patients were analyzed in their allocated group whatever the treatment received.

Baseline data are described using means and standard deviations (SD) for quantitative variables, and medians and interquartile ranges (IQR) for variables with asymmetric distributions. For qualitative variables, frequencies and percentages were computed.

Primary comparisons were between the OMT group (group A) and the sham OMT group+no additional treatment group pooled (group B+C).

The difference for the primary outcome between the two groups was evaluated at 6 months using a linear mixed longitudinal model estimating the difference in change from baseline between the 2 groups (coefficient for time × group interaction) and taking into account the correlation for data of a same patient (random effect). This difference was tested using the Student's *t*-test at a 5% level in order to test the non nullity of the coefficient of interest in the model.

Pairwise comparisons between all three groups were also performed at a 1.67% level to take into account the multiplicity induced by these three comparisons. To check consistency with the parametric analysis, Wilcoxon's tests with significance set at 5% were used for a non-parametric comparison of the difference between the two groups in the distribution of changes from baseline to month 6.

Final composite outcomes (M6) for neck and trapezius pain, headache and QOL scores were analyzed with the same strategy as the primary outcome.

The need for analgesics was analyzed using a mixed logistic regression model with a random intercept at the individual patient level.

The nlme package [25] from R software version 2.14 [26] was used for statistical analyses.

Results

Thirty-two patients were included between November 2009 and October 2010; 16 patients were randomized to osteopathic manipulative treatment (group A), eight patients to sham OMT (group B) and eight patients to usual care (group C). No patient dropped out of the study after randomization, and all 32 patients attended all the visits planned in the study until month 6. The last

Table 2. Change in the primary outcome measure (composite chest/back pain) between the first and the final visit in the three treatment groups and comparisons between groups.

	Composite chest/back pain in the OMT group (Group A) N = 16 Mean(SD)	Composite chest/back pain in the sham OMT group (Group B) N = 8 Mean(SD)	Composite chest/back pain in the usual care group (Group C) N = 8 Mean(SD)	Composite chest/back pain in the sham OMT or usual care group (Group B+C) N = 16 Mean(SD)	Mean change difference in composite chest/back pain between Group A and Group B+C [95%CI]	Mean change difference in composite chest/back pain between Group A and Group B [95% CI]	Mean change difference in composite chest/back pain between Group A and Group C [95% CI]	Mean change difference in composite chest/back pain between Group B and Group C [95% CI]
M0	6.60 (2.47)	7.94 (1.02)	6.23 (2.61)	7.08 (2.11)				
M3	4.00(3.44)	5.40 (2.07)	5.62 (2.86)	5.51 (2.41)	−1.08 [−3.34; 1.18]	−0.13 [−2.82; 2.57]	−2.09 [−4.79; 0.62]	−1.96 [−5.05;1.14]
M6	2.61 (2.95)	3.77 (3.65)	6.85 (1.26)	5.31 (2.08)	−2.20 [−4.81;0.42]; p = 0.1	0.19 [−2.70;3.08]; p = 0.9	−4.62 [−7.52; −1.72]; p = 0.002	−4.81 [−8.15; −1.47]; p = 0.006

SD: standard deviation.
95% CI: 95% confidence interval.

study visit took place on April 2011. Results for all 32 patients were included in the analysis (Figure 1).

Demographic and clinical factors are reported in Table 1.

Figure 2 and Table 2 show the changes in the primary outcome measure (composite chest/back pain) between the beginning and the end of the study in the experimental treatment and control groups. There was no statistically significant difference in the decrease of chest/back pain between the treatment group and the control group (difference = −2.20 IC95% [−4.81; 0.42], p = 0.098).

We performed prespecified ancillary analyses for the primary outcome (composite chest/back pain) in the three groups, differentiating between the sham OMT (group B) and no treatment (group C) groups (Figure 3 and Table 2). The primary outcome measure did not differ between patients who had received sham OMT and OMT (difference = 0.19 [−2.70 to 3.08], p = 0.9). However, chest/back pain was lower in the OMT (difference = −4.62 [−7.52 to −1.72], p = 0.002) and sham (difference: −4.81 [−8.15 to −1.47], p = 0.006) groups than in the usual care group.

No differences between the treatment group and the control group (group B+C) were found for the secondary outcome measures cervical pain, headache (Figure 4 and Table 3), or QOL.

When taking into account the mean VAS score and the mean number of days in pain in all arms of the study, the results were similar (Table S5). The difference of change from baseline for chest/back pain between the experimental group treated with OMT and the control group was −1.96 [−4.12; 0.22] for mean VAS [CI 95%]), p = 0.076.

All non-parametric analyses gave consistent results (not shown).

The need for analgesics did not differ significantly between groups (Table 4). Although it remained stable for patients with usual care and decreased for patients with OMT or sham treatment, the numbers of patients were too small for conclusions to be drawn.

No harm or unintended effect was reported due to treatment.

Twenty-six patients (81%) indicated that they had been interested in the study and six (19%) that they had been slightly interested. Fifteen of the 16 patients in the treatment arm were very satisfied (94%) and one was reasonably satisfied (6%); five of the eight patients in the sham group were very satisfied (62%), two were reasonably satisfied (25%) and one patient (12%) was not satisfied.

Discussion

Our pilot study is the first to demonstrate that it is feasible to evaluate OMT against the pain affecting CF patients. However, it did not show any difference in the decrease of pain between the group treated with OMT and the control group, though chest/back pain decreased more in patients receiving OMT and sham OMT than in those with no intervention. Our study was therefore not powered to be able to draw firm conclusions on the efficacy of OMT against the pain of patients with CF.

A sufficient number of patients were rapidly recruited (over 12 months rather than over the 18 months initially planned for) and none of the 32 patients dropped out of the study. This reflects the significant expectations that CF patients have for complementary medicine for pain relief. In a survey in French CF patients, 326 of 714 respondents (46%) had used CAM and 38% had experience of OMT [14]. In a survey on pain including 239 Italian adults with CF, 22.2% used non-pharmacological remedies including massage [8]. Hayes reported that 45% of 83 adult CF patients practiced chiropractic, yoga or massage for pain relief [6]. In a study of 97

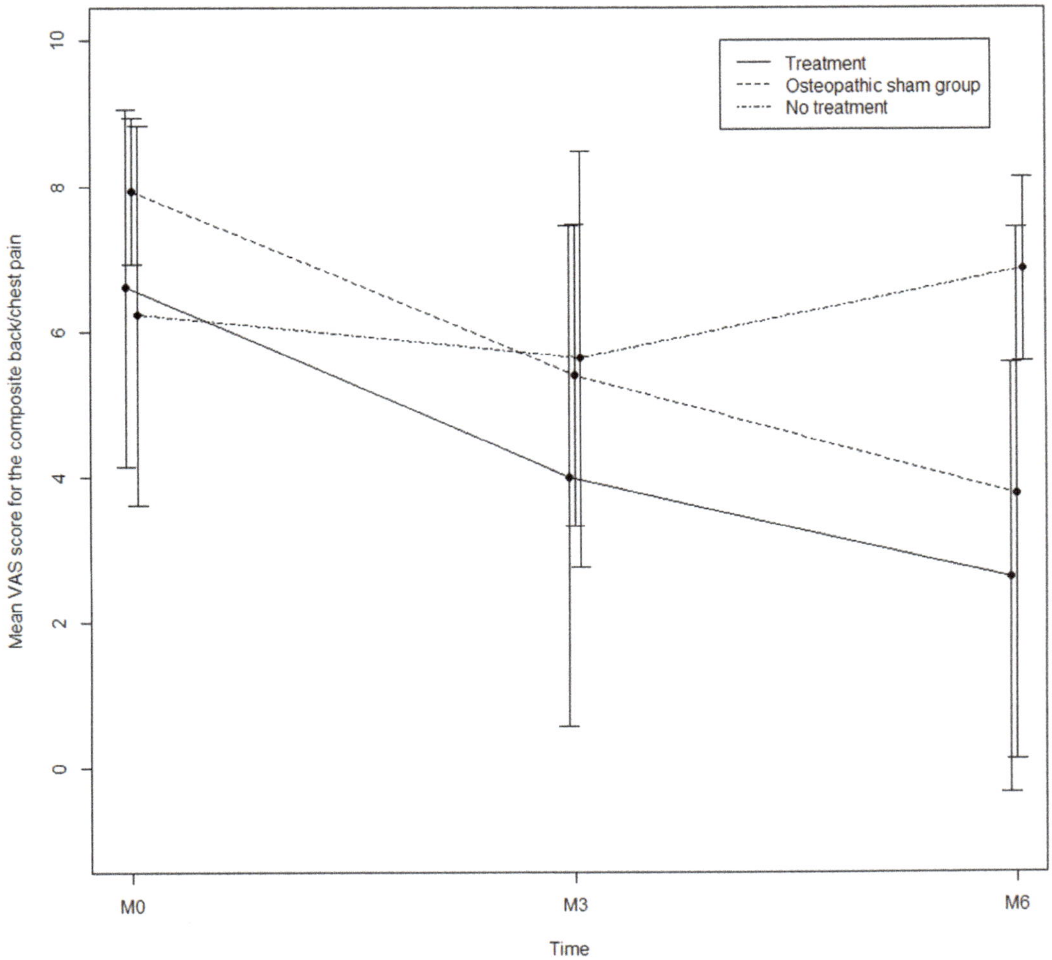

Figure 3. Composite chest/back pain at inclusion (M0), after 3 months (M3) and at the end of the study (M6) in the OMT group (A), the OMT sham group (B) and the group with only usual treatment (C). VAS: visual analog scale.

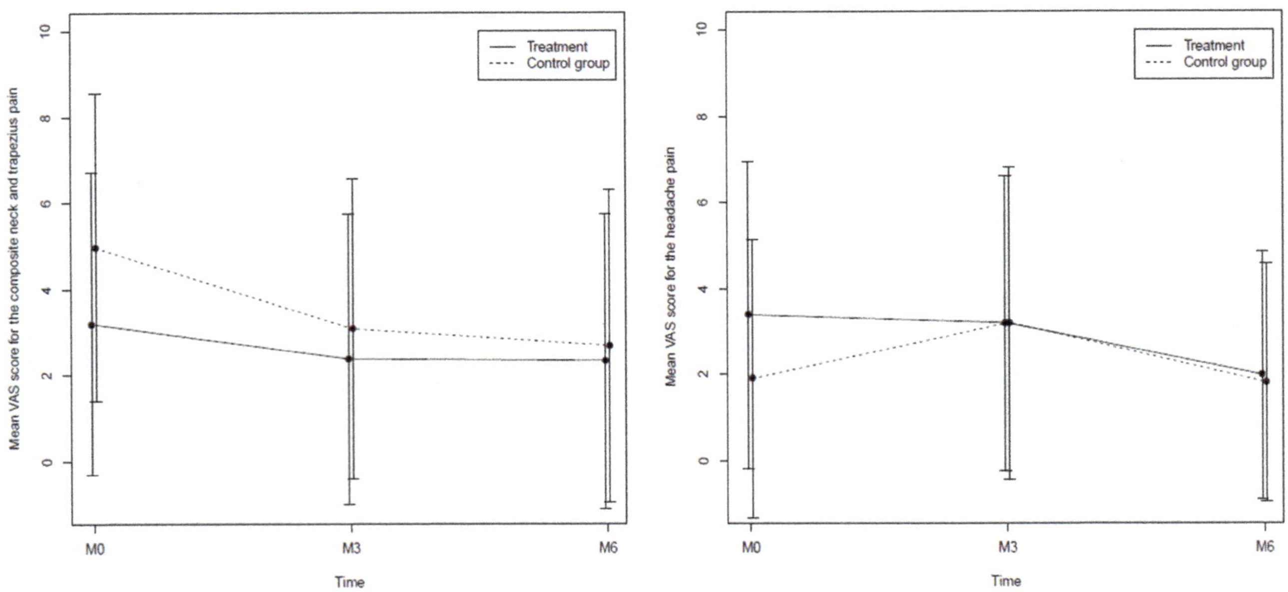

Figure 4. Composite neck/trapezius pain and headache at inclusion (M0), after 3 months (M3) and at the end of the study (M6) in the OMT group (A) and control group (B+C). VAS: visual analog scale.

Table 3. Mean neck/trapezius pain and headache between the first and the final visit for the treatment group and the control group.

	Composite neck/trapezius pain		Headache	
	OMT group (Group A) N = 16	sham OMT or usual care group (Group B+C) N = 16	OMT group (Group A) N = 16	Sham OMT or usual care group (Group B+C) N = 16
Mean (standard deviation)				
M0	3.20 (3.51)	4.97 (3.58)	3.39 (3.57)	1.91 (3.24)
M3	2.38 (3.37)	3.08 (3.48)	3.20 (3.42)	3.20 (3.63)
M6	2.33 (3.43)	2.69 (3.63)#	1.99 (2.88)	1.81 (2.76)##

#The difference (95% confidence interval) between Groups A and B+C was not significant: 1.51 (−0.97; 3.98)– p = 0.228.
##The difference (95% confidence interval) between Groups A and B+C was not significant: −1.30 (−3.27; 0.66)– p = 0.190.

pediatric CF patients, 77% used some method of CAM including manipulative techniques [15]. Only one study has evaluated the effects of manual mobilization techniques and massage therapy on pain: including 105 adults with CF, it reported positive results [27]; however, the study had limitations, and in particular there was no control group such that it could not reveal any placebo effect.

In our study, it is noteworthy that the majority of our patients were women. Indeed, in CF there is a female disadvantage in terms of survival and morbidity, called the "CF gender gap" [28], which might be due to the female sex hormone estrogen. Nevertheless, it is unclear from the literature whether women with CF are in greater pain than men with CF.

As complementary medical techniques become more mainstream, we anticipate that more adults with CF will attempt alternative therapies for pain relief. Our study is the first to assess a treatment of this type in CF patients. We chose to evaluate the effects of OMT on chest/back pain because pain at these sites is prevalent among adults with CF, affecting 15–72% of CF patients [4]. While some patients seek relief from their pain with osteopathic practitioners (but no more than a few times per year), this treatment is not currently approved in CF and is not covered by public health insurance in France. We opted for a monthly treatment regimen as the optimal OMT regimen is not known. Indeed, there are no existing studies on dose-response effects of OMT, nor are there any recommendations or studies on the optimal frequency of OMT. The only available data are descriptive and refer to the frequency of treatment in current practice [29]. Our choice for monthly treatments relied on expert opinions. Regarding the control group, we divided it into patients receiving usual care and those receiving sham OMT, so as to evaluate the feasibility of using sham OMT. Because sham treatment is difficult to implement in clinical trials of OMT [30], we chose to use light touch at the skull and at the sacrum which has been used as a placebo method in trials evaluating OMT [22–23]. Cranial palpation, equivalent to light touch, has been proposed as a sham OMT treatment option [31]. Although the results of a systematic review on the effects of craniosacral therapy suggest improvements on general wellbeing/quality of life and pain, the moderate quality of current studies and the scarcity of available data prevent any definitive conclusion regarding the clinical effectiveness of this type of OMT [32].

We found no statistically significant difference in the decrease of chest/back pain between patients treated with OMT and the control group. There was no statistically significant difference between patients receiving the OMT intervention treatment and those receiving the OMT sham treatment. However, chest/back pain decreased significantly more in patients receiving the OMT intervention treatment and in those receiving the osteopathic sham treatment than in patients only receiving usual routine care. There was also no difference between the intervention group and the control group with respect to neck/trapezius pain, headache, QOL scores or the need for analgesics. It has been reported that alternative medicine may be an especially successful placebo-generating health care system [33–34]. Clinical outcomes of OMT result from both OMT-specific and placebo mechanisms (e.g., importance of patient characteristics, practitioner characteristics, patient-practitioner interaction, length of patient encounter) [35].

A systematic review and meta-analysis of randomized, controlled trials assessed the effect of OMT on chronic low back pain: it concluded that OMT reduced low back pain significantly more than expected from placebo effects, and that the beneficial effects persisted for at least three months [36]. In a trial comparing standard medical therapies and OMT over a 12-week period in 155 patients, there was no statistically significant difference between the two groups in any of the primary outcome measures, but the OMT group required significantly less analgesic medication and used less physical therapy [37]. However, this study was

Table 4. Need for analgesics in the OMT group, the sham OMT group and the group with usual care.

Number of patients using analgesics (%)			
	OMT group (Group A) N = 16	sham OMT group (Group B) N = 8	Usual care group (Group C) N = 8
M0	10 (62)	5 (62)	4 (50)
M3	7 (44)	3 (37)	3 (37)
M6	4 (25)	2 (25)	4 (50)

not blinded, making it is difficult to distinguish the treatment effect from the placebo effect. In another trial, 91 subjects with chronic low back pain were randomized to OMT, sham manipulation, or a no-intervention control group [38]. As in our study, both the patients who received OMT and those who received the sham manipulation reported greater improvement in back pain than the no-intervention control subjects. It is unclear whether the benefits of OMT could be attributed to the manipulative techniques themselves or whether they were related to other non-specific aspects of OMT [38].

In conclusion, our pilot study shows that the assessment of the effects of OMT on chest and back pain in adults with CF is feasible. Patients have substantial expectations and hopes for such studies. The lack of any significant difference between the intervention OMT group and the control group might be related to the small number of patients, which also precludes any definitive conclusion about the greater decrease of pain in patients receiving OMT or sham OMT than in those with no intervention. This may raise the question of a placebo effect and highlights the importance of psychological factors and human relationships in the treatment of pain. Nevertheless, the results need to be interpreted with caution, due to the small number of patients in our pilot study and the multiplicity of the tests. Larger and more powerful studies are needed to determine whether OMT could be beneficial for CF patients who suffer chest and back pain.

Supporting Information

Table S1 Criteria for clinical decision about the severity of somatic dysfunction according to the three categories of tests.

Table S2 Different techniques of the Osteopathic Manipulative Treatment.

Table S3 Intervention used in the two OMT groups.

Table S4 Position of the patient and of the practitioner during the different techniques.

Table S5 Change in pain intensity and days in pain between the experimental OMT group (A) and the control group (B+C).

Checklist S1 CONSORT checklist.

Protocol S1 Trial protocol.

Methods S1 Supplementary methods.

Acknowledgments

We acknowledge Fawzia Aissat (Clinical Research Department, Hôpital Cochin APHP, Paris, France) who was the clinical research assistant in the study.

Author Contributions

Conceived and designed the experiments: DH LS FG RS EP RZP IB. Performed the experiments: DH LS DG. Analyzed the data: EP IB. Contributed reagents/materials/analysis tools: FG EP EP. Wrote the paper: DH IB RZP LS. Commented critically on each draft: FG DG RS EP.

References

1. Davies JC, Alton EWF, Bush A (2007) Cystic fibrosis. BMJ 335: 1255–1259.
2. Vaincre la Mucoviscidose, INED (2013) *Registre français de la mucoviscidose – Bilan des données 2011.* Paris, France: Vaincre la mucoviscidose.
3. Cystic Fibrosis Foundation (2012) *Cystic Fibrosis Foundation Patient Registry 2011 annual data report.* Bethesda, MD: Cystic Fibrosis Foundation.
4. Havermans T, Colpaert K, De Boeck K, Dupont L, Abbott J (2013) Pain in CF: Review of the literature. J Cyst Fibros 12: 423–430.
5. Sermet-Gaudelus I, De Villartay P, de Dreuzy P, Clairicia M, Vrielynck S, et al. (2009) Pain in children and adults with cystic fibrosis: a comparative study. J Pain Symptom Manage 38: 281–290.
6. Hayes M, Yaster M, Haythornthwaite JA, Riekert KA, McMillan KN, et al. (2011) Pain is a common problem affecting clinical outcomes in adults with cystic fibrosis. Chest 140: 1598–603.
7. Ravilly S, Robinson W, Suresh S, Wohl ME, Berde CB (1996) Chronic pain in cystic fibrosis. Pediatrics 98: 741–747.
8. Festini F, Ballarin S, Codamo T, Doro R, Loganes C (2004) Prevalence of pain in adults with cystic fibrosis. J Cyst Fibros 3: 51–57.
9. Flume PA, Ciolino J, Gray S, Lester MK (2009) Patient-reported pain and impaired sleep quality in adult patients with cystic fibrosis. J Cyst Fibros 8: 321–325.
10. Stenekes SI, Hughes A, Grégoire MC, Frager G, Robinson WM, et al. (2009) Frequency and self management of pain, dyspnea and cough in cystic fibrosis. J Pain Symptom Manage 38: 387–348.
11. Kelemen L, Lee AL, Button BM, Presnell S, Wilson JW, et al. (2012) Pain impacts on quality of life and interferes with treatment in adults with cystic fibrosis. Physiother Res Int 17: 132–141.
12. Abbott J, Hart A, Morton AM, Dey P, Conway SP, et al. (2009) Can health-related quality of life predict survival in adults with cystic fibrosis? Am J Respir Crit Care Med 179: 54–58.
13. Stern RC, Canda ER, Doershuk CF (1992) Use of nonmedical treatment by cystic fibrosis patients. J Adolesc Health 13: 612–615.
14. Agrario L, Naggiar C, Desmazes-Dufeu N, Hubert D (2006) Survey on complementary and alternative medicine in French patients with cystic fibrosis [abstract]. J Cyst Fibros 5 (Suppl 1), S90.
15. Tanase A, Zanni R (2008) The use of complementary and alternative medicine among pediatric cystic fibrosis patients. J Altern Complement Med 14: 1271–1273.
16. Huskisson EC (1974) Measurement of pain. Lancet 2(7889): 1127–1131.
17. World Health Organization. Benchmarks for training in traditional/complementary and alternative medicine: benchmarks for training in osteopathy. WHO Press, Geneva, Switzerland. 2010. Available:http://www.who.int/medicines/areas/traditional/BenchmarksforTraininginOsteopathy.pdf. Accessed on July 13, 2013.
18. Van Buskirk RL (1990) Nociceptive reflexes and the somatic dysfunction: a model. J Am Osteopath Assoc 90: 792–794, 797–809.
19. American Academy of Osteopathy (2002) Outpatient Osteopathic SOAP Note Form Series and Usage Guide. 2nd ed. Indianapolis, Ind: American Academy of Osteopathy. Available: http://www.academyofosteopathy.org/.
20. American Association of Colleges of Osteopathic Medicine. Authorized Osteopathic Thesaurus. Available: http://www.aacom.org/resources/bookstore/thesaurus/Pages/default.aspx. Accessed July 14, 2012.
21. Soubeiran L, Hubert D, Serreau R, Desmazes_Dufeu N, Zegarra-Parodi R (2011) Prevalence of somatic dysfunctions in adult patients with cystic fibrosis – a pilot study. J Phys Ther 4: 18–31.
22. Noll DR, Degenhardt BF, Morley TF, Blais FX, Hortos KA, et al. (2010) Efficacy of osteopathic manipulation as an adjunctive treatment for hospitalized patients with pneumonia: a randomized controlled trial. Osteopath Med Prim Care 4: 2. Available: http://www.ncbi.nlm.nih.gov/pmc/articles/PMC2848182. Accessed December 2, 2013.
23. Noll DR, Degenhardt BF, Fossum C, Hensel K (2008) Clinical and research protocol for osteopathic manipulative treatment of elderly patients with pneumonia. J Am Osteopath Assoc 108: 508–516.
24. Henry B, Aussage P, Grosskopf C, Goehrs JM (2003) Development of the Cystic Fibrosis Questionnaire (CFQ) for assessing quality of life in pediatric and adult patients. Qual Life Res 12: 63–76.
25. Pinheiro J, Bates D, DebRoy S, Sarkar D and the R Development Core Team (2011) nlme: Linear and Nonlinear Mixed Effects Models. R package version 3.1–102.
26. R Development Core Team (2011) R: A language and environment for statistical computing. R Foundation for Statistical Computing. Vienna, Austria. ISBN 3–900051–07–0. Available: http://www.R-project.org/.
27. Lee A, Holdsworth M, Holland A, Button B (2009) The immediate effect of musculoskeletal physiotherapy techniques and massage on pain and ease of breathing in adults with cystic fibrosis. J Cyst Fibros 8: 79–81.

28. Sweezey NB, Ratjen F (2014) The cystic fibrosis gender gap: Potential roles of estrogen. Pediatr Pulmonol 49: 309–317.
29. Degenhardt BF, Johnson JC, Gross SR, Hagan C, Lund G, et al. (2014) Preliminary findings on the use of osteopathic manipulative treatment: outcomes during the formation of the practice-based research network, DO-Touch.NET. J Am Osteopath Assoc 114: 154–170.
30. Licciardone JC, Russo DP (2006) Blinding protocols, treatment credibility, and expectancy: Methodologic issues in clinical trials of osteopathic manipulative treatment. J Am Osteopth Assoc 106: 457–463.
31. Sergueef N, Nelson KE, Glonek T (2002) The effect of cranial manipulation on the Traube-Hering-Mayer oscillation as measured by laser-Doppler flowmetry. Altern Ther Health Med 8: 74–76.
32. Jäkel A, von Hauenschild P (2012) A systematic review to evaluate the clinical benefits of craniosacral therapy. Complement Ther Med 20: 456–465.
33. Staud R (2011) Effectiveness of CAM therapy: understanding the evidence. Rheum Dis Clin North Am 37: 9–17.
34. Kaptchuk TJ (2002) The placebo effect in alternative medicine : can the performance of a healing ritual have clinical significance ? Ann Intern Med 136: 817–825.
35. Moulson A, Watson T (2006) A preliminary investigation into the relationship between cervical snags and sympathetic nervous system activity in the upper limbs of an asymptomatic population. Man Ther 11: 214–224.
36. Licciardone JC, Brimhall AK, King LN (2005) Osteopathic manipulative treatment for low back pain: a systematic review and meta-analysis of randomized controlled trials. BMC Musculoskelet Disord 6: 43. Available: http://www.ncbi.nlm.nih.gov/pubmed/16080794. Accessed December 2, 2013.
37. Andersson GB, Lucente T, Davis AM, Kappler RE, Lipton JA, et al. (1999) A comparison of osteopathic spinal manipulation with standard care for patients with low back pain. N Engl J Med 341: 1426–1431.
38. Licciardone JC, Stoll ST, Fulda KG, Russo DP, Siu J, et al. (2003) Osteopathic manipulative treatment for chronic low back pain: a randomized controlled trial. Spine 28: 1355–1362.

Permissions

All chapters in this book were first published in PLOS ONE, by The Public Library of Science; hereby published with permission under the Creative Commons Attribution License or equivalent. Every chapter published in this book has been scrutinized by our experts. Their significance has been extensively debated. The topics covered herein carry significant findings which will fuel the growth of the discipline. They may even be implemented as practical applications or may be referred to as a beginning point for another development.

The contributors of this book come from diverse backgrounds, making this book a truly international effort. This book will bring forth new frontiers with its revolutionizing research information and detailed analysis of the nascent developments around the world.

We would like to thank all the contributing authors for lending their expertise to make the book truly unique. They have played a crucial role in the development of this book. Without their invaluable contributions this book wouldn't have been possible. They have made vital efforts to compile up to date information on the varied aspects of this subject to make this book a valuable addition to the collection of many professionals and students.

This book was conceptualized with the vision of imparting up-to-date information and advanced data in this field. To ensure the same, a matchless editorial board was set up. Every individual on the board went through rigorous rounds of assessment to prove their worth. After which they invested a large part of their time researching and compiling the most relevant data for our readers.

The editorial board has been involved in producing this book since its inception. They have spent rigorous hours researching and exploring the diverse topics which have resulted in the successful publishing of this book. They have passed on their knowledge of decades through this book. To expedite this challenging task, the publisher supported the team at every step. A small team of assistant editors was also appointed to further simplify the editing procedure and attain best results for the readers.

Apart from the editorial board, the designing team has also invested a significant amount of their time in understanding the subject and creating the most relevant covers. They scrutinized every image to scout for the most suitable representation of the subject and create an appropriate cover for the book.

The publishing team has been an ardent support to the editorial, designing and production team. Their endless efforts to recruit the best for this project, has resulted in the accomplishment of this book. They are a veteran in the field of academics and their pool of knowledge is as vast as their experience in printing. Their expertise and guidance has proved useful at every step. Their uncompromising quality standards have made this book an exceptional effort. Their encouragement from time to time has been an inspiration for everyone.

The publisher and the editorial board hope that this book will prove to be a valuable piece of knowledge for researchers, students, practitioners and scholars across the globe.

List of Contributors

Dieter Böning, Angela Littschwager, Matthias Hütler and Ralph Beneke
Institut für Sportmedizin, Charité - Universitätsmedizin Berlin, Berlin, Germany

Doris Staab
Klinik für Pädiatrische Pneumologie und Immunologie, Charité - Universitätsmedizin Berlin, Berlin, Germany

Anne-Laure Michon, Brigitte Lamy and Hélène Marchandin
UMR 5119 ECOSYM, Equipe Pathogènes et Environnements, U.F.R. des Sciences Pharmaceutiques et Biologiques, Université Montpellier 1, Montpellier, France,
Laboratoire de Bactériologie, Hôpital Arnaud de Villeneuve, Centre Hospitalier Régional Universitaire de Montpellier, Montpellier, France,

Estelle Jumas-Bilak
UMR 5119 ECOSYM, Equipe Pathogènes et Environnements, U.F.R. des Sciences Pharmaceutiques et Biologiques, Université Montpellier 1, Montpellier, France,
Laboratoire d'Hygiène hospitalière, Centre Hospitalier Régional Universitaire de Montpellier, Montpellier, France

Raphaë l Chiron
Centre de Ressources et de Compétences pour la Mucoviscidose, Hôpital
Arnaud de Villeneuve, Centre Hospitalier Régional Universitaire de Montpellier, Montpellier, France

Matthew L. Workentine
Farncombe Family Digestive Health Research Institute, McMaster University, Hamilton, Ontario, Canada
Department of Medicine, McMaster University, Hamilton, Ontario, Canada

Christopher D. Sibley, Bryan Glezerson, Swathi Purighalla and Jens C. Norgaard-Gron
Department of Microbiology, Immunology and Infectious Diseases, University of Calgary, Calgary, Alberta, Canada

Michael D. Parkins and Harvey R. Rabin
Department of Microbiology, Immunology and Infectious Diseases, University of Calgary, Calgary, Alberta, Canada
Department of Medicine, University of Calgary, Calgary, Alberta, Canada
Adult Cystic Fibrosis Clinic, University of Calgary, Calgary, Alberta, Canada

Michael G. Surette
Farncombe Family Digestive Health Research Institute, McMaster University, Hamilton, Ontario, Canada
Department of Medicine, McMaster University, Hamilton, Ontario, Canada
Department of Biochemistry and Biomedical Sciences, McMaster University, Hamilton, Ontario, Canada
Department of Microbiology, Immunology and Infectious Diseases, University of Calgary, Calgary, Alberta, Canada

Mette Kolpen, Niels Høiby and Thomas Bjarnsholt
Department of Clinical Microbiology, Rigshospitalet, Copenhagen, Denmark
Department of International Health, Immunology and Microbiology, Faculty of Health Sciences University of Copenhagen, Copenhagen, Denmark

Michael Kühl
Marine Biological Section, Department of Biology, University of Copenhagen, Helsingør, Denmark
Plant Functional Biology and Climate Change Cluster, University of Technology Sydney, Sydney, Australia
Singapore Centre on Environmental Life Sciences Engineering, Nanyang Technological University, Singapore, Singapore

Christine Rønne Hansen and Tanja Pressler
Copenhagen CF Centre, Rigshospitalet, Copenhagen, Denmark

Lars Liengaard
Marine Biological Section, Department of Biology, University of Copenhagen, Helsingør, Denmark

Peter Østrup Jensen, Claus Moser and Arsalan Kharazmi
Department of Clinical Microbiology, Rigshospitalet, Copenhagen, Denmark

Matthew T. Cabeen
Department of Molecular and Cellular Biology, Harvard University, Cambridge, Massachusetts, United States of America

Liudmila Cebotaru and Daniele Rapino
Department of Ophthalmology, School of Medicine, The Johns Hopkins University, Baltimore, Maryland, United States of America
Department of Physiology, School of Medicine, The Johns Hopkins University, Baltimore, Maryland, United States of America

Valeriu Cebotaru
Department of Medicine, School of Medicine, The Johns Hopkins University, Baltimore, Maryland, United States of America

William B. Guggino
Department of Physiology, School of Medicine, The Johns Hopkins University, Baltimore, Maryland, United States of America

Hannah K. Bayes and Tom J. Evans
Institute of Infection, Immunology and Inflammation, College of Medical, Veterinary and Life Sciences, University of Glasgow, Glasgow, United Kingdom

Stephen Bicknell and Gordon MacGregor
West of Scotland Cystic Fibrosis Centre, Gartnavel General Hospital, Glasgow, United Kingdom

Jessica E. Char, Marlene H. Wolfe, Hyung-ju Cho, Il-Ho Park, Jin Hyeok Jeong and Eric Frisbee
Cystic Fibrosis Research Laboratory, Stanford University, Stanford, California, United States of America

Colleen Dunn, Zoe Davies, Carlos Milla and Richard B. Moss
Department of Pediatrics, Stanford University School of Medicine, Stanford, California, United States of America

Ewart A. C. Thomas
Department of Psychology, Stanford University, Stanford, California, United States of America

Jeffrey J. Wine
Cystic Fibrosis Research Laboratory, Stanford University, Stanford, California, United States of America
Department of Pediatrics, Stanford University School of Medicine, Stanford, California, United States of America
Department of Psychology, Stanford University, Stanford, California, United States of America

Celia N. Sanchez-Dominguez, Maria del C. Villalobos-Torres, Herminia G. Martinez-Rodriguez and Hugo A. Barrera-Saldaña
Departamento de Bioquimica y Medicina Molecular, Facultad de Medicina, Universidad Autonoma de Nuevo Leon, Monterrey, Nuevo Leon, Mexico

Miguel A. Reyes-Lopez
Laboratorio de Medicina de Conservacion, Centro de Biotecnologia Genomica, Instituto Politecnico Nacional, Reynosa, Tamaulipas, Mexico

Adriana Bustamante
Clinica de Fibrosis Quistica, Centro de Prevenciony Rehabilitacion de Enfermedades Pulmonares Cronicas (CEPREP), Facultad de Medicina y Hospital Universitario "Dr. Jose Eleuterio Gonzalez", Universidad Autónoma de Nuevo Leon, Monterrey, Nuevo Leon, Mexico

Ricardo M. Cerda-Flores
Facultad de Enfermeria, Universidad Autonoma de Nuevo Leon, Monterrey, Nuevo Leon, Mexico

Hugo L. Gallardo-Blanco
Departamento de Genetica, Facultad de Medicina, Universidad Autonoma de Nuevo Leon, Monterrey, Nuevo Leon, Mexico

Augusto Rojas-Martinez and Rocio Ortiz-Lopez
Departamento de Bioquimica y Medicina Molecular, Facultad de Medicina, Universidad Autonoma de Nuevo Leon, Monterrey, Nuevo Leon, Mexico
Centro de Investigacion y Desarrollo en Ciencias de la Salud, Universidad Autonoma de Nuevo Leon, Monterrey, Nuevo Leon, Mexico

Felice Amato, Sonia Giordano, Ausilia Elce, Giuseppe Castaldo and Rossella Tomaiuolo
CEINGE-Biotecnologie avanzate, Naples, Italy
Dipartimento di Medicina Molecolare e Biotecnologie Mediche, Università di Napoli Federico II, Naples, Italy

Manuela Seia
Laboratorio di Genetica Medica, Fondazione IRCCS Cà Granda - Ospedale Maggiore Policlnico, Mangiagalli e Regina Elena, Milan, Italy

Federica Zarrilli
CEINGE-Biotecnologie avanzate, Naples, Italy
Dipartimento di Medicina Molecolare e Biotecnologie Mediche, Università di Napoli Federico II, Naples, Italy
Dipartimento di Bioscienze e Territorio, Università del Molise, Isernia, Italy

Dominique Hubert
Adult CF Center and Pulmonology Department, Hôpital Cochin APHP, Paris, France
Université Paris Descartes, Sorbonne Paris Cité, Paris, France

Lucile Soubeiran, Fabrice Gourmelon and Raphaël Serreau
Clinical Research Department, Hôpital Cochin APHP, Paris, France

Dominique Grenet
Adult CF Center and Pulmonology Department, Hôpital Foch, Suresnes, France

Elodie Perrodeau
Clinical Epidemiology Center, Hôpital Hôtel Dieu APHP, Paris, France

Rafael Zegarra-Parodi
A.T. Still Research Institute, A.T. Still University, Kirksville, Missouri, United States of America

Isabelle Boutron
Clinical Epidemiology Center, Hôpital Hôtel Dieu APHP, Paris, France
Université Paris Descartes, Sorbonne Paris Cité, Paris, France

Katherine L. Tuggle and Michelle V. Fanucchi
Gregory Fleming James Cystic Fibrosis Research Center, University of Alabama at Birmingham, Birmingham, Alabama, United States of America
Department of Environmental Health Sciences, School of Public Health, University of Alabama at Birmingham, Birmingham, Alabama, United States of America

Susan E. Birket
Gregory Fleming James Cystic Fibrosis Research Center, University of Alabama at Birmingham, Birmingham, Alabama, United States of America
Department of Medicine, University of Alabama at Birmingham, Birmingham, Alabama, United States of America

Xiaoxia Cui, Joe Warren, Lara Reid, Andre Chambers, Diana Ji and Kevin Gamber
SAGE Labs, Inc., St. Louis, Missouri, United States of America

Jeong Hong
Gregory Fleming James Cystic Fibrosis Research Center, University of Alabama at Birmingham, Birmingham, Alabama, United States of America
Department of Cell, Developmental, and Integrative Biology, University of Alabama at Birmingham, Birmingham, Alabama, United States of America

Kengyeh K. Chu
Wellman Center for Photomedicine, Harvard Medical School, Massachusetts General Hospital, Boston, Massachusetts, United States of America
Department of Dermatology, Massachusetts General Hospital, Boston, Massachusetts, United States of America

Guillermo Tearney
Wellman Center for Photomedicine, Harvard Medical School, Massachusetts General Hospital, Boston, Massachusetts, United States of America
Department of Pathology, Massachusetts General Hospital, Boston, Massachusetts, United States of America

Li Ping Tang and James A. Fortenberry
Gregory Fleming James Cystic Fibrosis Research Center, University of Alabama at Birmingham, Birmingham, Alabama, United States of America

Ming Du
Gregory Fleming James Cystic Fibrosis Research Center, University of Alabama at Birmingham, Birmingham, Alabama, United States of America
Animal Resources Program, Office of the Vice President for Research, University of Alabama at Birmingham, Birmingham, Alabama, United States of America

Joan M. Cadillac
Animal Resources Program, Office of the Vice President for Research, University of Alabama at Birmingham, Birmingham, Alabama, United States of America

David M. Bedwell
Gregory Fleming James Cystic Fibrosis Research Center, University of Alabama at Birmingham, Birmingham, Alabama, United States of America
Department of Microbiology, University of Alabama at Birmingham, Birmingham, Alabama, United States of America

Steven M. Rowe and Eric J. Sorscher
Gregory Fleming James Cystic Fibrosis Research Center, University of Alabama at Birmingham, Birmingham, Alabama, United States of America
Department of Medicine, University of Alabama at Birmingham, Birmingham, Alabama, United States of America

Serena Schippa, Valerio Iebba, Floriana Santangelo, Antonella Gagliardi and Maria Pia Conte
Public Health and Infectious Diseases Department, Microbiology Unit, 'Sapienza' University of Rome, Rome, Italy

Riccardo Valerio De Biase, Antonella Stamato and Serenella Bertasi
Regional Cystic Fibrosis Centre, Paediatrics and Infant Neuropsychiatry Department, 'Sapienza' University of Rome, Rome, Italy

Marco Lucarelli and Serena Quattrucci
Department of Haematology and Cellular Biotechnologies, Sapienza University of Rome, Rome, Italy

Sara Zarei
Computational Science Research Center, San Diego State University, San Diego, California, United States of America

Ali Mirtar
Electrical and Computer Eng. Dep/University of California San Diego, San Diego, California, United States of America

Forest Rohwer
Department of Biology, San Diego State University, San Diego, California, United States of America

Peter Salamon
Department of Mathematics and Statistics, San Diego State University, San Diego, California, United States of America
Bradley S. Quon, Pearce G. Wilcox, S. F. Paul Man and Don D. Sin
Centre for Heart Lung Innovation, St. Paul's Hospital, University of British Columbia, Vancouver, British Columbia, Canada
Division of Respiratory Medicine, St. Paul's Hospital, University of British Columbia, Vancouver, British Columbia, Canada

David A. Ngan
Centre for Heart Lung Innovation, St. Paul's Hospital, University of British Columbia, Vancouver, British Columbia, Canada

Ha Won Lee, Jie Cheng, Mark Donowitz and William B. Guggino
Department of Physiology, Johns Hopkins University, School of Medicine, Baltimore, Maryland, United States of America

Olga Kovbasnjuk
Department of Medicine, Johns Hopkins University, School of Medicine, Baltimore, Maryland, United States of America

Randal C. Fowler and Nancy D. Hanson
Creighton University School of Medicine, Department of Medical Microbiology and Immunology, Center for Research in Anti-Infectives and Biotechnology, Omaha, Nebraska, United States of America

Markus Wettstein
Physiotherapy Institute, Inselspital, Bern University Hospital and University of Bern, Bern, Switzerland

Lorenz Radlinger
Bern University of Applied Sciences, Health, Bern, Switzerland

Thomas Riedel
Paediatric and Neonatal Intensive Care Medicine, Department of Paediatrics, Inselspital, Bern University Children's Hospital and University of Bern, Bern, Switzerland

Bruna Mendes Lourenço
Institute of Biological Sciences, Federal University of Pará, Belém, Pará, Brazil

João de Barros Barreto University Hospital, Federal University of Pará, Belém, Pará, Brazil

Kauê Machado Costa and Manoel da Silva Filho
Institute of Biological Sciences, Federal University of Pará, Belém, Pará, Brazil

Jeanine F. Amacher and Dean R. Madden
Department of Biochemistry, Geisel School of Medicine at Dartmouth, Hanover, New Hampshire, United States of America

Ruizhi Zhao
Department of Chemistry, Dartmouth College, Hanover, New Hampshire, United States of America
Norris Cotton Cancer Center, Dartmouth-Hitchcock Medical Center, Lebanon, New Hampshire, United States of America

Mark R. Spaller
Department of Chemistry, Dartmouth College, Hanover, New Hampshire, United States of America
Norris Cotton Cancer Center, Dartmouth-Hitchcock Medical Center, Lebanon, New Hampshire, United States of America
Department of Pharmacology and Toxicology, Geisel School of Medicine at Dartmouth, Hanover, New Hampshire, United States of America

James E. A. Zlosnik, Paul Y. Mori, Derek To, James Leung, Trevor J. Hird and David P. Speert
Centre for Understanding and Preventing Infection in Children, Department of Pediatrics, Faculty of Medicine, University of British Columbia, Vancouver, British Columbia, Canada

Veronica A. Peotta, Prasad Bhandary, Ugochi Ogu, Kenneth A. Volk and Robert D. Roghair
Department of Pediatrics, University of Iowa Carver College of Medicine, Iowa City, Iowa, United States of America

Xavier Puéchal
National Referral Center for Rare Systemic Autoimmune Diseases, Department of Internal Medicine, Hôpital Cochin, Assistance Publique-Hôpitaux de Paris, Université Paris Descartes, Paris, France
INSERM U1016, CNRS UMR 8104, Institut Cochin, Paris, France

Emmanuelle Génin
INSERM UMR-1078, Centre Hospitalier Universitaire, Brest, France

Thierry Bienvenu
Biochemistry and Molecular Biology Laboratory, Hôpital Cochin, Assistance Publique-Hôpitaux de Paris, Université Paris Descartes, Paris, France

Claire Le Jeunne
National Referral Center for Rare Systemic Autoimmune Diseases, Department of Internal Medicine, Hôpital Cochin, Assistance Publique-Hôpitaux de Paris, Université Paris Descartes, Paris, France

Daniel J. Dusser
Department of Respiratory Diseases, Hôpital Cochin, Assistance Publique-Hôpitaux de Paris, Université Paris Descartes, Paris, France

Judy M. Bradley
Institute of Nursing and Health Research, University of Ulster, Ulster, Northern Ireland

Paul Koker and Qiqi Deng
Boehringer Ingelheim Pharmaceuticals Inc, Ridgefield, Connecticut, United States of America

Petra Moroni-Zentgraf
Boehringer Ingelheim Pharma GmbH & Co KG, Ingelheim, Germany

Felix Ratjen
The Hospital for Sick Children, Toronto, Ontario, Canada

David E. Geller
Florida State University College of Medicine, Orlando, Florida, United States of America

J. Stuart Elborn
Centre for Infection and Immunity, Queen's University Belfast, Belfast, Northern Ireland

Nicole Scheuing, Reinhard W. Holl and Julia M. Hermann
Institute of Epidemiology and Medical Biometry, Central Institute for Biomedical Technology, University of Ulm, Ulm, Germany

Gerd Dockter
Cystic Fibrosis Centre, Saarland University Hospital for Pediatric and Adolescent Medicine, Homburg/Saar, Germany

Sibylle Junge
Clinic for Pediatric Pneumology and Neonatology, Hannover Medical School, Hannover, Germany

Cordula Koerner-Rettberg and Manfred Ballmann
Department of Pediatric Pulmonology, St. Josef Hospital Pediatric Clinic, Ruhr University Bochum, Bochum, Germany

Lutz Naehrlich
Department of Pediatrics, Justus-Liebig University Giessen, Giessen, Germany

Christina Smaczny
Medical Clinic I, Pneumology and Allergology, University Hospital Frankfurt/Main, Goethe University, Frankfurt/Main, Germany

Doris Staab
Division of Pulmonology and Immunology, Department of Pediatrics, Charité Berlin, Berlin, Germany

Gabriela Thalhammer
Department for Pediatric Pulmonology and Allergology, Medical University of Graz, Graz, Austria

Silke van Koningsbruggen-Rietschel
Cystic Fibrosis Centre Cologne, Childrens Hospital, University of Cologne, Cologne, Germany

Index